CHRONIC DISEASE EPIDEMIOLOGY, PREVENTION, AND CONTROL 5TH EDITION

For access to digital chapters,
visit the APHA Press bookstore (www.apha.org).

CHRONIC DISEASE EPIDEMIOLOGY, PREVENTION, AND CONTROL 5TH EDITION

Margaret B. Nolan, MD, MS
Mark V. Wegner, MD, MPH
Patrick L. Remington, MD, MPH

APHA PRESS
AN IMPRINT OF AMERICAN PUBLIC HEALTH ASSOCIATION

American Public Health Association
800 I Street, NW
Washington, DC 20001-3710
www.apha.org

Georges C. Benjamin, MD, MACP, Executive Director

Printed and bound in the United States of America
Book Production Editor: Maya Ribault
Typesetting: KnowledgeWorks Global Ltd.
Cover Design: Alan Giarcanella
Printing and Binding: Sheridan Books

Library of Congress Cataloging-in-Publication Data

Names: Nolan, Margaret B., editor. | Wegner, Mark V., 1972- editor. | Remington, Patrick L., editor. | American Public Health Association, issuing body.
Title: Chronic disease epidemiology, prevention, and control / editors, Margaret B. Nolan, Mark V. Wegner, and Patrick L. Remington.
Other titles: Chronic disease epidemiology and control.
Description: 5th edition. | Washington, DC : American Public Health Association, [2023] | Includes bibliographical references and index. | Summary: "In this edition, the focus on prevention of chronic disease is expanded through a deeper discussion of health equity and social determinants of health, as well as traditionally less-covered risk-factors such as sleep and oral health. Authors have considered chronic disease epidemiology, prevention and intervention programs and policies throughout the life course, along the continuum from health to illness, and from prebirth to death"-- Provided by publisher.
Identifiers: LCCN 2022053195 (print) | LCCN 2022053196 (ebook) | ISBN 9780875533360 (paperback) | ISBN 9780875533377 (adobe pdf)
Subjects: MESH: Chronic Disease--epidemiology | Chronic Disease--prevention & control | Risk Factors | Epidemiologic Methods
Classification: LCC RC108 (print) | LCC RC108 (ebook) | NLM QZ 185 | DDC 616/.044--dc23/eng/20230303
LC record available at https://lccn.loc.gov/2022053195
LC ebook record available at https://lccn.loc.gov/2022053196

Contents

Foreword

At the time of the release of the 4th edition of *Chronic Disease Epidemiology, Prevention, and Control,* there were reasons to be hopeful. The impacts of the Affordable Care Act were beginning to be seen, and high-quality health care coverage was becoming more available for millions of people. There were encouraging signs of the growing awareness of the steps that could be taken to reduce chronic disease. Cigarette use was down, the awareness of the dangers of obesity was higher than ever, and the public health and health care sectors were increasingly recognizing the impact of the social determinants of health. Nonetheless, the 4th edition Foreword expressed uncertainty about the future despite these promising signs.

As it turns out that uncertainty was well founded. Little did we know, within a few years we would be facing the devastating COVID-19 pandemic that was made much deadlier by the widespread presence of chronic disease within a large percentage of the population. We could not have guessed that this pandemic would worsen existing chronic conditions by making it more difficult for millions to seek treatment, access healthy food, and find ways to increase physical activity.

The 5th edition of *Chronic Disease Epidemiology, Prevention, and Control* comes at a time when more than a million people in the United States have died from COVID, many individuals have seen their chronic preexisting conditions exacerbated, and a still uncertain number are experiencing chronic post-COVID symptoms. Ironically, the focused attention on COVID in the media overshadowed the articles and public discussion of the prevention and treatment of obesity, heart disease, cancer, and other chronic conditions. Furthermore, personnel on the front lines of preventing and treating chronic conditions were sorely tested by the demands of the pandemic; they were pushed to their limits working long, stress-filled hours, often with inadequate resources and uneven public support.

Given these circumstances, the content of the new edition is even more important now. Chronic diseases have long been common and costly, increasingly so as older adults have become a larger proportion of the US population. By 2030, the number of Americans older than 65 years is expected to reach 72 million, up from 40 million in 2010.[1] In fact, those aged 65 years and older are members of the fastest-growing age group in the United States.[2] Virtually all of these older adults will develop one or more chronic diseases, leading to increased morbidity and/or mortality. And if, as expected, we experience other novel viruses and pandemics, the prevention and/or control of underlying chronic illnesses may yet again prove crucial to reducing severe illness and death from infectious disease.

Tackling chronic disease requires awareness of both the long-standing and the relatively new risks. While cigarette use is down, teens are using other tobacco-related products such as vaping devices.[3,4] Awareness of the risks related to obesity is relatively high, yet obesity levels are continuing to rise year after year.[5] It seems that every year there are new pharmaceutical or clinical interventions promising to reduce the onset or progression of chronic diseases, but we can't seem to adequately apply the effective medications we already have. For example, the percentage of people with hypertension who have their condition under control still hovers around 54%.[6] During the pandemic we saw a spike in chronic behavioral health issues, with depression, anxiety, and drug-related deaths increasing at alarming rates. The physical and behavioral health impacts from COVID are even worse among Black, Indigenous, and other people of color. For example, life expectancy for American Indians and Alaska Natives dropped by nearly 7 years between 2019 and 2020, from 71.8 to 65.2 years. That is compared to a life expectancy decrease of three years for the overall US population during the same period.[7]

The new edition recognizes the need for an up-to-date awareness and response. It heightens our understanding of the complexity of the issues by updating existing content and adding new areas of focus such as oral health and sleep deprivation.

While the pandemic has eroded gains, it is worth noting there are still reasons to be hopeful. Efforts to weaken the Affordable Care Act were largely unsuccessful. In fact, more and more states are expanding their Medicaid coverage.[8] Furthermore, the dramatic shift from fee-for-service to innovative value-based reimbursement and a whole-person approach to optimal health is continuing. More and more states are expanding such services as the community-based National Diabetes Prevention Program, home-based asthma risk reduction counseling, and medical equipment support. An increasing number of states are applying for Medicaid waivers that allow them to cover services to address needs such as home-delivered meals, transportation, housing supports, and care coordination provided by community health workers.

Yet despite these positive moves, we often still struggle to understand and implement the best approaches. As this edition highlights, tackling chronic disease prevention requires a well-informed and comprehensive approach. While we still need high-quality, effective clinical care, health education, and counseling, it is the "mezzo-level" or neighborhood factors that have the greater influence on the presence or absence of chronic illness. Income levels are correlated with many chronic illnesses, with those living in low-opportunity and low-wealth neighborhoods at greatest risk of experiencing ongoing health challenges. And existing structural and systemic racism continue to present real barriers for individuals and communities who struggle to achieve well-being. Many communities across the United States have come together to build on their assets during COVID and imagine a future where they are able to take advantage of opportunities to "bounce forward" from the pandemic as opposed to "returning to normal." That is, they seek to foster conditions where safe, stable, and affordable housing options were limited, access to healthy food were limited, and daily stressors—including racially based micro-aggression—weakened the overall immune system.

As was pointed out in the previous edition, we need a public health system that is able to demonstrate how risk factors that contribute to chronic disease can be mitigated, that has up-to-date tools including more real-time data and evidence-based approaches, that can build authentic partnerships with health care and other sectors, and that enables community residents and community power–building organizations to drive meaningful changes in their own communities. In an updated chapter, this edition rightly draws attention to the social, economic, and environmental factors that play a major role in causing and exacerbating or, alternatively, preventing the development of chronic illness. These factors ultimately contribute to the disparities in life expectancy between populations of color and White populations and between the rich and the poor.

The authors and editors of the current edition deserve credit for their crisp overview of the current knowledge and best practices, provided in frank detail. In this time of trauma, recovery, and change, reducing disease, promoting equity, and bending the cost curve will not come easily. We need to make these goals top priorities, adapt both the health care and the public health systems, and integrate them into a single health-oriented system while embracing the necessity of working beyond the walls of our clinical and governmental settings.

None of this is possible without adequate and sustainable resources. Yet, for many years, core funding for the public health system had been declining. A familiar pattern occurred during the COVID pandemic—namely, the infusion of lots of one-time-only funding in the midst of an immediate crisis, followed by a diminution or elimination of such funding and a return to the underfunded base.[9] However, the severity of the crisis has resulted—at least temporarily—in an increased awareness of the importance of shoring up the public health workforce and infrastructure. This allowed CDC to use billions of dollars in COVID funding to support these nondisease–specific, essential components of the public health system. Whether such practices survive the COVID era is yet to be determined.

As was true in past editions, this volume points the way to the future and is a useful summary and influential framework for our challenges. Its content is more meaningful than ever in the wake of the lessons from the COVID-19 pandemic—the reinforced awareness of the impact of structural racism and the heightened understanding that only through significant changes in social and economic conditions will we succeed in the widespread prevention of chronic disease. Now more than ever, we need audiences of this edition to include those partners outside of traditional public health and health care circles who play such a critical role in enabling communities to achieve health and well-being.

So, here is the ambitious goal of this latest edition. With chronic diseases growing in significance, it is intended to assist both public health and health care professionals in preventing and controlling these diseases. The ability to embrace and accept the urgency of this goal is within our power. Future generations will judge us harshly if we fail to learn the lessons from, and seize the opportunities to reduce chronic disease during, this extraordinary period in our history. They will note we saw the devastating, worldwide consequences of neglecting chronic illnesses (and their connection to infectious disease pandemics) and had the knowledge and experiences for this to be the turning point. The last few years have underlined this is a necessity and not just an option. The stakes are simply too great. We hope this edition contributes to the tasks in front of us—namely the challenges of not only reducing illnesses, premature deaths, and the costs associated with chronic disease but also for creating environments at the local, state, tribal, territorial, and federal levels that optimize equity, well-being, and the quality of life.

John Auerbach, MBA
Monica Valdes-Lupi, JD, MPH

REFERENCES

1. Colby SL, Ortman JN. Projections of the size and composition of the US population: 2014 to 2060. Report number P25-1143. US Census Bureau. March 3, 2015. Available at: https://www.census.gov/library/publications/2015/demo/p25-1143.html. Accessed September 12, 2023.
2. 2010 census shows 65 and older population growing faster than total US population [news release]. US Census Bureau. November 30, 2011. Available at: https://www.census.gov/newsroom/releases/archives/2010_census/cb11-cn192.html. Accessed December 7, 2022.
3. Wang TW, Gentzke AS, Creamer MR, et al. Tobacco product use and associated factors among middle and high school students—United States, 2019. *MMWR Surveill Summ.* 2019;68(12):1–22. Available at: http://dx.doi.org/10.15585/mmwr.ss6812a1. Accessed December 7, 2022.
4. Gentzke AS, Wang TW, Jamal A, et al. Tobacco product use among middle and high school students—United States, 2020. *MMWR Morb Mortal Wkly Rep.* 2020;69(50):1881–1888. Available at: http://dx.doi.org/10.15585/mmwr.mm6950a1. Accessed December 7, 2022.
5. Centers for Disease Control and Prevention. Surveillance systems: nutrition, physical activity, and obesity. Reviewed July 22, 2022. Available at: https://www.cdc.gov/obesity/data/surveillance.html#NPAO. Accessed December 7, 2022.
6. Farley TA, Dalal MA, Mostashari F, Frieden TR. Deaths preventable in the US by improvements in the use of clinical preventive services. *Am J Prev Med.* 2010;38(6):600–609. doi:10.1016/j.amepre.2010.02.2016
7. Arias E, Tejada-Vera B, Ahmad F. Provisional life expectancy estimates for January through June, 2022. National Center for Health Statistics. Vital Statistics Rapid Release No. 10. February 2021. Available at: https://www.cdc.gov/nchs/data/vsrr/VSRR010-508.pdf. Accessed December 7, 2022.

8. Kaiser Family Foundation. Status of state Medicaid expansion decisions: interactive map. July 27, 2023. Available at: https://www.kff.org/medicaid/issue-brief/status-of-state-medicaid-expansion-decisions-interactive-map. Accessed September 12, 2023.
9. Trust for America's Health. The impact of chronic underfunding on America's public health system: trends, risks, and recommendations, 2020. Available at: https://www.tfah.org/report-details/publichealthfunding2020. Accessed December 7, 2022.

Preface

Since the publication of the 1st edition of *Chronic Disease Epidemiology and Control* over 30 years ago, our understanding of the causes and consequences of chronic diseases has continued to progress. We have also recognized that some diseases are becoming more "chronic," due to advances in therapeutics, and that some chronic diseases have infectious origins, as a result of a better understanding of etiology and pathophysiology. Importantly, researchers have continued to identify effective programs and policies to reduce the risk of chronic disease, or to control their consequences. The addition of "prevention" to the previous edition—making it *Chronic Disease Epidemiology, Prevention, and Control*—reflected an increasing focus in public health and health care on the prevention of chronic diseases and their related risk factors. In this 5th edition, the focus on prevention is expanded further through a deeper discussion of health equity and the social determinants of health, as well as traditionally less-covered risk factors like sleep and oral health. Authors have been encouraged to look at chronic disease throughout the life course, along the continuum from health to illness and from prebirth to death.

Embarking upon this 5th edition two years into the COVID-19 pandemic has required us to look critically at the public health infrastructure in the United States, and the strengths and weaknesses of our health care systems. Disparities in chronic disease burden by race, ethnicity, socioeconomic status, and geography have never been so critical to address by implementing preventive health interventions or filling treatment gaps. We need to seize the world's current awareness of disease prevention, epidemiology, and control to inspire nontraditional public health partners to engage in community health–improvement efforts, such as private sector health care, business, media, academia, and community groups. Some health care systems are responding to this call with efforts to not only increase health care coverage and improve quality but also to develop incentives to reward population health improvement rather than simply rewarding more high-cost treatments.

In addition, information technology has continued to evolve and is now able to provide an overwhelming amount of information, which has become increasingly accessible with the near ubiquity of smartphones and other mobile devices. However, conflicting with the promise of better information for public health are concerns about patient privacy, confidentiality, and proprietary rights to health information technology.

With the changing landscape, this edition has been updated to help students and practitioners keep abreast of advances in chronic disease prevention and control by providing up-to-date and practical information about leading chronic diseases, conditions, and risk factors. This book is intended to support a broad range of chronic disease prevention and control activities; it is designed to serve as a quick reference guide for students or practicing public health and health care professionals who need to locate critical background information or develop appropriate interventions.

This book is intended for several audiences. First, it will be useful to professionals involved in the practice and teaching of chronic disease epidemiology, prevention, and control at all levels. In state public health agencies, this book will be helpful to staff involved in primary and secondary prevention of chronic diseases, including epidemiologists, physicians, nurses, health educators, and health promotion specialists. In local public health agencies, administrators, physicians, nurses, health educators, and sanitarians will find the text of value.

In academic institutions, the book will provide helpful background information on chronic diseases for students taking beginning and advanced public health courses. Although the book is intended primarily for a North American audience, there is literature drawn from all parts of the world, and we believe that much of the information covered will be applicable to countries and communities around the world.

Finally, the book will provide health care systems with important information about chronic disease prevention, especially as these systems seek to achieve the "Triple Aim" of health care—improving quality, reducing costs, and improving population health. Accountable care organizations are beginning to extend care into the community, using many of the evidence-based interventions described in this book.

The authors of the various chapters were selected for both their scientific expertise and their practical experience in carrying out chronic disease control programs at the community level. The new edition now includes 24 chapters and is organized into four major parts: I. Public Health Approaches; II. Upstream Risk Factors; III. Midstream Chronic Conditions; and IV. Downstream Chronic Diseases. In the new edition, we reflect feedback we have received informally from colleagues and have added two new chapters: "Sleep Behaviors and Disorders" and "Chronic Oral Diseases."

Chapter 1 provides a historical review of chronic disease control, a brief explanation of the current status of chronic disease control programs, and a discussion of the prospects and challenges for chronic disease control during the next decade and beyond. Chapters 2 and 3 briefly review the methods used in chronic disease epidemiology and surveillance and provide a framework for the interpretation of the information in the following chapters. Chapter 4 provides an overview of chronic disease intervention methods, providing a theoretical grounding for interventions that address the diseases and risk factors discussed in later chapters. It also summarizes some of the important features of successful interventions and provides practical examples. Finally, Chapter 5 provides an overview of approaches that can be used in the health care system to not only better manage chronic diseases but also to prevent them, focusing on health behaviors and even social and economic determinants.

In Part II, Chapters 6 through 10 focus on upstream and potentially modifiable risk factors for chronic diseases. The chapters in this section examine the important areas of tobacco use, diet and nutrition, physical inactivity, and alcohol use. In Part III, Chapters 11 through 14 focus on those chronic disease conditions that often result from high-risk behaviors and substantially increase the risk of chronic diseases. These conditions include obesity, diabetes, high blood pressure, and high blood cholesterol. In Part IV, Chapters 15 through 24 describe major downstream chronic diseases: sleep disorders, cardiovascular disease, cancer, chronic lung diseases, mental disorders, chronic neurological disorders, arthritis and other musculoskeletal diseases, liver disease, kidney disease, and oral diseases.

A standard format has been used for all chapters that focus on specific risk factors and chronic diseases to allow the reader quick and easy access to information. Each chapter begins with a brief introduction, reviewing the significance of the chronic disease, condition, or risk factor, and its underlying biological or physiological processes. The next section addresses descriptive epidemiology by examining high-risk groups (person), geographic variation (place), and secular trends (time). The third section describes the causes of the disease, condition, or risk factor under consideration. The final section discusses evidence-based interventions for prevention and control. When available, specific examples of practical and effective public health interventions are described as well as recommendations for future research and demonstration. A list of resources for additional information on chapter topics has been compiled during the editing process and appears at the end of the text book.

This book is not intended to provide a complete and final review of chronic disease epidemiology, prevention, and control. Because the field is so broad, with overlapping issues, any division of the topic becomes somewhat arbitrary. There are literally thousands of different chronic diseases. We have chosen to focus on those that account for a large proportion of morbidity and mortality in the adult population and to emphasize risk factors that can be modified through public health interventions.

Future research will continue to expand our understanding of chronic disease epidemiology, prevention, and control. Epidemiological studies will identify new risk factors and quantify their effects. Intervention studies underway will expand the array of interventions available for public health practitioners. Additionally, the COVID-19 pandemic has forever changed the way we understand the relationship between acute infectious disease and chronic disease, with long COVID and other sequelae of COVID-19 becoming a new priority for research and practice.

Chronic disease epidemiology, prevention, and control is a rapidly expanding field, and much has changed in the six years since the 4th edition was published. We are indebted to the contributors of this 5th edition for volunteering their time and talents as scholars in the field and to Lilah Andrew for help coordinating all aspects of the work.

There is a compelling and increasing need for health professionals with knowledge and expertise in chronic disease prevention and control. We hope this book will become a useful resource for public health and health care professionals as they are called on to meet new public health challenges.

Margaret B. Nolan, MD, MS
Mark V. Wegner, MD, MPH
Patrick L. Remington, MD, MPH

I. PUBLIC HEALTH APPROACHES

1

Current Issues and Challenges in Chronic Disease Prevention and Control

Peter A. Briss, MD, MPH, and Karen A. Hacker, MD, MPH

LEARNING OBJECTIVES

After completing this chapter, readers should be able to

1. Describe the morbidity, mortality, and cost related to chronic disease.
2. Describe key upstream and downstream causes of chronic disease and how they interrelate.
3. Understand the relationships between social determinants of health, health disparities, and the morbidity, mortality, and cost related to chronic disease.
4. Identify and apply evidence-based resources for chronic disease prevention.

INTRODUCTION

In the early 20th century major public health advances transformed communities and led to remarkable increases in life expectancy for Americans. At the same time the population grew rapidly and the geographic distribution and demographic composition of the American population became more urban, older, and more diverse, heralding shifts in the burden of disease from primarily acute causes to chronic ones.

Chronic diseases remain the major causes of US morbidity and mortality; long-standing challenges persist, and new challenges are here. The COVID-19 pandemic has had a major impact on those with chronic disease and will likely have additional implications for the future. Public health again is taking innovative steps to create healthier physical and social environments, support health and healthful behaviors, and encourage the transformation of health care delivery to support population health.

This book provides readers with an up-to-date overview of the major chronic diseases, conditions, and risk factors and the scientific and programmatic principles related to chronic disease prevention and control, including current challenges and opportunities.

Context

About a century ago an epidemiologic transition[1] resulted in declines in infectious causes of death. Heart disease became the leading cause of death by 1933. Since that time, despite much progress, heart disease has remained the leading cause of death in the first quarter of the 21st century, even during the COVID-19 pandemic.

The transition from primarily infectious disease to primarily chronic disease causes of death and the related demographic transition from a predominantly young to an older population both continued into the 21st century in the United States. These changes were driven historically by economic development and technological advances leading to improvements in nutrition, education, sanitation, safety, housing, perinatal and newborn survival, and other factors that reduce death rates. The changes also increased life expectancy and altered the characteristics of the population, including the age distribution. As of 2020 the median age of the US population was 38.2 years,[2] compared to 29.5 years in 1960 and just 22.9 years in 1900. In addition, more than 52 million adults—16% of the population—are age 65 or older, compared with just 3 million adults (<4% of the population) in 1900.[3,4] Age is a leading nonmodifiable risk factor for chronic disease. As the population ages, even if disease incidence, prevalence, and mortality rates stay constant, the number of people living with (and dying from) these diseases will increase. Thus, the age structure of the population has a large impact on the burden of chronic diseases and on public health and health care practice.

Major demographic shifts in the composition of the American population are again underway, with a still aging and increasingly diverse population. Three states—California, Hawaii, and Maryland—and the District of Columbia now have a population that is less than 50% White,[5] i.e., "majority minority."

New challenges are also here. COVID-19 has shown that interactions between chronic and infectious diseases can be more complex than is suggested by a too simplified view of the classical epidemiologic transition. It has exposed the gaps in both the health care and public health systems and has affected people with chronic diseases particularly severely. Given preexisting disparities in chronic disease occurrence and living conditions such as food and housing insecurity, COVID-19 disproportionately affected certain populations—namely, African Americans, American Indians, and Hispanic persons.

Lack of health equity and systemic racism are also long-standing issues that have recently been brought into urgent focus by events like the murder of George Floyd in 2020. These structural issues require immediate public health attention and have been identified by the Centers for Disease Control and Prevention (CDC) as issues that need to be addressed as a core element of public health efforts.[6]

Definition of Chronic Disease

There is not a single universally accepted definition of *chronic disease*. Many definitions have been proposed.[7] Definitions typically share characteristics, including a long course (months to lifelong), but vary on others, including whether they are noninfectious, reversible, result in functional limitations, or produce a need for medical care.

For the purpose of this chapter, we adopt a US Department of Health and Human Services (USDHHS, or simply HHS) definition of a chronic condition: one that lasts a year or more and requires ongoing medical attention and/or limits activities of daily living.[8]

In addition, for public health practice, a distinction is often made between infectious and chronic diseases. This boundary is blurry, however. Many infections (e.g., HIV, Epstein-Barr virus, hepatitis B, hepatitis C, *Helicobacter pylori*, human papillomavirus,[9] now possibly SARS-CoV-2 [see last paragraph of next section]) can cause chronic diseases.

PUBLIC HEALTH IMPACT

From the early 20th century to about 2014, Americans experienced increasingly longer lives. Life expectancy at birth rose from 47.3 years in 1900 to 78.9 in 2014,[10] after which there was some retrenchment that has been attributed to "deaths of despair," prior to a very large 1.8-year decline in 2020 that was largely related to COVID-19. Life expectancy at birth for Americans in 2020 was 77 years.[11] Progress against individual diseases, conditions, and risk behaviors has been impressive. For example, smoking prevalence among adults in the United States has declined by about two-thirds from 42.4% in 1965[12] to 12.5% in 2020.[13] Coronary heart disease death rates have sharply declined since the 1960s, from a peak of 483 deaths per 100,000 population in 1968[14] to 92 per 100,000 in 2020.[15] Age-adjusted death rates from cancer have shown gradual declines since 1990,[16] with similar gradual declines in cancer incidence since 1992.[17]

Despite great public health progress evident in Americans' living longer, healthier lives, Americans do not live as long as people in peer countries. For example, among 34 countries in the Organisation for Economic Cooperation and Development (OECD), the United States ranked 23rd in life expectancy at birth, behind countries like Japan (84 years) and Switzerland (84 years), and just kept pace with lower-income countries such as Estonia (78.4 years) and Turkey (78.3 years).[18] These outcomes are occurring despite the fact that the United States spends more per capita on health care services than any other country in the world (about triple the OECD average) and about a third more than Switzerland, the next highest spender.[18] At the same time the United States lags considerably behind other high-income countries in investments in health promotion and disease prevention, as well as in other public health and social services interventions that keep people well.[19]

The advances mentioned previously improved quality of life and helped usher in longer lives. However, changes over time also brought additional threats to health, among them tobacco use, overconsumption of food with low nutritional value, and reduced physical activity. These, along with excessive alcohol use, are the leading "actual" causes of death in the United States[20] in the 20th and 21st centuries, contributing to all the major chronic disease killers: heart disease, cancer, stroke, chronic obstructive lung disease, and diabetes. These behaviors contribute to nearly 40% of all deaths in the United States[20] and are part of the reason US life expectancy lags behind that of other countries and chronic diseases affect such a large portion of the population. In addition, the contribution of these behaviors to morbidity and diminished quality of life is unquestioned.

Chronic diseases, including heart disease, cancer, obesity, and diabetes, and chronic conditions, such as nicotine addiction and high blood pressure, are among the most common, costly, and preventable health problems in the United States. Chronic diseases represented 7 of the top 10 causes of death in both 2019 and 2020, and cancer and heart disease remained the first and second leading causes of death in the United States both before and after the COVID-19 pandemic.[11]

Every year more than 600,000 people die of heart disease and almost half of Americans have one or more of the three major risk factors for heart disease: uncontrolled high blood pressure, high cholesterol, or smoking.[21] About 1.7 million cases of cancer are diagnosed annually, and about 600,000 Americans die of this disease every year.[22] In 2019 some 1.4 million American adults were diagnosed with diabetes. Currently about 37 million Americans (11.3%) are living with diabetes and, of these, about 23% are undiagnosed. Another 96 million Americans have prediabetes, a condition that puts them at high risk of developing diabetes.[23] In 2017 and 2018 more than 42% of adults were obese (defined as body mass index [BMI] $\geq$ 30 kg/m^2), up from 30.5% in 2000, and more than 9% were severely obese (BMI $\geq$ 40 kg/m^2).[24] In addition, nearly one in five (19.3%) youths age 2 to 19 years is obese (BMI $\geq$ 95th percentile).[25] The prevalence of cigarette smoking has steadily declined since the 1960s, but 12.5% of adults in the United States continue to smoke.[13] Chronic diseases are a substantial cause of morbidity as well as mortality, with arthritis the most common cause of disability in the United States. Of the almost 59 million adults with doctor-diagnosed arthritis, almost 26 million have trouble with usual activities because of the condition.[26] Finally, among the most common chronic conditions in the United States might be "multiple chronic conditions." About 60% of US adults have one or more chronic conditions, and two in five adults have two or more.[27]

Mental and substance use disorders have arguably received short shrift in both the health care and public health systems, yet these conditions are increasingly recognized as intertwined with the prevention and control of other chronic diseases. In 2020 an estimated 52.9 million US adults (21%) had a mental disorder in the past year, among them 14.2 million adults with serious mental illness. Of Americans age 12 years and older, 40.3 million (14.5%) had a substance use disorder in the past year, with alcohol being the most common substance. Of the 28.3 million Americans with an alcohol use disorder, 6.5 million also had another substance use disorder. Nearly eight million Americans age 18 years and older had both a mental disorder and a substance use disorder.[28] In addition, about 38.5 million Americans were found to binge drink,[29] many of whom would not be considered to have an alcohol use disorder. Nonetheless, binge drinking contributes to substantial injury, violence, and premature death. Mental health and substance use challenges are not limited to adults. In 2021 the US Surgeon General issued an advisory calling attention to the "urgent public health issue" of mental health challenges in children and youth that were increasing before, and exacerbated by, the COVID-19 pandemic.[30]

People with mental or substance use disorders have higher mortality and lower life expectancy than people without these disorders. Serious mental disorders can shorten life expectancy by 10 years or more.[31] Chronic diseases or chronic disease risk factors often occur alongside mental disorders or substance use disorders. People with mental disorders are more likely to smoke cigarettes and have obesity, diabetes, or heart disease than people without these disorders, and an estimated 50% of people with chronic physical diseases have comorbid mental disorders.[32]

Our highly specialized health care system often separates treatment of mental health and physical health needs, poorly serving people with comorbid physical and mental disorders. This gap results in poor management and persistence of the physical condition, greater likelihood of disability, higher health care utilization and costs, and premature death.[32]

Mental and substance use disorders challenge the ability of public health and health care to effectively prevent, treat, and manage chronic (and other) diseases. These challenges reinforce the need to more effectively address the social determinants of health and other upstream causes of chronic diseases, including mental disorders, to support healthful environments and behaviors for all people and to integrate medical and health services within the health care system to improve management of both physical and mental health conditions.

In addition to causing significant morbidity and mortality, chronic conditions are increasingly costly, estimated to contribute to 90% of the nation's $4.1 trillion per year health care expenditures.[27,33] These costs are largely borne by public and private health insurers, governments, and businesses, which means they are paid by all of us, whether through taxes, insurance premiums, employer health insurance contributions, or out-of-pocket payments. Obviously, these direct costs do not show the full picture of suffering, lost wages and employment, disability, premature death, reduced productivity, and lack of economic competitiveness attributable to chronic disease.

While the foregoing text clearly demonstrates the burden of chronic disease in the United States, in addition it appears that many chronic conditions have worsened during the COVID-19 pandemic. Obesity may have risen because of less access to healthy foods and fewer opportunities for physical activity.[34] Substance use and mental conditions have increased.[35] Diabetes may be being diagnosed more frequently in people who have had COVID-19.[36] Use of health care services declined, especially early in the pandemic, for preventive, routine, and even emergency care.[37] Finally, some people have experienced relatively long-term symptoms following COVID-19,[38] some of which might become chronic conditions in their own right.

EPIDEMIOLOGY

Upstream Causes, Social Determinants, and Downstream Causes

As McGinnis and Foege first noted in 1993,[20] the leading actual causes of death in the United States are the behaviors that give rise to the diseases that lead to premature death. These are tobacco use, poor nutrition, lack of physical activity, and excessive alcohol use. These behaviors often reflect easy, accessible choices and may be aggressively promoted. Advertising, marketing, and promotion; community design; readily available prepared, packaged, and restaurant foods; and the lack of safe public spaces in which to be physically active—these all help shape the choices we make and the behaviors we are most likely to adopt.

The factors that influence health (Figure 1-1) were described by Frieden[39] as falling into five categories, or levels of a pyramid, organized from greatest to least impact. The base of the pyramid includes "socioeconomic factors," including the "social determinants of health." These factors affect large numbers of people, contribute powerfully to poor health, and can, if ameliorated or mitigated, dramatically improve the health of large numbers of people. They are also unequally distributed across society, with those individuals with the least resources being those most negatively affected.

Social determinants are also present at the next level of the Frieden pyramid, including "environmental" or "community" factors. These can influence health directly or can help people adopt and maintain healthful behaviors. Improving these environmental or community factors and creating nudges that make healthy choices easy, or even the default choice, are public health strategies that may deliver large health impacts and return on investment.

At higher levels of the health impact pyramid, there are "long-lasting protective interventions," often occurring at intersections of public health and health care, where outreach is critical to engage large populations for delivery of one-time or long-acting interventions. These interventions can prevent diseases from developing in the first place (e.g., polyp removal to prevent colon cancer, or vaccinations), detect diseases

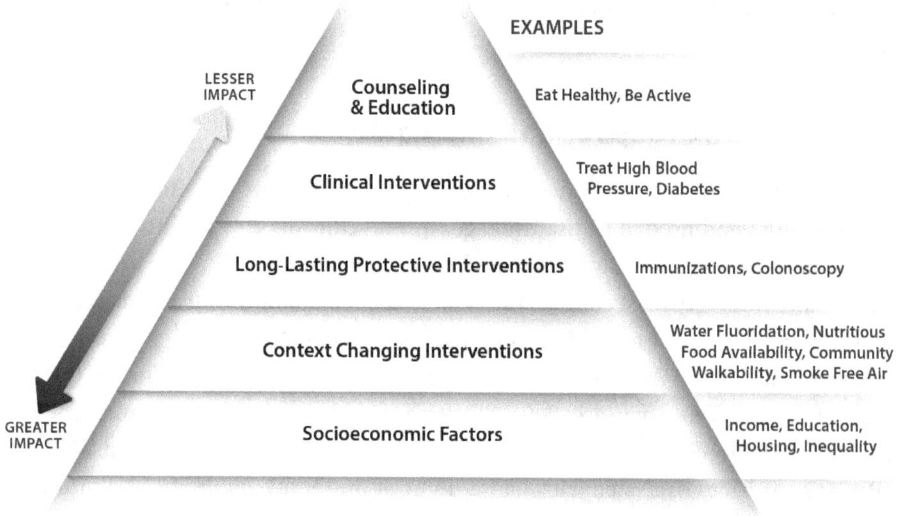

Source: Adapted from Frieden.[39]

Figure 1-1. The Health Impact Pyramid

early when they can be treated and often cured more cheaply and effectively (e.g., cervical cancer early detection), and effectively manage risk factors to avert disease (e.g., smoking cessation). To have a population health impact, long-lasting protective interventions must reach widely into the population, even as interventions are delivered to individuals.

"Clinical interventions" and "counseling and educational interventions" (the fourth and fifth levels of the pyramid) require the greatest investment of resources and the greatest commitment on the part of individuals to obtain the interventions and follow through on the recommendations or treatment. Although they can be highly effective on a case-by-case basis, these interventions tend to have lesser impact, reach, and return on investment than more upstream approaches at the population level.

Chronic disease prevention and public health more generally tend to work most effectively when addressing social determinants of health, in the "context changing" and "long-acting" levels, where governmental public health has the clearest mandate, population impact is great, fewer resources are required, and individuals are more strongly supported in achieving and maintaining behaviors that keep them well. Nonetheless, public health also has a role in monitoring and addressing the socioeconomic factors at the base of the pyramid that have such a profound impact on health status and in strengthening the effective delivery of quality health care services where the existing burden of disease must be treated cost effectively. The levels of the pyramid are not in competition with one another and instead represent a menu of choices requiring careful selection of appropriate choices at multiple levels to best meet community needs and preferences.

Disadvantaged Groups and Health Equity

Health equity is achieved when every person has the opportunity to attain his or her full health potential and no one is disadvantaged from achieving this potential because of social position or other socially determined circumstances.[40]

Death and disability rates are elevated among socioeconomically disadvantaged populations and some racial and ethnic populations (particularly Blacks, Hispanics, and American Indians).[41] Woolf and colleagues have demonstrated that during the last decade of the 20th century nearly 900,000 premature deaths could have been averted in the United States by eliminating the disparity in death rates between Blacks and Whites.[42]

Poverty has been associated with higher rates of morbidity, disability, and mortality for centuries. Possible explanations for these higher rates include the disproportionate burden of individual risk factors associated with poverty, but also a constellation of social determinants including inadequate or crowded housing, poor education, substandard medical care, exposure to hazardous environments, racial discrimination, and stressful life events.[43] In the United States there are also substantial disparities by geography. For example, in 2014 life expectancy at birth varied by as much as 20.1 years by US county. The lowest life expectancies for both sexes were concentrated in the southeastern states, Appalachia, and some counties in the Dakotas that typically included Native American reservations.[44] Similar geographic patterns also often occur for specific diseases.

The COVID-19 pandemic underscored how differences in race/ethnicity, occupation, poverty, and other factors have significant impacts on health and illness.[45] Specifically, it showed that disadvantages in housing, personal space, access to safe places for physical activity, food and nutrition security, and health care, among many other factors, resulted in worsened health outcomes.[46]

The Life Course Perspective

Many of the issues addressed in this chapter, such as aging of the population, social determinants of health, and inequities, are not related to point-in-time insults but reflect harmful or protective effects at critical periods in development or those that may accumulate over time. *Life course epidemiology* has been defined as "the study of long-term effects on later health or disease risk of physical or social exposures during gestation, childhood, adolescence, young adulthood and later adult life."[47] Much has already been learned about factors in early life that influence later life trajectories; yet, much remains to be learned about what works to influence the life course in a healthier direction and how best to intervene early to facilitate longer, healthier lives.

EVIDENCE-BASED APPROACHES AND INTERVENTIONS

Although chronic diseases have major negative effects on morbidity, mortality, and quality of life, they can be prevented or delayed and their effects ameliorated at every stage. Some gains can be realized quickly, but most take time and persistence over the long term. Effective strategies are available in both community and clinical settings.

Effective program planning involves assessing the community, setting priorities and objectives, selecting interventions that address community conditions and priorities, implementing interventions, and evaluating results.[48]

Goals

The goals of chronic disease prevention and control are to improve health, life expectancy, and quality of life so that people live longer, healthier lives, free of disability, with morbidity at the end of life compressed into as brief a time as possible. Although such improvements could off-load considerable burden from the health care delivery system, a substantial burden of disease requires medical intervention, and many health care services work effectively to prevent and control chronic diseases. Thus, health care approaches to improving health system performance are an important component of chronic disease prevention and control. Berwick identified a widely used set of goals for achieving health system quality called the triple aim, which includes (1) increasing the effective delivery of quality clinical preventive, management, and treatment services; (2) reducing the costs of health care delivery; and (3) improving population health.[49] These goals become easier as public health achieves success in improving the overall health of the population and as health care payment models move from paying for volume of services to paying for improvements in health.

It is not enough for these goals to be achieved only among advantaged populations. Because health equity is achieved when every person has the opportunity to attain his or her full health potential, chronic disease prevention and control must assure that all populations reduce their disease burden and that efforts reduce existing inequities.

Strategies

With these goals in mind, chronic disease prevention and control focuses on

- Assuring social conditions and environments in which people can be healthy;
- Preventing the development of risk behaviors (e.g., cigarette smoking and excessive alcohol use);
- Promoting the development of healthful behaviors (e.g., regular physical activity, healthy diet, and adequate sleep);

- Identifying and eliminating modifiable risk behaviors and factors when they do occur (e.g., tobacco use cessation and exposure to secondhand smoke);
- Screening for and reducing disease risks (e.g., screening for high blood pressure and various cancers);
- Enabling community delivery of structured lifestyle interventions to help people manage disease once it occurs and prevent progression and complications; and
- Treating disease to prevent progression, disability, and premature death.

A commonly used taxonomy names these levels of intervention health promotion, primary prevention, secondary prevention, and tertiary prevention; these levels relate to the populations targeted by the interventions (healthy people, those with risk factors, asymptomatic people with adverse biologic changes, and those with disease, respectively). This classification scheme is not unique to chronic disease prevention but applies to disease prevention generally.

Strategies to prevent and control chronic disease can be organized into domains, among them epidemiology and surveillance, environmental approaches, health systems interventions, and linking community and clinical services.[50] These strategies especially require attention to improve the social determinants of health that set the stage for chronic disease development (i.e., the lower levels of the pyramid shown in Figure 1-1).

Epidemiology and Surveillance

Epidemiology and surveillance involve monitoring the occurrence and distribution of diseases, conditions, and risk factors across a population. They require expertise to collect data and to develop and deploy effective interventions, identify and address gaps in program delivery, and monitor and evaluate progress in achieving program goals. Work in these areas provides essential data and information to define and prioritize public health problems, identify places and populations most affected, guide solutions, and monitor progress. Information and insights are not collected for their own sake but must be effectively communicated to educate decision makers, practitioners, and the public about the high rates of disease, disability, and death and the high health care costs associated with chronic diseases. They are also utilized to help choose and promote effective interventions and to communicate successes in addressing chronic diseases and/or remaining gaps and unmet needs.

Environmental Approaches

Environmental approaches promote health directly and support and reinforce healthful behaviors at national, state, and community levels, and in settings such as schools, childcare and senior programs, worksites, and businesses. They include improvements in the social determinants of health and some approaches to improving health equity.

This strategic area works to address areas like improving the physical environment (e.g., reducing air pollution), ensuring food and nutrition security (e.g., expansions in access to and availability of healthy foods and beverages), improving the built environment (e.g., providing safe and convenient places for physical activity), implementing tobacco-free policies (that reduce availability, affordability, and use of tobacco and eliminate exposure to secondhand smoke), improving social connectedness, and improving clinical community linkages (discussed further below). These kinds of approaches are often advanced through policy and regulatory processes that change the context in which people live, work, and play. These tend to be cost-effective approaches that can have lasting effects on population health.

Health Systems Interventions

Health systems interventions improve the quality of clinical preventive services and other health care of public health importance and increase their effective use to prevent disease, detect diseases early, reduce or eliminate risk factors, and mitigate or manage complications. Interventions that increase access to and build demand for quality preventive services can also reduce disparities in access to care and care-related health outcomes. This is particularly true in an era of health care reform that facilitates system improvements in the service of improving population health.

Although health care interventions can be powerful drivers of population health and have, for example, driven much progress in cardiovascular outcomes,[51] they typically generate smaller health improvements than policies and environmental changes and are complements to, and not replacements for, more upstream and community approaches. Indeed, health care is estimated to contribute only around 20% or less of variation in health outcomes.[52] Nonetheless, clinical and other preventive services that detect diseases early and better manage risk factors play a critical role in chronic disease prevention and health promotion and offer the promise of improving quality of life and reducing health care costs.

Linking Community and Clinical Services

Strategies that link community and clinical services help ensure that people with or at high risk of chronic diseases have access to clinical resources they need to prevent or manage these diseases. In addition, the health care system can help link people with social needs (that interfere with their health) to needed services. With these linkages in place, people can improve their quality of life, delay or avert the onset or progression of disease, avoid complications, and reduce the need for more health care. Community programs that provide these benefits include chronic disease self-management programs, the National Diabetes Prevention Program, and a variety of fall prevention, arthritis self-management, and diabetes self-management programs. From the clinical setting, people can be linked to services related to nutrition, housing, and transportation, for example, that address the need for, or reduce barriers to, health care.[53] To be most effective, these bidirectional services need to allow communication between clinical and community providers and to be appropriately reimbursed.

Population-Wide and High-Risk Approaches

The British epidemiologist Geoffrey Rose contrasted population-wide and high-risk approaches to disease prevention.[54] The former attempts to move the distribution of risk factors to healthier levels in the whole population, whereas the latter attempts to reduce risk among the most affected. Rose and others have argued that the population-wide approach has important advantages. The common risk factors for chronic diseases are usually distributed among a large proportion of the population, and the largest number of the cases of chronic disease arises from the populations that possess intermediate- and low-risk profiles (because that is where the bulk of the population is). The implication for prevention is that small changes in risk in the total population will result in a greater overall disease reduction than greater changes in a specified and relatively smaller group at high risk.

High-risk approaches require correct classification of people at high risk but can support efficiently targeting people with highest need. For example, targeting Diabetes Prevention Program activities to people at highest risk improves the efficiency and cost-effectiveness of that program.[55] In general, health professionals and decision makers select from a menu of interventions that address major chronic diseases, conditions, and risk behaviors based on a range of factors including effectiveness, cost-effectiveness, preventable burden, acceptability, and feasibility, among others. For the major chronic diseases, both population-wide and high-risk approaches are generally warranted.

Evidence-Based Information Sources

Many key information sources are now available that assist with documenting the burden of disease, prioritizing health issues and interventions, establishing appropriate goals and targets, and understanding the effectiveness and sometimes cost-effectiveness of programs, policies, and interventions (see Table 1-1). However, better evidence and more action are needed.

Evidence Gaps and Translation Gaps

The sources in Table 1-1 provide substantial evidence to support action on many topics, but there are many remaining knowledge gaps that need to be filled to allow more and faster progress toward preventing and controlling chronic disease. For example, there is

Table 1-1. Sources of Evidence to Support Decision-Making

Source	Comments
Burden of Disease	
CDC and NCHS National Vital Statistics System (NVSS) https://www.cdc.gov/nchs/nvss/index.htm	Regularly provides state-level information on risk behaviors, including the "actual" causes of death, and other issues at the state level.
CDC PLACES https://www.cdc.gov/places/index.html	Provides localized US data at county, census tract, and zip code levels using model-based estimates for 27 self-reported chronic disease-related behaviors and chronic conditions using data from the Behavioral Risk Factor Surveillance System.
America's Health Rankings https://www.americashealthrankings.org County Health Rankings https://www.countyhealthrankings.org	Provides state and local data on community health published annually by the United Health Foundation and the Robert Wood Johnson Foundation, respectively.
The Global Burden of Disease (GBD) study https://www.healthdata.org/research-analysis/gbd	Provides information on leading causes of morbidity, mortality, and disability for more than 200 countries worldwide.
Setting Goals and Targets	
Healthy People 2030 https://health.gov/healthypeople/objectives-and-data/browse-objectives https://health.gov/healthypeople/objectives-and-data/leading-health-indicators	Sets health goals and objectives for the nation that are frequently adapted for use in individual states. Provides a subset of high-priority objectives (leading health indicators), most of which are related to chronic diseases, conditions, and risk factors.
Health care quality data for the following:	Can be used for benchmarking and goal setting and to promote improvement on a range of health care issues.
Health plans: National Committee for Quality Assurance (NCQA) https://www.ncqa.org	
Hospitals: The Joint Commission https://www.jointcommission.org	
Group practices and providers: Medicare https://www.medicare.gov/care-compare	
Intervention Selection	
Cochrane Collaboration https://www.cochrane.org	Provides good-quality systematic reviews, primarily related to health care. A Cochrane Collaboration Public Health Group addresses some nonclinical or public health-related issues.
Campbell Collaboration https://www.campbellcollaboration.org	Provides good-quality systematic reviews, primarily in education, crime and justice, international development, and social welfare.

(Continued)

Table 1-1. (Continued)

Source	Comments
Intervention Selection	
Evidence-based cancer control programs: National Cancer Institute https://ebccp.cancercontrol.cancer.gov/index.do	Provides information on programs that have good supporting evidence. Includes additional supporting information related to cancer prevention and control.
Links Evidence and Recommendations	
US Preventive Services Task Force (USPSTF) https://www.uspreventiveservicestaskforce.org/uspstf	Provides reviews and recommendations for clinical prevention in the US.
National Institute for Health and Care Excellence (NICE) https://www.nice.org.uk	Provides reviews and recommendations related to health care for the UK.
The Guide to Community Preventive Services https://www.thecommunityguide.org	Provides recommendations for community prevention in the US.
Other Selected High-Quality Evidence Resources	
Office of the US Surgeon General https://www.hhs.gov/surgeongeneral/reports-and-publications/index.html	Periodically issues reports summarizing evidence and making recommendations on the prevention of tobacco use in addition to a broad range of other topics.
National Academies of Science, Engineering, and Medicine https://www.nationalacademies.org	Issues reports summarizing evidence and making recommendations on a broad range of health and medical topics.

Note: CDC = Centers for Disease Control and Prevention; NCHS = National Center for Health Statistics.

much left to learn about how best to address structural racism and implicit bias, health equity, and the social determinants of health. At the same time, many chronic disease areas such as tobacco-use prevention and cardiovascular disease prevention and control have numerous known effective interventions that are inadequately resourced (e.g., state tobacco funding relative to CDC-recommended levels)[56] or inadequately delivered (e.g., effective prevention and treatment for hypertension control).[57] Much more work is needed to find effective ways to fill these and other translation gaps.

Improving Reach and Impact

Even the most effective public health efforts and programs fail to reach many people who could benefit from them. Examples include the nearly 40% of the population who are still not covered by comprehensive smoke-free air laws[58] and the still large numbers of the 96 million Americans with prediabetes who are not yet reached by the National Diabetes Prevention Program.

Much more work is needed to continue to expand the reach of programs, services, and health-promoting environments, both in the general population and in the most affected groups. Better coordination of public health programs, the movement of individually oriented efforts outside clinical contexts (e.g., the National Diabetes Prevention Program and tobacco quitlines), and delivery of programs in ways other than one-on-one and face-to-face are also likely to improve reach and efficiency.

MOVING FORWARD

COVID-19 and the Health Debt

As noted, chronic disease causes enormous avoidable death, suffering, and economic cost in the United States, and the COVID-19 pandemic has worsened the status quo. Heart disease, cancer, chronic obstructive pulmonary disease, obesity, and other chronic diseases are risk factors for COVID-19 morbidity and mortality. COVID-19 has also worsened chronic diseases, creating what has been called a health debt.[59] The pandemic has in some cases reduced healthful behaviors or increased unhealthful ones. It has reduced utilization of and access to health care for non-COVID conditions. It may have led to increases in some chronic diseases such as obesity and diabetes. Post-COVID conditions—that is, new, returning, or ongoing health problems people can experience four or more weeks after first being infected with the virus that causes COVID-19[38]—may eventually be seen as new chronic diseases in their own right. All these issues are likely to disproportionately affect those individuals with the greatest social and economic hardship at baseline. Pre-pandemic disparities have been amplified as a result of the pandemic. To address the resulting health debt, we will need to redouble our efforts across the spectrum of chronic disease prevention and control to meet this urgent situation.

Health Equity and Social Determinants of Health

Racial and ethnic minorities experience poorer health status because of a variety of factors, including upstream social determinants of health such as racism,[60] lower income, and less formal education or lower-quality education, and downstream conditions such as reduced access to quality health care. Challenges to public health and health care will include growing a culturally diverse workforce, expanding team care (including community health workers[61] and traditional healers), understanding and accommodating cultural attitudes toward health and disease, overcoming linguistic barriers, and improving overall cultural humility.

Multicomponent approaches, frequently involving both whole-population and targeted strategies, seem likely to best address equity and social determinants. It will likely require specific attention to narrowing disparities as jurisdiction-wide trends improve, assuring that gaps between individuals based on race/ethnicity, gender, geography, poverty, sexual orientation, and other factors can simultaneously narrow. Therefore, whole-population efforts will often need to be complemented with targeted efforts. CDC's Racial and Ethnic Approaches to Community Health (REACH)[62] is an example of a program that serves populations with higher rates of disease using broad policy approaches and more specific individual-level approaches. Results have shown that disparities in risk factors and conditions can be reduced or eliminated with concentrated effort and effective interventions. A key challenge is how to scale and sustain such programs to achieve large and lasting impacts.

Health equity in chronic disease outcomes will require addressing the upstream social determinants of health that currently keep all people and communities from achieving their full health potential. This will require learning lessons from communities that have successfully innovated to address these grand public heath challenges. It will also require equal opportunities for health promotion and disease prevention. (For more detail on health equity and social determinants of health, see Chapter 6.)

Health Care System Improvements

Improvements in health care systems provide an enormous opportunity to accelerate progress in chronic disease prevention and control. Even before the pandemic many gaps existed in the delivery of high-quality health care. For example, there are estimated to be more than 90 million US adults who have hypertension that is not currently adequately controlled.[63] Numerous approaches are being tested to improve the quality of clinical care, reduce health care costs, and improve health outcomes.

Because individuals spend most of their time outside the health care system and health is greatly influenced by what happens outside the health care setting, public health and health care—community as well as clinic—will need to collaborate to ensure that health care systems are performing at their highest levels and that community conditions are as health-promoting as possible. In addition, likely much is to be learned from some of the novel approaches that emerged from attempting to better reach out to populations with health care needs during the COVID-19 pandemic. The use of telemedicine, teledentistry, and some types of home-based testing, for example, has the potential to improve access to and outcomes of care. These new approaches deserve additional work to improve fitness for purpose, reach, and impact, and to assure that all populations have the capacity to access them.

Surveillance

Surveillance is needed to identify chronic disease successes and challenges, to support interventions, and to identify continuing unmet needs.

Although public health surveillance is essential and has had many successes, it also has many long-standing challenges. Surveillance provides excellent information on many topics at the national level; data at state and especially substate levels are often sparse. Information is frequently not available quickly enough, data from various sources are insufficiently connected, data are insufficiently available to the broad range of potential users, and there is frequently inadequate information to help address equity (e.g., adequate information on race, ethnicity, or poverty). The COVID-19 pandemic has highlighted those challenges but has also provoked new investments and illuminated creative ways forward, like increasing connectedness of various data sources and creative uses of health care data. Efforts are underway at multiple levels of public health and health care to help address some of these issues.[64] (For more on surveillance, see Chapter 3.)

An Aging Population

Because of longer lives and lower birth rates than ever before, average ages of the population are increasing in the United States and worldwide.[65] For example, the proportion of adults older than age 65 nearly quadrupled from 1900 to 2019 (4.1%–16%) and is projected to be almost 22% by 2040. Several states and territories, among them Florida, Maine, Vermont, West Virginia, and Puerto Rico, already have more than 20% of their populations older than 65.[66] Because older people use more health care and social services than younger people, the public health successes that led to an aging population have resulted in strains on public health, health care, and social service resources. Public health efforts to address these challenges will need to particularly focus on helping people maintain their health and function as they age. This will involve prioritizing prevention, addressing the social determinants of health in a way that assures health equity, and moving services from clinic to community settings while linking people to those services.

Global Health and Chronic Disease

Infections and other acute conditions, including COVID-19, obviously continue to exact a tremendous toll on the health of persons living in low-, middle-, and high-income countries. However, all countries are also simultaneously experiencing chronic disease epidemics. The World Health Organization (WHO) estimates that chronic diseases—especially cardiovascular disease, cancer, chronic respiratory diseases, and diabetes—cause 71% of all deaths worldwide and about 77% of these deaths occur in low-income and middle-income countries.[67] These chronic diseases represent an enormous toll in premature mortality that will continue to increase unless major changes take place in health policy, training, and resource allocation.

To raise awareness about the burden and preventability of the chronic disease epidemic in the developing world, in 2014 WHO set voluntary goals with the intent of reducing chronic disease death rates from cardiovascular diseases, cancer, and diabetes: to reduce sodium intake, tobacco use, inadequately treated high blood pressure, and the rise of obesity and diabetes, while increasing physical activity, treatment intended to prevent heart attacks and strokes, and the availability of essential medicines and basic technologies to treat major chronic diseases.[68]

In addition to developing policies and health system priorities that address these health problems, there need to be improvements in the training received by health care and public health workers. The current medical and public health workforce in developing countries is inadequate in terms of numbers and has primarily been trained to address acute health problems. Effective care for older patients and populations requires ongoing attention to lifestyle behaviors and coordinated care for complex, chronic conditions that often require multiple specialties and interventions across a variety of settings. Although the science, strategies, and public health approaches described in this book are based on evidence from high-income nations, many are likely also to apply in a range of global settings.

The Public Health Workforce

The skills and other attributes required for a successful public health workforce continue to evolve. Much of the public health workforce remains non-Hispanic White, especially at managerial and executive levels.[69] Additional diversity would improve the ability to serve an increasingly diverse US population. For some time skills have been required in epidemiology, public health management, and community organization, but new skills are always being added. Current examples include cross-jurisdictional collaboration, quality improvement, bridging health care and public health, including public health and primary care integration, evidence-based public health practice, multisectoral collaboration related to social determinants of health and other issues, traditional and new communication, and informatics, among others. However, assessments of the workforce engaged in institutional public health routinely identify major deficiencies in the education, training, and experience of the practitioners in this workforce.[70]

In 2002 the Institute of Medicine (IOM) published a report, "Who Will Keep the Public Healthy? Educating Public Health Professionals for the 21st Century," that identified the training needs of the public health workforce now and into the future.[71] This report called for greater funding and support for training and developing the public health workforce to meet current and emerging skill needs. Some progress is being made, including creative approaches to using distance learning and relatively new undergraduate training in public health.

However, barriers remain in attracting and retaining the public health workforce, as well as providing funding, support, initial training, and continuing education; these barriers have only been exacerbated by the stresses of the COVID-19 pandemic.[72] Workforce gaps can be especially acute for high-demand professionals like epidemiologists, informaticians, laboratory scientists, and nurses.[69] Despite progress in some areas, achieving the ability to attract, train, and retain the public health workforce we need will continue to be a challenge for the foreseeable future.

Multisector Approaches

Chronic disease prevention and control is never accomplished by one actor alone—especially in relation to issues that must be squarely addressed in complex community contexts including equity, social determinants of health, and health behaviors. Chronic disease prevention and control works most effectively when there is the following: broad buy-in to the goals; involvement from multiple sectors, actors, and institutions at the local, state, and federal level and; the political and social will to undertake the most effective strategies. Public health plays a significant role in addressing these issues but requires a broad range of collaborations to succeed. Collaborative partners include government and nongovernmental organizations, health care organizations, insurers, nonprofit organizations, community and faith-based groups, schools, businesses, and others. Success is most likely when appropriate interventions are undertaken at multiple levels (federal, state, and local), in multiple sectors (including housing, education, business, transportation, and health care, among others), and across settings.

Local coalitions and community groups are particularly important, especially when addressing equity and social determinants of health, and especially in communities where trust was not adequately developed or has frayed. Communications need to be mutual, respectful, and long term to be fully successful.[73]

As IOM has noted, "In a society as diverse and decentralized as that of the United States, achieving population health requires contributions from all levels of government, the private business sector, and the variety of institutions and organizations that shape opportunities, attitudes, behaviors, and resources affecting health."[74]

CONCLUSION

Progress in chronic disease prevention and control will require sustained effort to address upstream issues such as the social determinants of health and health equity, health behaviors like tobacco use, and downstream issues like hypertension control. It will require hard work across sectors and organizations and at all levels of society. It will not be easy, but it is a challenge worth taking on.

DISCUSSION QUESTIONS

1. How do systemic racism and health disparities contribute to chronic disease burden, and what approaches to health equity might be part of the solution?
2. What are promising ways that US health outcomes might be brought more into line with those achieved in higher-performing peer countries?

3. What might be promising ways to better prevent or treat the very common issue of multiple chronic conditions?
4. What more might be done to better address the syndemics of chronic physical and mental health conditions?

ACKNOWLEDGMENTS

The findings and conclusions in this chapter are those of the authors and do not necessarily represent the official position of the Centers for Disease Control and Prevention.

We thank Dr. Ursula Bauer for her work on the previous edition of this chapter.

REFERENCES

1. Omran AR. The epidemiologic transition: a theory of the epidemiology of population change. 1971. *Milbank Q.* 2005;83(4):731–757. doi:10.1111/j.1468-0009.2005.00398.x
2. US Census Bureau. 2016–2020 American Community Survey 5-year estimates. Table B01002: median age by sex. Available at: https://data.census.gov/cedsci/table?hidePreview=true&tid=ACSDT5Y2020.B01002. Accessed January 4, 2023.
3. US Census Bureau, 2016–2020 American Community Survey 5-year estimates. Table S0101: age and sex. Available at: https://data.census.gov/cedsci/table?q=2020%20census%20age. Accessed January 4, 2023.
4. Federal Interagency Forum on Aging-Related Statistics. Older Americans 2012: key indicators of well-being. Available at: https://agingstats.gov/docs/PastReports/2012/OA2012.pdf. Accessed January 4, 2023.
5. US Census Bureau. Race and ethnicity in the United States: 2010 census and 2020 census. August 12, 2021. Updated February 5, 2022. Available at: https://www.census.gov/library/visualizations/interactive/race-and-ethnicity-in-the-united-state-2010-and-2020-census.html. Accessed January 4, 2023.
6. Centers for Disease Control and Prevention, Office of Minority Health and Health Equity. Impact of racism on our nation's health. Updated April 8, 2021. Available at: https://www.cdc.gov/healthequity/racism-disparities/impact-of-racism.html. Accessed January 4, 2023.
7. Goodman RA, Posner SF, Huang ES, Parekh AK, Koh HK. Defining and measuring chronic conditions: imperatives for research, policy, program, and practice. *Prev Chronic Dis.* 2013;10:E66. doi:10.5888/pcd10.120239
8. US Department of Health and Human Services. Multiple chronic conditions: a strategic framework. 2010. Available at: https://www.hhs.gov/sites/default/files/ash/initiatives/mcc/mcc_framework.pdf. Accessed January 4, 2023.
9. Institute of Medicine. *The Infectious Etiology of Chronic Diseases: Defining the Relationship, Enhancing the Research, and Mitigating the Effects: Workshop Summary.* Washington, DC: National Academies Press; 2004. doi:10.17226/11026

10. Arispe IE, Gindi RM, Madans JH. Health, United States, 2019. 2021. National Center for Health Statistics. Available at: https://stacks.cdc.gov/view/cdc/100685. Accessed January 4, 2023.
11. Murphy SL, Kochanek KD, Xu JQ, Arias E. Mortality in the United States, 2020. National Center for Health Statistics. 2021. NCHS data brief 427. Available at: https://stacks.cdc.gov/view/cdc/112079. Accessed January 4, 2023.
12. American Lung Association. Overall tobacco trends. Available at: https://www.lung.org/research/trends-in-lung-disease/tobacco-trends-brief/overall-tobacco-trends. Accessed January 4, 2023.
13. Cornelius ME, Loretan CG, Wang TW, Jamal A, Homa DM. Tobacco product use among adults—United States, 2020. *MMWR Morb Mortal Wkly Rep.* 2022;71(11):397–405. doi:10.15585/mmwr.mm7111a1
14. Centers for Disease Control and Prevention, National Center for Health Statistics. Compressed Mortality File CMF 1968–1978. CDC WONDER online database, Series 20, No. 2A, 2000. Available at: http://wonder.cdc.gov/cmf-icd8.html. Accessed January 4, 2023.
15. Centers for Disease Control and Prevention, National Center for Health Statistics. About underlying cause of death, 1999–2020. CDC WONDER online database. 2021. Available at: http://wonder.cdc.gov/ucd-icd10.html. Accessed January 4, 2023.
16. National Center for Health Statistics. Health, United States, 2019. Table 005. Available at: https://www.cdc.gov/nchs/hus/contents2019.htm. Accessed January 4, 2023.
17. National Cancer Institute. Cancer trends progress report: incidence. Updated October 2022. Available at: https://progressreport.cancer.gov/diagnosis/incidence. Accessed January 4, 2023.
18. United Health Foundation. America's Health Rankings. 2020 annual report: international comparison. Available at: https://www.americashealthrankings.org/learn/reports/2020-annual-report/international-comparison. Accessed January 4, 2023.
19. Bradley EH, Taylor LA. *The American Health Care Paradox: Why Spending More Is Getting Us Less.* New York, NY: Public Affairs Books; 2013.
20. McGinnis JM, Foege WH. Actual causes of death in the United States. *JAMA.* 1993;270(18):2207–2212.
21. Fryar CD, Chen T, Li X. Prevalence of uncontrolled risk factors for cardiovascular disease: United States, 1999–2010. NCHS Data Brief 103. National Center for Health Statistics. 2012. Available at: https://www.cdc.gov/nchs/data/databriefs/db103.pdf. Accessed January 4, 2023.
22. Centers for Disease Control and Prevention. Cancer data and statistics. Updated June 6, 2022. Available at: https://www.cdc.gov/cancer/dcpc/data/index.htm. Accessed January 4, 2023.
23. Centers for Disease Control and Prevention. National diabetes statistics report: estimates of diabetes and its burden in the United States. Updated June 29, 2022. Available at: https://www.cdc.gov/diabetes/data/statistics-report/index.html. Accessed January 4, 2023.
24. Hales CM, Carroll MD, Fryar CD, Ogden CL. Prevalence of obesity and severe obesity among adults: United States, 2017–2018. NCHS Data Brief 360. National Center for Health Statistics.

2020. Available at: https://www.cdc.gov/nchs/products/databriefs/db360.htm. Accessed January 4, 2023.

25. Fryar CD, Carroll MD, Afful J. Prevalence of overweight, obesity, and severe obesity among children and adolescents aged 2–19 years: United States, 1963–1965 through 2017–2018. NCHS Health E-Stats. 2020. Available at: https://www.cdc.gov/nchs/data/hestat/obesity-child-17-18/overweight-obesity-child-H.pdf. Accessed January 4, 2023.
26. Theis KA, Murphy LB, Guglielmo D, et al. Prevalence of arthritis and arthritis-attributable activity limitation—United States, 2016–2018. *MMWR Morb Mortal Wkly Rep*. 2021;70(40): 1401–1407. doi:10.15585/mmwr.mm7040a2
27. Buttorff C, Ruder T, Bauman M. *Multiple Chronic Conditions in the United States.* Santa Monica, CA: RAND Corporation; 2017. Available at: https://www.rand.org/pubs/tools/TL221.html. Accessed January 4, 2023.
28. Substance Abuse and Mental Health Services Administration. Key substance use and mental health indicators in the United States: results from the 2020 National Survey on Drug Use and Health. 2021. HHS publication PEP21-07-01-003, NSDUH series H-56. Rockville, MD: Center for Behavioral Health Statistics and Quality, Substance Abuse and Mental Health Services Administration. Available at: https://www.samhsa.gov/data/sites/default/files/reports/rpt35325. Accessed January 4, 2023.
29. Bohm MK, Liu Y, Esser MB, et al. Binge drinking among adults, by select characteristics and state—United States, 2018. *MMWR Morb Mortal Wkly Rep*. 2021;70(41):1441–1446. doi:10.15585/mmwr.mm7041a2
30. Office of the Surgeon General. Protecting youth mental health: the US surgeon general's advisory. US Department of Health and Human Services. 2021. Available at: https://www.hhs.gov/sites/default/files/surgeon-general-youth-mental-health-advisory.pdf. Accessed January 4, 2023.
31. Chesney E, Goodwin GM, Fazel S. Risks of all-cause and suicide mortality in mental disorders: a meta-review. *World Psychiatry*. 2014;13(2):153–160. doi:10.1002/wps.20128
32. Manderscheid R, Kathol R. Fostering sustainable, integrated medical and behavioral health services in medical settings. *Ann Intern Med*. 2014;160(1):61–65. doi:10.7326/M13-1693
33. Centers for Medicare & Medicaid Services. National health expenditure data: historical. Updated December 15, 2022. Available at: https://www.cms.gov/Research-Statistics-Data-and-Systems/Statistics-Trends-and-Reports/NationalHealthExpendData/NationalHealthAccountsHistorical. Accessed January 4, 2023.
34. Lin AL, Vittinghoff E, Olgin JE, Pletcher MJ, Marcus GM. Body weight changes during pandemic-related shelter-in-place in a longitudinal cohort study. *JAMA Netw Open*. 2021;4(3):e212536. doi:10.1001/jamanetworkopen.2021.2536
35. Czeisler MÉ, Lane RI, Petrosky E, et al. Mental health, substance use, and suicidal ideation during the COVID-19 pandemic—United States, June 24–30, 2020. *MMWR Morb Mortal Wkly Rep*. 2020;69(32):1049–1057. doi:10.15585/mmwr.mm6932a1
36. Barrett CE, Koyama AK, Alvarez P, et al. Risk for newly diagnosed diabetes >30 days after SARS-CoV-2 infection among persons aged <18 years—United States, March 1, 2020–June 28, 2021. *MMWR Morb Mortal Wkly Rep*. 2022;71(2):59–65. doi:10.15585/mmwr.mm7102e2

37. Czeisler MÉ, Marynak K, Clarke KEN, et al. Delay or avoidance of medical care because of COVID-19-related concerns—United States, June 2020. *MMWR Morb Mortal Wkly Rep.* 2020;69(36):1250–1257. doi:10.15585/mmwr.mm6936a4
38. Centers for Disease Control and Prevention. Long COVID or post-COVID conditions. Updated December 16, 2022. Available at: https://www.cdc.gov/coronavirus/2019-ncov/long-term-effects/index.html. Accessed January 4, 2023.
39. Frieden TR. A framework for public health action: the health impact pyramid. *Am J Public Health.* 2010;100(4):590–595. doi:10.2105/AJPH.2009.185652
40. Centers for Disease Control and Prevention, National Center for Chronic Disease Prevention and Health Promotion. Health equity. Updated December 8, 2022. Available at: https://www.cdc.gov/chronicdisease/healthequity/index.htm. Accessed January 4, 2023.
41. Adler NE, Rehkopf DH. US disparities in health: descriptions, causes, and mechanisms. *Annu Rev Public Health.* 2008;29:235–252. doi:10.1146/annurev.publhealth.29.020907.090852
42. Woolf SH, Johnson RE, Fryer GE Jr, Rust G, Satcher D. The health impact of resolving racial disparities: an analysis of US mortality data. *Am J Public Health.* 2004;94(12):2078–2081. doi:10.2105/ajph.94.12.2078
43. Murray CJ, Kulkarni SC, Michaud C, et al. Eight Americas: investigating mortality disparities across races, counties, and race-counties in the United States [published correction appears in *PLoS Med.* 2006 Dec;3(12):e545]. *PLoS Med.* 2006;3(9):e260. doi:10.1371/journal.pmed.0030260
44. Dwyer-Lindgren L, Bertozzi-Villa A, Stubbs RW, et al. Inequalities in life expectancy among US counties, 1980 to 2014: temporal trends and key drivers. *JAMA Intern Med.* 2017;177(7):1003–1011. doi:10.1001/jamainternmed.2017.0918
45. Centers for Disease Control and Prevention. Health equity. Updated July 1, 2022. https://www.cdc.gov/coronavirus/2019-ncov/community/health-equity/racial-ethnic-disparities/index.html. Accessed January 4, 2023.
46. Abrams EM, Szefler SJ. COVID-19 and the impact of social determinants of health. *Lancet Respir Med.* 2020;8(7):659–661. doi:10.1016/S2213-2600(20)30234-4
47. Kuh D, Ben-Shlomo Y, Lynch J, Hallqvist J, Power C. Life course epidemiology [published correction appears in *J Epidemiol Community Health.* 2003 Nov;57(11):914]. *J Epidemiol Community Health.* 2003;57(10):778–783. doi:10.1136/jech.57.10.778
48. Zaza S, Briss P, Harris K, eds. *The Guide to Community Preventive Services.* New York, NY: Oxford University Press; 2005.
49. Berwick DM, Nolan TW, Whittington J. The triple aim: care, health, and cost. *Health Aff (Millwood).* 2008;27(3):759–769. doi:10.1377/hlthaff.27.3.759
50. Bauer UE, Briss PA, Goodman RA, Bowman BA. Prevention of chronic disease in the 21st century: elimination of the leading preventable causes of premature death and disability in the USA. *Lancet.* 2014;384(9937):45–52. doi:10.1016/S0140-6736(14)60648-6
51. Ford ES, Ajani UA, Croft JB, et al. Explaining the decrease in US deaths from coronary disease, 1980–2000. *N Engl J Med.* 2007;356(23):2388–2398. doi:10.1056/NEJMsa053935
52. Hood CM, Gennuso KP, Swain GR, Catlin BB. County health rankings: relationships between determinant factors and health outcomes. *Am J Prev Med.* 2016;50(2):129–135. doi:10.1016/j.amepre.2015.08.024

53. Magnan, S. Social determinants of health 101 for health care: five plus five. *NAM Perspectives*. National Academy of Medicine. 2017. doi.org/10.31478/201710c
54. Rose G. *The Strategy of Preventive Medicine*. New York, NY: Oxford University Press; 1992.
55. Zhuo X, Zhang P, Kahn HS, Gregg EW. Cost-effectiveness of alternative thresholds of the fasting plasma glucose test to identify the target population for type 2 diabetes prevention in adults aged ≥45 years. *Diabetes Care*. 2013;36(12):3992–3998. doi:10.2337/dc13-0497
56. Centers for Disease Control and Prevention, Office on Smoking and Health, National Center for Chronic Disease Prevention and Health Promotion. Smoking and tobacco use: best practices for comprehensive tobacco control programs—2014, Centers for Disease Control and Prevention. 2014. Updated June 28, 2022. Available at: https://www.cdc.gov/tobacco/stateandcommunity/guides/index.htm. Accessed January 17, 2023.
57. US Department of Health and Human Services. The surgeon general's call to action to control hypertension. US Dept of Health and Human Services, Office of the Surgeon General. 2020. Available at: https://millionhearts.hhs.gov/files/SG-CTA-on-Hypertension-508.pdf. Accessed January 4, 2023.
58. American Nonsmokers Rights Foundation. Percent of US state populations covered by 100% smokefree air laws. Updated January 1, 2023. Available at: https://no-smoke.org/wp-content/uploads/pdf/percentstatepops.pdf. Accessed January 17, 2023.
59. Ruth L, Alongi J, Robitscher J. Confronting the health debt: the impact of COVID-19 on chronic disease prevention and management. Health Affairs Blog. September 17, 2021. Available at: https://www.healthaffairs.org/do/10.1377/forefront.20210914.220940. Accessed January 4, 2023.
60. Centers for Disease Control and Prevention. Minority health: science and research. Updated November 1, 2021. Available at: https://www.cdc.gov/minorityhealth/racism-disparities/research-articles.html. Accessed January 4, 2023.
61. Centers for Disease Control and Prevention, National Center for Chronic Disease Prevention and Health Promotion. Community health worker resources. Updated July 11, 2022. Available at: https://www.cdc.gov/chronicdisease/center/community-health-worker-resources.html. Accessed January 4, 2023.
62. Centers for Disease Control and Prevention, National Center for Chronic Disease Prevention and Health Promotion. REACH. Updated September 8, 2022. Available at: https://www.cdc.gov/chronicdisease/resources/publications/factsheets/reach.htm. Accessed January 4, 2023.
63. US Department of Health and Human Services, Million Hearts. Estimated hypertension prevalence, treatment, and control among US adults. Updated March 22, 2021. Available at: https://millionhearts.hhs.gov/data-reports/hypertension-prevalence.html. Accessed January 4, 2023.
64. Centers for Disease Control and Prevention. Public health surveillance data: data modernization initiative. Updated December 15, 2022. Available at: https://www.cdc.gov/surveillance/data-modernization/index.html. Accessed January 4, 2023.
65. Centers for Disease Control and Prevention. Trends in aging—United States and worldwide. *MMWR Morb Mortal Wkly Rep*. 2003;52(6):101–106.
66. Administration for Community Living. 2020 profile of older Americans. May 2021. Available at: https://acl.gov/sites/default/files/Aging%20and%20Disability%20in%20America/2020ProfileOlderAmericans.Final_.pdf. Accessed January 4, 2023.

67. World Health Organization. Noncommunicable diseases. Updated September 16, 2022. Available at: https://www.who.int/news-room/fact-sheets/detail/noncommunicable-diseases. Accessed January 4, 2023.
68. World Health Organization. Noncommunicable disease surveillance, monitoring and reporting: NCD global monitoring framework. Available at: https://www.who.int/teams/ncds/surveillance/monitoring-capacity/gmf. Accessed January 4, 2023.
69. Sellers K, Leider JP, Gould E, et al. The state of the US governmental public health workforce, 2014–2017. *Am J Public Health*. 2019;109(5):674–680. doi:10.2105/AJPH.2019.305011
70. Bogaert K, Castrucci BC, Gould E, et al. The Public Health Workforce Interests and Needs Survey (PH WINS 2017): an expanded perspective on the state health agency workforce. *J Public Health Manag Pract*. 2019;25(suppl 2); Public Health Workforce Interests and Needs Survey 2017(2 suppl):S16–S25. doi:10.1097/PHH.0000000000000932
71. Gebbie K, Rosenstock L, Hernandez LM, eds. *Who Will Keep the Public Healthy? Educating Public Health Professionals for the 21st Century*. Washington, DC: National Academies Press; 2003.
72. Stone KW, Kintziger KW, Jagger MA, Horney JA. Public health workforce burnout in the COVID-19 response in the US. *Int J Environ Res Public Health*. 2021;18(8):4369. doi:10.3390/ijerph18084369
73. Hacker KA, Briss PA, Richardson L, Wright J, Petersen R. COVID-19 and chronic disease: the impact now and in the future. *Prev Chronic Dis*. 2021;18:E62. doi:10.5888/pcd18.210086
74. Institute of Medicine. *The Future of the Public's Health in the 21st Century*. Washington, DC: National Academies Press; 2003:17.

2

Epidemiologic Methods for Chronic Disease Prevention and Control

Lin Zhao, MD, MPH, and Patrick L. Remington, MD, MPH

LEARNING OBJECTIVES

After completing this chapter, readers should be able to

1. Define and interpret basic terms and methods used in the epidemiology of chronic disease.
2. Identify the features of epidemiologic study designs and describe their strengths and limitations in chronic diseases.
3. Compute and interpret measures of association between a risk factor and a health outcome and evaluate causal inferences between risk factors and health.
4. Describe major sources of bias and confounding and identify limitations of the methods.

INTRODUCTION

The field of epidemiology has been invaluable in understanding the burden from, and causes of, chronic diseases and in measuring the effects of interventions to prevent and treat chronic diseases. Chronic diseases are distinguished from other health problems by their multiple and interrelated causes, often rooted in early life and related to multiple health factors, including individual behaviors, health care, social and economic factors, and the environment. As public health advances have reduced the burden from infectious diseases, chronic diseases have become the leading causes of death and disability in the United States. As of 2020 heart disease remains the leading cause of death in the United States among both men and women, followed closely by cancer.[1] In addition, many people are surviving with chronic diseases, as most are controlled through health care or lifestyle interventions, rather than being cured or becoming rapidly fatal.

The purpose of this chapter is to provide a brief overview of the methods that can be used to understand not only the epidemiology of chronic diseases, conditions, and risk factors but also the methods that can be used to evaluate the effectiveness of strategies to prevent, detect, and treat chronic disease in the population. After reading this chapter, you will be able to understand the epidemiologic methods used to study and control chronic diseases discussed in the following chapters.

CHRONIC DISEASE EPIDEMIOLOGY

For diseases of known infectious origin, such as AIDS, influenza, and COVID-19, the presence of a single, known, necessary cause (e.g., a virus) helps to focus epidemiologic research and intervention strategies. For injuries, the cause is often acute and leads to immediate health consequences. By contrast, a wide variety of chronic diseases lack such unifying causal agents and often develop over the life course.

For most chronic diseases, the causal process is prolonged and typically complex. Many modest influences, rather than a single predominant cause, contribute to the chances of developing disease. The prolonged duration of these diseases, which often includes a pre-symptomatic phase and subsequent development of chronic disease conditions, provides numerous overlapping opportunities for intervention. For most chronic diseases, the large number of modest risk factors and the diverse opportunities for intervention make their control difficult and typically require a multifaceted approach.

Another important consideration for chronic disease is the meaning of "control" or what it is we are trying to prevent. Chronic disease often affects quality of life long before it affects duration of life, if it affects duration at all. People with diabetes, for example, do have higher mortality, but only many years after diagnosis. In the interim, however, they may experience blindness, kidney failure, painful foot ulcers, leg amputation, or premature heart disease, all as a direct result of having diabetes. "Controlling" diabetes implies not only prolonging life but also, as important, improving the quality of life while one is living with diabetes. Both disease-specific and general measures of quality of life have been developed and validated,[2] and these measures are being used increasingly to describe both the course (natural history) of disease and the effect of various methods of control.

The public and health policymakers frequently underestimate the health and economic burden from chronic diseases. Research has demonstrated that the public is more concerned about diseases and exposures that are unknown or out of one's individual control. For example, although three behaviors (tobacco use, poor nutrition, and physical inactivity) account for nearly two-thirds of preventable deaths in the United States,[3] and the number of deaths attributable to social factors is comparable to that of pathophysiological causes in the United States,[4] the public often perceives much greater risk from AIDS, homicide, and environmental pollution (so-called involuntary risks).[5] There is much to do for chronic disease epidemiologists to convey the disease burden to the public and policymakers.

DESCRIPTIVE EPIDEMIOLOGY

Descriptive epidemiology makes use of available data to examine the distribution of diseases in populations by person, place, and time. This type of information can be used to assess the burden of disease, identify high-risk groups, or monitor trends over time.

Statements such as "602,350 deaths in the US are caused by cancer in 2020" are an easy way to communicate burden to the general public and to policymakers. However, the absolute number of people affected is almost entirely dependent on the size of the population under consideration. Therefore, other measures, like the rate of the disease, must be used when one is making comparisons across populations and over time. The principal rates used in chronic disease epidemiology are incidence and prevalence:

Incidence (or incidence rate) is defined as the number of new cases that occurred during a given time interval divided by the population at risk at the beginning of the time interval. In practice, the incidence rate is typically used to describe the number of new cases that develops in a year in a specified population.

Cumulative incidence refers to the number of new cases over a defined period divided by the "person-time experience of the population"—that is, the number of persons multiplied by the period (multiple years) over which they were monitored; this is often called "person-years."

Prevalence is the number of individuals with a given disease at a given point in time divided by the population at risk for that disease at that time. The prevalence of disease is influenced by the incidence (more new cases yield more existent cases) and persistence of the disease (the longer a disease lasts, the more people carrying the disease at the time of measurement).

Person Factors

Rates of risk factors or diseases can be compared for various subpopulations, such as those defined by age, gender, race, ethnicity, or education. The risk of most chronic diseases increases dramatically with increasing age. Thus, age is perhaps the most important characteristic to consider when one is comparing rates across populations. One way epidemiologists compare rates by age is by breaking up the population into age groups that are narrow enough to detect age-related patterns in the data. For chronic diseases, 10-year age groups are usually adequate. A second way to ease comparison of rates is to adjust the rate to a standard population. This, in effect, combines many age-specific rates into a single age-adjusted rate.

The above-mentioned methods can also be used to compare and adjust other person characteristics, like sex, ethnicity/race, and education.

Place Factors

Rates calculated from an area with a small population are subject to a large amount of variation from year to year, especially for rare diseases. When rates are calculated for small areas, such as a county, the numerator of the rate will usually be small. When a numerator is smaller than 20, rates are "unstable" and may vary by chance alone. If only a few cases are detected a year early or a year late, the incidence rate calculated for a particular year may appear much higher or much lower than it is on average over a longer period. Such rates are not representative of the region and time and cannot be used for comparison. For this reason, one should calculate rates from cases diagnosed over several years to increase the number of cases in the numerator of the incidence rate, thereby increasing the precision of the calculated rate.

The use of these methods can be seen in the maps of cancer mortality for the United States by geographic area (Figures 2-1 and 2-2).[6] These maps compare the cancer mortality rates by health service area (HSA) and by state from 2015 to 2019. First, notice that five years of data were combined to produce more reliable rates. In addition, these rates are age-adjusted (to the US population in 2000) to account for differences in the ages of the populations. Most important to note is that a smaller geographic area shows more detailed health information within a state. Thus, when choosing the size of an area to study a chronic disease, epidemiologists need to consider the balance of too small a geographic area that does not have enough population to generate reliable data versus too large an area that omits the health disparity within the region.

Time Trends

Disease rates change over time. For many chronic diseases, epidemiologists are interested in long-term trends or patterns in the number of cases or the rate. Plotting the incidence rate of a disease over years shows long-term trends in the occurrence of the disease. Health officials use these trends to assess the impact of interventions, guidelines, or the environmental events that may cause an increase or decrease in the occurrence of a disease.

Comparing Rates Across Populations

Once rates have been calculated for various populations or population subgroups, these rates can be compared by using risk ratios. The *risk ratio* (or *relative risk*) of a disease is the ratio of the incidence proportion in people with the risk factor (e.g., smoking) to the incidence proportion in people without the risk factor. Risk ratio is useful to identify risk factors and high-risk groups. An example is provided in the analytic epidemiology section.

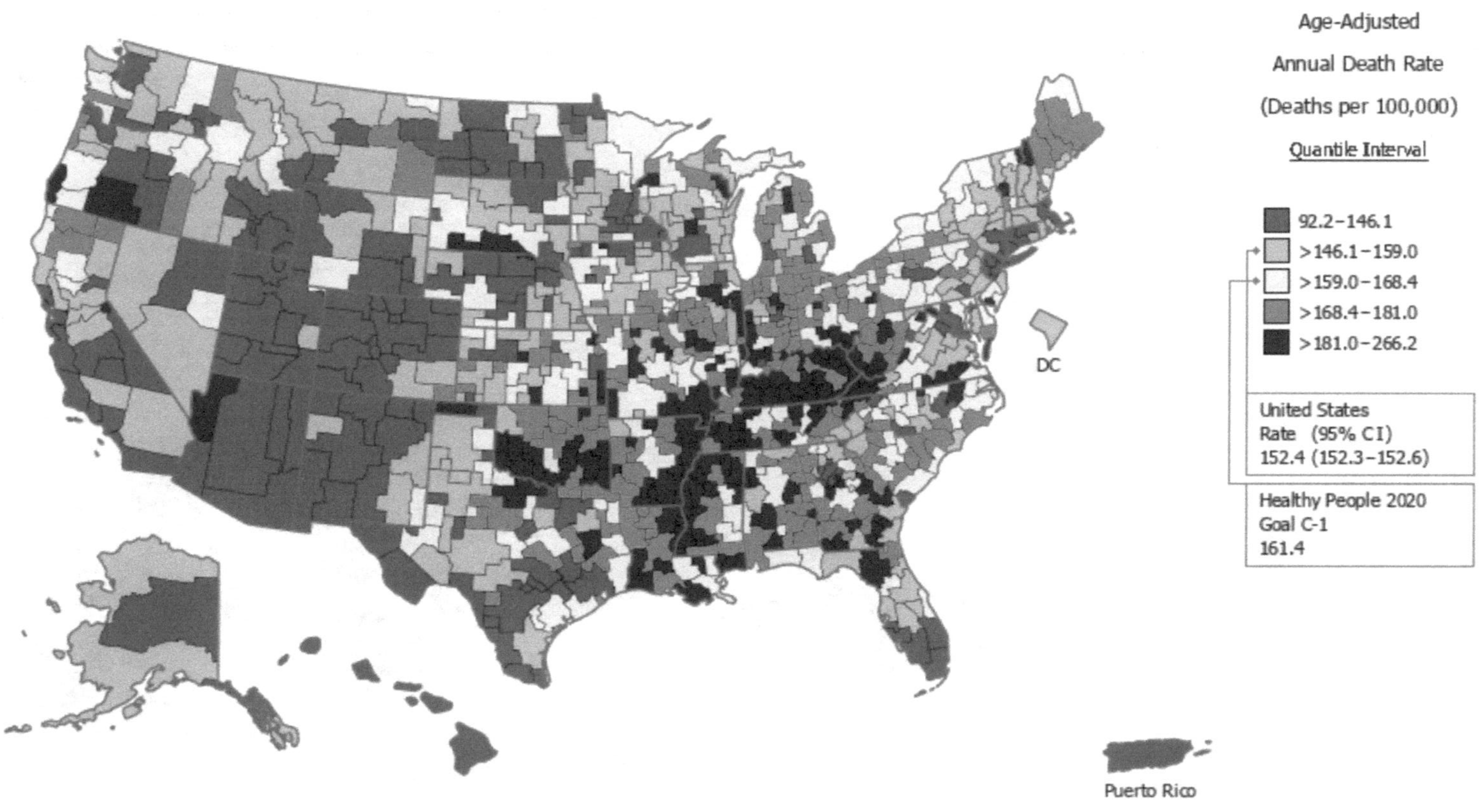

Source: Based on NCI.[6]

Note: CI = confidence interval. Maps were calculated on the NCI Cancer Mortality Maps website. Rates are age-adjusted to the 2020 US population.

Figure 2-1. Cancer Mortality Rates by Health Service Area, United States, 2015–2019

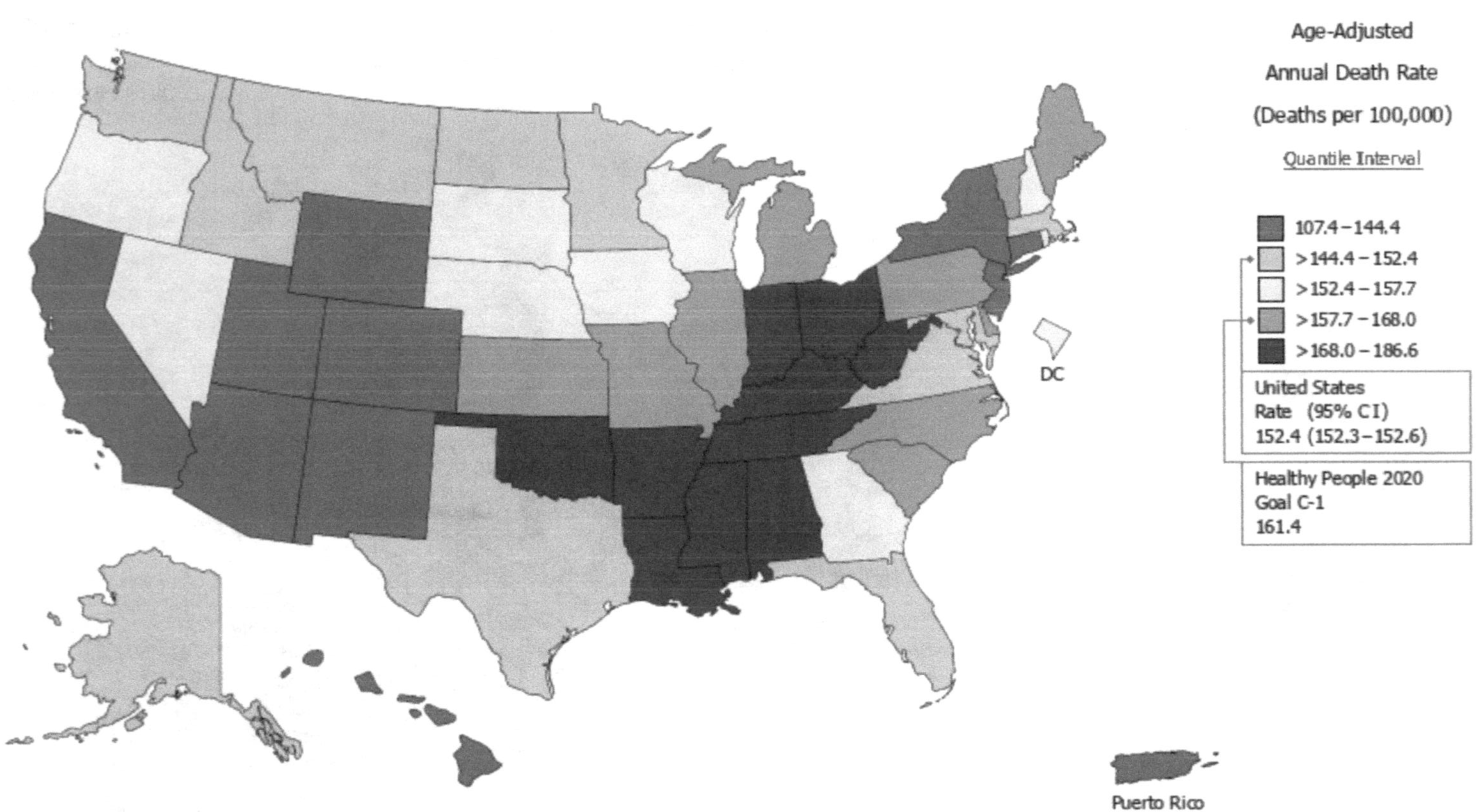

Source: Based on NCI.[6]

Note: CI = confidence interval. Maps were calculated on the NCI Cancer Mortality Maps website. Rates are age-adjusted to the 2020 US population.

Figure 2-2. Cancer Mortality Rates by State, United States, 2015–2019

An alternative to the ratio measure is the rate difference, or when considering prevention, the *absolute risk reduction* (ARR), which is calculated by subtracting the rate from baseline rate. ARR allows clinicians to calculate the *number need to treat* (NNT), which is the reciprocal of ARR (1/ARR). This measure provides a simple way to judge the actual impact of a treatment or preventive service in a population.

ANALYTIC EPIDEMIOLOGY

Analytic epidemiology is used to understand the "determinants" (i.e., causes) of chronic diseases—with a focus on those determinants that can be modified. One of the most important and challenging roles for analytic epidemiology is to differentiate between factors that are simply associated with chronic diseases and those factors that actually cause those chronic diseases.

Analytic epidemiology can be used not only to identify modifiable risk factors but also to estimate the morbidity and mortality that might be prevented by interventions. Experimental evidence can evaluate the effects of intervention measures and use those results to design new and better programs for controlling chronic diseases. Even when there are strong theoretical reasons to expect benefit, an evaluation is needed to prove the intervention reduces mortality or improves quality of life in a real-life setting. Every intervention has a downside, either through undesired consequences or by consuming excess resources. Calculating the proportion of a disease that is attributable to a particular risk factor may help to quantify the effect of an intervention used to address that factor (cost-effective analysis).

STUDY DESIGNS IN CHRONIC DISEASE EPIDEMIOLOGY

Observational Studies

Many medical research questions started with careful observations by health care providers of what they see during clinical practice. Those observations are documented in case reports or case series. Case reports and case series describe a particular clinical phenomenon in one or a few patients. They provide a comprehensive and detailed description of the case(s) under observation. They serve to generate hypotheses that can be tested by studies designed to have a comparison/control group.

By contrast, observational studies such as cohort or case-control studies, allow researchers to compare the effects of an exposure on disease, and vice versa.

Cohort Studies

In a cohort study, exposed and unexposed participants are identified and then observed over time for the development of disease. Having obtained measures of disease

Table 2-1. Incident Rates of Cervical Carcinoma in Situ and Rate Ratios Among Ever-Smokers and Nonsmokers: European Prospective Investigation Into Cancer and Nutrition (EPIC) Study

Smoking Status	Person-Years of Observation	No. of CIS Cases	Incidence Rate of CIS (per 1,000 person-years)	Rate Ratio (HR)
Nonsmokers	1,581,045	325	0.206	1.0 (Reference)
Ever-smokers	1,125,354	468	0.416	2.0

Source: Based on Roura et al.[7]

Note: CIS = carcinoma in situ; HR = hazard ratio. Data from 308,036 women selected for the EPIC study. Crude rate ratios are slightly different from those in the published manuscript, which were adjusted for age.

occurrence (incidence rates or cumulative incidence) for both exposed and unexposed groups, the influence of exposure can be quantified as either the ratio of disease in those exposed compared to those unexposed (the relative risk) or the difference between disease rates among those who are exposed versus unexposed (the rate difference), as discussed earlier.

Table 2-1 is an example comparing incident rates of cervical carcinoma in situ (CIS) among smokers versus nonsmokers.[7] A total of 308,036 European women were followed up for a median of nine years. Incident rates and the rate ratio were calculated. In this case, the rate ratio is also called the hazard ratio.

The advantage of a *prospective* cohort study is the opportunity to actively and intensively measure the exposures of interest before the period of disease induction, leaving less room for bias. For example, instead of having participants recall dietary fat intake over many years (*retrospective* cohort study), intake could be calculated more accurately if periodic direct measurements were made. However, for rare diseases and those with a prolonged period between exposure and the manifestation of adverse effects (typical of chronic diseases), prospective studies must be extremely large and prolonged, and therefore they are very expensive.

Case-Control Studies

A case-control study is another type of observational study that can be used to investigate the causes of chronic diseases. Case-control studies recruit participants on the basis of their health outcomes (e.g., disease); this design intentionally oversamples persons who have developed the disease of interest. In case-control studies, researchers identify a sample of people with the disease, or case patients (often, all available case patients), and a sample of people without the disease, or control participants, from the same population that yielded the case patients.

The historical exposures that may have influenced disease risk are ascertained for all participants, and the frequency of exposure among case patients is compared with that among control participants. Such studies cannot yield incidence rates or cumulative incidence because the population at risk is not comprehensively defined; the control participants are typically a sample of that source population, but the sampling fraction is unknown. An estimate of the ratio of incidence rates or risks can be obtained, however, by calculating the ratio of the odds of exposure among cases (the number exposed divided by the number not exposed) to the odds of exposure among controls, referred to as the odds ratio (OR). The odds ratio is intended to approximate the relative risk. No estimate of the risk difference can be obtained from a case-control study.

The obvious advantages of case-control studies are the relative speed with which they can be conducted, because the latent period is all in the past, and the small number of participants who have to be enrolled. In contrast to a cohort study, in which many participants who never develop the disease must be monitored, a case-control study includes only a small but adequate fraction of the non-diseased population. For example, with the smoking as a risk factor for cervical cancer study, human papillomavirus (HPV) infection is a known risk factor/cause for cervical cancer and might influence the result. It would be labor and money intensive to test HPV serology for all 308,036 women who participated in the study. To solve this problem, a nested case-control study was conducted to test only a subset of the original population of HPV serology and confirm that smoking is an independent risk factor for cervical cancer (OR = 1.7).[7]

The principal weakness of case-control studies is the vulnerability to bias arising from the fact that the disease has occurred before risk factor information was ascertained. The strengths and limitations of prospective and case-control studies are summarized in Table 2-2.

Table 2-2. Strengths and Limitations of Various Study Designs

Study Type	Strengths	Limitations
	Experimental Studies	
Randomized clinical trial	• Controls for bias by random assignment	• High cost • Not practical for many exposures (e.g., lifestyle, environmental, socioeconomic) • Not practical for long latency periods
	Observational Studies	
Prospective cohort	• Opportunity to measure risk factors before disease occurs • Can study multiple disease outcomes • Can yield incidence rates as well as relative risk estimates	• Often expensive • Requires large number of participants • Requires long follow-up period
Case-control	• Useful for rare diseases • Relatively inexpensive • Relatively quick results	• Possible bias in measuring risk factors after disease has occurred • Possible bias in selecting control group • Identified cases may not represent all cases

Experimental Studies

Experimental studies are designed to evaluate interventions of disease treatment and prevention. One big challenge of experimental studies is to choose appropriate comparison groups. Comparison groups tend to vary in their appropriateness for disease intervention studies. Least convincing are comparisons with national data or populations in other studies. Previous data on the same population are most appropriate if the disease can be shown to have been stable for a long period and if there are no other reasons for a change in disease incidence. The best control groups are those that can be shown to be similar to the intervention population and from which disease information is collected concurrently.

Randomized Controlled Trials

Randomized controlled trials (RCTs) are considered the most scientifically rigorous type of epidemiological study. In an RCT, participants are randomly assigned to either receive or not receive a preventive or therapeutic procedure. The disease course or mortality patterns are then observed over time to assess the effectiveness of the preventive or therapeutic procedure. One key objective of an RCT is to draw specific conclusions about the intervention. If the health of the population receiving the intervention improves, the investigators must demonstrate that a similar population that did not receive the intervention did not improve, at least to the same extent.

One way to improve the comparability between the intervention group and the control group is to use randomization when assigning study participants. Randomization protects the study from biases that might be introduced by the investigator into the assignment process and allows even distribution of variables (or characteristics of the participants) that the investigators are not aware might influence the outcome.

Validity of the Study

Despite the increasing sophistication of research studies, uncertainty continues to exist in our understanding of the causes and consequences of chronic diseases. As mentioned at the beginning of the chapter, the causal processes for many chronic diseases are prolonged and complex. There are many modest influences, rather than a single predominant cause, that contribute to the probability of developing a chronic disease. It is possible that errors in measurement or in selection of study participants lead to spurious results. When interpreting a study, epidemiologists often ask themselves whether the observed association is valid or not. Two of the most important factors to consider are bias and confounding.

Bias

Bias is defined as any systematic error in the design, conduct, or analysis of a study that results in a mistaken estimate of an exposure's effect on the risk of disease. There are two major categories of bias: selection bias and information bias.

Selection bias, as the name indicates, comes from error during the selection process regarding how the participants enter the study. A faulty sampling mechanism, caused by such problems as nonresponse or refusal to participate, could produce a sample that has a higher or lower disease risk. For example, when we choose control participants from a hospital, health problems that led to their hospitalization may be associated with the exposure of interest. Similarly, when we choose control participants by telephone screening, omitting households without telephones could introduce a bias. Note that the only kind of sampling distortion that matters is the selection that influences disease risk.

Information bias is when the information gathered from study participants regarding exposures and/or outcomes is incorrect. Information bias is also called misclassification bias. Although efforts should be made to minimize such bias, errors in classification of exposure are unavoidable. Past exposures such as dietary intake, alcohol use, or physical activity are impossible to measure perfectly, even if we know what aspect of such exposures was the most relevant to disease causation. In many instances, the errors in exposure classification can be assumed to be similar for those who do and do not develop disease. This situation, referred to as nondifferential misclassification of exposure, results in a predictable bias in which the measure of association (such as odds ratio or relative risk) will be biased toward the null value of no association (1.0 for ratio measures, 0 for difference measures). This means that virtually all reported associations between exposure and disease will be diluted to some degree or missed entirely.

When the patterns of misclassification are different for the study groups, this is referred to as differential misclassification. This can occur when exposure is classified differently for diseased and non-diseased participants or when disease is classified differently for exposed and unexposed participants. Now the distortion in the measure of association can be in either direction (exaggerated or understated), depending on the precise pattern of error. A particular worry in case-control studies is the possibility of recall bias, which is a particular type of differential misclassification. Recall bias exists when the recall of exposure information is different for case patients than for control participants, presumably because the illness experience of the case patients has in some way altered their memory or reporting of past events. For example, case patients may overreport their past exposures to explain their illness, whereas control participants tend to overlook or ignore their past exposures. In either situation, the reported exposures of case patients are artificially greater than the reported exposures of control participants, and the relative risk is falsely elevated.

Table 2-3. Example of Effect of Adjusting to Control for Confounding Effects of Age in Breast Cancer Death Rates for Whites and Blacks, United States, 2020

Race	No. Deaths	Population	Rate	Age-Adjusted Rate
Black	6,500	24,514,353	26.5	25.4
White	34,121	128,628,889	26.5	18.7

Confounding

One reason for uncertainty is the possibility for *confounding*, in which the influence of an exposure of interest is mixed with the effect of another. This arises when a risk factor for the disease of interest is also associated with the exposure of interest. One of the most common confounders in practice is age. For example, when studying breast cancer mortality rates among Black and White women in the United States in 2020, simply comparing the "crude" rates suggests that the rates are the same (26.5 deaths/100,000; Table 2-3). However, this is because Black women are, on average, younger than White women. When age (the confounder) is taken into effect (by "adjusting" the rates), one sees that the rates among Black women are, in fact, higher than those among White women (25.4 vs. 18.7 deaths/100,000). In research studies, confounders can include age or any other factor that is associated with both the exposure of interest and the outcome under study.

In an experiment or RCT these potential confounders can be balanced among the study groups through the design of the study and the random way the exposure is assigned. Conversely, in an observational study, potential confounders must be measured and adjusted statistically. The strategy involves creating groups that are similar with respect to the potential confounder and examining the impact of the exposure of interest within each of those groups. For example, age is a common confounder for many chronic diseases. Older age is associated with osteoporosis, for example. Also, as people age they tend to have higher blood pressure. In an observational study, although we might find people with hypertension also have osteoporosis, until we stratify their age group, or adjust age when examining this association, we cannot conclude that hypertension causes osteoporosis.

Causal Inference

We understand that association does not equal causation. After taking bias and confounding into consideration, what else do we need to make a causal inference? The Bradford Hill criteria are often cited as a checklist for causality in epidemiological studies.[8] These criteria have value, but only as general guidelines, and are as follows:

- Temporality: The exposure must precede the disease. This is the only absolute criterion for causality. Prospective study design helps establish the case for temporality.

- Strength of association: Stronger associations are less likely to be the result of some subtle confounding or bias, presuming major distorting influences would be more readily recognized than small ones.
- Biological gradient: A dose–response curve, in which the risk of disease increases with increasing exposure, indicates an association is probably not the result of a confounder or other bias. This criterion is generally valid, but the absence of a perfect dose–response pattern does not negate the possibility of a causal explanation because true thresholds or ceilings of effects may exist. Conversely, the presence of a dose–response gradient may be the result of a strong confounder that closely tracks the exposure.
- Consistency of association: The association is observed across diverse populations and circumstances, making a particular bias unlikely to explain a series of such observations.
- Plausibility: Evidence from other disciplines suggests that the agent is biologically capable of influencing the disease. This is useful supportive evidence when it is available, but the lack of advancements in the other biological sciences should not be used to negate an epidemiological observation.
- Coherence: The evidence should not be contradictory to the known biology and natural history of the disease (similar to the plausibility criterion).
- Experimental evidence: When attainable, experimental evidence for causality—obtained by removing or randomly assigning exposure—is very strong because both known and unknown confounders are controlled when exposure is randomly allocated.
- Analogy: When other similar agents have been established as causes of disease, then the credibility of theories regarding a new disease operating in a similar manner is enhanced. This is the epidemiological counterpart to plausibility; however, the supportive evidence comes from other areas of epidemiology rather than from other disciplines.
- Specificity of association: The exposure causes one rather than many diseases, and the disease is associated with one rather than many exposures, suggesting that the association is not the result of bias. This is the weakest of the criteria for chronic diseases and might as well be eliminated because we now know that many, perhaps most, exposures that influence one health outcome affect others (e.g., tobacco, radiation, diet) and that virtually all diseases have multiple causes.

In practice, the establishment of evidence for causality is largely through the elimination of noncausal explanations for an observed association. Consider, for example, the evidence that alcohol use may increase the risk of breast cancer. A series of further studies might confirm this relationship is valid and not a result of confounding or other biases such as detection bias (in which disease is more thoroughly diagnosed among alcohol users) or nonresponse bias. By whittling away alternative explanations, the hypothesis that asserts alcohol use causes breast cancer becomes increasingly credible. It is the job of critics to propose and test noncausal explanations; so when the association has withstood a series of such challenges, the case for causality is strengthened.

The danger of formalizing the process of declaring causality based on a checklist or any other mechanistic process is that it can lead to endless debates about the degree of certainty and can impede needed public health actions. Those who argue causality must be established with absolute certainty before interventions can begin fail to appreciate that their two alternatives—action and inaction—each have risks and benefits. Decisions must therefore be grounded on evidence that exposure causes diseases and must consider the costs of intervention, the potential for the intervention to produce adverse side effects, and the potential costs of failing to act.

For example, the tobacco companies have until recently argued that the association between smoking and disease is uncertain. In a technical sense, we will always have some degree of uncertainty, especially with no definitive data from large numbers of participants randomly assigned to be smokers and nonsmokers. We have no doubt, however, that the evidence indicates a need to intervene because smoking has no clear health benefits and scientists have exhausted all reasonable noncausal explanations for the strong associations observed between smoking and several diseases. Nonetheless, to the extent tobacco companies continue to argue that the evidence for causality is not definitive, they create enough controversy to distract some policy makers from supporting needed interventions. Establishing causality is an important goal for epidemiological research, but absolute proof is not needed to justify action.

CHRONIC DISEASE AND PUBLIC HEALTH

In the traditional role of epidemiology as the basic science of public health, quantitative considerations of preventable disease can help us make a rational choice. Relative risk estimates indicate how strongly exposure and disease are associated, but this measure does not directly indicate the benefits that could be gained through modifying the exposure. How can we predict what benefits one or more of these interventions might yield in the community? This is where estimates of population-attributable risk may be particularly useful. When presented with an array of potential causal factors for disease, we need to evaluate how much might be gained by reducing or eliminating each of the hazards.

Attributable Risk

Attributable risk is a measure of how much of the disease burden could be eliminated if the exposure were eliminated. The attributable risk represents the proportion of disease among exposed people that actually results from the exposure. This issue might arise in a court case in which an exposed individual claims the agent to which he or she was exposed caused the disease. Note that we are presuming the associations reflect causality for the purposes of estimation. The attributable risk among exposed individuals is calculated as follows:

$$[\text{relative risk} - 1]/\text{relative risk}$$

Thus, a relative risk of 2.0 (risk is doubled by exposure) yields an attributable proportion among exposed people of 0.5. This suggests a 50% chance that the disease resulted from the exposure in this study population.

Population-Attributable Risk

Of still greater potential value is the incorporation of information on how common the exposure is. Although some exposures exert a powerful influence on individuals (i.e., a large relative risk), they are so rare that their public health impact is minimal. Conversely, some exposures have a modest impact but are so widespread that their elimination could have great benefit. To answer the question "What proportion of disease in the total population is a result of the exposure?" the population-attributable risk or etiologic fraction is used. The population-attributable risk can be calculated in two ways. First, if the rate in the exposed and unexposed population is known, then the population-attributable risk is

$$[\text{rate (total population)} - \text{rate (unexposed)}]/[\text{rate (total population)}].$$

The population-attributable risk is more commonly calculated with information only about the relative risk (usually obtained from research studies) and exposure in the population (often obtained from surveys). It is calculated as follows:

$$[P_e\,(\text{relative risk} - 1)]/[1 + P_e\,(\text{relative risk} - 1)],$$

where P_e represents the proportion of the population that is exposed.

The population-attributable risk is most commonly used to estimate the proportion of disease caused by a certain risk factor, such as the proportion of lung cancer caused by smoking. Assuming that the relative risk of lung cancer attributable to cigarette smoking is 15 and that 30% of the population are smokers, the population-attributable risk is 0.81, or 81%. This would suggest that 81% of the lung cancer burden in the population is caused by cigarette smoking and could be eliminated if the exposure were eliminated.

Population-attributable risk could also be used to estimate the proportion of a risk factor attributable to various "upstream" determinants. For example, research has shown that children exposed to smoking in the movies are at increased risk of becoming regular smokers.[9] If one assumes that this is a causal relationship, about 35% of smoking among adolescents could be attributed to exposure to smoking in the movies.

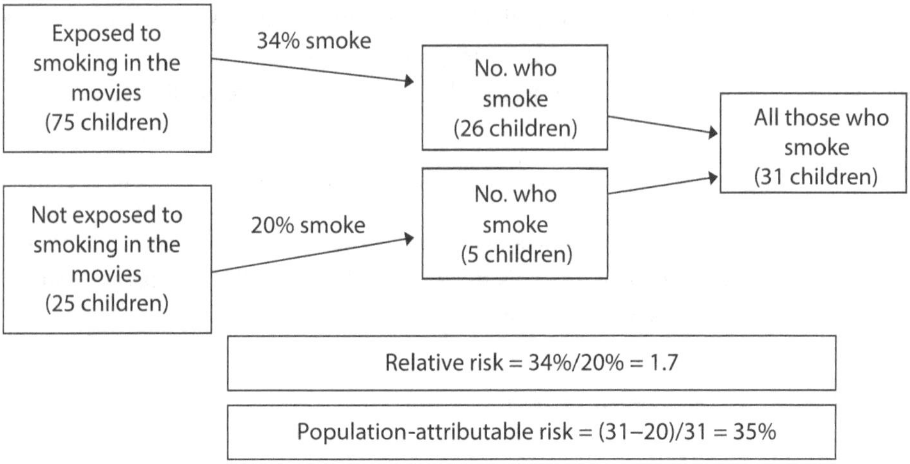

Figure 2-3. Risks of Becoming a Smoker Among 100 Children Exposed or Not Exposed to Smoking in the Movies

Intuitively, the 35% figure sounds very high, which would cast doubt on the assumption of a causal relationship. It is also important to note, because of the effects of interactions between various risk factors, population-attributable risk estimates for a given disease can sometimes add up to more than 100%. The relationship between risk, relative risk, and population-attributable risk is illustrated in Figure 2-3 as a hypothetical example for 100 children:

- Risk: Of all children exposed to smoking in the movies, 34% become smokers, compared with only 20% of children not exposed to smoking in the movies.
- Relative risk: Children exposed to smoking in the movies are 1.7 times more likely to become smokers.
- Population-attributable risk: Among adolescents, 35% of smoking results because of smoking in the movies.

Although population-attributable risk estimates provide a useful estimate of the public health burden, they may be unrealistic as absolute goals because only rarely can a risk factor be completely eliminated.

Interactions

Interactions among exposures, also known as *effect modification*, in the causation of disease are of particular importance in our fully understanding etiology. Effect modification occurs when the effect of one exposure on disease risk is modified by the presence of another exposure. In the purest form, which is rarely observed, each of two exposures

Table 2-4. Example of Interaction Between Smoking and Human Papillomavirus Exposure on the Risk of Cervical Cancer in a Case-Control Study

	No HPV		HPV	
Smoking Status	**Rate**	**Relative Risk**	**Rate**	**Relative Risk**
Nonsmoker	31.7% (76/240)	Reference	41.5% (83/200)	1.3
Smoker	48.6% (104/214)	1.5	85.5% (153/179)	2.7

Source: Based on Roura et al.[7]

Note: HPV = human papillomavirus.

alone may have little effect on disease, but when the two are combined a synergism occurs, causing an increase in disease. Conversely, two exposures that can each influence disease risk independently may be antagonistic, so in combination they have a smaller effect on disease risk.

In epidemiologic studies interaction is measured as a combined effect of exposures that is larger than would be expected by simply adding the effects of the two separate exposures. Interaction is most easily detected by comparing the disease risk in groups with all combinations of exposure to the group exposed to neither agent. For example, looking at the same study of cigarette smoking and cervical cancer, we see that HPV exposure has increased the risk of cervical cancer for women who smoke and are also exposed to HPV (Table 2-4). The risk of cervical cancer among nonsmokers who are exposed to HPV (relative risk = 1.3) is slightly less than for smokers who are not exposed to HPV (relative risk = 1.5). However, an additive effect is observed among smokers who are exposed to HPV (relative risk = 2.7).

This measure of interaction has direct implications for developing intervention and prevention programs. If two factors interact, then the benefit of removing a given exposure will be greater if the other exposure is also present. For example, eliminating smoking has even more benefit for a group of workers exposed to HPV than for individuals who are not exposed to HPV.

Evidence-Based Public Health Interventions

Many factors enter into decisions about public health interventions, including certainty of causality, amenability to intervention, and social and political issues. Developing evidence-based interventions requires going beyond epidemiology to use other disciplines, such as behavioral and social sciences, environmental health sciences, health management, and policy analysis. Several important methods and tools are available to epidemiologists and practitioners to assist in determining when public health action is warranted.

It is often necessary to use these because exposure–disease relationships in chronic disease epidemiology typically show relatively weak associations, in which the relative risk estimate is not too different from the null value of 1.0. As noted earlier in the description of population-attributable risk, even when a risk factor is weak, if it is highly prevalent in the population, the public health impact can be large. Therefore, we have great interest in determining when even relatively weak associations provide the basis for public health intervention, which can come only from a series of well-designed studies.

Systematic reviews use explicit and comprehensive (systematic) methods to identify, select, and critically assess all relevant research on the issue under consideration. To avoid bias, systematic reviews usually begin with a protocol stating in advance how the review will be carried out (searching for data, appraising, and combining study data).

Meta-analysis is most useful for combining the results of multiple, small RCTs whose results are generally consistent, yet imprecision is a problem in each individual trial. The method is less useful in situations in which intervention trials have found truly heterogeneous results through different methods or because the relationship of interest varies across populations. Partly for that reason, one must be careful not to be overwhelmed by the impressively large numbers that can be accrued in a meta-analysis. Although the improved precision is a strength, one must also consider the validity of combining results across studies and whether the estimated size of the effect is large enough to warrant action.

Most government agencies, in both executive and legislative branches, and voluntary health organizations use *expert panels* when examining epidemiological studies and their relevance to health policies and interventions. Ideally, the goal of expert panels is to provide peer review by scientific experts of the quality of the science and scientific interpretations that underlie public health recommendations, regulations, and policy decisions. If conducted well, peer review can provide an important set of checks and balances for the regulatory process. Optimally, the expert review process has the following common properties: experts are sought in epidemiology and related disciplines (e.g., clinical medicine, biomedical sciences, biostatistics, economics, ethics); panels typically consist of 8 to 15 members and meet in person to review scientific data (written guidance is provided to panel members); panel members should not have financial or professional conflicts of interest; and draft findings from expert panels are frequently released for public review and comment before final recommendations.

CONCLUSION

In this chapter we have discussed the issues that help to determine whether associations are causal, the role of intervention research in disease control, and the uses of epidemiologic evidence to make public health decisions. We have also outlined several types of epidemiological study designs and the biases that can complicate interpretation of results.

Such information will serve as a foundation to help you navigate through issues of chronic disease epidemiology and control in the following chapters.

DISCUSSION QUESTIONS

1. Pick one chronic disease, condition, or risk factor from this book and describe its epidemiology (time, person, and place) to a friend or colleague.
2. Describe an instance where you might use a cohort study to better understand the etiology of a chronic disease. Do the same for when you would use a case-control study.
3. Describe how you would apply the causal criteria to one chronic disease.
4. Describe some of the challenges that might arise when trying to implement evidence-based public health policies.

REFERENCES

1. Centers for Disease Control and Prevention, National Center for Health Statistics. Leading causes of death. Updated September 6, 2022. Available at: https://www.cdc.gov/nchs/fastats/leading-causes-of-death.htm. Accessed January 5, 2023.
2. McDowell I, Newell C. *Measuring Health: A Guide to Rating Scales and Questionnaires*. 3rd ed. New York, NY: Oxford University Press; 2006.
3. Mokdad AH, Marks JS, Stroup DF, Gerberding JL. Actual causes of death in the United States, 2000 [published correction appears in *JAMA*. 2005 Jan 19;293(3):298] [published correction appears in *JAMA*. 2005 Jan 19;293(3):293–294]. *JAMA*. 2004;291(10):1238–1245. doi:10.1001/jama.291.10.1238
4. Galea S, Tracy M, Hoggatt KJ, Dimaggio C, Karpati A. Estimated deaths attributable to social factors in the United States. *Am J Public Health*. 2011;101(8):1456–1465. doi:10.2105/AJPH.2010.300086.
5. Tinker T, Vaughan E. Risk communication. In: Nelson DE, Brownson RC, Remington PL, Parvanta C, eds. *Communicating Public Health Information Effectively: A Guide for Practitioners*. Washington, DC: American Public Health Association; 2002:185–203.
6. National Cancer Institute. State cancer profiles. Available at: https://statecancerprofiles.cancer.gov/map/map.noimage.php. Accessed January 5, 2023.
7. Roura E, Castellsagué X, Pawlita M, et al. Smoking as a major risk factor for cervical cancer and pre-cancer: results from the EPIC cohort. *Int J Cancer*. 2014;135(2):453–466. doi:10.1002/ijc.28666
8. Hill AB. The environment and disease: association or causation? *Proc R Soc Med*. 1965;58(5):295–300.
9. Charlesworth A, Glantz SA. Smoking in the movies increases adolescent smoking: a review. *Pediatrics*. 2005;116(6):1516–1528. doi:10.1542/peds.2005-0141.

3

Chronic Disease Surveillance

Mark V. Wegner, MD, MPH, Lena C. Swander, MPH, Shelby L. Vadjunec, MPH, and Patrick L. Remington, MD, MPH

LEARNING OBJECTIVES

After completing this chapter, readers should be able to

1. Define *public health surveillance.*
2. Describe the data sources used for chronic disease surveillance.
3. Describe the types of analyses used for chronic disease surveillance.
4. Understand how to disseminate chronic disease surveillance data to have the best impact on the population of interest.
5. Understand how information gathered from chronic disease surveillance can be used to influence policy decisions.

INTRODUCTION

Public health surveillance is the systematic, ongoing collection, management, analysis, and interpretation of data. As shown in Figure 3-1, functional capacity for data collection, analysis, interpretation, and dissemination linked to public health programs through human and data system inputs constitutes a public health surveillance system.[2] Surveillance information is then used in the program cycle from program planning, implementation, and evaluation. In addition, public health surveillance systems provide early warnings for emergencies, enable the evaluation of the impact of interventions, and inform public health policy and strategic priorities.[3]

Historically, public health surveillance systems were structured around infectious diseases, then expanded to a host of other topics over the last century (Table 3-1). The last 30 years are marked by increased application of public health surveillance toward monitoring chronic diseases, partly because of their associated rapidly increasing health care costs and rising disease incidence.

In 2020 the COVID-19 pandemic thrust public health surveillance systems into the spotlight as never before. The pandemic emphasized just how crucial accurate and

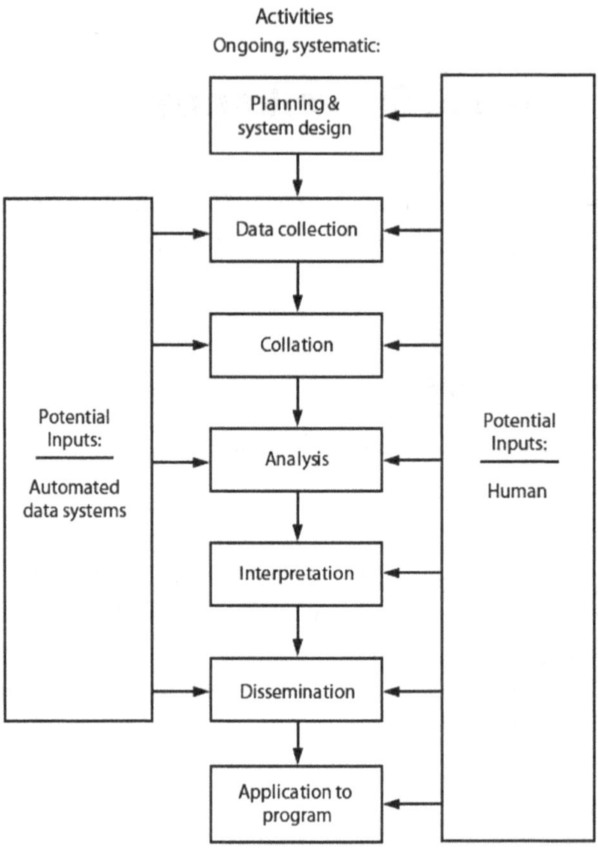

Source: Adapted from CDC.[1]

Figure 3-1. Optimal Balance of Human and Automated Inputs Into Ongoing, Systematic Public Health Surveillance System Activities

timely surveillance data are to inform prevention and control measures and develop a rapid and effective response to both infectious and chronic disease public health threats.

This chapter describes three basic elements of chronic disease surveillance systems: (1) data sources, (2) data analysis and interpretation, and (3) dissemination of data to public health programs and target audiences. The chapter concludes by emphasizing the importance of linking surveillance data to chronic disease prevention and control efforts.

DATA SOURCES

Data sources that public health surveillance systems rely on changed dramatically over the last few decades, ranging from improvements in data repositories to the advent of new interoperable systems exchanging real-time health data.[4] Data sources we explore in

Table 3-1. Trends in the Application of Surveillance to Public Health From 1900 to Present

Period	Application	Examples
1900s	Individual contacts of infected patients	Surveillance of individuals who came in contact with a case of smallpox is conducted.
1950s	Communicable diseases	Cases of polio are reported to the public health agency as part of a communicable disease control program.
1970s	Select chronic diseases	Cancer registries are established as part of the Surveillance, Epidemiology, and End Results Program.
1990s	Behavioral, occupational, and environmental risk factors	Trends in the prevalence of cigarette smoking, determined through telephone surveys, are used to plan tobacco control programs.
2000s	Bioterrorism and preparedness Built environment	Syndromic surveillance for early detection of outbreaks is conducted. Surveillance programs look at both health status and the communities in which individuals live.
2010s	Electronic health records and meaningful use	Surveillance is enhanced with more real-time data and data on results of clinical procedures.
2020s	COVID-19 pandemic	Surveillance tracking dashboards receive daily updates for confirmed and suspected COVID-19 cases and deaths. Mobile applications are utilized for contact tracing.

this chapter include notifiable diseases and national surveillance, sentinel and syndromic surveillance, chronic disease registries, health surveys, health services data, vital statistics or records, health policy surveillance, and census data (Table 3-2). Note that chronic disease surveillance may use data from one or more sources. For example, prescription drug monitoring programs are databases that collect information about dispensed prescription drugs and can provide health authorities timely information about prescribing and patient behaviors. These systems can rely on data from vital statistics, administrative claims, law enforcement reports, telephone surveys, and pharmacy reporting of dispensing events.[5]

Public health practitioners need access to multiple data sources to draw a comprehensive picture of chronic disease burden. Many data sources are owned and managed directly by public health agencies whose data governance scope and structure often differ. In some agencies, access is regulated by application processes where data users must explain their research or analytical needs. In others, data users may need to sign data-use agreements or confidentiality statements certifying that they use the data only for specific purposes. Unfortunately, data sharing and access are common barriers faced by public health agencies. Barriers range from those that are technical in nature (e.g., lack of metadata and standards) to economic (e.g., lack of funding and resources), or even legal (e.g., ownership and copyright).[6] Data governance and access policies are also an important part of Public Health Accreditation Standards.[7] Therefore, public health

Table 3-2. Selected Chronic Disease Data Sources and Surveillance Systems

Data System	Definition	Example	Strengths	Limitations
Notifiable diseases and national surveillance[a,b,c]	System of standardized criteria for reportable and notifiable diseases and conditions (infectious and noninfectious).	State-based lead poisoning reporting systems	• Data are available at the local level. • Usually coupled with a public health response (e.g., lead paint removal). • Detailed information can be collected to aid in designing control programs. • Laboratory-based systems are inexpensive and effective.	• Requires participation by community-based clinicians. • Clinician-based systems have low reporting rates. • Active reporting systems are time consuming and expensive.
Sentinel and syndromic surveillance[b,c]	System that collects symptoms and diagnoses to inform trends and population health, usually collected and reported by health care professionals, laboratories, and public health agencies.	Sentinel Event Notification System for Occupational Risks (SENSOR)	• Low-cost system to monitor selected diseases. • Usually coupled with a public health response (e.g., asbestos removal following report of mesothelioma). • Provides information on risk factors and disease severity.	• Requires motivated reporting providers. • May not be representative.
Registries[b,c]	System that collects information on people with a specific condition, disease, care, or other defined parameter.	Cancer registries	• Data increasingly available throughout the United States. • Includes accurate tissue-based diagnoses. • Provides stage-of-diagnosis data.	• Systems are expensive. • Data are affected by patient out-migration from one geographic unit to another. • Risk factor information is seldom available.
Health surveys[b,c]	Standardized tool or instrument of questions to collect information about the health of individuals through a variety of modes such as interviews, self-reports, or clinical measurements or tests.	BRFSS telephone surveys	• Monitors trends in risk factor prevalence. • Can be used for program design and evaluation.	• Information is based on self-reports. • May be too expensive to conduct at the local level. • May not be representative because of nonresponse (e.g., telephone surveys).

(Continued)

Table 3-2. (Continued)

Data System	Definition	Example	Strengths	Limitations
Health services data[b,c]	Utilization, claims, and other administrative procedures documented under the provision of health care services such as hospitalization stays, surgeries, and diagnoses.	Hospital discharge systems	• Reflects regional differences on disease hospitalization rates. • Can capture cost information. • Data are readily available. • One of the few sources of morbidity data.	• Often lacks personal identifiers. • Rates may be affected by changing patterns of diagnosis related to reimbursement mechanisms. • Difficult to separate initial from recurrent hospitalizations.
Vital statistics or records[a,b,c]	Reports and certificates of life events collected and maintained by the government.	Death certificates	• Data are widely available at the local, state, and national levels. • Population-based. • Can monitor trends in age-adjusted disease rates. • Can target areas with increased mortality rates.	• Cause of death information may be inaccurate (e.g., lack of autopsy information). • No information about risk factors.
Health policy surveillance	Systematic collection of policies and laws of public health significance.	The Policy Surveillance Program: A Law Atlas Project	• Longitudinal policy data can provide quasi-experimental and other more rigorous chronic disease intervention evaluation designs.	• Difficult collection (e.g., legal information often found in text files or PDFs and not standardized). • Usually observing policy as text only when collecting, not documenting or describing implementation of policies.
Census data[a,b,c]	Actual counts and estimations of the US population, including the 5 US territories.	Poverty rates by county	• Required to calculate rates. • Important predictors of health status. • Available to all communities and readily available online.	• Collected infrequently (every 10 years). • May undercount certain populations (e.g., the poor, homeless persons).

Note: BRFSS = Behavior Risk Factor Surveillance System.

[a]Data available from most local public health agencies.

[b]Data available from most state departments of health.

[c]Data available from many US federal agencies (e.g., Centers for Disease Control and Prevention, National Cancer Institute, Health Care Financing Administration).

agencies should use their data collection systems, analytics, and data dissemination plans to help secure accreditation.

Notifiable Diseases and National Surveillance

The Centers for Disease Control and Prevention (CDC) and the Council of State and Territorial Epidemiologists (CSTE), the latter an organization consisting of public health epidemiologists employed by state, territorial, and local agencies, identify and list national notifiable diseases and conditions. The majority of these national notifiable diseases and conditions are infectious diseases or food-borne outbreaks.[8] However, among the diseases considered notifiable are five noncommunicable diseases: cancer, carbon monoxide poisoning, elevated lead blood levels, acute pesticide-related illness and injury, and silicosis.

Data collection on cases with notifiable diseases and conditions starts with local, state and territorial public health department reporting. Local laws and regulations specify which diseases and conditions are considered reportable. If a reportable disease or condition is on the national notifiable list, states and territories voluntarily report those cases to CDC.

In 1996 CSTE voted to include cigarette smoking prevalence as a nationwide surveillance indicator. This was the first time that a behavioral risk factor, rather than a disease or condition, was considered for national surveillance. CSTE selected a health survey—the Behavioral Risk Factor Surveillance System—as the data source for this indicator, which marked a transition to more flexible national surveillance methods. Cigarette smoking prevalence national surveillance goals included monitoring trends in tobacco use, guiding prevention resource allocation, and evaluating public health interventions.

In 1998 CSTE, CDC, and the National Association of Chronic Disease Directors developed a uniform set of chronic disease surveillance indicators.[9] The set of chronic disease indicators underwent multiple revisions and now includes 124 indicators organized in 18 health topic areas. CDC's Division of Population Health maintains publicly available online tools where anyone can access indicator data and information.[10]

Sentinel and Syndromic Surveillance

Sentinel surveillance describes a network of health care providers or hospitals recruited by public health agencies to regularly report specified health events.[11] Sentinel surveillance lends itself well to observing communicable diseases—for example, by monitoring the spread of influenza-like illness.[12] This type of surveillance can be used in school settings, child-care centers, hospitals, or other organizations serving certain populations. When resources for more active surveillance are unavailable, sentinel surveillance serves as a useful tool, especially when used in communities with a high risk of disease.

Some states have occupational respiratory disease sentinel surveillance programs for work-related conditions. The National Institute for Occupational Safety and Health funds select states for programs that depend on sentinel providers to report detailed information about people diagnosed with diseases such as work-related asthma and silicosis.[13]

Syndromic surveillance tracks patient symptoms, lab results, and/or vitals using electronic health data from participating health care facilities on an integrated, shared platform. Syndromic surveillance has been used as an early warning system for opioid overdoses, flu and COVID surges, e-cigarette- or vaping-associated lung injury, and natural disasters. This type of surveillance has also been used for routine monitoring of cardiovascular and chronic diseases from inpatient encounters.

Chronic Disease Registries

Chronic disease registries are essential for monitoring trends. State law frequently mandates collecting chronic disease surveillance, and a registry entity is usually charged with fulfilling this responsibility. Detailed information about each patient can be collected, such as disease classification, demographics, stage at diagnosis, or treatments provided. Given the scope and complexity of the data collection and processing, registries require considerable financial resources to implement and maintain.

Cancer registries are the most common type of registry used for chronic disease surveillance. Hospitals, pathology laboratories, physician offices, and clinics collect patient data after cancer diagnosis or treatment and report to the registry. Data include demographics, detailed tumor information (e.g., primary site, histology, diagnostic confirmation, stage of disease at diagnosis, distant metastases at time of diagnosis, date of diagnosis, patient's residence at diagnosis, behavior, grade), and treatment information (date and type of cancer-directed first-course treatment).

Population-based cancer registries, which collect information on all people residing in a specific geographic area, were first established in Connecticut in 1936, their aim to identify and better understand regional differences in cancer incidence rates.[14] The Surveillance, Epidemiology, and End Results (SEER) program of the National Cancer Institute, established in 1972, is composed of individual population-based registries in 22 separate geographic areas, covering approximately 48% of the US population. SEER provides data on national trends in cancer incidence and mortality and is used by researchers to conduct epidemiologic studies.[15]

In October 1992 Congress passed the Cancer Registries Amendment Act, establishing the National Program of Cancer Registries. As a result of this law, CDC provides annual financial support to state and territorial health departments and select universities to establish and improve population-based cancer registries. CDC provides 46 states, the District of Columbia, Puerto Rico, the US Pacific Island jurisdictions, and the Virgin Islands with support for cancer registries—areas that together represent 97% of the US population.[16]

Other chronic disease registries include traumatic brain injury, stroke, birth defects, and Alzheimer's and other dementia registries. The National Institutes of Health highlight registries at the national level.[17] Since the 1990s states have maintained statewide registries for traumatic brain injury to identify individuals and facilitate and coordinate their rehabilitation.[18]

After Georgia senator Paul Coverdell died suddenly from a stroke in 2000, the US Congress directed CDC to implement state-based registries of all acute strokes. CDC funded and provided technical assistance to nine states to develop, implement, and enhance systems for collecting data on patients experiencing an acute stroke. As of 2022, there were more than one million stroke patients in the Paul Coverdell National Acute Stroke Registry.[19]

Health Surveys

Public health practitioners and researchers collect data on health behaviors, conditions, and service utilization using a variety of health surveys (Table 3-3). Many surveys utilized in chronic disease surveillance systems are self-report, meaning respondents select their own responses. Important self-report surveys to monitor chronic diseases and risk factors at the national, state, and territorial levels include the Behavioral Risk Factor Surveillance System (BRFSS), the Youth Risk Behavior Surveillance System (YRBSS), the National Health and Nutrition Examination Survey (NHANES), the National Health Interview Survey (NHIS), and the Pregnancy Risk Assessment Monitoring System (PRAMS).

BRFSS is one of the most frequently utilized surveys in chronic disease surveillance.[2] It is the nation's premier system of health-related phone surveys, collecting data in all 50 states, the District of Columbia, and three US territories.[20] CDC established BRFSS in 1984, and it became a national surveillance system in 1993.[21] State health department

Table 3-3. Important Chronic Disease Health Surveys by Geographically Representative US Sample Level and Type of Information Collected

		Type of Information Collected	
Geographically Representative Sample	Survey Name	Self-Report Survey	Physical Exam and Biologic Samples
National	National Health and Nutrition Examination Survey	yes	yes
National	National Health Interview Survey	yes	
State and territory	Behavioral Risk Factor Surveillance System	yes	
State and territory	Youth Risk Behavior Surveillance System	yes	
State	Survey of the Health of Wisconsin	yes	yes
State and territory	Pregnancy Risk Assessment Monitoring System	yes	

interviewers, contracted telephone call centers, and universities collect responses from more than 400,000 noninstitutionalized US adults 18 years or older each year. Interviews take about 15 to 20 minutes, and individuals are selected using random digit–dialed phone sampling. BRFSS survey questions address a variety of behaviors, events, and chronic conditions. In addition to core questions, jurisdictions can add optional modules or questions relevant to their local health issues.

BRFSS data users should be cognizant of frequently faced survey challenges and biases, like low response rates and reaching linguistically diverse populations.[22–24] Users should also be aware of survey methodology modifications. For example, in 2011 CDC added cell phone sampling because of decreasing landline coverage in households.[25] CDC also changed its weighting methodology that same year. These changes had significant implications for survey estimates. As a result, BRFSS data before 2011 are not directly comparable to subsequent years.

CDC also supports YRBSS. Jurisdictions across the United States administer anonymous surveys to a representative sample of 9th- to 12th-grade students. YRBSS monitors tobacco use, alcohol and other drug use, sexual behaviors, unhealthy dietary behaviors, inadequate physical activity, and behaviors that contribute to unintentional injuries and violence.

Some surveys combine self-report with physical measurements and biologic samples, like CDC's NHANES. Estimating rates of undiagnosed conditions are a particular strength of NHANES. The National Center for Health Statistics at CDC created NHANES in the 1960s to monitor the health status of the US population. In 1999 NHANES became an annual survey of a nationally representative sample of approximately 5,000 persons. Survey staff conduct health interviews in respondents' homes. Physical measurements and collection of biologic samples occur in mobile centers. Some states and local jurisdictions model their surveying techniques after NHANES. One of the first adaptations, the Survey of the Health of Wisconsin, started at the University of Wisconsin-Madison in 2008. The university still maintains and collects self-report survey data combined with physical measurements and biologic samples.[26]

NHIS is also a principal source of chronic disease information. Like BRFSS, NHIS is a cross-sectional interview survey. However, unlike BRFSS, NHIS is conducted at the household level and in person. NHIS data users should be mindful of survey methodology, which has been updated about every 15 to 20 years since 1957.

Finally, CDC and states, territories, and local health departments support PRAMS, a population-based survey on women and infants at high risk for health problems. Developed in 1987, PRAMS is the principal surveillance system for data about pregnancy and the first few months after birth.[27] Using birth certificate lotteries to randomly sample women who have had a recent live birth, PRAMS conducts its program using a combination of mailing and telephone surveying. Each survey site samples between 1,300 and 3,400 women annually.

Health Services Data

Many data on chronic diseases are collected as part of routine administration, such as hospital discharge and claims. Hospital discharge data—hospitalizations, emergency department visits, and outpatient visits—are the most widely available health services data. Hospital discharge data are often used to characterize morbid conditions associated with chronic diseases and to predict short-term and long-term mortality.[28] Information is collected from the medical abstracts and billing records of each patient discharged from the hospital. The United States uses the *International Classification of Diseases,* Tenth Revision, *Clinical Modification* for coding of patient diagnoses and procedures.[29]

Unfortunately, the usefulness of administrative databases is limited by incomplete records, unreliable or invalid coding, missing important clinical variables, and underreporting or undercoding for certain diagnoses or procedures; in addition, the databases are typically stored in an unwieldy form. Measurement errors associated with hospital discharge data arise chiefly in the coding process, which requires coders to know clinical diagnoses and the organization of the *International Classification of Diseases* coding scheme. Thus, misclassification may occur either unintentionally if providers lack understanding of diagnostic coding and grouping or intentionally if providers code with an eye toward maximizing reimbursement via particular diagnosis-related groups.[30] Also, although diagnoses are often listed on the face sheet of the medical record, the principal diagnoses may be cited inaccurately when the hospital discharge form is completed.

Another limitation is inherent in the fact that these data capture events that occur only in a hospital. Thus, the growing number of procedures that historically required hospitalization but can now be performed in outpatient settings would not be captured. In addition, information on injuries may be missed by this system if the injury is either serious enough that the patient dies before being admitted to a hospital or not serious enough to warrant a hospital stay.[31]

The principles of surveillance can also be applied by state and national agencies to monitor the quality of health care.[32] For example, consumers and purchasers of health care use Healthcare Effectiveness Data and Information Set (HEDIS) data to assess the performance of managed health care plans.[33] Developed and maintained by the National Committee for Quality Assurance, HEDIS addresses six performance domains: effectiveness of care, access or availability of care, utilization and risk-adjusted utilization, health plan descriptive information, and measures reported using electronic clinical data systems.[34] It is one of the most widely used sets of health care performance measures in the United States.

With the increased use of electronic health records (EHRs) comes a continuing opportunity to improve public health surveillance capabilities. Some states have piloted surveillance on the basis of automated data feeds from hospitals and providers to their surveillance systems and found improved efficiency and timely data reporting, as well as including clinical information related to the reported disease. Enhancing current methods, as well as developing new ones, for tracking and reporting chronic diseases and forming agreements or policies with health care systems or EHR vendors will be necessary for systemic utility and integration of EHR clinical data and public health surveillance.

The usefulness of EHRs can be extended to many data systems, among them birth registries—collecting parental information and the data needed for the birth certificates—and chronic disease registries. Additionally, patients in health care settings fill out questionnaires collecting behavioral, socioeconomic, cultural, and environmental information. All this information is important for public health surveillance.

Vital Statistics or Records

Information collected at the time of birth and death are often used for chronic disease surveillance to monitor prevalence of disease and overall health status, develop programs to improve public health, and evaluate the effectiveness of interventions. Vital statistics measure the impact of health insurance, access to care, and prenatal care on birth outcomes and monitor deaths attributable to injury, cancer, heart disease, diabetes, and other conditions.[35] Mortality records are often used most in chronic disease surveillance and constitute the oldest disease surveillance data systems.

In the United States mortality data are collected through the vital registration system. After a person dies, a physician or coroner completes the death certificate. The physician or coroner lists the immediate cause of death (e.g., pneumonia), the sequence of events that led to the death (e.g., lung cancer), other contributing causes (e.g., tobacco use), and the manner of death, which specifies the context surrounding the death, such as accidents, suicide, homicide, or natural causes. The disease or condition that triggered the chain of events that eventually caused the death is considered to be the "underlying cause of death."[36,37] In the example cited previously, lung cancer would be listed as the underlying cause, tobacco use and pneumonia would be listed as contributing causes, and the manner of death would be natural cause.

One important limitation of using mortality data for surveillance is that death certificates are occasionally incomplete. Physicians do not receive extensive training in completing death certificates, and the physician or coroner who is completing the certificate may not know the entire clinical history of the deceased person or may not have the time or capacity to properly complete the certificate. States register the death certificates and transmit the files to the National Center for Health Statistics (NCHS) for processing, and in return the states receive their files coded (using *International Classification of Disease* codes). NCHS uses SuperMICAR, a coding software, to sift through the text fields the coroner or medical examiner provides to the state.[38] With the advent of electronic reporting, the text in the fields is typed; however, the clinical information from the physician establishing the cause of death might not be. In cases in which the event could not be coded by SuperMICAR, professional coders are employed. The NCHS manual has examples of how difficult it can be for coders to read doctors' handwriting, yet many attestations that doctors provide remain handwritten and faxed into the reporting system. In some instances, the manner of death may not be determined even after autopsy and forensic investigation and is therefore coded as "Could Not Be Determined."[39]

In most states mortality data are readily accessible for chronic disease surveillance. State-specific data are collected and maintained by vital statistics departments in a standard format. CDC has developed training and guidelines for the use of mortality data.[40] In addition, these mortality data are easily accessible online. Birth certificate data can be used to identify the presence of some chronic conditions during pregnancy, such as hypertension, diabetes, and cardiac disease; however, hospital discharge or other data sources may perform better than vital statistics for identifying some chronic diseases in pregnancy.[41]

In addition to death and birth certificates, state vital records systems collect marriage, divorce, and abortion data. Although state registrars are mandated to report on death and birth data[42] for surveillance purposes, depending on data governance disposition, those systems are available for research scientists and analysts to report on disease processes.

Maternal and birth screening is another important feature of national and state public health surveillance. At birth all babies are screened with a heel stick (blood card), hearing test, and pulse oximetry before they leave the hospital. Newborn screening began in the early 1960s when Dr. Robert Guthrie developed a blood test for the metabolic disorder phenylketonuria, which causes devastating brain damage and death if left untreated.[43] Ever since, more tests have been developed to screen newborns for a variety of severe conditions. Currently, the Department of Health and Human Services' Recommended Uniform Screening Panel includes 35 core conditions and 26 secondary conditions; however, each state may mandate different newborn screening panels according to the state department of health.[44]

Health Policy Surveillance

Because the core functions of public health include assessment, assurance, and policy development, identifying and supporting policies enacted to protect the health of the people is as important as collecting and analyzing health data and enforcing laws and regulations. Policies consist of any laws, regulations, or procedures from federal, state, and local health departments that influence health either by reducing the disease burden and risk factors or by promoting environmental and social determinant changes. The development of policy surveillance systems helps keep track of policies and offers a venue for impact and outcome evaluation. In addition, policy surveillance systems can help conduct more sophisticated research on the determinants of health based on hypotheses that can be tested in intervention studies. A few efforts are underway to develop public health policy surveillance systems,[45] and websites such as Temple University's Law Atlas can be useful for tracking laws and policies of public health significance.[46]

The analysis of the impact of health policies can be quantitative or qualitative. Measures based on policies are diverse, as they can range from yes-or-no questions to more sophisticated measures. Time- and location-based variations may be necessary "policy inputs" in analytics to address needed behavior changes.[47]

Census Data

Every 10 years the US government conducts a census of the entire US population. In addition to counting the population, the census collects detailed information on individual and household characteristics such as age, race, education, occupation, insurance coverage, income, and disability. These census data are essential to provide denominators for calculating rates in populations, to compare disease burden and trends among regions or over time, and to generate geographic characteristics associated with social determinants of health.

Despite efforts to enumerate the entire population, however, the census misses some people. To improve the timeliness of population information, the US Census has instituted the American Community Survey (ACS). ACS uses monthly samples, combining data over multiple years, when necessary, to create small-area data on topics such as educational attainment, income, ancestry, and housing. This information was previously collected in the "long form" of the decennial census. More timely small-area population estimates are especially important for population groups whose numbers are changing rapidly and for areas that may experience large, sustained population changes because of natural disasters, economic changes, or other causes (see Chapter 2 for more information on small-area analyses in chronic disease epidemiology). Given declining response rates, ACS started to combine computer-assisted telephone interviews and computer-assisted personal interviews to the mailed data collection strategy. ACS provides housing-unit data and also includes group quarters, which consist of military barracks and school dormitories. The strength of the ACS data resides more in ACS capabilities to estimate sociodemographic characteristics (percentage, means, or median estimates) of geographical areas than for population total for rate calculation.[48] However, it is standard practice to use the ACS single age, sex, and race estimates to compute age-adjusted rates over time.

In conclusion, chronic disease surveillance can be conducted by using a wide variety of existing data sources. When using these data, public health practitioners must understand the advantages and limitations inherent in each system. Despite these limitations, a comprehensive surveillance system—using a wide variety of chronic disease data—can serve as a resource to improve the health of the entire population.[49]

DATA ANALYSIS AND INTERPRETATION

Chronic disease surveillance systems should analyze and interpret data from a variety of sources. Sound analysis and interpretation requires knowledge of chronic disease pathology, epidemiology, and the relationships among risk factors, morbidity, and mortality. Responsible analysis and interpretation also requires a thorough understanding of the data sources and statistics.

Thanks to technological advancements, chronic disease surveillance is more portable than ever before. Most large data sets can now be accommodated on laptops and mobile devices. Chronic disease surveillance source data as well as interactive query systems and dashboards are frequently available online at the national, state or territorial, and local levels.[50–52]

Chronic disease surveillance relies heavily on descriptive epidemiology. Descriptive epidemiology searches for patterns in health behaviors and conditions across *person*, *place*, and *time*. Considering needs and priorities, public health agencies often develop a set of indicators to monitor change in their communities and evaluate long-term programmatic impact.[53] Brief examples of these types of analyses follow.

Person-Based Analyses

There are many personal characteristics relevant to chronic disease that analysts can examine. Analyses frequently begin by investigating differences between age, sex, educational attainment, income level, and race/ethnicity categories. These variables are commonly used when investigating health disparities, since health outcomes and conditions can vary markedly between them. Other personal characteristics include occupation, health-related behaviors such as smoking or alcohol consumption, and family history.

Many chronic disease surveillance activities use survey data to examine differences in health behaviors and diseases across personal characteristics. When using survey data, analysts must pay attention to the sampling frame and remember to use appropriate statistical methods when estimating and interpreting prevalence rates (e.g., stratification and weighting procedures). Table 3-4 shows age-adjusted diabetes prevalence estimates in Wisconsin using BRFSS data. In the entire sample, 590 total respondents indicated

Table 3-4. Age-Adjusted Diabetes Prevalence by Race/Ethnicity: BRFSS, Wisconsin, 2020

Race/Ethnicity	Sample Size	% (95% CI)
American Indian, non-Hispanic	31	14.4 (8.3-20.4)
Black, non-Hispanic	43	12.4 (8.0-16.8)
Hispanic/Latino	13	11.0 (6.3-15.7)
White, non-Hispanic	492	6.9 (6.1-7.8)
Other, non-Hispanic	11	5.2 (1.9-8.5)

Note: BRFSS = Behavioral Risk Factor Surveillance System; CI = confidence interval.

that a health care provider told them they had diabetes. This sample attempted to represent the 4.5 million Wisconsin noninstitutionalized adult residents in 2020.[54] Notice that because of the low sample size among non-Hispanic, American Indian, Black, and Hispanic/Latino respondents, the 95% confidence intervals around the diabetes estimates are much wider than they are for White, non-Hispanic respondents.[55]

Place-Based Analyses

Chronic disease surveillance place-based analyses often compare health behaviors, diseases, or conditions between geographies. Place-based information may be used to target a specific intervention in a region.[56] For example, a state health department may wish to compare its obesity prevalence estimates to those of the neighboring states, or across the entire nation, to inform or benchmark the department's control or prevention goals. Figure 3-2 shows the differences in obesity prevalence between states in the United States.

Place-based analyses should account for differences in age structure between and among geographies by using age-adjusted (i.e., age-standardized) rates. Analysts should also consider that geographic differences in chronic disease rates may result from differences in diagnostic practices or disease definitions. Chronic disease surveillance place-based analyses are often limited because of low case counts in small regions, such as cities, villages, or towns. In recent years public health researchers have begun using small-area estimation methods to produce county, census tract, and zip code tabulation area chronic disease measure comparisons. One publicly available example of such work is PLACES: Local Data for Better Health, a project supported by CDC and the Robert Wood Johnson Foundation.[57] See Chapter 2 for a more detailed discussion of the challenges created by working with small numbers of cases and how to handle these types of analyses.

A specialized form of place-based analysis involves cases that appear to cluster in a geographic area. Investigating clusters poses a continuing challenge to state and local public health officials. Public health agencies can receive hundreds of inquiries about suspected cancer clusters every year as concerned members of the public or clinicians witnessing a series of specific cancer diagnoses in their area may look for answers.[58]

Systematic protocols, guidelines, and procedures exist to aid public health agencies in reported disease cluster investigations. One example is CDC's Guidelines for Examining Unusual Patterns of Cancer and Environmental Concerns.[59] Conducting a cancer cluster epidemiologic investigation involves defining the population at risk, ascertaining all cases, estimating rate ratios (i.e., observed vs. expected), and assessing exposure and biological plausibility. Because of the rigor applied in CDC guidelines, only a small fraction of cancer cluster inquiries eventually meet the statistical and etiologic criteria to support an investigation. Despite the many challenges involved in investigating

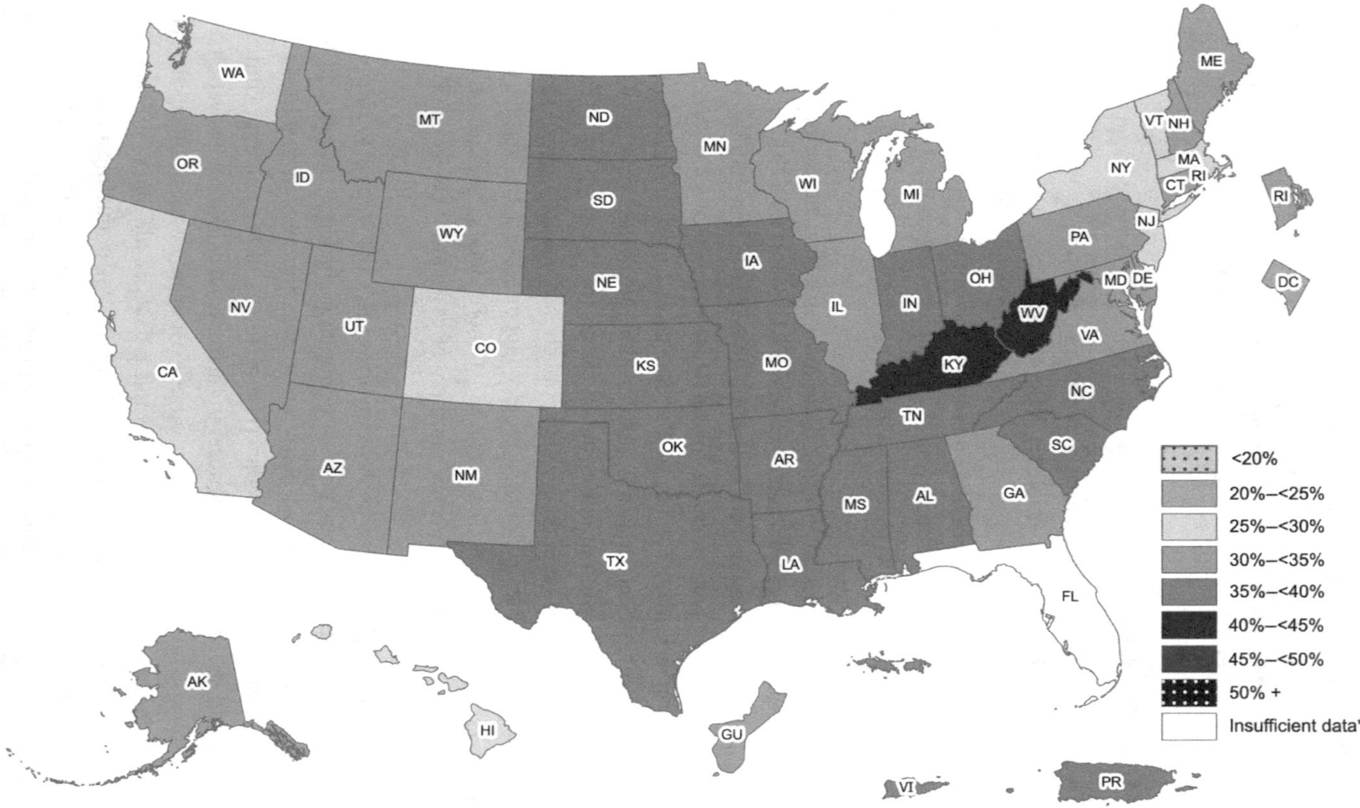

Source: Based on CDC.[20]

Note: BRFSS = Behavioral Risk Factor Surveillance System.

Figure 3-2. Obesity Prevalence in the United States and Territories: BRFSS, 2020

suspected cancer clusters, CDC guidelines encourage state and local health agencies to place emphasis on transparent and effective communication to remain responsive and build community trust.

Time-Based Analyses

Robust chronic disease surveillance systems monitor trends over time in diseases and related health behaviors. The epidemic curve has traditionally been used for infectious disease surveillance to detect outbreaks, to better characterize transmission patterns, and to determine appropriate intervention strategies. Similarly, in chronic disease surveillance, trends in variables such as per capita cigarette sales can be used to monitor the effectiveness of interventions following the implementation of a statewide tobacco control program.[60]

Like place-based analyses, time-based analyses must consider changes in the age structure of the population as well as changes in diagnostic practices or disease definitions over time. Both time-based and place-based analyses can be used for specific population subgroups. For example, as mammography began to be widely implemented in the mid- to late 1980s and improvements in treatment were achieved in the 1990s, a significant gap developed in breast cancer mortality between White women and Black women in the United States (Figure 3-3). Although more recently the rates of breast cancer appear to be declining among both White women and Black women in the United States, the rate of decline for Black women began later and has been less

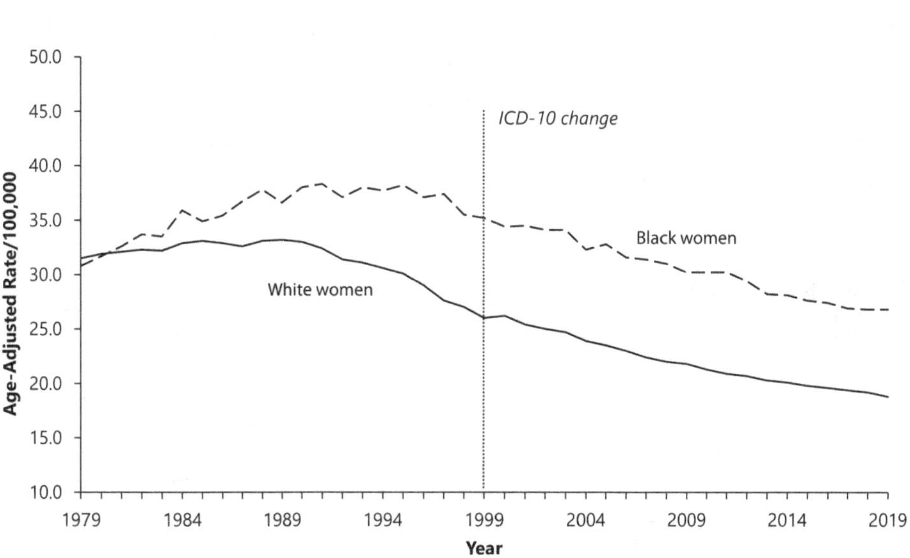

Source: Based on CDC.[50]

Figure 3-3. Trends in Age-Adjusted Breast Cancer Mortality in the United States by Race, 1980–2019

pronounced than the decline for White women, and a large disparity persists. These findings have important implications in the development of programs to ensure that all demographic groups have equal access to advances in public health knowledge.

DISSEMINATION

The final step in chronic disease surveillance is to disseminate the information that has been collected. The increasing amount of surveillance data described previously provides a wealth of information to public health agencies. However, care must be taken to avoid simply analyzing the data and reporting the results in agency reports that are long and contain technical jargon. To be impactful, the information should be linked to program priorities, and the reports used to promote public health practice or as a vehicle for setting priorities for action.

In the past, public health surveillance systems typically produced communicable disease reports that were distributed to health care providers. Recent advances in surveillance and increasing focus on chronic disease requires public health practitioners to create and disseminate surveillance reporting to a broader constituency, including policymakers, voluntary health organizations, professional organizations, and the general public. In light of this, information should be communicated through several channels using different strategies to reach multiple audiences.

Epidemiologists working in public health agencies are frequently asked to disseminate the results of a surveillance report, often by publishing the information in a health department report. To increase application of surveillance findings to disease prevention and health promotion programs, a basic framework for communicating surveillance information can be used (Table 3-5).[61,62] Once the analysis has been completed, this framework has five additional steps: establishing messaging, setting communication objectives, defining audiences, selecting channels, and evaluating impact. These steps are discussed next in the sections that follow.

Table 3-5. Steps in Communicating Public Health Surveillance Information

Step	Question	Action
1	What are the results?	Conduct analyses.
2	What is the key takeaway point?	Establish messaging.
3	What should be accomplished?	Set objectives.
4	Who needs to hear the message?	Define audiences.
5	What is the best way to deliver the message?	Select channels.
6	Was communication successful?	Evaluate impact.

Source: Adapted with permission of Oxford University Press.[61]

Establishing Messaging

Perhaps the most important step in disseminating health and surveillance information is to establish messaging. Like businesses, public health agencies have a product (i.e., information) that they need to sell (i.e., communicate). An epidemiologist must convince audience members that it is worth their time to read, understand, and act on the information. In this endeavor it is important to remember that an important adage in marketing is the message "less is more."

Many reports produced by public health agencies are long, technical, and full of information. These reports might be mailed to the media, policymakers, or health care providers who, in turn, rarely take time to read through the report to find the important information. To capture their attention, the main points of the report must be obvious and simple to understand. Fortunately, established tools and guidance are available for helping to craft plain language communications.[63]

Population health rankings are an effective, yet sometimes controversial, approach to call attention to differences in population health data, including mortality rates and chronic disease risk factors. Implementations of this concept, such as the America's Health Rankings and the County Health Rankings, are often used as a catalyst for improving health by drawing attention to the areas that need improvement through an easily interpretable synthesis of objectively measured community health data.[64] Ranking the health of places increases interest in the results, enabling organizations reporting the information to craft messages not only to explain the observed differences but also to suggest ways to improve health through community action.

Setting Communication Objectives

Why is the information being reported? Public health agencies often report information without any specific goal, but simply "because it is there." Other times, the purpose is to educate the general public about a health issue. Educating the public is a worthwhile but challenging goal, given the complexity of the message and the inability to shape the message for the target audience.

Defining Audiences

Once the objective for communicating the information has been established, one can define the target audience. Local health departments and health care providers have traditionally been the long-standing audience of communicable disease surveillance information, as these professionals have been responsible for implementing disease control strategies. In addition, physicians tend to be the source of these reports, and so reporting back to them has shown the usefulness of the system and helped maintain their continued reporting.

The audience for public health surveillance information is much broader today, however, and includes policymakers, voluntary health organizations, professional organizations, and the general public. For example, a state health department's data reveal high blood pressure prevalence rates are increasing in the state; men in particular and people living in communities with low socioeconomic status are affected at higher rates than found in the general public. This one finding can be tailored to effectively reach multiple defined audiences. It could, for instance, be communicated to the general public or to men specifically, increasing awareness of the importance of taking antihypertensive medications and engaging in self-monitoring blood pressure. It might also be targeted to health care systems and pharmacists to adopt standardized hypertension treatment protocols. Communication could also be tailored for local coalitions and community-based organizations to hold blood pressure measurement events within those communities of low socioeconomic status. Finally, it could be communicated to health insurers or payers to cover the cost of self-measured blood pressure monitors and cuffs so that patients can continuously monitor their own blood pressure at home to detect any issues before they arise.

Selecting Channels

A *channel* is the medium through which messages travel to reach the target audience. Various channels are available to convey a message, and they continue to evolve. Traditional channels include professional journals, direct mail, television, radio, newspapers, blogs, and statistical bulletins. Now channels also include social media, webpages, press releases, infographics, factsheets, and dashboards, among others.

Careful selection of proper communication channels (more than one may be used concurrently) increases the likelihood that the information will reach the target audience and be effectively delivered. This requires a thorough understanding, based on market research, of how those individuals obtain their information. For example, children and teachers might best be reached through the school system newsletter. Policymakers might be reached through a direct mailing to their offices or via a constituent organization. Doctors might be reached through a state medical society journal. For most audiences, it is also helpful to disseminate a message through an effective presence on the internet, as internet access has become nearly universal and, with the rise of smartphones and social media, is often the most accessible and first source individuals turn to for information.

Comparing chronic disease surveillance findings with other societal harms is a creative way to present information and increase media coverage. For example, in support of a comprehensive smoking ban in Wisconsin, it was pointed out that in Wisconsin in a given year, the number of people who die from secondhand smoke exposure (a harm viewed by many as an insignificant risk not requiring government intervention) and the number of people who die in motor vehicle accidents (a cause of death well recognized as a significant public health issue requiring government regulation) is approximately the same at about 800 individuals per year.

Evaluating Impact

The final step in data dissemination is to evaluate how widely the information was circulated and whether the information led to the intended outcome. The dissemination can be measured by determining the number of reports distributed, the readership of a journal, the coverage in the media, or the number of views on a particular website. To assess the accuracy and appropriateness of the messages as they were picked up by the media, internet searches can be performed to find all articles on the topic of interest in a defined geographic area following a dissemination campaign. These articles can also be reviewed by the program staff to assess the geographic distribution and extent of the media coverage. Another step that could help determine the practical impact of public health efforts would be to evaluate any policy changes that were enacted following a campaign.

These methods can provide early indicators of success of public health campaigns. However, one major drawback of evaluating efforts aimed at reducing chronic disease is that because of the slow progression from risk factors to physiologic changes to symptoms to eventual disease development, demonstrating definitive proof of disease reduction may take decades, whereas the typical political cycle is only every two to six years. Thus, if the political winds shift, potentially effective programs may be cut before they have had a chance to demonstrate their impact. In addition, evaluations of societal change and impact on disease are often expensive, time consuming, and difficult to interpret.

CONCLUSION

Data collection, analysis, and dissemination are vital components of a chronic disease surveillance system. The final link in surveillance is the application of the data to prevention and control.[65] Unfortunately, the long latency period of most chronic diseases often results in a perceived lack of urgency in developing and implementing control measures. For example, at the onset of the COVID-19 pandemic, media attention was intense and considerable amounts of resources were deployed to develop an effective vaccine in unprecedented time. By contrast, it has been nearly 60 years since the first Surgeon General's Report on Smoking and Health was released, definitively linking smoking to cancer and other serious chronic diseases. Yet, about half of the states in the United States still lack comprehensive smoke-free laws. In those states where legislation has passed, it has come only after heavy sustained effort and occasionally compromises on issues for which the strong weight of the evidence rests on the side of public health. Building up a definitive library of evidence and scientific data in support of a public health issue does not in and of itself constitute a "public health surveillance system" unless these data are disseminated in such a way that they can have an impact on public health policies aimed at controlling chronic disease.

With chronic disease prevalence continuously rising and recent evidence that people with chronic conditions are at higher risk for developing more severe illness and outcomes from COVID-19, chronic disease programs and surveillance efforts continue to play a necessary role in state, local, and tribal departments of health. This role must continue to be strengthened by enhancing the links between clinical medicine and public health, ensuring integration and better utilization of EHRs, and reframing how health care systems are the focus for chronic disease prevention and management. These improvements could provide more timely and necessary data, indicate how chronic diseases interrelate with the social determinants of health and other risk factors, and more clearly demonstrate to policymakers and other funders the importance of allocating sufficient state and federal resources to address the significant chronic disease issues that exist in our society.

DISCUSSION QUESTIONS

1. What are the advantages and disadvantages of each source of chronic disease surveillance data? What types of analyses do each of the data sources best lend themselves to address?
2. How has chronic disease surveillance changed over time?
3. What are the main challenges to chronic disease surveillance and what are potential solutions to overcome them?

REFERENCES

1. Thacker SB, Qualters JR, Lee LM. Public health surveillance in the United States: evolution and challenges. *MMWR Morb Mortal Wkly Rep.* 2012;61(3):3–9. Available at: https://www.cdc.gov/mmwr/preview/mmwrhtml/su6103a2.htm. Accessed May 4, 2023.
2. Lee LM, Thacker SB. Public health surveillance and knowing about health in the context of growing sources of health data. *Am J Prev Med.* 2011;41(6):636–640.
3. World Health Organization. Surveillance in emergencies. Available at: https://www.who.int/emergencies/surveillance. Accessed January 6, 2023.
4. Lee LM, Thacker SB. Public health surveillance and knowing about health in the context of growing sources of health data. *Am J Prev Med.* 2011;41(6):636–640.
5. Centers for Disease Control and Prevention. Leveraging prescription drug monitoring program (PDMP) data in overdose prevention and response. 2021. Available at: https://www.cdc.gov/drugoverdose/pdf/Leveraging-PDMPs-508.pdf. Accessed January 6, 2023.

6. van Panhuis WG, Paul P, Emerson C, et al. A systematic review of barriers to data sharing in public health. *BMC Public Health*. 2014;1144(14). https://doi.org/10.1186/1471-2458-14-1144
7. Public Health Accreditation Board. Standards and measures for initial accreditation. Version 2022. Available at: https://phaboard.org/wp-content/uploads/Standards-Measures-Initial-Accreditation-Version-2022.pdf. Accessed January 6, 2023.
8. Centers for Disease Control and Prevention. National Notifiable Diseases Surveillance System (NNDSS): search results year. 2022. Available at: https://ndc.services.cdc.gov/search-results-year. Accessed January 6, 2023.
9. Centers for Disease Control and Prevention. Indicators for chronic disease surveillance—United States, 2013. *MMWR Morb Mortal Wkly Rep*. 2015;64(1). Available at: https://www.cdc.gov/mmwr/pdf/rr/rr6401.pdf. Accessed January 6, 2023.
10. Centers for Disease Control and Prevention. Chronic disease indicators. 2022. Available at: https://www.cdc.gov/cdi/index.html. Accessed January 6, 2023.
11. Centers for Disease Control and Prevention. VPD surveillance manual, Chapter 19: enhancing surveillance. Available at: https://www.cdc.gov/vaccines/pubs/surv-manual/chpt19-enhancing-surv.html. Accessed January 6, 2023.
12. Centers for Disease Control and Prevention. Overview of influenza surveillance in the United States. 2016. Updated October 14, 2022. Available at: http://www.cdc.gov/flu/weekly/overview.htm. Accessed January 6, 2023.
13. Centers for Disease Control and Prevention. State-based occupational respiratory disease surveillance. Updated April 12, 2012. Available at: https://www.cdc.gov/niosh/topics/surveillance/ords/statebasedsurveillance.html. Accessed January 6, 2023.
14. Austin DF. Cancer registries: a tool in epidemiology. In: Lillienfeld AM, ed. *Reviews in Cancer Epidemiology*. Vol. 2. New York, NY: Elsevier North Holland; 1983:118–140.
15. National Cancer Institute, Surveillance Epidemiology and End Results (SEER) Program. About the Seer program. Available at: https://seer.cancer.gov/about. Accessed January 6, 2023.
16. Centers for Disease Control and Prevention. National Program of Cancer Registries (NPCR): about the program. 2018. Updated August 25, 2022. Available at: http://www.cdc.gov/cancer/npcr/about.htm. Accessed January 6, 2023.
17. National Institutes of Health. List of registries. Updated December 1, 2022. Available at: https://www.nih.gov/health-information/nih-clinical-research-trials-you/list-registries. Accessed January 6, 2023.
18. Langlois JA, Rutland-Brown W. *Traumatic Brain Injury in the United States: The Future of Registries and Data Systems*. Atlanta, GA: Centers for Disease Control and Prevention, National Center for Injury Prevention and Control; 2005.
19. Centers for Disease Control and Prevention. Paul Coverdell Stroke Program. Updated September 30, 2020. Available at: http://www.cdc.gov/dhdsp/programs/stroke_registry.htm. Accessed January 6, 2023.
20. Centers for Disease Control and Prevention. Behavioral Risk Factor Surveillance System (BRFSS) FAQs. 2018. Available at: https://www.cdc.gov/brfss/about/brfss_faq.htm. Accessed January 6, 2023.
21. Centers for Disease Control and Prevention. BRFSS history. 2014. Available at: https://www.cdc.gov/brfss/about/about_brfss.htm. Accessed January 6, 2023.

22. Kempf AM, Remington PL. New challenges for telephone survey research in the twenty-first century. *Annu. Rev. Public Health*. 2007;28:113–126.
23. Blumberg SJ, Luke JV. Reevaluating the need for concern regarding noncoverage bias in landline surveys. *Am. J. Public Health*. 2009;99(10):1806–1810.
24. Rolle-Lake L, Robbins E. Behavioral Risk Factor Surveillance System. Updated February 17, 2022. In: StatPearls [Internet]. Treasure Island, FL: StatPearls Publishing; 2022. Available at: https://www.ncbi.nlm.nih.gov/books/NBK553031. Accessed January 6, 2023.
25. Centers for Disease Control and Prevention, Division of Health Informatics and Surveillance. Methodologic changes in the Behavioral Risk Factor Surveillance System in 2011 and potential effects on prevalence estimates. June 12, 2012. Available at: http://www.cdc.gov/surveillancepractice/reports/brfss/brfss.html. Accessed March 16, 2023.
26. University of Wisconsin–Madison School of Medicine and Public Health. Survey of the Health of Wisconsin (SHOW). Available at: http://www.show.wisc.edu. Accessed January 6, 2023.
27. Centers for Disease Control and Prevention. Frequently asked questions about PRAMS. Updated April 22, 2022. Available at: https://www.cdc.gov/prams/about/prams-faq.htm. Accessed January 6, 2023.
28. Quail JM, Lix LM, Osman BA, Teare GF. Comparing comorbidity measures for predicting mortality and hospitalization in three population-based cohorts. *BMC Health Serv Res*. 2011;11:146.
29. National Centers for Health Statistics. *International Classification of Diseases*, Tenth Revision, Clinical Modification (ICD-10-CM). Reviewed October 17, 2022. Available at: https://www.cdc.gov/nchs/icd/icd-10-cm.htm. Accessed March 17, 2023.
30. National Opinion Research Center. *The Value of Hospital Discharge Databases*. Bethesda, MD: National Opinion Research Center; 2005.
31. Schoenman J, Sutton J, Elixhauser A, Love D. Understanding and enhancing the value of hospital discharge data. *Med Care Res Rev*. 2007;64(4):449–468.
32. Chassin MR, Hannan EL, DeBuono BA. Benefits and hazards of reporting medical outcomes publicly. *N Engl J Med*. 1996;334(6):394–398.
33. Iglehart JK. The National Committee for Quality Assurance. *N Engl J Med*. 1996;335(13):995–999.
34. National Committee for Quality Assurance. HEDIS and performance measurement. Available at: https://www.ncqa.org/hedis. Accessed January 6, 2023.
35. The Annie E. Casey Foundation, National Association for Public Health Statistics and Information Systems. More better faster: strategies for improving the timeliness of vital statistics. April 2013. Available at: https://www.aecf.org/resources/more-better-faster. Accessed March 16, 2023.
36. Kirscher T, Anderson RE. Cause of death: proper completion of the death certificate. *JAMA*. 1987;258(3):349–352.
37. Centers for Disease Control and Prevention. *Physicians' Handbook on Medical Certification of Death*. Atlanta, GA: Centers for Disease Control and Prevention; 2003. DHHS publication (PHS) 2003-1108.
38. National Centers for Health Statistics. SuperMICAR. Updated November 6, 2016. Available at: http://www.cdc.gov/nchs/nvss/mmds/super_micar.htm. Accessed January 6, 2023.
39. National Centers for Health Statistics. ICD-10-CM Official Guidelines for Coding and Reporting FY 2016. 2016. Available at http://www.cdc.gov/nchs/data/icd/10cmguidelines_2016_final.pdf. Accessed January 6, 2023.

40. National Centers for Health Statistics. National Vital Statistic System: training and instruction materials. Updated February 10, 2022. Available at: https://www.cdc.gov/nchs/nvss/training-and-instructional-materials.htm. Accessed January 17, 2023.
41. Devlin HM, Desai J, Walaszek A. Reviewing performance of birth certificate and hospital discharge data to identify births complicated by maternal diabetes. *Matern Child Health J.* 2009;13(5):660–666.
42. State of Wisconsin. Chapter 69: collection of statistics. Updated 2021–2022. Available at: http://docs.legis.wisconsin.gov/statutes/statutes/69.pdf. Accessed January 6, 2023.
43. Koch J. *Robert Guthrie—the PKU Story: A Crusade Against Mental Retardation.* Pasadena, CA: Hope Publishing House; 1997.
44. Advisory Committees on Heritable Disorders in Newborns and Children. Recommended uniform screening panel. Health Resources and Services Administration. Updated August 2022. Available at: https://www.hrsa.gov/advisory-committees/heritable-disorders/rusp/index.html. Accessed January 6, 2023.
45. Brownson RC, Chriqui JF, Stamatakis KA. Understanding evidence-based public health policy. *Am J Public Health.* 2009;99(9):1576–1583.
46. Temple University. The Policy Surveillance Program: A LawAtlas Project. Available at: https://lawatlas.org. Accessed January 6, 2023.
47. Chriqui JF, O'Connor JC, Chaloupka FJ. What gets measured, gets changed: evaluating law and policy for maximum impact. *J Law Med Ethics.* 2011;39(suppl 1):21–26.
48. US Census Bureau. Design and methodology report. American Community Survey. 2014. Updated December 12, 2022. Available at: https://www.census.gov/programs-surveys/acs/methodology/design-and-methodology.html. Accessed January 6, 2023.
49. Roos LL, Mustard CA, Nicol JP, et al. Registries and administrative data: organization and accuracy. *Med Care.* 1993;31(3):201–212.
50. Centers for Disease Control and Prevention. CDC WONDER online database. 2022. Available at: http://wonder.cdc.gov. Accessed January 6, 2023.
51. Wisconsin Department of Health Services. WISH (Wisconsin Interactive Statistics on Health) Query System. 2019. Available at: https://www.dhs.wisconsin.gov/wish/index.htm. Accessed January 6, 2023.
52. Chicago Health Atlas. Available at: http://www.chicagohealthatlas.org. Accessed January 6, 2023.
53. Rogers T, Chappelle EF, Wall HK, Barron-Simpson R. *Using DHDSP Outcome Indicators for Policy and Systems Change for Program Planning and Evaluation.* Atlanta, GA: Centers for Disease Control and Prevention; 2011.
54. Wisconsin Department of Health Services. WISH population portal. 2022. Available at: https://www.dhs.wisconsin.gov/wish/population/form.htm. Accessed January, 2023.
55. Wisconsin Department of Health Services. WISH: Behavioral Risk Factor Survey module. Updated March 29, 2022. Available at: https://www.dhs.wisconsin.gov/wish/brfs/index.htm. Accessed January 6, 2023.
56. Brownson RC, Smith CA, Jorge NE, Deprima LT, Dean CG, Cates RW. The role of data-driven planning and coalition development in preventing cardiovascular disease. *Public Health Rep.* 1992;107:32–37.

57. Centers for Disease Control and Prevention. PLACES: local data for better health. Updated December 9, 2022. Available at: https://www.cdc.gov/places/index.html. Accessed January 6, 2023.
58. Trumbo CW. Public requests for cancer cluster investigations: a survey of state health departments. *Am. J. Public Health.* 2000;90:1300–1302.
59. Centers for Disease Control and Prevention. Guidelines for examining unusual patterns of cancer and environmental concerns. Updated December 8, 2022. Available at: https://www.cdc.gov/nceh/cancer-environment/guidelines/. Accessed June 19, 2023.
60. Bandi P, Remington PL, Moberg DP. Progress in reducing cigarette consumption: the Wisconsin tobacco control program, 2001–2003. *Wis Med J.* 2006;105(5):45–49.
61. Remington PL. Communicating epidemiologic information. In: Brownson RC, Petitti DB, eds. *Applied Epidemiology: Theory to Practice.* New York, NY: Oxford University Press; 1998: 323–348.
62. Goodman R, Remington PL. Disseminating surveillance information. In: Teutsch SM, Churchill RE, eds. *Principles and Practice of Public Health Surveillance.* New York, NY: Oxford University Press; 1993.
63. Centers for Disease Control and Prevention. Health literacy: guidance and tools. Updated September 3, 2021. Available at: https://www.cdc.gov/healthliteracy/developmaterials/guidancestandards.html. Accessed January 6, 2023.
64. Remington PL, Catlin BB, Gennuso KP. The county health rankings: rationale and methods. *Popul Health Metr.* 2015;13(11):1–12.
65. Thacker SB, Berkelman RL. Public health surveillance in the United States. *Epidemiol Rev.* 1988;10:164–190.

4

Community-Based Interventions

Robert J. McDermott, PhD, MS, Alyssa B. Mayer, PhD, MPH,
Mary P. Martinasek, PhD, MPH, Claudia Aguado Loi, PhD, MPH,
Sandra D. Vamos, EdD, Mahmooda K. Pasha, PhD, MPH, and
Justin T. McDaniel, PhD, MBA

LEARNING OBJECTIVES

After completing this chapter, readers should be able to

1. Describe the determinants of chronic diseases as they differentially affect various subgroups in the population.
2. Explain what is meant by a social-ecological approach to chronic disease prevention and control and how various levels of intervention are used separately and in combination to promote public health.
3. Describe the application of various models in understanding and influencing health-related behaviors that affect the risk of chronic disease development.
4. Discuss how family, friends, and social networks influence health-related behaviors and, in turn, the risk of chronic diseases.
5. Assess the roles of various settings as venues for delivery of health promotion programs for prevention and control of chronic diseases.
6. Enumerate the benefits of and approaches to community-level planning, community-based programs, community engagement, and community partnerships for chronic disease prevention and control.
7. Describe the role of advocacy and lobbying in public health program development and policymaking.
8. Evaluate the role of health literacy in chronic disease prevention and control.

INTRODUCTION

Heart disease, cancer, and diabetes are the leading chronic diseases in the United States; these diseases, along with stroke, chronic respiratory illness, Alzheimer's disease, and chronic kidney disease represent the most common and economically threatening of all health problems.[1] Fortunately, most of these problems are largely preventable or can have their severity markedly reduced. Whereas the risk factors for most of these chronic diseases and conditions are well known, preventing their occurrence is an arduous task for public health authorities. This challenge stems from the fact that many chronic diseases have their origins in social, cultural, environmental, and behavioral factors, thereby making their causes (and potential interventions) both complex and multilevel.

Interventions to prevent or control chronic diseases can involve efforts at any system level—individuals, communities, or larger societal systems—however, if the various levels combine in an organized manner, they become multilevel, comprehensive programs. Moreover, interventions can address prevention efforts at the pre-pathogenesis stage (before disease onset) or at the pathogenesis stage (early or late disease onset).

- Pre-pathogenesis prevention efforts include primary prevention (e.g., reducing the risk of disease through exercise, healthy eating, nonsmoking).
- Pathogenesis prevention efforts include (1) secondary prevention (e.g., early detection of breast cancer through mammograms for women, colon cancer screening for men and women aged ≥45 years, blood pressure checks for persons of all ages) and (2) tertiary prevention (e.g., management of disease to minimize confounding complications through carefully monitored insulin intake for diabetes management, adherence to a prescribed diet, or moderate-to-vigorous exercise several days per week for patients who have had a heart attack).

Interventions for altering a health risk profile may address behaviors at the individual level such as altering a poor diet, reducing or eliminating tobacco use, moderating alcohol consumption, and increasing physical activity. These interventions take shape as health-promoting messages or through evidence-based interventions. These can come from print and electronic media (internet and social media) or from one-to-one education through health care providers, prevention specialists, lay and peer educators, health navigators, teachers, employers, members of a faith-based community, or a host of other individuals. Group education can provide an avenue to deliver information while encouraging and motivating individuals to change their behaviors.

Other chronic disease interventions focus on system-level changes, including policy development or change, economic incentives, and specific actions within the health care system. Examples of these interventions include food product labeling of nutrition content, enactment of tobacco excise taxes to reduce purchases by novice users, and insurance coverage for physical examinations and early detection screening, among other actions.

Multilevel interventions seek to change many aspects of the environment that contribute to chronic disease development. These interventions include multiple activities that prioritize change at the individual level and the larger system level. There are several instances of such interventions in the literature. For example, Kim et al.[2] implemented more than one intervention to promote colorectal cancer screening at the individual patient level using patient reminders and at the larger clinic system through provider education, patient navigation services, and provider feedback and assessment.

Comprehensive interventions also may address root causes of some chronic diseases, such as poverty, low literacy and education, or poor access to health care. Additionally, they may seek social support for positive health behaviors. These interventions often involve health advocacy groups and empower coalitions of individuals and community organizations to act.

MULTIPLE DETERMINANTS OF CHRONIC DISEASE

To be effective, chronic disease prevention and control efforts must consider the multiple determinants of chronic disease, including lifestyle and health risk behaviors, the health care system, the physical environment, and social and economic factors. The next sections describe the influence of these chronic disease determinants.

Biological and Genetic Determinants

Biological determinants across the life course, such as genetics and family predisposition, play a role in chronic disease development. Whereas some chronic diseases, such as breast or ovarian cancer, directly result from genetic mutations such as BRCA1 or BRCA2[3] and allow for early prevention efforts, the root causes of other chronic diseases, such as type 1 diabetes, are not as well understood, and are possibly explained by an interaction of environmental and genetic factors. Family history, for example, increases the risk of several chronic diseases, including heart disease, cancer, asthma, and diabetes, but they can be attributed to myriad risk factors, where a biological explanation is only part of the puzzle. Experts known as epigeneticists suggest that chronic diseases may arise as a result of the accumulation of risk factors that influence how our inherited genes are expressed.[4] Epigenetics, a field introduced a century ago, has received a rapid increase in attention in the last two decades. Epigenetic studies demonstrate how genes are expressed through interactions with the environment and individual behaviors. For example, smoking behaviors can change the pathophysiology of the brain, muscle development, and lung functioning.[4,5]

Behavioral Determinants

More than half of all American adults, nearly 129 million people, had 1 of 10 selected chronic disease conditions (arthritis, cancer, chronic obstructive pulmonary disease, coronary heart disease, asthma, diabetes, hepatitis, hypertension, stroke, and weak or failing kidneys) in 2018. In addition, approximately 27% of the population had two or more co-occurring chronic conditions, a slight rise since 2012.[6] Women, non-Hispanic Whites, older adults, adults receiving Medicaid, and rural Americans bear most of the comorbidity burden in the United States. Many chronic disease conditions can be prevented, have their onset delayed, or have their symptoms significantly reduced through modest changes in individual behaviors. Four behaviors in particular—physical inactivity, poor nutrition, smoking, and excessive alcohol use—account for much of the illness and early death caused by chronic diseases. Despite this, more than half of adults do not meet the recommendations for physical activity.[7] Furthermore, just 10% to 12% of adults eat the recommended daily servings of fruits and vegetables,[8,9] only one in four adults and one in five high school students engage in recommended levels of physical activity,[9] and 38.5 million Americans, or nearly 16.6%, report binge drinking during the past 30 days.[10] About 50.6 million US adults (20.8%) report current use of a tobacco-related product, including cigarettes (14.0%), e-cigarettes (4.5%), cigars (3.6%), smokeless tobacco (2.4%), and pipes (1.0%). Most tobacco-related product users (80.5%) use combustible products (cigarettes, cigars, or pipes), and 18.6% use two or more products.[11] Public health authorities believe that implementing comprehensive, evidence-based interventions at the population level, along with ongoing regulation of tobacco products, will reduce tobacco-related diseases and deaths.[11]

Many chronic diseases are associated with overweight and obesity, and Americans have experienced significant increases in obesity during the past three decades. According to Hales et al.,[12] the age-adjusted prevalence of American adults who are obese has increased from 30.5% in 2000 to 42.2% in 2018. Obesity increases the risk of developing associated chronic diseases, including hypertension, dyslipidemia (e.g., high total cholesterol or high levels of triglycerides), type 2 diabetes, coronary heart disease, stroke, gallbladder disease, osteoarthritis, sleep apnea, respiratory problems, mental disorders (e.g., depression, anxiety), and several cancers, notably cancers of the endometrium, breast, and colon.[13]

Adults are not alone in experiencing obesity. Overall, obesity among children remains high and has continued to increase since 2012. Based on data from 2017 to 2018,[14] 13.4% of children aged 2 to 5 years, 20.3% of children aged 6 to 11 years, and 21.2% of youths aged 12 to 19 years were obese (i.e., had a body mass index [BMI] in the 95th percentile for age and sex). Despite these increasing rates, children aged 2 to 19 years from a household with higher education and income are reported to have lower obesity rates (10.9%) than children in the lowest income group.[14]

These health risk behaviors come with a cost. Annual medical costs for a person who is obese are $3,429 higher than for someone of normal weight.[15] Direct medical costs associated with obesity totaled nearly $147 billion in 2008.[13] Medical costs for heart disease and stroke are estimated at $216 billion per year.[16] Smoking, excessive alcohol use, and physical inactivity are also expensive, costing $225 billion, $249 billion, and $117 billion a year in medical costs, respectively.[1] Taken together, these risk behaviors and resulting chronic disease conditions are the largest economic drivers of the nation's $3.8 trillion in annual health care cost.[13] Of the $3.8 trillion, 90% occurs for chronic and mental health conditions that often result from risk behaviors.[17]

Health Care Determinants

Access to high-quality health care is an important determinant of health at the individual and community level. Medicare, the federal health insurance program for people aged 65 years and older and people with permanent disabilities, contributes to the reimbursement for hospital and physician visits, prescription drugs, and other services. Medicare spending in 2018 accounted for 15% of the federal budget. Medicare reimbursements to the health care system accounted for 20% of total national health spending in 2017, 25% of spending on hospital care, and 23% of spending on physician services.[18] The cost of treating chronic diseases contributes significantly to these costs.

Since 2015, the Affordable Care Act (ACA) requires that every health plan cover all costs related to preventive services. Under Section 2713 of ACA, private health plans must provide coverage for a range of preventive services and may not impose cost-sharing (such as co-payments, deductibles, or coinsurance) on patients receiving these services.[19] The adult-targeted preventive services for chronic disease covered under ACA are ones that are evidence based and related to screening for breast, cervical, colorectal, and lung cancer, as well as skin cancer counseling, and screenings related to cardiovascular disease (including hypertension and hyperlipidemia), type 2 diabetes, obesity, and osteoporosis.[18]

Environmental Determinants

The environment can affect health, not only from traditional exposures in the air, water, or food but also from how we design and build our communities. During the past few years, Americans have witnessed many discussions in both scholarly literature and the popular press about the obesity epidemic. One cause attributed to the rise in obesity is the role of our built environment—those aspects of a person's surroundings that contribute favorably or unfavorably to that individual's particular health initiatives. These elements broadly encompass one's local environment (e.g., inside the home and school) and one's surroundings, such as neighborhoods, urban development, land use, transportation, industry, and agriculture.

An environment with accessible and safe sidewalks, nearby parks, and such entities as bike trails and community swimming pools encourage people to engage in physical activity. Likewise, aesthetically pleasing stairways at work, signs reminding people to use the stairs, and such amenities as showers and facilities for changing clothes at work after exercising are pro-health surroundings. In contrast, an environment that lacks aesthetics and is unsafe (e.g., sidewalks in need of repair, no sidewalks, heavy vehicular traffic, poor lighting, criminal activity) discourage people from being active. A person's home environment also has an important influence on activity level—a point that has become more evident with the presence of multi-television households, computers, and other electronic and smart devices such as tablets, smartphones, and video games, all of which contribute to sedentary behavior.

The built environment also influences what one chooses nutritionally. Menu choices in schools, restaurants, and worksite cafeterias may offer healthy choices, but perhaps too often, less healthy alternatives. Neighborhoods lacking grocery stores or convenient farmers' markets may be devoid of fresh fruit and vegetable options, thereby forcing people to purchase what is cheap or available regardless of its nutritional value. The many linkages between the built environment and obesity have resulted in diverse considerations for health promotion programming.[20] We also see similar associations where certain built environment conditions influence populations to assume adverse behaviors such as smoking and excessive alcohol use.[21]

Given the unequal distribution of health outcomes across different neighborhoods and, more broadly, across counties, states, and rural or urban areas throughout the United States—no doubt attributable to differential access to services and exposure to environmental risk factors for disease or injury—public health interventions are best implemented after a thorough investigation of high-priority areas. One way to identify areas in need of intervention is with the use of geographic information systems (GIS) and various mapping methodologies,[22] such as choropleth maps with graduated symbols representing magnitudes of disease burden in different areas or spatial clustering/hotspot maps. For example, McDaniel et al.[23] examined the geographic distribution of county-level disability rates among American children aged 5 to 17 years between 2012 and 2016. The prevalence of disability was higher in federally designated regions of socioeconomic deprivation, such as the Mississippi Delta region and the Appalachian region; they further showed that the most rural areas in those regions were the most disproportionately affected. They were able to make recommendations about geographically targeted interventions in those regions (i.e., for specific counties), especially interventions that were culturally relevant and resource mindful.

An additional study of disability prevalence among older military veterans expanded on this approach, created a descriptive county-level choropleth map, and determined hotspots/clusters of counties with high disability prevalence rates.[24] It identified clusters of counties, particularly in the southern United States, with relatively high rates of disability but no in-county access to a Veterans Affairs (VA)–owned medical facility. These results advanced discussion about the urgent need for geographically placed disability services in identified counties, as well as recommendations about VA health care policy. Capitalizing on the proliferation and availability of GIS software programs for research and practice purposes is important for the identification of geographic areas in need of tailored interventions.

Social Determinants

For at least three decades, public health professionals have viewed individual behaviors (e.g., smoking, alcohol and other substance abuse, sexual activity, physical activity, nutrition) as contributing to most of the suboptimal health of Americans. As a consequence, most interventions focus on change at the individual level. Although individual behaviors are clearly determinants of health status, focusing on the individual presents a limited and inefficient view of change on a population scale.

Population health is the science of variations in health status among segments of a society or culture. Population health scientists study the indicators of health behavior and health status as they relate to a social determinants perspective. These indicators encompass social, economic, political, and environmental factors. Therefore, issues such as level of education, health literacy, language, employment, social or economic stressors, access to health care, transportation, housing, income inequality, discrimination or social inclusion, and exclusion stemming from sex, race, or age are relevant matters. Policymakers and health professionals often blame persons at high risk for poor health on their own "lifestyles" or "choices" when, in fact, their available lifestyle choices are limited and their behaviors are strongly influenced by their social, economic, cultural, or physical environment.[1] The many observed health disparities are largely a result of these social determinants. Richard Besser, president and CEO of the Robert Wood Johnson Foundation, has noted: "We talk about choice being such a big part of health, but the choices you make depend on the choices you have."[25]

If the United States is to reduce the burden of chronic disease and eliminate health disparities, there will need to be better understanding of the relationship between individual health behaviors and social context. Advertising, pricing, and retail practices of the food, alcohol, and tobacco industries that target vulnerable populations strongly influence health choices. We have seen the effects of tobacco marketing that preys on teens and on low-income communities' accessibility to nicotine products for several years.[1,26] For example, Morton et al.[27] reported higher tobacco outlet density and increased tobacco retail in census tracts of low-socioeconomic-status populations. In addition, the lack of public transportation may deter persons with less income and people on fixed incomes from meeting health care appointments. Whereas improvement in school graduation rates could reduce disparities in health, especially among the most disadvantaged, public health agencies, legislatures, and policymakers rarely make the school dropout problem a priority for altering the status quo in health matters. Strong alliances among public health authorities, policymakers, and educators may favorably influence population health.

LEVELS OF INTERVENTION: A SOCIAL-ECOLOGICAL PERSPECTIVE

A social-ecological perspective considers that health decisions are influenced by numerous factors (Figure 4-1).[28] Therefore, this perspective addresses individual as well as social and environmental factors as the foci of chronic disease interventions.

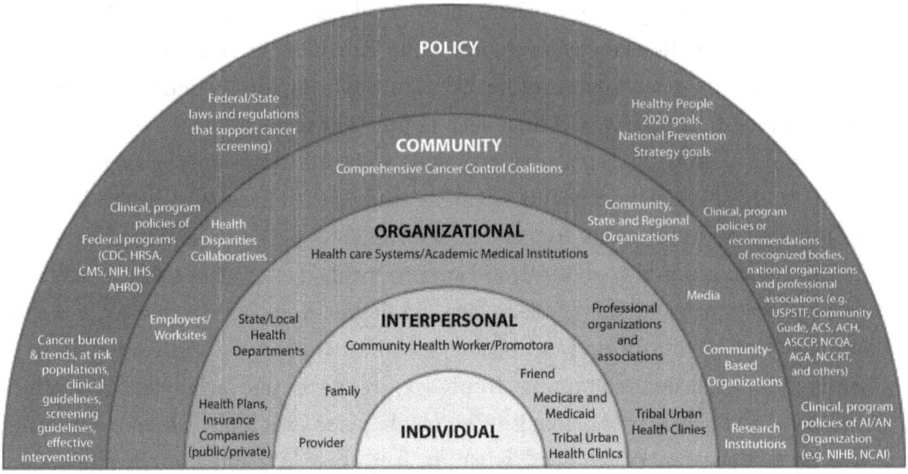

Source: Reprinted from CDC.[28]

Figure 4-1. Social-Ecological Model

Whereas individual health behaviors are popular targets of interventions, they often result in a victim-blaming culture that fails to respect the influence of the social and physical environments that may need to be modified. Use of an ecological approach acknowledges the interaction of an individual and the environment and considers the following elements that influence health behavior:

- Intrapersonal factors: altering knowledge, attitudes, skills, and future behavioral intentions at the level of the individual person.
- Interpersonal factors: understanding and accessing the relationships that people have with other individuals in their social network such as friends, peers, coworkers, family members, neighbors, and others from whom behavioral patterns and behavioral norms are acquired.
- Organizational factors: using organizations such as schools, faith-based groups, worksites, or health care facilities to direct, influence, or support health behavior change and help to define health behavior norms.
- Community factors: catalyzing interest within an area with geographic or political boundaries to leverage power structures to achieve a particular set of health objectives, perhaps to address the most serious health problems among persons typically in the weakest position to advocate on their own behalf (e.g., the rural poor, members of underrepresented minorities, less educated, physically or mentally challenged).
- Policy factors: advocating, organizing, and analyzing policies and procedures, regulations, and laws that favorably influence the fight against chronic diseases.

INTRAPERSONAL APPROACHES TO CHRONIC DISEASE INTERVENTION

Intrapersonal models or theoretical frameworks assume that people can be motivated to take individual action that changes their health knowledge, attitudes, skills, behavioral intentions, and eventual behavior. Although there are many such approaches, four frameworks are presented here for their potential utility in chronic disease prevention and intervention: the Health Belief Model, the Transtheoretical Model, the Theory of Planned Behavior, and the Control Model.

Health Belief Model

The Health Belief Model was one of the first attempts of behavioral scientists to use theory to study preventive health behaviors. The model was developed by a group of social psychologists at the US Public Health Service in the 1950s to explain the failure of people to participate in programs designed to prevent or detect disease.[29] According to the original model, the likelihood of individuals taking preventive action to avoid disease is enhanced if they perceive themselves to be susceptible to the disease, perceive the consequences of contracting the disease to be at least of moderate severity, recognize the benefits of choosing a preventive action, view the benefits as being superior to the costs and barriers of adopting the behavior, and receive cues to action—that is, internal or external messages that affect their readiness to take action. In the 1980s, another component was added to the Health Belief Model: self-efficacy, or the belief that one can perform the activity of interest.

A simple application of the Health Belief Model can be seen in the following example of a 45-year-old woman with average breast cancer risk deciding whether to seek a baseline mammogram, a health behavior in the category of secondary prevention. The American Cancer Society[30] recommends that women with average risk of developing breast cancer have a baseline screening mammogram at age 45, with annual mammograms thereafter until age 55, and then at least a biennial procedure until age 70. This 45-year-old woman may see herself as susceptible (e.g., past her 44th birthday, no previous baseline mammogram). She may see breast cancer as being severe (e.g., in the event of disease, possible mastectomy, physical disfigurement, loss of self-esteem, and even death). She may perceive the benefits of mammography (e.g., early detection of disease and, consequently, easier intervention if disease is present, peace of mind if there is no disease) to outweigh any perceived costs or barriers (e.g., fear of disease, fear or embarrassment related to the procedure). Her motivation may be inspired by cues to action (e.g., reminder postcard, email, text message, recommendation by a physician, message seen or heard through mass/social media, learning that an acquaintance just had a mammogram or recently received a breast cancer diagnosis). Finally, her likelihood of following through is enhanced if she possesses the confidence and ability (i.e., self-efficacy) to ask her physician about receiving a baseline mammogram, to know where to obtain one, to feel comfortable with calling for an appointment or scheduling online, and to know she can get herself to the facility.

Whereas the Health Belief Model has been used largely to explain the failure of people to adopt preventive behaviors, the model can be useful for intervening at points along the way to develop targeted messages and other intervention strategies (i.e., changing perceptions of susceptibility and severity, assessing benefits and costs or barriers accurately, creating frequent and effective cues to action to which women will respond, and increasing women's confidence to follow through in receiving the procedure).

Transtheoretical Model and Stages of Change

The Transtheoretical Model, often referred to as the Stages of Change Model, was developed by Prochaska and DiClemente[31] through their work on understanding how people quit smoking. The essence of the model is that not everyone is at an equivalent stage of readiness to change health behavior, and thus interventions need to take on different characteristics to be responsive to these various stages.

The model comprises a series of stages, the exact number of which may vary. In the *precontemplation stage*, there is no intention to change behavior, perhaps not even any awareness that change is an alternative or something that can result in an improvement of health or lifestyle. In the *contemplation stage*, an individual may recognize that change is a possibility but is still thinking about making the change or adaptation and has not fully committed to doing so. In the *preparation stage*, people may gather information about the consequences of altering their lifestyle, affirming the need to change, and possibly deciding to do so at a specified time in the future, usually in the next 30 days. At the *action stage*, the person actually implements the change, shifting the plan from one that is theoretical to one that is operational—a period that may last up to six months. If the action stage becomes routinized, one moves on into the *maintenance stage*, in which the behaviors initiated previously are consolidated into one's typical lifestyle. At this point, people can go in one of two possible directions: they can enter the *termination stage*, in which the former problem behavior is no longer perceived as being acceptable; or they can move into the *relapse stage*, in which there is recidivism and a resumption of former, less healthy behavior.

With respect to planning and designing interventions, taking a person's stage of readiness to change into account can enhance the likelihood of moving the person along the behavioral continuum and ultimately improving the chances of success. For example, addressing the needs of a person who has a long history of physical inactivity and is contemplating change is quite different than intervening with someone who is in the preparation stage or who has moved back and forth between that stage and the action stage.

Whereas the contemplative individual may require encouragement to evaluate the pros and cons of behavior change and identification of positive outcomes and expectations, the person who has already tested the waters, so to speak, may instead need to find social support, receive specific suggestions for overcoming obstacles to cementing the change, and seek satisfaction from small, incremental successes in the direction of the desired behavior. It is important to realize that this model is more circular or spiraling in nature than linear. People may advance a stage but then regress. Moreover, individuals may go through multiple cycles of contemplation, preparation, and action before reaching a terminal stage or exiting the system altogether. Understanding what stage people are in will assist intervention efforts.

Theory of Planned Behavior

The Theory of Planned Behavior posits that individual behavior is driven by behavioral intentions.[32,33] Behavioral intentions are influenced by a person's collective attitudes about the behavior in question, the subjective norms with respect to carrying out the behavior, and the person's perception of the ease with which the behavior can be carried out (behavioral control). This theory has its roots in Fishbein's model of behavioral intentions[34] and the theory of reasoned action.[35,36]

With the Theory of Planned Behavior, one's attitude toward a behavior (e.g., daily exercise) is the sum of all the positive feelings (e.g., doing something good for one's health, feeling better about oneself, accepting exercise as a popular activity) or negative feelings (e.g., exercise exhausts me, exercise is inconvenient, exercise will make me sore) about performing a behavior. This sum comes from determining one's beliefs about the consequences arising from a behavior and an evaluation of the desirability of these consequences. A person's overall attitude is the sum of the individual consequences and the desirability assessments for all expected consequences of the behavior.

The beliefs underlying a person's subjective norms are called normative beliefs. The subjective norm is defined as a person's perception of whether people important to him or her value a behavior and think the person should engage in it. The opinion of any significant other is weighted by the motivation that the person has to comply with the wishes of that significant other. The overall subjective norm is the sum of the individual perceptions and the motivation assessments for all significant others who may influence the person considering a behavior.

Behavioral control is a person's perception of the difficulty of carrying out the behavior (e.g., skills, available time, sacrifice of other activities for this particular behavior). In the Theory of Planned Behavior, the control that people have over their behavior is a continuum of behaviors from ones that are easily carried out to ones requiring much time, effort, resources, and so on. The link between behavior and behavioral control in this model should be between behavior and actual behavioral control rather than perceived behavioral control. However, the difficulty of assessing actual behavioral control has resulted in behavioral scientists using perceived control as a proxy measure for actual behavior.

Health Locus of Control Model

Locus of control refers to a person's expectations about where control over events in life resides. In a health context, it means who or what is responsible for that which happens to one's health. Expectancy, which concerns future events, is an important part of the locus of control construct. Locus of control is grounded in expectancy value theory; that is, if a person values a particular outcome and believes that carrying out a particular behavior will result in that outcome, then that person is more likely to pursue that behavior.

Rotter[37] classified beliefs concerning who or what influences things along a continuum from completely internal control to completely external control. Whereas internal control is the expectancy that future events are largely under the control of the individual, external control refers to the belief that future events are outside individual control, such as under the control of others or attributable entirely to fate or chance.

Since its introduction in the 1960s, the locus of control construct has seen many permutations and iterations through the work of behavioral scientists in numerous fields. However, health behavior researchers have used the locus of control idea extensively. Among the most widely used health-specific measure is the Multidimensional Health Locus of Control Scale.[38]

In practice, people who believe that their health status is largely within their own control are more likely to embrace preventive, positive health behaviors. Persons perceiving their locus of control to be more external are less inclined to take on preventive actions, concluding that a higher power, fate, luck, or other influences, including regulatory measures, will determine their health outcomes. Public health workers attempting to influence health behavior choices regarding vaccine acceptance, for example, may have better success with a target group that possesses more of an internal locus of control. Conversely, changing policies or using a systems approach, such as mandatory mask wearing for prevention of transmission of novel viruses, may be more effective for individuals with an external locus of control.

INTERPERSONAL APPROACHES TO CHRONIC DISEASE INTERVENTION

Models of interpersonal health behavior assume that the interpersonal environment is one of the most powerful avenues of influence for health-related behavior and health status. Moreover, mechanisms that link individuals' social contexts with health effects revolve around two social processes: social support and social influence. The next section describes the interactions of individuals, environments, and corresponding health behaviors.

Social Cognitive Theory

Social cognitive theory is one interpersonal-level theory that has been used in multiple chronic disease prevention and control studies. Social cognitive theory addresses both the psychosocial dynamics influencing health behavior and methods for promoting behavioral change. With this theory, human behavior is explained in terms of a triadic, dynamic, and reciprocal model in which behavior, personal factors (including cognitions), and environmental influences all interact.[39] Critical factors include the individual's ability to monitor behavior, to anticipate the outcomes of behavior (including overcoming the obstacles in performing a given behavior), to self-determine or self-regulate behavior, and to reflect on and analyze experiences.[39]

Social cognitive theory emphasizes the importance of enhancing a person's behavioral capability (knowledge and skills) and self-confidence (self-efficacy) to engage in a particular health behavior. Self-efficacy, one of the most important constructs in this theory, has been demonstrated to predict the initiation of a new health behavior, the continuation of the target behavior, and the maintenance of complex health behaviors. The most powerful and consistent way of enhancing self-efficacy is through mastery of a task. Successful social cognitive theory interventions engage participants in small steps of an enacted behavior, with self-monitoring as well as feedback from others. Bandura[39,40] also developed several theory constructs that are important to understand and intervene in health behavior. These constructs include reciprocal determinism, environments and situations, observational learning, behavioral capability, reinforcement, outcome expectations, outcome expectancies, self-control of performance, and managing emotional arousal.

Social cognitive theory has wide applicability for different audiences, as it has been used to promote condom use among young adults,[41] to take actions to reduce occurrence of dental caries,[42] and to promote physical activity.[43] By recognizing the importance of the environment, people, and behavior, social cognitive theory provides a framework for designing, implementing, and evaluating comprehensive behavioral change programs.

Family-Based Interventions

Family-based interventions draw on the enhancement of existing close social network linkages and often entail education and interventions that affect the health and self-care behavior of persons with chronic disease. Family interventions affect not only the patient but also the family and its environment. Interventions can improve coping, communication, and understanding of negative emotion; in turn, they can aid in decreasing relationship stress and anxiety around a chronic illness.[44]

Family-based approaches to chronic disease prevention and control emphasize the context of the disease to include the physical environment, relationships, education, and personal needs in a more comprehensive care program. For example, two systematic reviews on the effects of family interventions in diabetes outcomes found that glycemic control[45] and quality of life[46] improved with family assistance.

The family environment can contribute to childhood obesity as children assimilate the behaviors and beliefs of their parents. Ethical family interventions focused on sound nutrition and physical activity practices can influence the entire family and serve to reduce childhood obesity. However, advocates of broad-based interventions must be sensitive to balancing ethical responsibility and equity.[47]

Social Support and Social Networks

The web of social relationships that people form constitutes their social network. The powerful influence that social relationships have on health has elicited a great deal of interest among public health researchers and practitioners. An understanding of the impact of social relationships on health status, health behaviors, and health decisions has the potential to influence the design of interventions for more effective chronic disease prevention and health promotion.

One important function of social relationships is to provide functional social support, which House[48] defines as consisting of four distinct supportive behaviors: (1) emotional support, (2) instrumental support, (3) informational support, and (4) appraisal support. By comparison, a social network is the web of relationships surrounding individuals. Whereas the provision of social support is one important function of these networks, not all social networks are necessarily supportive.[49] Social networks can be described by the following characteristics[50]:

- Homogeneity: how alike network members are in terms of demographic characteristics such as age, race, and socioeconomic status.
- Geographic dispersion: the extent to which network members live near each other.
- Density: how well network members know each other and how often they interact.
- Intensity: the emotional closeness of people within a network.
- Formality: the extent to which relationships are embedded in organizational structures within a social network.
- Complexity: how many functions are served by relationships within a network.
- Reciprocity: whether or not resources and support are both given and received among members in a network.

Having a strong social network accompanied by social support was found to be effective for enhancing diabetic self-management.[51] Creating social networks among older adults who may not be familiar with nor have access to online social media sites is important for reducing health costs related to chronic disease management. Additionally, social support coming from families may be especially helpful and acceptable to older adults.[52]

Friends and Social Networks

Another type of social network intervention entails developing new social network linkages through mentor programs, buddy systems, and self-help groups. Groups such as Alcoholics Anonymous, Overeaters Anonymous, and Weight Watchers provide access to new social networks designed to provide cognitive, instrumental, and emotional support for lifestyle change.[53]

Peer groups are particularly important for interventions focused on adolescents. Studies of adolescent friendship networks show that peer influence plays a key role in risk behaviors associated with chronic disease development.[54,55] Specifically, Farhat[56] documented that adolescents' social networks moderate the pathway from weight stigma to negative health behaviors.

In addition, Montgomery et al.[57] demonstrated that school-based social networks were driven by either homophilic social selection or a drive for popularity. Adolescents in a denser than average network tended to have lower health risk behaviors, suggesting that behaviors such as smoking, drinking, and other substance use were mitigated by social networks, with limited evidence to support that they were similarly effective with respect to physical activity and eating behaviors.

Positive orientation to school and academic achievement are also consistently protective factors for health; in contrast, poor health behaviors are linked to lower academic achievement among children and adolescents.[58] This connection between health and academic achievement has been formalized into a framework that acknowledges the reciprocal influences among children, school, and the broader community and the impact these connections have on health-related behaviors and risk factors for chronic disease.[59]

In the 21st century social networks have expanded to include social media as well. Depending on audience focus, contemporary multipronged interventions may leverage entities such as Facebook, Instagram, Twitter, Pinterest, mobile apps, blogs, emails, and text messaging, as well as more traditional print and electronic media. Having theory-based interventions that resonate with the target audience but have the necessary constructs for behavioral change is important for engagement and therefore for outcome assessment and better health control.

Community Health Workers

Community health workers are lay members of communities who perform volunteer or compensated work for the local health care system and in the Indigenous community.

Community health workers usually share ethnicity, language, socioeconomic status, and life experiences with the community members they serve. They have been identified by many titles, such as community health advisers, lay health advisers or advocates, coaches, *promotores(as),* outreach educators, community health representatives, peer health promoters, peer navigators, and peer mentors.[60]

Community health workers are respected and trusted members of social networks to whom individuals turn for advice, support, and other types of aid. They can access underserved communities affected by health and economic disparities, and they are therefore a valuable asset to public health education and chronic disease prevention efforts. Community health workers provide direct support to members in a network as well as link people in the network to each other and to outside resources. They have collaborated with researchers on numerous and diverse community-based interventions in urban neighborhoods, rural counties, residential institutions for the elderly, migrant farmworker communities, and churches, but they are especially recognized for their work in Latinx communities as *promotores(as).* These Indigenous workers have engaged in educational movements and social activism in the United States and Latin America since the 1960s and in recent decades have moved into health promotion and disease prevention interventions in some of the most underserved communities in the United States.[61] These community health workers also have been instrumental in providing language translation in clinical settings to improve access to health care within immigrant and ethnic communities. In summary, community health workers have emerged as an effective resource in chronic disease prevention programs.

ORGANIZATIONAL-LEVEL VENUES FOR INTERVENTION

Health Care System

The health care setting is an effective venue for providing screening and follow-up services that help to control chronic diseases. Historically, the health care setting has been used for clinical preventive services such as blood pressure monitoring, diabetes control, cardiovascular health assessment, cancer screening, and various other secondary prevention measures. However, it is also an ideal, although often underutilized, venue for patient education, including primary prevention. Research firmly establishes that physician advice given in the health care setting provides a powerful and motivational message for health behavior change.[62,63]

An intervention that has shown effectiveness without being especially burdensome on health care providers or patients is known as a "brief intervention." Brief interventions usually last for 5 to 60 minutes and consist of counseling and education. Sometimes there are multiple sessions, perhaps initiated by a primary care provider, but then transitioned

Box 4-1. Examples of Brief Interventions for Health Promotion

- When taking a blood pressure reading, sharing information about the causes and problems of high blood pressure and talking about exercise and proper diet as ways to reduce blood high pressure.
- When taking a medical history or conducting a routine physical examination, encouraging a patient at risk of developing diabetes to talk about the foods the patient eats, offering nutrition advice, and talking about practical ways to shop for food and prepare healthy meals.
- When taking a medical history or conducting a routine physical examination, mentioning that just 150 min of brisk walking per week can reduce one's risk of obesity and several chronic disease conditions compounded by obesity.
- When treating an infant or child with a respiratory infection, talking to the mother who smokes to find out if she knows about passive smoking, recommending ways of reducing the child's exposure to smoking, and asking if she is thinking about quitting.
- When taking a medical history or conducting a routine physical examination, urging adults to obtain a screening mammogram, prostate examination, colonoscopy, and other screenings as recommended for women or men in selected age groups.
- When taking a medical history or conducting a routine physical examination, finding out from patients who drink alcohol if they are drinking in a harmful way, and if they are, addressing the need to adjust their drinking to a healthier level, perhaps conveying factual information about the health effects of alcohol.

to a health education specialist to carry on the intervention. However, a brief intervention can be as limited as 30 seconds and consist of just one "teachable moment" session conducted by an alert and opportunistic health care provider. The content, duration, and number of sessions may depend on the provider, the patient's receptivity and readiness to change, the setting, and previous patient–provider rapport. The brief intervention can be leveraged at any point in the health promotion–disease prevention–treatment continuum depending on the patient's readiness to change.

There are a number of circumstances that lend themselves to brief interventions such as the ones listed in Box 4-1. However, a creative and alert health care provider will be able to note many other opportunities to intervene.

Schools

Schools are excellent venues for primary and secondary prevention. Philosophically, schools ought to convey health education along with the many other essential subjects that compose responsive education. Youth attend school for 12 or more years and are a captive audience for educators and health professionals to convey prevention messages and for health care providers to conduct selective health screenings. Moreover, establishing healthy habits in youth can help prevent many chronic health problems later in life that are attributable to unhealthy eating, sedentary lifestyle, sexual risk-taking, and other health-related issues. In addition to teaching health education, schools can offer services that promote health and monitor key health indicators in children and youth (e.g., height, weight, BMI, blood pressure, immunizations).

The Whole School, Whole Community, Whole Child (WSCC) model depicted in Figure 4-2 includes 10 components and illustrates a multitude of health-promoting opportunities in the school setting for youth as well as adults.[59,64] Many public health care providers work with school systems, thereby offering an opportunity for an effective partnership.

Prevention research focused on children and youth has yielded several evidence-based interventions that have applicability in school health education curricula. Several initiatives have emanated from the Prevention Research Centers (PRCs) promoted by the Centers for Disease Control and Prevention (CDC). PRCs constitute a national network of community–academic research partnerships situated in either a school of public

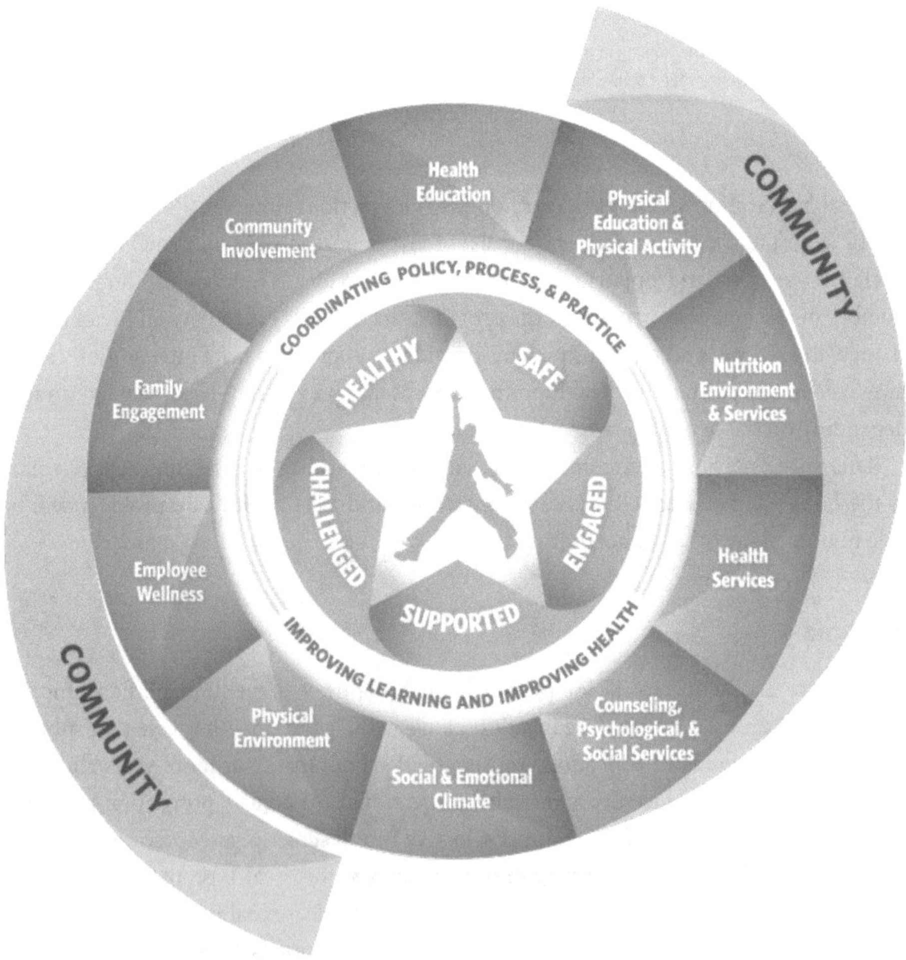

Source: Reprinted from CDC.[64]

Figure 4-2. Whole School, Whole Community, Whole Child Model

health or a medical school.[65] These centers are funded by CDC in five-year cycles to engage in community-based participatory prevention research and translate this research into public health policy and practice. Each PRC comprises academic and community partners that develop chronic disease prevention initiatives that fit the local context.[65] Community partners include health departments, school boards, and community-based organizations and residents who collaborate with the PRC to form long-term partnerships engaged in community-based research and action.[65] Three programs especially worth noting include one aimed at smoking cessation among adolescents (Quit & Fit: Improving Health Among Rural Teens)[65] and two targeting physical activity and healthy eating for elementary- and middle-school children (Coordinated Approach to Child Health [CATCH] and Planet Health).[66,67] These three programs share the following features[65]:

- Focus on chronic disease prevention and health promotion
- Identification of staff and resources that facilitate program implementation and dissemination
- Stakeholder involvement (e.g., teachers, students, other school personnel, parents, nonprofit organizations, professional organizations) during all phases of program development and dissemination
- Planning for dissemination of programs
- Rigorous evaluation

Workplaces

The workplace provides a ready channel for health promotion interventions. Because chronic diseases collectively are the leading cause of death in the United States, worksite wellness programs can reach a large population of employed individuals with a focus on addressing risk factors for chronic disease in the individual, supporting individual and family stressors, and providing health protection benefits such as occupational safety and health interventions. Building a workplace health program should involve a coordinated, systematic, and comprehensive approach (Figure 4-3).[68] These combined organizational efforts are designed to develop comprehensive and essential elements of effective workplace programs and policies.

Employers feel confident in the programs they implement and report reduced cost, absenteeism, and health-related productivity losses. The Total Worker Health model[69] provides guidance from program initiation to program evaluation of worksite wellness programs. The model encompasses four overarching areas: organizational culture and leadership, program design, program implementation, and resources and program evaluation. ACA, which includes the Prevention and Public Health Fund, supports a focus on prevention and wellness, offering opportunities to strengthen the public's health through

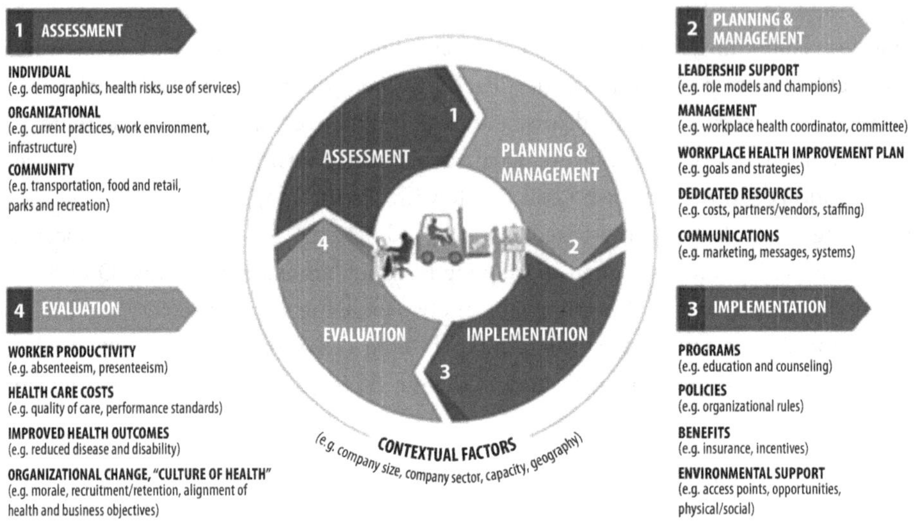

Source: Reprinted from CDC.[68]

Figure 4-3. Workplace Health Model

workplace wellness initiatives. Under ACA, employers can reduce the coverage amount they charge employees who participate in a workplace wellness program; this amounts to up to 30% of the cost of health coverage.

With the increased desire by public health professionals to mitigate chronic disease development and employers to decrease costs, interest in businesses adopting wellness programs surged. Researchers found that for every dollar spent on wellness programs, associated medical costs were reduced by approximately $3.27, and absenteeism costs were reduced by approximately $2.73.[70]

COVID-19 disrupted workers and employers alike worldwide, resulting in emergent changes in work practices (e.g., working from home, virtual teamwork) and emergent changes for workers (e.g., social distancing, stress, unemployment). In addition, the potential moderating factors (demographic characteristics, individual differences, and organizational norms) that COVID-19 generated disparately affected workers.[71]

Faith-Based Organizations

Faith-based organizations such as ones whose communities assemble at churches, synagogues, mosques, temples, and other entities have a long history of supporting health promotion programs in areas such as general health education, screening for and management of high blood pressure and diabetes, weight loss, smoking cessation, cancer prevention and control, geriatric care, nutritional guidance, and mental health care. In addition, these organizations have promoted immunization to at-risk and underserved populations, welcomed migrants threatened by discrimination and violence, and intervened to contain infectious diseases.[72]

Most health program initiatives in these organizations in the United States serve Christian communities. Powers et al.[73] used a faith-based, multilevel, social-ecological model for a health promotion initiative in one underserved rural area. It focused on having faith communities adopt policies requiring healthy options for meals and snacks and implement environmental changes to promote healthy eating and physical activity. Participants reported significant improvements in healthy eating encouragement, shopping practices, and vegetable consumption. A multilevel intervention prompted faith communities to become healthier places and individuals to adopt healthy lifestyles.

Black Americans are disproportionately affected by health problems and experience more health disparities and inequities that White Americans. In response, more faith-based organizations offer structured health promotion activities in what is sometimes referred to as their health ministry. Black American pastors now find themselves serving not only as preachers but also as teachers, politicians, and agents of health-related behavior change. Public health practitioners can support these efforts by identifying health priorities, facilitating access to evidence-based interventions, and offering technical assistance with the implementation of health promotion programs. For example, interventions developed for Black American organizations now address the broad range of chronic diseases identified earlier as well as other emerging issues. However, there is limited awareness of these interventions and how to access them. Other challenges include maintaining qualified volunteers, garnering financial resources, and having technical assistance needs met that support education, screening, and referral initiatives.[74]

COMMUNITY-LEVEL INTERVENTIONS

The term *community* is defined in numerous ways, but in public health it is used to describe a group of people with diverse characteristics who are linked by social ties, share common perspectives, and engage in joint action.[75,76] Communities may be bound geographically (e.g., a neighborhood, city, or other place); by shared values, issues, and characteristics (e.g., sexual orientation, language, ethnic heritage); or virtually through social media and networks. In all cases a shared identity and interdependency are extremely important. Neighborhoods and other social groups that do not share a sense of identity, norms and values, or common activities are not considered communities. This section examines community intervention strategies, including community-level activities, involvement of community members, and community-based participatory research (CBPR).

Community interventions are designed to be multilevel and educate and empower the community instead of individual members, enhance their ability to tackle problems, and modify the community environment or structure to make it easier for people to adopt healthy practices. Adolescent obesity prevention programs could focus on nutrition, specifically healthy food options. This may involve strategies at the individual level, community level, and policy or environmental level. At the individual level one aspect consists of increasing awareness of healthy food choices, making the choices more appealing and in line with the wants and needs of the individual; at the community level this may engage school- or community-based settings like recreation centers and school booster clubs; and at the environmental or policy level this could involve institutional policy change that results in healthy food choices being listed on the menu, priced lower than unhealthy options, shown in close proximity to the consumer, and promoted or given more visibility through communication channels and materials.[77,78]

Guiding actions for improving community intervention effectiveness include elements of building trust and partnerships, followed by codesign, implementation, and evaluation[75,79–81]:

- Assessing community needs and priorities.
- Acknowledging and building on community partners' skills and assets.
- Looking to and building on existing evidence-based programs, policies, and system-level interventions.
- Aligning intervention activities with community members' perceived needs, knowledge, attitudes, values, and constraints.
- Integrating activities within the community structure (e.g., by offering programs through local businesses, faith-based organizations, or other community-based organizations).
- Offering a broad range of activities to reach large numbers of community members, build community capacity, and modify the community to facilitate change.
- Implementing the intervention for a sufficient period of time and with adequate resources to make change realistic and sustainable (i.e., providing an adequate intervention dose).
- Monitoring activities to identify and remedy problems quickly.

As the next section demonstrates, it also is essential to involve community members in all phases of the intervention.

Community Engagement

Many public health organizations (e.g., CDC, National Institutes of Health, Institute of Medicine) have endorsed community engagement to increase intervention effectiveness.[82,83] Involving community members in goal setting, program design, and program implementation has been shown to improve health and psychosocial outcomes and improve the long-term sustainability of interventions.[82,84,85] In a meta-analysis of more than 9,000 primary studies, O'Mara-Eves et al.[82] found that community engagement improved program impact on health behaviors, health consequences, self-efficacy, and perceived social support. Interventions were especially effective when community members were engaged in delivering the intervention.

Community engagement can take many forms, ranging from asking community members for information and advice to equal sharing of all program decisions. A full partnership between public health professionals and local community members can lead to empowerment of individuals, enhance the community's capacity to identify and solve its own problems, and result in more effective management of health issues and economic, social, and political forces in the community.[75] Community participation also increases its sense of ownership of the intervention. This, in turn, may provide better access to community leaders, lead to changes in community norms, enhance local problem-solving skills, and increase the likelihood that the intervention will be sustained. Community members' help tailoring the intervention to fit the norms and values of the community ensures that it will be culturally sensitive and relevant.

Community-Based Participatory Research

One form of community engagement that has gained recognition in the past 30 years is community-based participatory research (CBPR), a collaborative process in which community members and public health researchers work together as equal partners in the research process to tackle community health problems.[75] The fundamental principles of CBPR include that it is participatory, engages community members and researchers in a collaborative process to which each contributes equally, is a co-learning process, involves local capacity building and systems development, empowers participants, and results in a balance between research and action.[86,87]

CBPR offers public health researchers and their community partners many benefits. This collaborative approach

- Ensures culturally and logistically appropriate research;
- Enhances recruitment capacity;
- Generates professional capacity and competence in stakeholder groups;
- Results in productive conflicts followed by useful negotiation;
- Increases the quality of outputs and outcomes over time;
- Increases the sustainability of project goals beyond funded time frames and during gaps in external funding; and
- Creates system changes and new, unanticipated projects and activities.

Despite these benefits, CBPR is also challenging to conduct. Of special importance is trust and mutual commitment between public health researchers and community members. Trust is subject to overall power relations in the community and the larger society, members' previous experiences with research and researchers, the priority issues facing the community, and the ability to negotiate relationships between the CBPR researchers and community participants.[75] Community members engaged in CBPR report difficulty understanding the research language, protocols, and rules (e.g., institutional review board approvals, study design issues). Thus, time is needed to develop both trust and understanding to support this approach.

Unfortunately, relatively few chronic disease prevention and control programs have taken advantage of community-level interventions and strategies. Nevertheless, CBPR enables context-specific and culturally appropriate intervention designs that ensure that existing barriers are addressed, and that community stakeholders and intended end-users are involved in the design of educational materials and messages that target the unique needs and knowledge gaps of marginalized groups, thereby playing a role in reducing health disparities.[61] The CDC-sponsored Prevention Research Centers,[65,66] noted earlier, do offer several examples of successful CBPR projects, some of which have been sustained in communities.

Community Coalitions

Community coalitions with public health–related missions are formal, semipermanent, action-oriented partnerships comprising community members, representatives of government agencies, policymakers, and academic partners that focus on promoting policy, systems, and environmental change.[88–91] Coalitions identify specific community-level health problems, assess existing needs and resources, develop and implement formal strategies for addressing these problems, and ultimately work to improve the health and well-being of the community.[91–94] In addition, coalitions can be powerful agencies for connecting health and human service providers in underserved communities often closed off to other, more formal public agencies, benefiting individual health as well as the overall health care delivery system.[95]

> The coalition is composed of community members; it focuses mainly on local issues rather than national issues; it addresses community needs, building on community assets; it helps resolve community problems through collaboration; it is community-wide and has representatives from multiple sectors; it works on multiple issues; it is citizen influenced if not necessarily citizen driven; and it is a long term, not ad hoc, coalition.[96]

Community coalitions evolved from the experiences of civic engagement and community building in the 1960s and 1970s and are now a well-established strategy for addressing a diverse array of local health and social conditions focused on the social determinants of health using a social-ecological perspective.[90,97] Evolving in structure and scope over the past 30 years, coalitions have formed around issues including physical activity, nutrition, substance abuse, obesity, tobacco cessation, asthma, maternal and child health, diabetes, cancer screening, and youth development[90]; at times these efforts have been disseminated to other coalitions statewide and even across the United States.

Coalition impact is often measured by documenting progress and providing ongoing feedback to the community, seeking out technical assistance for action planning and effective strategizing, obtaining ongoing funding for sustained coalition activities, and identifying measurable outcomes. A theoretical basis for evaluating coalition effectiveness was formalized by Butterfoss and Kegler[98] in their Community Coalition Action Theory (CCAT). In a systematic review assessing coalition effectiveness by Kegler et al.,[90] the CCAT was the most often cited formal model used to evaluate these partnerships. The CCAT builds on ideas from interorganizational relations, as well as community development, community participation, citizen participation, political science, and group processes.[90] The CCAT is based on several models of partnership building that focus on community building and community development, as well as those that focus on the structure of these types of organizations.[88,99]

The CCAT was developed for the purpose of integrating the relevant characteristics of these partnership models into a comprehensive picture of coalition structure and function.[98] This theory comprises 14 constructs that exist within three stages—formation, implementation, and maintenance—formalizing how coalitions function as they plan, implement, and monitor community-based initiatives.[91,98] Elements of the CCAT that have stood the test of time, proving integral to the success of coalitions in recent decades, include formalized rules and procedures, effective leadership, active participation of coalition members, membership that pulls from diverse sectors of the community, collaboration with outside agencies, and group cohesion.[100,101] However, whereas the CCAT addresses many aspects of coalition structures and processes, research over the past decade has sought a more comprehensive model for monitoring and evaluating the impact and sustainability of these diverse and ever-evolving partnerships.[101–104] Further work to develop a more universally accepted model for coalition functioning using a social-ecological approach could provide future partnerships with a blueprint for effective implementation and evaluation of diverse community-based health promotion initiatives.[101]

The increasing use of coalitions as a powerful health promotion strategy parallels the growth of large-scale community-level health promotion and chronic disease prevention efforts such as the Robert Wood Johnson Foundation's Active Living by Design, Kaiser Permanente's Healthy Eating Active Living Zones initiative, and Communities That Care, a community-wide substance abuse prevention program for youth that is now in its third decade of project implementation and evaluation.[89,100,104–106]

From the time of its authorization by Congress in 1984, and for more than the three decades since, CDC has sponsored a network of academic research centers to conduct community-based, applied public health research to address chronic diseases and other leading causes of death and disability. Known as the Prevention Research Centers

(PRC) Program, there are currently 26 PRCs across the country. A cornerstone of the PRC Program is community-engaged research that includes partnerships between academic research centers and community advisory boards.[107] These and other examples of effective and sustained community-based initiatives, whose primary goals are to contribute to targeted, long-term health outcomes at the community level, provide evidence of the power of community coalitions at promoting policy, systems, and environmental change to what are often the most underserved populations in the United States.

Advocacy and Lobbying in Public Health

In general, *advocacy* relates to activism surrounding a particular issue. Public health advocacy traditionally seeks to influence public opinion, and where possible, policymakers as well. Advocacy is a central tenet of public health. Health advocacy includes educating policymakers and the public about evidence-based policies and practices. Public health advocates have been largely responsible for the enactment of such measures as clean indoor air regulations, seatbelt laws, fair housing rights and obligations, safe drinking water, and nutrition labeling.

Whereas *lobbying* contains some form of advocacy, not all advocacy is lobbying. A major difference between lobbying and advocacy is that lobbying is a type of advocacy specific to influencing a legislator to take a particular action. That is, lobbying may include written and oral communication for or against specific legislation. It is important that local health department officials are able to distinguish between advocacy and lobbying because they may not be permitted to lobby state and federal legislators directly. One thing that public health officials can do is encourage the public to contact legislators about pending issues, that is, engage in what is known as *grassroots advocacy*. Citizens can both lobby and practice advocacy, and it is wise to become familiar with the legislative system as it influences public health decisions. The National Association of County and City Health Officials (NACCHO)[108] provides excellent guidance on advocacy and lobbying activities as shown in Table 4-1.

Media advocacy is "the strategic use of mass media in combination with community organizing to advance healthy public policies."[109] Whereas most communication strategies address individuals as consumers by delivering focused information to help people decrease their risks of injury and illness, media advocacy focuses on raising the voices of populations for systems change from a policy level, with the policymakers as the audience.[110] Learning to use media to address system-level factors can empower communities to participate in the political process.

As in other forms of advocacy, a variety of tasks and approaches are used to create a shift in public opinion to bring about policy change: community organizing, agenda setting, framing, engaging in public demonstrations, and working with groups to reach opinion leaders to change public policies and address social inequities.

Table 4-1. Examples of Education, Advocacy, and Lobbying Activities

Education and Advocacy	Lobbying
Explaining workforce challenges your health department is facing and discussing how higher salaries, loan repayment, or additional funding could help.	Asking a member of Congress or their staff to cosponsor legislation that would create new funding for the public health workforce.
Describing to a member of Congress how local health departments administer flu vaccinations and why vaccinations are important for preventing the spread of flu.	Urging a member of Congress to vote for legislation that expands insurance coverage of flu vaccines.
Providing legislators educational materials that emphasize success stories from your local health department programs. The materials include information about what federal funding supports programs at your health department and examples of what you could do with more funding.	Providing legislators materials that ask them to support a specific amount of funding for specific programs in the upcoming annual appropriations bill.
Tweeting statistics about your diabetes programs, how local health departments are helping reduce diabetes rates, and how additional resources can assist your local health department to reduce diabetes rates.	Tweeting a message urging Congress to vote for or against legislation for diabetes prevention programs in local health departments.
Sending a weekly e-newsletter discussing factual information on opioid abuse in your community and outlining programmatic efforts that are proven to reduce this public health issue.	E-mailing a "call to action" to members of your organization to encourage them to contact their legislator in favor of opioid prevention legislation.

Source: Reprinted with permission of NACCHO.[108]

Successful chronic disease control programs rely on involvement from the community. The organization of community members helps to prioritize problems and strategies to address them, thereby increasing the opportunities for change. The Community Organization Model empowers community members to tell their story, helps to establish a shared agenda, increases ownership of health-related issues, and mobilizes people for accomplishing favorable change through collaborative decision-making and problem-solving initiatives. Successful community organization is a key component of many of the population-based interventions for chronic disease control (see Resources section at the end of this book).

How advocacy groups and communities frame an issue is of critical importance. Framing uses symbols, metaphors, and stories to define an issue, to suggest who is responsible for the problem, and to propose solutions. Media advocates try to frame public health issues in ways that direct attention to environmental or system-level factors responsible for the problem and suggest policy solutions rather than hold individual "victims" responsible for it.

Mass media also are used to place pressure on decision makers. As with media coverage designed to garner public support, media advocates frame policy positions to make them attractive to policymakers and use a variety of techniques to keep their issue in the news (e.g., by framing an event as a milestone, a breakthrough, or a controversial topic). Because policy battles often wage for years, media advocates must identify new opportunities to reintroduce an issue and keep it in the media spotlight over prolonged periods of time.[108]

The growth in popularity of social media sites has provided additional platforms for advocacy and political pressure. According to Mendoza-Herrera et al.[111]

> Social media can encourage citizen participation, optimize health systems, be an interactive space for science dissemination, support health policies, and promote healthy behaviors. This perspective emphasizes the benefits and limitations of social media, considering that they could effectively address public health nutrition problems.

HEALTH POLICY AND LEGAL INTERVENTIONS

Effective health policies can have a substantial impact on the public's health.[112] Public health policies include laws, regulations, written standards, ordinances, resolutions, and organizational and institutional practices designed to guide individual and group behavior that have an impact on population health.[112] Examples include economic incentives, taxes, business regulations, and other laws that protect the public or special population groups, such as workers. Laws requiring drivers to wear seatbelts, sanctions for illegal drug use, and environmental protection standards are well-known examples.

Policy changes have been deemed more effective than behavior change programs and more easily sustained for lengthy periods of time when external funding has ended.[113] In fact, policy initiatives have brought about some of the most important public health victories in the United States in the past century. Declining lead exposure rates, reduced rates of smoking, improvements in motor vehicle safety, and increased vaccination rates have resulted from legislation, regulation, litigation, or a combination of these three actions.

Federal policies can have a significant population effect. Consider, for example, the effect of ACA on health care access, especially for chronic disease prevention and control. Unfortunately, many promising public health policies have yet to be enacted. Considering the importance to public health of policy change for reducing chronic diseases and other health problems, tools are available to help public health professionals identify, tailor, and promote policy change and evaluate its impact (see Resources section at the end of this book).

Multilevel Approaches to Chronic Disease Control

Comprehensive interventions for controlling chronic diseases require primary, secondary, and tertiary prevention approaches. Moreover, these strategies must be directed at the individual, interpersonal, organizational, community, and policy levels. A relevant example is tobacco use, still one of the leading causes of death among Americans. Because of tobacco's important negative health consequences, a multilevel or comprehensive intervention to control tobacco must involve a number of approaches:

- Primary prevention education programs for youths in school settings
- Education programs for physicians, dentists, and other health care providers to inspire patient education in care settings through brief interventions and other mechanisms
- Free or low-cost cessation programs for smokers before the onset of disease (secondary prevention)
- Health insurance cost reductions for nonsmokers as an economic incentive to eliminate tobacco use
- Tobacco excise taxes to bring an economic disincentive to continue use and raise revenue to finance care for affected individuals (tertiary prevention)
- Rigorous enforcement of age restriction for purchase of cigarettes
- Partnering with national and local voluntary organizations (e.g., American Heart Association, American Lung Association, American Cancer Society) for advocacy of anti-tobacco programs and policies
- Clean indoor air legislation
- Restriction of smoking in public places
- A watchful eye on alternative forms of tobacco use (vaping, hookah pipes, etc.) and the targeting of youth or other vulnerable populations through advertising

Whereas each one of these initiatives may have a modest influence on smoking and tobacco consumption, none is as singularly effective as a comprehensive program. Arguably, multilevel anti-tobacco programs have changed the cultural norm in the United States in the nearly six decades since the surgeon general's first report on smoking and health and are beginning to do so in other countries that have had a history of high tobacco consumption.

Given the demographic transition of age distribution, population growth and the dynamics of chronic diseases, coordinated chronic disease prevention strategies are gaining momentum from state health departments. The purpose of coordinated approaches is to work with state and community partners to implement chronic disease prevention and health promotion strategies. These multipronged approaches are warranted, given the increased prevalence of multiple chronic conditions in the population.

EXAMPLES OF COMMUNITY-LEVEL HEALTH PLANNING APPROACHES

The frameworks used in chronic disease prevention and control can provide structure to the planning process for an overall cohesive plan and a foundation for critical analysis.[114]

Although various intervention planning frameworks exist, most comprise similar principles. Successful program planning in the community involves time and resources for identifying key stakeholders, understanding the culture of the community, and gathering necessary data. Program planning processes to combat chronic diseases need to be carried out for ongoing implementation and interventions need to address agreed-upon priorities. Having both short-term and long-term goals is important; accomplishing short-term goals demonstrates small wins that can inspire continued effort, and having long-term goals helps to maintain focus and direction. A logic model can be utilized for the process to keep the community members aligned and offer a reminder of where we are in the process.[115]

One innovative approach to monitoring health status and planning health interventions at the community level is the Mobilizing Action Toward Community Health project,[116] an initiative that

- Uses relevant criteria to calculate county-level health rankings for each of the 50 states;
- Develops partnerships and models for increasing involvement and accountability for population health improvements; and
- Develops incentive-based models to encourage implementation of community-level programs and policies to improve population health.

The criteria (physical and mental health measures) used for determining county health rankings provide estimates of a community's overall health-related quality of life and enable public health authorities to assess priorities for intervention. This initiative led to the development of the County Health Ranking and Roadmaps, an initiative that ranks the health of all 3,000 US counties and provides an "action model" for community health improvement.

Numerous planning models provide frameworks for implementing community-level interventions for chronic disease prevention and control through behavioral change. The following models illustrate popular and tested strategies: PRECEDE-PROCEED, Mobilizing Action through Planning and Partnerships (MAPP), Intervention Mapping, and Community-Based Prevention Marketing (CBPM).

PRECEDE-PROCEED Framework

The PRECEDE-PROCEED framework reflects an ecological and educational approach to intervention planning that acknowledges both the real and perceived needs of the community while following a systems approach to improving health and quality of life.[114,117] The PRECEDE-PROCEED framework has two main components, each having a series of phases. The first component is PRECEDE (predisposing, reinforcing, and enabling constructs in educational/ecological diagnosis and evaluation) and comprises four phases:

- Phase 1: social assessment and situational analysis—During this phase, one assesses the real and perceived needs of the community of interest. Data include both social indicators and subjective problems and priorities reflective of the community of interest.
- Phase 2: epidemiological assessment—During the epidemiological assessment, one specifies and prioritizes health issues in addition to the etiologic genetic, behavioral, and environmental risk factors.
- Phase 3: educational and ecological assessment—Once the key health issue and etiologic factors have been prioritized and selected, the educational and ecological assessment explores and prioritizes the predisposing, enabling, and reinforcing factors that influence the selected behavioral and environmental risk factors.
- Phase 4: administrative and policy assessment and intervention alignment—During this phase, one identifies the program components, interventions, and policy, organizational, and administrative resources needed to effect changes determined in Phases 1 through 3.

The second component is PROCEED (policy, regulatory, and organizational constructs in educational and environmental development) and comprises the following phases:

- Phase 5: implementation—During this phase, one assesses organizational readiness and capacity before program implementation.
- Phase 6: process evaluation—One assesses that the intervention is implemented according to plan and makes any necessary midcourse adjustments.
- Phase 7: impact evaluation—One assesses the immediate effects of the intervention on factors related to the health problem of interest.
- Phase 8: outcome evaluation—Phases 6 through 8 pertain to intervention evaluation. During these phases, the planning team determines the evaluation plan and design considering program processes (Phase 6), short-term impacts (Phase 7), and longer-term outcomes (Phase 8).

Mobilizing Action through Planning and Partnerships

Mobilizing Action through Planning and Partnerships (MAPP) is a planning framework developed in 2000 by NACCHO in cooperation with the Public Health Practice Program Office at CDC.[118,119] The guiding principles in the MAPP planning model include systems thinking, dialogue, shared vision, data, partnerships and collaboration, strategic thinking, and celebration for success. The MAPP planning model consists of four core assessments that drive the planning process (Figure 4-4).[119] The main purposes of these

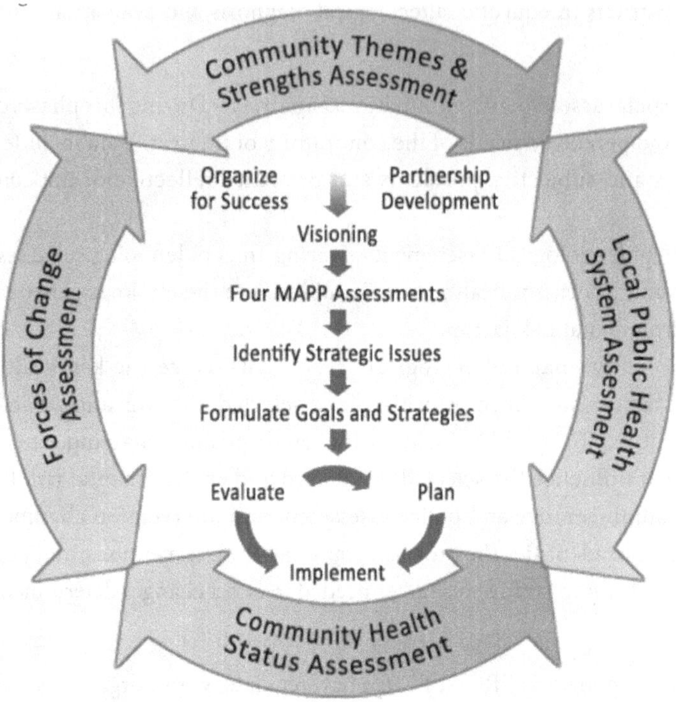

Source: Community Toolbox.[119] Reprinted under the terms of the CC BY license (https://creativecommons.org/licenses/by/4.0).

Figure 4-4. Mobilizing for Action Through Planning and Partnerships (MAPP) Model

four assessments are to provide insight concerning gaps between community wants and current circumstances, to provide information for identifying strategic issues, and to provide information for developing goals and strategies. These assessments are as follows:

- Community themes and strengths: This assessment provides the planning team with an understanding of the perceived strengths and needs of the selected community.
- Local public health system: Assessment of the local public health system comprises a capacity assessment in addition to an overview of how essential services are being provided to the community.
- Community health status: Like the previously described planning models, the community health status assessment provides the planning team with the community health and quality-of-life status for determining health priorities.
- Forces of change: The forces-of-change assessment provides the planning team with information on legislation, technology, and other issues that may affect the priority health issue, the community functioning, or the operations of the public health system.

Intervention Mapping

Bartholomew and Mullen[120] and Fernandez et al.[121] describe intervention mapping as a systematic and cumulative process for developing, implementing, and sustaining public health interventions. The steps and procedures of the intervention mapping framework facilitate the development of theory-based interventions based on the literature and population-specific data. Intervention mapping is a tool to serve as a blueprint for the design, implementation, and evaluation of an intervention once the planners have identified the health issue, behavioral and environmental risk factors, and associated determinates. There are six core steps in the intervention mapping framework:

- Assessing need: The first step in the intervention mapping process entails performing a needs assessment to describe the individuals who have or are at risk for a health problem needing intervention within a community.
- Preparing matrices-of-change objectives: This stage requires stating expected program outcomes for health-related behavior and environmental conditions. Behavioral and environmental conditions are then subdivided into performance objectives and ranked by importance and changeability. This information informs the creation of matrix-of-change objectives for each level of the intervention.
- Selecting theory-informed intervention methods and practical applications: Once program ideas are developed, the theoretical methods that influence change are identified, informing the creation of intervention strategies.
- Producing program components and materials: Working with intended program participants, program components, including delivery channels, themes, and program materials, are developed. Program materials are then pretested.
- Planning program adoption, implementation, and sustainability: Program outcomes and performance objectives are stated; determinants of program adoption, implementation, and sustainability are specified; and matrices-of-change objectives are developed to ensure that interventions are aligned with program adoption, implementation, and sustainability.
- Planning for evaluation: The research team writes evaluation questions about performance objectives and determinants based on the matrices developed in step 2. Indicators and measures are developed on the basis of these questions, and the team writes an evaluation plan.

Community-Based Prevention Marketing

Community-based prevention marketing (CBPM) recognizes the importance of addressing determinants at the individual, interpersonal, organization, and community and societal levels to bring about desired change. CBPM blends aspects of community organization and social marketing into a planning framework that empowers communities to evaluate a health concern systematically and then work with researchers to bring about change.[122] At the heart of CBPM is social marketing. Social marketing applies principles of commercial marketing to achieve behavioral change for social good.[123] It is a consumer-oriented approach that uses a strategic decision-making process to design and implement an integrated intervention plan. When driven by a community-based organization or coalition of organizations, social marketing builds on the power of local wisdom and control by providing community groups with an effective framework to set goals, select target populations, develop and implement strategies to bring about behavior change, and optimize service delivery.[124]

CBPM has been used to promote prevention efforts related to several public health issues through the application of three forms of the framework. CBPM frameworks have been used to design behavior change programs (CBPM for Program Development),[124–127] policy strategies (CBPM for Policy Development),[78,128,129] and systems science approaches (CBPM for Systems Change).[130] Together, these frameworks enable a community coalition to select, tailor, implement, and evaluate multilevel evidence-based interventions involving programs, policies, or systems.

Overall, the CBPM framework follows an eight-step process:

1. Mobilize the community.
2. Identify the problem and changes required to remedy it.
3. Select a subgroup or audience segment to give the greatest priority in planning intervention.
4. Conduct research.
5. Develop a marketing plan strategy organized around the four Ps: product, price, place, and promotion.
6. Develop and pretest intervention materials and strategies.
7. Monitor and evaluate the plan.
8. Implement the program.

ENHANCING HEALTH LITERACY: THE KEY TO ALL CHRONIC DISEASE INTERVENTIONS

Low health literacy constitutes a significant challenge for public health. Health literacy includes a broad range of skills needed in everyday settings, whereby communication and decision-making coupled with an understanding of health and medical concepts and context across the life course are all important.[131] Reading a medicine or nutrition label, using an asthma inhaler, and managing diabetes represent a few examples in which health literacy skills are both relevant and required to function. Given the complexity of chronic disease, health literacy is an important lens for understanding health promotion constructs.

Other definitions of health literacy have been advanced since the World Health Organization introduced the concept in its 1998 glossary of health promotion terms.[132] Health literacy has expanded from a narrow medical concept to a much broader multidimensional concept associated with skills and factors contributing to individual competencies, social empowerment, provider responsibilities, and organizational capacity. Health literacy refers not only to the abilities or traits of individuals but also to the health-related systems and providers of information and services within those systems.[133] As a complex concept needed in chronic disease prevention, self-management, and treatment, it involves the ability to access, comprehend, evaluate, communicate, and act on health information.[134] Recognizing the cross-cutting significance of health literacy to meet health objectives for the nation, it appears as a key focus in Healthy People 2030.[135] Healthy People 2030 now addresses both personal health literacy and organizational health literacy, which together help to "eliminate health disparities, achieve health equity and attain health literacy to improve the health and well-being of all." The personal health literacy definition put forth refers to health literacy as "the degree to which individuals have the ability to find, understand, and use information and services to inform health-related decisions and actions for themselves and others." Organizational health literacy is the "degree to which organizations equitably enable individuals to find, understand, and use information and services to inform health-related decisions and actions for themselves and others."

The Institute of Medicine[136] reports that almost half of Americans have difficulty understanding and acting on health information. Persons with lower health literacy and chronic disease have less knowledge of their illness management than those with higher levels and, consequently, may

- Have reduced access to services and information (e.g., free cancer screening clinics, community health services).
- Be less likely to act on important public health alerts (influencing health outcomes).
- Make less use of secondary prevention and diagnostic services (e.g., mammograms, Papanicolaou tests).
- Be more likely to misunderstand instructions about prescription medication and make medication errors.
- Be unable to manage chronic conditions (e.g., diabetes, high blood pressure, asthma).
- Overuse hospitals and emergency rooms.

Greater health literacy has been associated with reductions in risk behaviors linked to chronic disease,[137] decreased rates of hospitalizations,[138,139] and higher self-reported health status.[140] Lower health literacy relates to poorer health outcomes and higher health care costs. Economists estimate that low health literacy costs the US economy between $106 billion and $238 billion annually in the form of additional health care and sick days' pay.[141] Chronic disease interventions targeting low health literacy have been cost-effective.

For example, one study revealed that implementing a health literacy–focused intervention to promote breast and cervical cancer screenings among Korean American women overdue for these tests saved on average $236 per patient when compared to usual care.[142] A program to teach low-income parents how to treat common childhood illnesses at home resulted in significant decreases in emergency department visits, days off school for children, and days off work for the caregivers.[143] Moreover, parents are high users of web-based health information for their children's health.[144] This has implications for digital health interventions (e.g., mobile apps, videos, web-based platforms). For some parents, excessive and stressful health-seeking behavior via the internet can occur as part of the parenting for a chronically ill child,[145] a behavior known as cyberchondria.[146] A systematic review of digital health interventions to improve health literacy among parents of children up to 12 years of age with health conditions found health literacy increases parents' health knowledge and behavior and also has a beneficial impact on their children's health outcomes.[147]

The relevance of health literacy for the complex dimensions of chronic diseases is evident for prevention, self-management, and treatment efforts. Health literacy plays many roles at the individual, provider, and system levels. For example, to manage long-term conditions on a daily basis, individuals must be able to understand the diagnoses, instructions for self-care, and medical regimens; interpret and translate health information, often for multiple outputs and multiple comorbidities; plan and make lifestyle adjustments for comorbidities; know when and where to access screenings, health care, services, and products when necessary; and communicate any health needs, concerns, and questions.

Health literacy is also a function of the complexity of the health care system, consisting as it does of providers and organizations. To enhance health literacy, as a key to all chronic disease interventions, we must reframe health literacy as solely an individual attribute and consider broad contextual and system-level factors. With the growing interest to identify organization factors (e.g., organization policies, institutional practices, navigation, culture and language, communication), Rudd et al.[133] developed Health Literacy Environment of Hospital and Health Centers (HLE2), which is a revised tool that can support or inhibit people's access to information, care, and services. It is also important for health-related personnel to have a range of skills and strategies to respond to patients with varying health literacy needs and to reduce the complexity of medical care and related situational factors to protect the safety and promote the health of patients and health consumers alike.[148] More specifically, those who provide information and services require health literacy skills to help people find what they need, decide which information and services are appropriate for different situations, understand how to provide the appropriate information and services, and communicate effectively with others. Furthermore, "systems can be health literate by providing equal, easy, and shame-free access to and delivery of health care and information."[149]

In the early days of the COVID-19 pandemic, health care personnel increased their reliance on telemedicine to reduce risks to patients and providers alike. Although well intentioned, this reliance exposed another health disparity existent not only in the United States but also elsewhere—namely, variation in "digital literacy."[150] Use of telemedicine may, for example, systematically exclude some elderly persons, economically challenged individuals, and persons without a device or signal that facilitates communication with providers. Given such issues, the Calgary Charter on Health Literacy[149] outlines the key principles that support development of curricula, initiatives, and tools to improve the health literacy of the public and of those who work in any capacity in health care or related systems.

Health literacy as an emerging field of research and practice has the potential to increase understanding of both chronic diseases and health promotion in the global context.[131] Thus, increasing the health literacy of the population is an important endeavor. Health literacy is an intervention in emerging strategies, initiatives, and specific policies taking place through an increasing number of national action plans around the world. One such action plan is the US National Action Plan to Improve Health Literacy,[151] which outlines goals that will improve health literacy and strategies for achieving them. The plan's focus on "education for health literacy perspective" is a supportive instructional and capacity-building global resource initiative found in emerging action plans, research, and policies around the world.[152,153] The scope of promising health literacy research, policy, and practice developments continues to expand throughout the United States and around the globe.

MOVING FORWARD

Chronic diseases financially burden the US health care system and reduce the overall quality of life for many Americans. As described in this chapter, intervention science for chronic disease prevention has increased its precision, making it possible for many disease threats to be prevented, to be delayed, or to have their overall impact lessened. Today there is excellent surveillance of diseases and an improved understanding of the interrelationships involving individual, social, environmental, and political factors. Moreover, there are sophisticated models, theories, and frameworks for intervening at the individual, interpersonal, organizational, community, and policy levels.

As noted in this chapter, the most promising of these interventions are multilevel ones that simultaneously address complex disease causes. A challenge moving forward is to assist state and local public health authorities in adapting multilevel interventions to the extent that budget and human resources allow. More case studies and applications of interventions are necessary to test the adaptability of previous findings in diverse settings. However, the evidence base gained to date through an abundance of demonstration projects can now be enlarged in scale to translate and disseminate these findings to broader audiences and address the major chronic disease issues facing Americans. Key to assimilating knowledge of disease threats by the public is the advancement of health literacy skills at multiple stages of life.

DISCUSSION QUESTIONS

1. Select a chronic disease problem of interest (e.g., high cancer diagnosis resulting in part from inadequate cancer screenings; high incidence of complications from type 1 diabetes; high percentages of school-aged youth who are obese or overweight), and then develop a prevention and intervention plan for a local health department and its community that encompasses as many of the features described in this chapter as you possibly can.
2. Select a health problem of interest that has a strong behavioral component and illustrate how each of at least two models could be used to improve understanding of the points of intervention to reduce the health problem's occurrence or severity.
3. Examine the various assets in your local community that play an actual or potential role in the prevention and control of a chronic disease problem of interest. Investigate how or to what extent these assets interact and identify mechanisms for removing barriers and improving overall performance for chronic disease prevention and control.
4. Evaluate settings and mechanisms for assessing and improving health literacy in your community, paying particular attention to such groups as school-aged children, young adults, parents and families, older adults, policymakers, and health care providers.

REFERENCES

1. Centers for Disease Control and Prevention. About chronic diseases. Updated July 21, 2022. Available at: http://www.cdc.gov/chronicdisease/about. Accessed January 8, 2023.
2. Kim K, Polite B, Hedeker D, et al. Implementing a multilevel intervention to accelerate colorectal cancer screening and follow-up in federally qualified health centers using a stepped wedge design: a study protocol. *Implement Sci.* 2020;15:96.
3. National Cancer Institute. BRCA gene mutations: cancer risk and genetic testing. 2020. Available at: https://www.cancer.gov/about-cancer/causes-prevention/genetics/brca-fact-sheet. Accessed January 8, 2023.
4. Centers for Disease Control and Prevention. What is epigenetics? 2020. Updated August 15, 2022. Available at: https://www.cdc.gov/genomics/disease/epigenetics.htm. Accessed January 8, 2023.
5. McCartney DL, Stevenson AJ, Hillary RF, et al. Epigenetic signatures of starting and stopping smoking. *EBioMedicine.* 2018;37:214–220.
6. Boersma P, Black LI, Ward BW. Prevalence of multiple chronic conditions among US adults, 2018. *Prev Chronic Dis.* 2020;17:E106.

7. Centers for Disease Control and Prevention. Exercise or physical activity. Updated December 15, 2022. Available at: http://www.cdc.gov/nchs/fastats/exercise.htm. Accessed January 8, 2023.
8. Centers for Disease Control and Prevention. *State Indicator Report on Fruits and Vegetables, 2018.* Atlanta, GA: CDC; 2018. Available at: https://www.cdc.gov/nutrition/downloads/fruits-vegetables/2018/2018-fruit-vegetable-report-508.pdf. Accessed January 8, 2023.
9. American Cancer Society. Cancer risk, prevention, and screening. Available at: https://www.cancer.org/healthy.html. Accessed January 8, 2023.
10. Bohm MK, Liu Y, Esser MB, et al. Binge drinking among adults, by select characteristics and state—United States, 2018. *MMWR Morb Mortal Wkly Rep*. 2021;70:1441–1446.
11. Cornelius ME, Wang TW, Jamal A, et al. Tobacco product use among adults—United States, 2019. *MMWR Morb Mortal Wkly Rep*. 2020;69(46):1736–1742.
12. Hales CM, Carroll MD, Fryar CD, Ogden CL. Prevalence of obesity and severe obesity among adults: United States, 2017–2018. *NCHS Data Brief*. 2020;(360):1–8.
13. Centers for Disease Control and Prevention. Adult obesity causes and consequences. Updated March 21, 2022. Available at: https://www.cdc.gov/obesity/adult/causes.html. Accessed January 8, 2023.
14. Centers for Disease Control and Prevention. Childhood obesity facts. Updated May 17, 2022. Available at: https://www.cdc.gov/obesity/data/childhood.html. Accessed January 8, 2023.
15. Biener A, Cawley J, Meyerhoefer C. The high and rising costs of obesity to the US health care system. *J Gen Intern Med*. 2017;32(suppl 1):S6–S8.
16. Benjamin EJ, Virani SS, Callaway CW, et al. Heart disease and stroke statistics—2018 update: a report from the American Heart Association. *Circulation*. 2018;137:e67–e492.
17. Martin AB, Hartman M, Lassman D, Catlin A. National healthcare spending in 2019: steady growth for the fourth consecutive year. *Health Aff (Millwood)*. 2020;40(1):1–11.
18. Cubanski J, Neuman T, Freed M. The facts on Medicare spending and financing. Henry J. Kaiser Family Foundation. August 20, 2019. Available at: http://kff.org/medicare/fact-sheet/medicare-spending-and-financing-fact-sheet. Accessed January 8, 2023.
19. Henry J. Kaiser Family Foundation. Preventive services covered by private health plans under the Affordable Care Act. 2016. Updated October 26, 2022. Available at: http://kff.org/health-reform/fact-sheet/preventive-services-covered-by-private-health-plans. Accessed January 8, 2023.
20. Vargas CM, Stines EM, Granado HS. Health-equity issues related to childhood obesity: a scoping review. *J Public Health Dent*. 2017;77(suppl 1):S32–S42.
21. Schulz M, Romppel M, Grande G. Built environment and health: a systematic review of studies in Germany. *J Public Health (Oxf)*. 2018;40(1):8–15.
22. Kazda MJ, Beel ER, Villegas D, et al. Methodological complexities and the use of GIS in conducting a community needs assessment of a large US municipality. *J Community Health*. 2009;34:210–215.
23. McDaniel JT, Davis T, Yahaya M, Nuhu K. Descriptive epidemiology of childhood disability prevalence by sex in the Mississippi Delta and Appalachian regions. *J Sch Health*. 2019;89(12):969–976.

24. McDaniel JT. Geographic distribution of disability among older veterans, United States, 2013–2017. *Prev Chronic Dis.* 2020;17:E35.
25. Powder J. Spreading the health. Global Health Now. Available at: https://globalhealthnow.org/2018-03/spreading-health. March 29, 2018. Accessed January 8, 2023.
26. Gentzke AS, Wang TW, Cornelius M, et al. Tobacco product use and associated factors among middle and high school students—National Youth Tobacco Survey, United States, 2021. *MMWR Surveill Summ.* 2022;71(SS-5):1–29.
27. Morton C, Want Y, Peterson A. Investigating the spatiotemporal relationship between neighborhood demographics and tobacco outlet density. Washington, DC: Society for Social Work and Research. January 17, 2020. Available at: https://sswr.confex.com/sswr/2020/webprogram/Paper40671.html. Accessed January 8, 2023.
28. Centers for Disease Control and Prevention. Models and frameworks for the practice of community engagement. Available at: https://www.atsdr.cdc.gov/communityengagement/pce_models.html. Accessed March 19, 2023.
29. Hochbaum GM. *Public Participation in Medical Screening Programs: A Socio-Psychological Study.* Washington, DC: US Government Printing Office; 1958.
30. American Cancer Society. American Cancer Society recommendations for early detection of breast cancer. Available at: https://www.cancer.org/cancer/breast-cancer/screening-tests-and-early-detection/american-cancer-society-recommendations-for-the-early-detection-of-breast-cancer.html. Accessed January 8, 2023.
31. Prochaska JO, DiClemente CC. Stages and processes of self-change of smoking: toward an integrative model of change. *J Consult Clin Psychol.* 1983;51(3):390–395.
32. Ajzen I. From intentions to actions: a theory of planned behavior. In: Kuhl J, Beckmann J, eds. *Action Control: From Cognition to Behavior.* Berlin, Germany: Springer; 1985:11–39.
33. Ajzen I. The theory of planned behavior. *Organ Behav Hum Decis Process.* 1991;50(2):179–211.
34. Fishbein M. Attitude and the prediction of behavior. In: Fishbein M, ed. *Readings in Attitude Theory and Measurement.* New York, NY: Wiley; 1967:477–492.
35. Ajzen I, Fishbein M. Attitudinal and normative variables as predictors of specific behavior. *J Pers Soc Psychol.* 1973;27(1):41–57.
36. Fishbein M, Ajzen I. *Belief, Attitude, Intention, and Behavior: An Introduction to Theory and Research.* Reading, MA: Addison-Wesley; 1975.
37. Rotter JB. Generalized expectancies for internal versus external control of reinforcement. *Psychol Monogr.* 1966;80(1):1–28.
38. Wallston KA, Wallston BS, DeVellis R. Development of the Multidimensional Health Locus of Control (MHLC) Scales. *Health Educ Monogr.* 1978;6(2):160–170.
39. Bandura A. *Social Learning Theory.* Englewood Cliffs, NJ: Prentice Hall; 1977.
40. Bandura A. *Social Foundations of Thought and Action.* Englewood Cliffs, NJ: Prentice Hall; 1986.
41. Whiting W, Pharr JR, Buttner MP, Lough NL. Behavioral interventions to increase condom use among college students in the United States: a systematic review. *Health Educ Behav.* 2019;46(5):877–888.
42. Kabiri B, Hidarnia AR, Alavijeh MM, et al. Family-centered social cognitive factors preventing primary tooth caries in children based on intervention mapping approach. *Biomed Res Int.* 2021;2021:6626090.

43. Lee CG, Park S, Lee SH, et al. Social cognitive theory and physical activity among Korean male high-school students. *Am J Mens Health.* 2018;12(4):973–980.
44. Rahia DR. Family-based intervention to manage anxiety and depression in chronic illness patients. In: *5th ASEAN Conference on Psychology, Counselling, and Humanities (ACPCH 2019).* London, UK: Atlantis Press; 2020:310–313.
45. Chrvala CA, Sherr D, Lipman RD. Diabetes self-management education for adults with type 2 diabetes mellitus: a systematic review of the effect on glycemic control. *Patient Educ Couns.* 2016;99(6):926–943.
46. Cunningham AT, Crittendon DR, White N, et al. The effect of diabetes self-management education on HbA1c and quality of life in African-Americans: a systematic review and meta-analysis. *BMC Health Serv Res.* 2018;18(1):1–13.
47. Smith HJ, Piotrowski JI, Zaza S. Ethics of implementing US Preventive Services Task Force recommendations for childhood obesity. *Pediatrics.* 2021;148(1):e2020048009.
48. House JS, Umberson D, Landis KR. Structures and processes of social support. *Ann Rev Sociol.* 1988;14:293–318.
49. Song L, Pettis PJ, Chen Y, Goodson-Miller M. Social cost and health: the downside of social relationships and social networks. *J Health Soc Behav.* 2021;62(3):371–387.
50. Glanz K, Rimer B, Viswanath K. *Health Behavior and Health Education: Theory, Research, and Practice.* 4th ed. San Francisco, CA: Jossey-Bass; 2008.
51. Bustamante AV, Vilar-Compte M, Lagunas AO. Social support and chronic disease management among older adults of Mexican heritage: a US-Mexico perspective. *Soc Sci Med.* 2018;216:107–113.
52. Lindsay Smith G, Banting L, Eime R, et al. The association between social support and physical activity in older adults: a systematic review. *Int J Behav Nutr Phys Act.* 2017:14(1):1–21.
53. Medline Plus. Living with a chronic illness—reaching out to others. 2022. Available at: https://www.nlm.nih.gov/medlineplus/ency/patientinstructions/000602.htm. Accessed January 8, 2023.
54. Shoham DA, Tong L, Lamberson PJ, et al. An actor-based model of social network influence on adolescent body size, screen time, and playing sports. *PLoS One.* 2012;7(6):e39795.
55. Simpkins SD, Schaefer DR, Price CD, Vest AE. Adolescent friendships, BMI, and physical activity: untangling selection and influence through longitudinal social network analysis. *J Res Adolesc.* 2013;23(3):537–549.
56. Farhat T. Stigma, obesity and adolescent risk behaviors: current research and future directions. *Curr Opin Psychol.* 2015;5:56–66.
57. Montgomery SC, Donnelly M, Bhatnagar P, et al. Peer social network processes and adolescent health behaviors: a systematic review. *Prev Med.* 2020;130:105900.
58. Michael SL, Merlo CL, Basch CE, et al. Critical connections: health and academics. *J Sch Health.* 2015;85(11):740–758.
59. Lewallen TC, Hunt H, Potts-Datema W, et al. The Whole School, Whole Community, Whole Child model: a new approach for improving educational attainment and healthy development for students. *J Sch Health.* 2015;85(11):729–739. doi:10.1111/josh.12310
60. Centers for Disease Control and Prevention. Community health worker resources. Available at: https://www.cdc.gov/chronicdisease/center/community-health-worker-resources.html. Accessed January 8, 2023.

61. Rodriguez NM, Casanova F, Pages G, et al. Community-based participatory design of a community health worker breast cancer training intervention for South Florida Latinx farmworkers. *PLoS One*. 2020;15(10):e0240827.
62. Hooker SA, Punjabi A, Justesen K, et al. Encouraging health behavior change: eight evidence-based strategies. *Fam Pract Manag*. 2018;25(2):31–36.
63. Van der Pol M, Hennessy D, Manns B. The role of time and risk preferences in adherence to physician advice on health behavior change. *Eur J Health Econ*. 2017;18(3):373–386.
64. Centers for Disease Control and Prevention. Whole School, Whole Community, Whole Child (WSCC). Available at: https://www.cdc.gov/healthyschools/wscc/index.htm. Accessed April 14, 2022.
65. Centers for Disease Control and Prevention. Prevention Research Center profiles, 2019–2024. Available at: https://www.cdc.gov/prc/center-descriptions/index.htm. Accessed January 8, 2023.
66. Centers for Disease Control and Prevention. Prevention Research Centers [stories and highlights of notable accomplishments]. Updated November 10, 2022. Available at: https://www.cdc.gov/prc/index.htm. Accessed January 8, 2023.
67. CATCH Global Foundation. Coordinated Approach to Child Health (CATCH). 2021. Available at: https://catch.org. Accessed January 8, 2023.
68. Centers for Disease Control and Prevention. Workplace health model. 2016. Available at: https://www.cdc.gov/workplacehealthpromotion/model/index.html. Accessed April 14, 2022.
69. Centers for Disease Control and Prevention. Essential elements of effective workplace programs. 2015. http://www.cdc.gov/niosh/twh/essentials.html. Accessed January 8, 2023.
70. Baicker K, Cutler D, Song Z. Workplace wellness programs can generate savings. *Health Aff (Millwood)*. 2010;29(2):304–311.
71. Kniffin KM, Narayanan J, Anseel F, et al. COVID-19 and the workplace: implications, issues, and insights for future research and action. *Am Psychol*. 2021;76(1):63–77.
72. Morabia A. Faith-based organizations and public health: another facet of the public health dialogue. *Am J Public Health*. 2019;109(3):341.
73. Powers A, Brock RW, Funderburk K, et al. Multilevel faith-based public health initiative in rural Alabama, 2017. *Prev Chronic Dis*. 2019;16:E117.
74. Holt CL, Graham-Phillips AL, Mullins CD, et al. Health ministry and activities in African American faith-based organizations: a qualitative examination of facilitators, barriers, and use of technology. *J Health Care Poor Underserved*. 2017;28(1):378–388.
75. Wallerstein N, Minkler M, Carter-Edwards L, et al. Improving health through community engagement, community organization, and community building. In: Glanz K, Rimer B, Viswanath K, eds. *Health Behavior: Theory, Research, and Practice*. 5th ed. San Francisco, CA: John Wiley and Sons; 2015:277–300.
76. Yuen T, Park AN, Seifer SD, Payne-Sturges D. A systematic review of community engagement in the US environmental protection agency's extramural research solicitations: implications for research funders. *Am J Public Health*. 2015;105(12):e44–e52.
77. Alfonso M, Martinasek M, Khaliq M. Social marketing and consumer-based approaches in public health. In: Shi L, Johnson JA, eds. *Novick & Morrow's Public Health Administration*. Burlington, MA: Jones & Bartlett Publishers; 2020:449–472.

78. Bryant CA, Courtney A, McDermott RJ, et al. A social marketing approach for increasing community coalitions' adoption of evidence-based policy to combat obesity. *Soc Mar Q.* 2014;20(4):219–246.
79. Nápoles AM, Stewart AL. Transcreation: an implementation science framework for community-engaged behavioral interventions to reduce health disparities. *BMC Health Serv Res.* 2018;18:710.
80. Savage C, Aboul-Enein BH, Bernstein J. Perspectives of health promotion and primary prevention of cardiovascular disease: revisiting the social ecological model. *Evid Based Med Public Health.* 2015;2:e911.
81. Haggis C, Sims-Gould J, Winters M, et al. Sustained impact of community-based physical activity interventions: key elements for success. *BMC Public Health.* 2013;13:892.
82. O'Mara-Eves A, Brunton G, Oliver S, et al. The effectiveness of community engagement in public health interventions for disadvantaged groups: a meta-analysis. *BMC Public Health.* 2015;15:129.
83. Hicks S, Duran B, Wallerstein N, et al. Evaluating community-based participatory research to improve community-partnered science and community health. *Prog Community Health Partnersh.* 2012;6(3):289–299.
84. Newton S, Asbroek GT, Hill Z, et al. Maximizing community participation and engagement: lessons learned over 2 decades of field trials in rural Ghana. *Emerg Themes Epidemiol.* 2021;18(1):19.
85. Brunton G, Thomas J, O'Mara-Eves A, et al. Narratives of community engagement: a systematic review-derived conceptual framework for public health interventions. *BMC Public Health.* 2017;17(1):944.
86. Smith SA, Whitehead MS, Sheats JQ, et al. Community-based participatory research principles for the African American community. *J Ga Public Health Assoc.* 2015;5(1):52–56.
87. Israel BA, Schulz AJ, Parker EA, Becker AB. Review of community-based research: assessing partnership approaches to improve public health. *Annu Rev Public Health.* 2005;19(1): 173–202.
88. Butterfoss FD, Morrow AL, Webster JD, Crews C. The coalition training institute: training for the long haul. *J Public Health Manag Pract.* 2003;9(6):522–529.
89. Cheadle A, Atiedu A, Rauzon S, Schwartz P, et al. A community-level initiative to prevent obesity: results from the Kaiser Permanente's Healthy Eating Active Living Zones initiative in California. *Am J Prev Med.* 2018;54(suppl 1):S150–S159.
90. Kegler MC, Halpin SN, Butterfoss FD. Evaluation methods commonly used to assess effectiveness of community coalitions in public health: results from a scoping review. *New Dir Eval.* 2020;165:139–157.
91. Motley M, Holmes A, Hill J, et al. Evaluating community capacity to address obesity in the Dan River region: a case study. *Am J Health Behav.* 2013;37(2):209–217.
92. Butterfoss FD, Goodman R, Wandersman A. Community coalitions for prevention and health promotion. *Health Educ Res.* 1993;8(3):315–330.
93. McLeroy KR, Kegler M, Steckler A, et al. Community coalitions for health promotion: summary and further reflections. *Health Educ Res.* 1994;9(1):1–11.
94. Whitt M. *Fighting Tobacco: A Coalition Approach to Improving Your Community's Health.* Lansing, MI: Michigan Department of Public Health; 1993.

95. Anderson LM, Adeney KL, Shinn C, et al. Community coalition-driven interventions to reduce health disparities among racial and ethnic minority populations. *Cochrane Database Syst Rev*. 2015;6:CD009905.
96. Wolff T. Community coalition building—contemporary practice and research: introduction. *Am J Comm Psych*. 2001;29(2):165–172. doi:10.1023/A:1010314326787
97. Butterfoss FD, LaChance LL, Orians CE. Building allies coalitions: why formation matters. *Health Promot Pract*. 2006;7(2 Suppl):23S–33S.
98. Butterfoss FD, Kegler MC. The Community Coalition Action Theory. In: DiClemente RJ, Crosby RA, Kegler MC, eds. *Emerging Theories in Health Promotion Practice and Research*. San Francisco, CA: Jossey Bass; 2009:451–510.
99. Minkler M, Estrada J, Thayer R, et al. Bringing healthy retail to urban "food swamps": a case study of CBPR-informed policy and neighborhood change in San Francisco. *J Urban Health*. 2018;95(6):850–858.
100. Gloppen KM, Arthur MW, Hawkins JD, Shapiro VB. Sustainability of the Communities That Care prevention system by coalitions participating in the Community Youth Development Study. *J Adolesc Health*. 2012;51(3):259–264.
101. Mayer AB, McDermott RJ, Bryant CA, et al. Sustainability of community-based health promotion coalitions: putting theory into practice. *Health Behav Policy Rev*. 2017;4(5):511–520.
102. Shelton R, Griffith D, Kegler M. The promise of qualitative research to inform theory to address health equity. *Health Educ Behav*. 2018;44:815–819.
103. Yin R. *Case Study Research Design and Methods*. Thousand Oaks, CA: Sage Publications; 2014.
104. Brownson R, Brennan L, Evenson K, Leviton L. Lessons from a mixed-methods approach to evaluating Active Living by Design. *Am J Prev Med*. 2012;43(suppl 4):S271–S280. doi:10.1016/j.amepre.2012.07.002
105. Hawkins JD, Oesterle S, Brown EC, et al. Results of a type 2 translational research trial to prevent adolescent drug use and delinquency: a test of Communities That Care. *Arch Pediatr*. 2009;163(9):789–798. doi:10.1001/archpediatrics.2009.141
106. Hawkins JD, Oesterle S, Brown EC, et al. Youth problem behaviors 8 years after implementing the communities that care prevention system: a community-randomized trial. *JAMA Pediatr*. 2014;168(2):122–129.
107. Centers for Disease Control and Prevention. About the PRC program. Available at: https://www.cdc.gov/prc/about-prc-program/index.htm. Accessed January 8, 2023.
108. National Association of County and City Health Officials. The NACCHO advocacy toolkit. February 2023. Available at: https://www.naccho.org/uploads/downloadable-resources/Advocacy-Toolkit-February-2023.pdf. Accessed September 26, 2023.
109. Wallack L. The role of mass media in creating social capital: a new direction for public health. In: Smedly BD, Syme SL, eds. *Promoting Health: Intervention Strategies From Social and Behavioral Research*. Washington, DC: National Academies Press; 2000:337–365.
110. Dorfman L, Krasnow ID. Public health and media advocacy. *Annu Rev Public Health*. 2014;35:293–306.
111. Mendoza-Herrera K, Valero-Morales I, Ocampo-Granados ME, et al. An overview of social media use in the field of public health nutrition: benefits, scope, limitations, and a Latin American experience. *Prev Chronic Dis*. 2020;17:E76.

112. Centers for Disease Control and Prevention. Public health policy. 2019. Available at: https://www.cdc.gov/publichealthgateway/policy/index.html. Accessed January 8, 2023.
113. Moreland-Russell S, Brownson R. *Prevention, Policy, and Public Health.* New York, NY: Oxford University Press; 2015.
114. Community Toolbox. PRECEDE–PROCEED model. Available at: http://ctb.ku.edu/en/table-contents/overview/other-models-promoting-community-health-and-development/preceder-proceder/main. Accessed January 8, 2023.
115. Community Toolbox. Developing a logic model or theory of change. Available at: http://ctb.ku.edu/en/table-of-contents/overview/models-for-community-health-and-development/logic-model-development/main. Accessed January 8, 2023.
116. Centers for Disease Control and Prevention. Mobilizing Action Toward Community Health (MATCH) project. Available at: https://www.cdc.gov/hrqol/featured-items/match.htm. Accessed January 8, 2023.
117. Green LW, Kreuter M. *Health Program Planning: An Educational and Ecological Approach.* 4th ed. Columbus, OH: McGraw Hill; 2005.
118. National Association of County and City Health Officials. Mobilizing for Action through Planning and Partnerships. 2016. Available at: www.naccho.org/mapp. Accessed January 8, 2023.
119. Community Toolbox. Section 13. MAPP: Mobilizing for Action through Planning and Partnerships. Available at: https://ctb.ku.edu/en/table-of-contents/overview/models-for-community-health-and-development/mapp/main. Accessed January 8, 2023.
120. Bartholomew LK, Mullen PD. Five roles for using theory and evidence in the design and testing of behavior change interventions. *J Public Health Dent.* 2011;71:S20–S33.
121. Fernandez ME, Ruiter RAC, Markham CM, Kok G. Intervention mapping: theory- and evidence-based health promotion program planning: perspective and examples. *Front Public Health.* 2019;7:209.
122. Khaliq M, Boddupalli S, Parvanta C, Bryant C. Community-based prevention marketing (CBPM): evolution from programming to policy development to systems change. In: Fourali C, French J eds. *The Palgrave Encyclopedia of Social Marketing.* London, UK: Palgrave Macmillan, Cham; 2021.
123. McKenzie-Mohr D. Introduction to community-based social marketing. Tools of Change Website. Available at: https://toolsofchange.com/en/programs/community-based-social-marketing/#:~:text=Definition,for%20the%20greater%20social%20good. Accessed March 19, 2023.
124. Bryant CA, Courtney AH, McDermott RJ, et al. Promoting physical activity among youth through community-based prevention marketing. *J Sch Health.* 2010;80(5):214–224.
125. Bryant CA, Forthofer MS, Brown KRM, et al. Community-based prevention marketing: the next steps in disseminating behavior change. *Am J Health Behav.* 2000;24(1):61–68.
126. Bryant CA, Brown KM, McDermott RJ, et al. Community-based prevention marketing: a framework for facilitating health behavior change. *Health Promot Pract.* 2007;8(2):154–163.
127. Bryant CA, Brown KM, McDermott RJ, et al. Community-based prevention marketing: a new planning framework for designing and tailoring health promotion interventions.

In: DiClemente R, Crosby RA, Kegler MC, eds. *Emerging Theories in Health Promotion Practice and Research: Strategies for Improving Public Health.* 2nd ed. San Francisco, CA: Jossey-Bass; 2009.

128. Biroscak BJ, Khaliq M, Truong S, et al. Social marketing and policy making: tools for community-based policy advocacy. *Soc Mar Q.* 2015;21(4):249–259.
129. Mayer A, Lefebvre R, McDermott R, et al. Social marketing approach for increasing community coalitions' adoption of evidence-based policy to combat obesity. In: Brennan L, Binney W, Parker L, Watne T, eds. *Behavior Change Models: Theory and Application for Social Marketing.* Cheltenham, UK: Edward Elgar Publishers; 2015.
130. Biroscak B, Bryant CA, Khaliq M, et al. Using systems dynamics modeling to evaluate a community-based social marketing framework: a computer simulation study. *J Soc Mark.* 2019;9(1):53–76.
131. Vamos S, Frankish J. Health literacy and non-communicable diseases. In: McQueen D, ed. *Oxford Bibliographies in Public Health.* New York, NY: Oxford University Press; 2013.
132. Nutbeam D. Health promotion glossary. *Health Promot Int.* 1998;13(4):349–364.
133. Rudd RE, Oelschlegel S, Grabeel KL, et al. *The HLE2 Assessment Tool.* Boston: Harvard T.H. Chan School of Public Health; 2019. Available at: https://cdn1.sph.harvard.edu/wp-content/uploads/sites/135/2019/05/april-30-FINAL_The-Health-Literacy-Environment2_Locked.pdf. Accessed January 8, 2023.
134. Poureslami I, Nimmon L, Rootman I, Fitzgerald M. Health literacy and chronic disease management: drawing from expert knowledge to set an agenda. *Health Promot Int.* 2017;32(4):743–754.
135. US Department of Health and Human Services (USDHHS). *Health Literacy in Healthy People 2030.* Atlanta, GA: USDHHS; 2021.
136. Nielsen-Bohlman L, Panzer AM, Kindig DA, eds. *Health Literacy: A Prescription to End Confusion.* Institute of Medicine. Committee on Health Literacy. Washington, DC: National Academies Press; 2004.
137. Rootman I, Gordon-El-Bihbety D. A vision for a health literate Canada: report of the Expert Panel on Health Literacy. Canadian Public Health Association. 2008. Available at: https://www.cpha.ca/sites/default/files/uploads/resources/healthlit/report_e.pdf. Accessed March 19, 2023.
138. Cho YI, Arozullah AM, Crittenden KS, Lee SYD. Effects of health literacy on health status and health service utilization amongst the elderly. *Soc Sci Med.* 2008;66(8):1809–1816.
139. Nielsen-Bohlman L, Panze AM, Kindig DA, eds. *Health Literacy: A Prescription to End Confusion.* Washington, DC: National Academies Press; 2004.
140. Organisation for Economic Co-operation and Development (OECD). *OECD Skills Outlook 2013: First Results from the Survey of Adult Skills.* Washington, DC: OECD Publishing; 2013.
141. Eichler K, Wieser S, Bruegger U. The costs of limited health literacy: a systematic review. *Int J Public Health.* 2009;54(5):313–324.
142. Schuster AL, Frick KD, Huh B-Y, et al. Economic evaluation of a community health worker-led health literacy intervention to promote cancer screening among Korean American women. *J Health Care Poor Underserved.* 2015;26(2):431–440.

143. Herman A, Jackson P. Empowering low-income parents with skills to reduce excess pediatric emergency room and clinic visits through a tailored low literacy training intervention. *J Health Commun.* 2010;15(8):895–910.
144. Kubb C, Foran HM. Online health information seeking by parents for their children: systematic review and agenda for further research. *J Med Internet Res.* 2020;22(8): e19985.
145. Barke A, Doering BK. Development of an instrument to assess parents' excessive web-based searches for information pertaining to their children's health: the "Children's Health Internet Research, Parental Inventory" (CHIRPI). *J Med Internet Res.* 2020;22(4):e16148.
146. McMullan RD, Berle D, Arnáez S, Starcevic V. The relationships between health anxiety, online health information seeking, and cyberchondria: systematic review and meta-analysis. *J Affect Disord.* 2019;245:270–278.
147. Mörelius E, Robinson S, Arabiat D, Whitehead L. Digital interventions to improve health literacy among parents of children aged 0 to 12 years with a health condition: systematic review. *J Med Internet Res.* 2021;23(12):e31665.
148. Batterham RW, Hawkins M, Collins PA, et al. Health literacy: applying current concepts to improve health services and reduce health inequalities. *Public Health.* 2016;132:3–12.
149. Centre for Literacy. *The Calgary Charter on Health Literacy: rationale and core principles for the development of health literacy curricula.* 2011:3. Available at: http://www.centreforliteracy.qc.ca/sites/default/files/CFL_Calgary_Charter_2011.pdf. Accessed January 8, 2023.
150. Bejarano G. Digital literacy, health inequities, and the COVID-19 pandemic. *Am J Public Health.* 2022;112(4):588–589.
151. US Department of Health and Human Services (USDHHS). *National Action Plan to Improve Health Literacy.* Washington, DC: USDHHS; 2010:5.
152. Vamos S, Okan O, Sentell T, Rootman I. Making a case for "education for health literacy": an international perspective. *Int J Environ Res Public Health.* 2020;17:1436.
153. Vamos S, McDermott RJ. Rebranding school health: the power of health literacy. *J Sch Health.* 2021;91(8):670–676.

5

The Role of Health Care Systems in Chronic Disease Prevention and Control

Karina A. Atwell, MD, MPH, and Maureen A. Smith, MD, PhD, MPH

LEARNING OBJECTIVES

After completing this chapter, readers should be able to

1. Understand the burden of chronic diseases on health care systems.
2. Describe how the Affordable Care Act has influenced health care system reform initiatives.
3. Identify the component of the Chronic Care Model, and the Expanded Chronic Care Model.
4. Describe how health systems can address chronic diseases at various levels of the prevention spectrum (e.g., primary, secondary, tertiary).

INTRODUCTION

A rapidly aging population in the United States combined with advances in medicine and public health is leading to increased life expectancy and a growing burden of chronic disease on health systems and communities. In 2018 there were 24.6% (61 million) of adults with one chronic condition and 27.2% (68 million) with two or more chronic conditions.[1] People living with multiple chronic conditions (MCC) account for a disproportionate share of health care utilization and costs, 64% of all clinician visits, 70% of all inpatient stays, 83% of all prescriptions, 71% of all health care spending, and 93% of Medicare spending. Nearly all hospital readmissions among Medicare beneficiaries occur among those with MCC. The prevalence of MCC is greater among low-income individuals and racial/ethnic minorities, who also develop MCC at earlier ages.[2]

People with multiple or complex chronic conditions have more complicated health needs, including frequent monitoring and evaluation, and multiple care providers across different health environments. As an individual's number of chronic conditions increases, that individual's risk for dying, incurring avoidable hospitalizations, and experiencing poor day-to-day functioning also rises. In addition, these conditions contribute to frailty and disability, which often complicate access to health care, interfere with self-management, and necessitate reliance on caregivers.[3] Many chronic diseases act synergistically, such as diabetes and depression, compounding the risk for poor outcomes.[4]

Risk factors for chronic illness are multiple and interrelated; have roots in individuals, families, and communities; and require coordinated strategies across multiple levels and sectors for improvement. These issues are driving substantial change in how health care systems, public health, and other sectors are addressing the chronic disease epidemic.[5] Most nations across the globe are strategizing ways to address the growing burden of chronic disease in their populations. Although this chapter focuses on US health care system approaches, there is much to learn from other countries who are ahead of the United States in this feat.

The unbalanced distribution of costs and opportunities for chronic disease management and prevention across a population serviced by a health care system can be outlined in a population pyramid (Figure 5-1).[6] At the top of the pyramid are those 5% of patients with the most complex and advanced disease, highest risk, and highest costs. They have multiple chronic conditions, typically with at least one under poor control or at end stages for which acute care and tertiary prevention measures are the mainstay of management. This subset of the population requires the most intensive and frequent care, often through specialized complex case management. This group can consume 50% or more of the total cost of care within the health system.

The next 15% of the pyramid is the chronic care population; individuals in this group usually have at least one chronic condition, often under suboptimal control. These patients

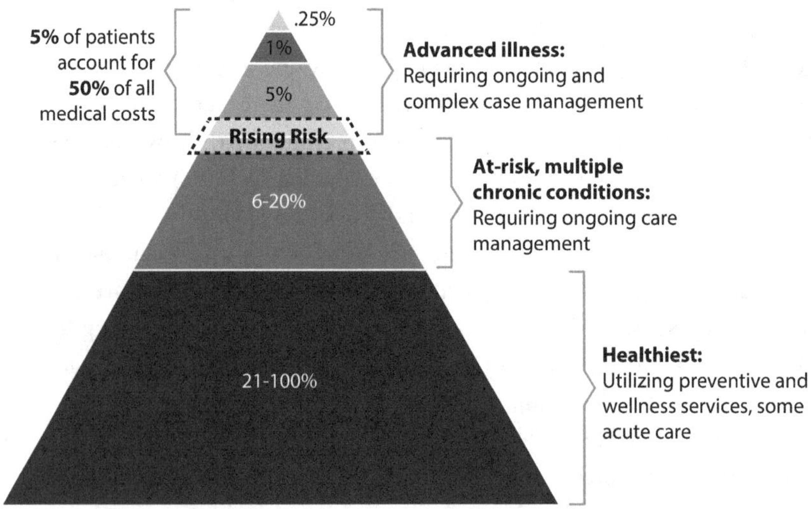

Source: Reprinted from Marks and Levin.[6]

Figure 5-1. Population Pyramid Depicting How a Health System Might Characterize Its Population of Patients as It Relates to Chronic Disease Status, Risk, Health Care Needs, and Costs

require frequent monitoring and are at risk for progression and complications of their chronic disease(s). They also require ongoing care management, albeit less intense than that required for the most complex 5% of the population.

The bottom 80% of the pyramid represents the generally "well" or "still healthy" share of the population. These individuals tend to interact with the health system only for acute care and preventive services but may be at risk for developing chronic diseases because of one or a combination of lifestyle, hereditary, socioeconomic, and environmental factors. This group presents opportunities for primary and early secondary prevention through timely evidence-based screening and health promotion counseling.

As health care systems shoulder the strain of chronic disease care for the top 20% of this pyramid, there is a recognized need to transform the ways in which this care is delivered to achieve better and equitable outcomes at lower costs.[7] Given that most chronic conditions and their subsequent complications are preventable, there is also expanding interest in health care system approaches that target health promotion and disease prevention (the bottom 80% of the pyramid), activities once considered mainly in the arena of public health.

This broader reach demands a true population health perspective. *Population health* refers to the "distribution of health outcomes within a population, the health determinants that influence distribution, and the policies and interventions that impact the determinants."[8] It spans the breadth of wellness and prevention, management of chronic disease, care of the frail and elderly, and end-of-life transitions. Population health rests on four pillars (Figure 5-2): chronic care management, quality and safety, public health, and health policy.[7] As its own pillar, the model acknowledges the critical role chronic disease plays in population health. It also reinforces the opportunities health care systems have to affect all four pillars of population health.

This population health lens expands the scope of health care systems beyond their historical reactionary "sick care" delivery models targeting the individual patient, which have proved ineffective, fragmented, and poorly incentivized for preventing and managing chronic disease. To meet the goals of successful population health management, health care systems must not only better manage their chronic disease patients but also invest in strategies to preserve wellness and minimize the impact of illness for their entire population. Health care leaders see population health as an essential element of health reform. Provisions of the Affordable Care Act (ACA) encouraging transformative models of care delivery and "value over volume" have motivated health systems to broaden their scope for how to best manage and prevent chronic disease and its complications at the population level.[9]

Collaboration among health care systems, public health, and communities in tackling chronic disease has also been prioritized within heath care reform and other leading national health improvement initiatives, including Healthy People 2030 and the four domains of chronic disease prevention (epidemiology and surveillance,

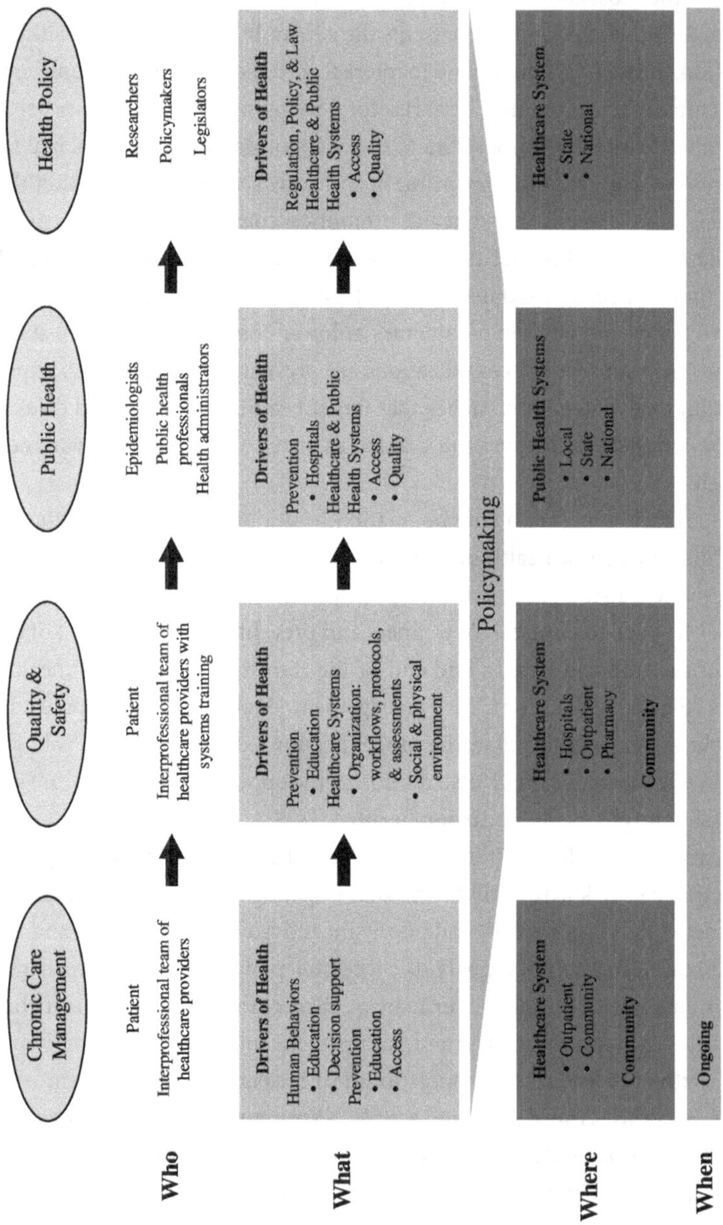

Source: Nash.[7] Reprinted with permission of the Governance Institute.

Figure 5-2. The Four Pillars of Population Health

environmental approaches, health care system interventions, and community–clinical links), the latter established by the Centers for Disease Control and Prevention (CDC).[10] This call for partnership signals the recognition that health is dependent on many factors beyond the walls of the health care system. Among the various contributing health factors that affect an individual's and a community's health, the County Health Rankings Model of Population Health attributes only about 20% to the health care system.[11] To effectively and equitably address chronic disease burden, health care systems need to deploy integrated approaches with public–private partnerships and other stakeholders that bundle strategies and interventions, address many risk factors and conditions simultaneously, create population-wide changes, and target the population subgroups most affected.[10]

HEALTH CARE REFORM: INCENTIVES FOR IMPROVED CHRONIC DISEASE CONTROL AND PREVENTION

In addition to its more familiar health insurance coverage reforms, the ACA contains numerous provisions that directly target how health care is organized, delivered, and paid for in the United States. These provisions directly and indirectly affect chronic disease prevention and management. Building on existing reform models in both the private and the public sectors, the law takes multiple complementary approaches to addressing the health system's long-standing issues in effectively tackling chronic disease.

Centers for Medicare and Medicaid Services Innovation Center

The ACA created many new resources to establish a foundation for accelerated public- and private-sector innovation in health care delivery. One example is the Centers for Medicare and Medicaid Services Innovation Center (CMMI). This center was established to identify, test, and spread new payment and service delivery models to reduce expenditures while maintaining or improving quality of care for beneficiaries of Medicare, Medicaid, and the Children's Health Insurance Program. The US Secretary of Health and Human Services was granted authority to expand innovations if evidence shows actual cost reductions or improvements in outcomes. When the ACA was enacted, the Congressional Budget Office estimated that the Innovation Center, with its $10 billion of direct funding over 10 years, would save $1.3 billion between 2010 and 2019. Recognizing the critical role of states in providing, purchasing, and regulating health care services, CMMI established the State Innovation Models Initiative to help states achieve better health outcomes at lower cost. These grants provide federal dollars and technical assistance for a wide range of health system transformation efforts, with 38 total awardees, including 34 states, three territories, and the District of Columbia.[12]

Since its inception CMMI has designed, implemented, and tested over 40 payment and service delivery models. The models can be generally categorized by their delivery and payment approaches and the beneficiaries covered:

- Accountable care: Models are built around accountable care organizations (ACOs) which hold groups of providers responsible for cost and quality of care for a population of patients.
- Episode-based payment initiatives: Providers are held accountable for costs and quality for certain conditions or "episodes of care" during a specified period of time.
- Primary care transformation: Models are built around the medical home structure and improved investments in primary care.
- Initiatives to speed the adoption of best practices: Models include cross-sector collaboration focused on preventing disease and addressing upstream factors that affect health.
- Initiatives to accelerate the development and testing of new payment and service delivery models: State-based and locally developed models address care for Medicare, Medicaid, and dually eligible beneficiaries and Children's Health Insurance Program beneficiaries.[13]

We explore some of these initiatives in more depth next.

Accountable Care Organizations

One of the most notable incentives to shift toward population health–minded systems is the promotion of ACOs. An ACO is an entity formed by health care providers across various practice settings who agree to collectively take responsibility for the quality and total costs of care for a population of patients. Beginning in 2012 the ACA established the Medicare Shared Savings Program to encourage the development of ACOs. If participating ACOs meet quality benchmarks, such as with diabetes care or depression screening, and keep spending for their attributed patients below budget, they receive half the savings that result, with the rest going to the Centers for Medicare & Medicaid Services (CMS), which administers the program. Effective chronic disease care and prevention is a cornerstone to achieving benchmarks and realizing cost savings within an ACO structure.

Participation by health care systems in ACOs is promising. In 2022 there were 483 shared-savings ACOs serving nearly 11 million beneficiaries.[14] In 2020 there was a total shared savings of $2.3 billion.[15] ACOs have contributed to slowing the growth in health care costs, demonstrated improved care coordination and quality, promoted the shift to value-based care, increased the use of preventative care, and improved the ability of health care systems to respond to emergencies. For example, interviews with ACOs detail how investments in data infrastructure, care coordination, and training combined with financial flexibility afforded by value-based payment models allowed them to more effectively respond to the needs of patients during the COVID-19 emergency.[16]

Provider Payment Reform

CMMI also plays a critical role in testing new payment models for reimbursement of health care services. The Quality Payment Program was created by Congress as part of the Medicare Access and CHIP Reauthorization Act of 2015 (MACRA). MACRA allowed CMS to shift away from fee-for-service models and instead reward high-value, high-quality Medicare clinicians with payment increases, at the same time reducing payments to those clinicians who are not meeting performance standards. One example is an approach known as bundled payment—a single reimbursement for all services required for a given medical condition or procedure episode of care. Ideally, this should incentivize the various providers involved in a patient's care to collaborate and strive for efficient and effective outcomes, including prevention of complications and disease progression.

As of 2020 bundled payment models have shown reduced Medicare fee-for-service payments for most of the clinical episodes of care evaluated while maintaining quality of care. Overall, Medicare has experienced net losses, but evaluators expect that the model's financial sustainability will improve because of significant design changes to CMS made in 2021.[17]

Primary Care Transformation

Although primary care is fundamental to a well-functioning health system, the United States has undervalued and underinvested in it for decades. The disregard of primary care is largely a consequence of the prevailing fee-for-service reimbursement approach in which providers have inherent financial incentives to provide more care and procedures over care management and other cost-saving services targeting chronic disease.

There is considerable evidence that comprehensive, coordinated, and well-targeted primary care can improve outcomes and reduce costs.[18] These characteristics are embodied in the patient-centered medical home (PCMH), a model of care that emphasizes more comprehensive care coordination, care teams, patient engagement, and population health management. Several of the ACA's reforms seek to transform primary care by way of the medical home model across various care environments. The ACA is also supporting health care systems and states to experiment with ways to improve quality by testing models that integrate primary care more seamlessly with other health care services, such as behavioral health and long-term care. This integration is key to successful management of chronic disease, in particular for the most costly and complex patients. Examples of primary care transformation initiatives include the Comprehensive Primary Care Initiative, which tests a new way to deliver and pay for care that is designed to improve access, coordination, and chronic disease management while engaging patients and their caregivers. This initiative supports health homes targeting low-income Medicaid beneficiaries with complex needs, such as chronic conditions, mental health issues, or substance abuse problems. The federal government pays 90% of the costs of these additional services for two years with the expectation that the state will sustain the program thereafter.[19]

For various reasons, none of the models completed so far have been found to meet the statutory criteria of lower spending or improved quality, and none have been expanded nationwide.[20] These early primary care–focused models do offer important lessons, however, and some of the promising characteristics tested continue to be incorporated and refined in new CMMI transformation models.

A major theme emerging from this work to transform primary care is the critical role of technical and financial support in building the capacity of physician practices to function as medical homes. Each of the ACA-supported transformation initiatives includes some level of support for practices to address common challenges, including providing timely collection, reporting, and use of data for care management and quality improvement; shifting the practice culture to enable effective teamwork; and acquiring information about patients from settings outside the clinical setting. Overall, federal investments have stimulated extraordinary collaboration and dialogue among payers, both private and public, and providers on how to reorganize primary care to achieve the aims of improved population health and decreased costs.[9]

Looking Ahead

In 2021 the CMS Innovation Center set a strategic goal for its next 10 years: to transform the health system into one that achieves equitable outcomes through high-quality, affordable, person-centered care (Figure 5-3). As part of this, the Center is committed to

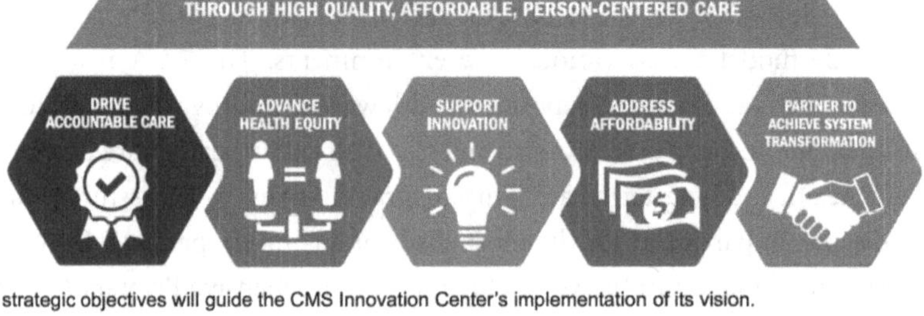
A HEALTH SYSTEM THAT ACHIEVES EQUITABLE OUTCOMES
THROUGH HIGH QUALITY, AFFORDABLE, PERSON-CENTERED CARE
DRIVE ACCOUNTABLE CARE
ADVANCE HEALTH EQUITY
SUPPORT INNOVATION
ADDRESS AFFORDABILITY
PARTNER TO ACHIEVE SYSTEM TRANSFORMATION
Five strategic objectives will guide the CMS Innovation Center's implementation of its vision.

Source: Reprinted from CMS Innovation Center.[19]

Figure 5-3. CMS Innovation Center's Strategic Objectives

designing models that are inclusive of a variety of providers who care for underserved populations, ultimately increasing beneficiaries' access to high-quality care.[20]

THREE LEVELS OF INVOLVEMENT FOR HEALTH CARE SYSTEMS IN CHRONIC DISEASE PREVENTION AND CONTROL

The spectrum of prevention introduced in Chapter 1 is a helpful framework for exploring the ways in which health care systems influence chronic disease management and prevention. Health promotion (primary prevention) activities encourage healthy living and limit the initial onset of chronic diseases. Early detection efforts (secondary prevention) include screening at-risk populations and applying strategies for proactive management of existing diseases to prevent complications. Complex care management and care coordination approaches for high-risk populations with multiple comorbidities or complications of chronic disease encompass tertiary prevention. These three levels of health care system activities are explored next, starting with tertiary prevention efforts and moving upstream.

Level 1: Chronic Disease Management: The Chronic Care Model

Effectively managing disease and minimizing complications requires a well-coordinated, interdisciplinary approach. One well-recognized framework for achieving comprehensive chronic disease management is the Chronic Care Model (CCM; Figure 5-4).[21] The basis for the CCM stemmed from a review of interventions to improve care for various

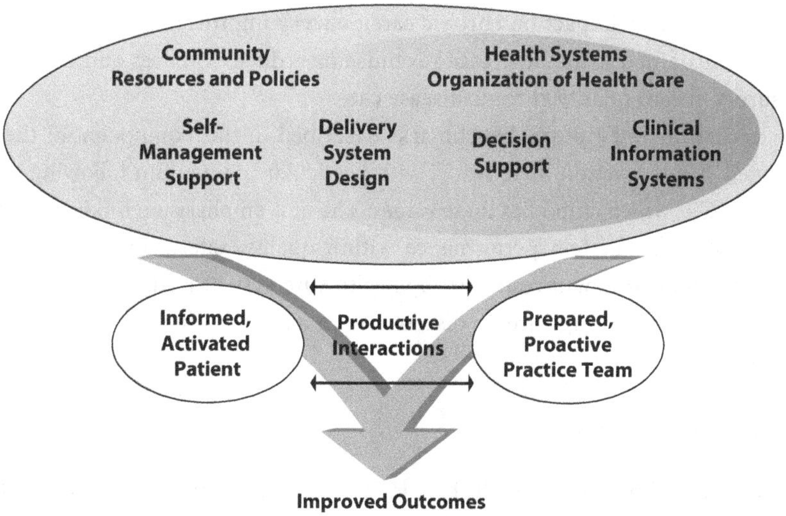

Source: Wagner.[21] Reprinted with permission of American College of Physicians.

Figure 5-4. The Chronic Care Model

chronically ill populations. This review concluded that multicomponent practice changes in four categories led to the greatest improvements in health outcomes: increasing providers' expertise and skill, educating and supporting patients, making care delivery more team-based and -planned, and making better use of registry-based information systems.[21]

The CCM's six interrelated components are health care organization, clinical information systems, delivery system redesign, decision support, self-management support, and community resources. The first four components of the CCM address practice strategies. The final two are specifically patient-centered.[22] In the CCM improved functional and clinical outcomes for disease management are the result of productive interactions between informed, activated patients and the prepared, proactive practice team of clinicians and other health care professionals.[23] Each of the CCM components is explored next.

Components of the Chronic Care Model

Organization of Health Systems

The structure, goals, and values of a health care system and its relationships with purchasers, payers, and other service providers form the foundation for the CCM. The ideal system has a culture in which the optimal management of chronic disease and practice improvement are key values. Leadership is committed and visibly involved, supports transformational change, and creates incentives for providers and patients to improve care and adhere to evidence-based practice. Facilitation of communication and data-sharing between care environments is emphasized. The reimbursement environment has a major impact on chronic care delivery improvements, which are more likely to be sustained if they increase revenues or reduce expenses and if purchasers and insurers reward quality chronic disease care.[23]

The leadership and cultural benchmarks described in this component of the CCM have gained steady traction nationwide, with particular momentum following the passage of the ACA, which embodies these values. The new emphasis on linking reimbursement to health care system performance within quality, safety, and health outcome measures has ignited new investments by health care system leaders in assessing how their systems are managing chronic disease and in adopting improvement strategies to address identified gaps.

Delivery System Design

Improving the health of people with chronic illness requires a shift from systems that are essentially reactive—responding mainly once a person is sick—to one that is proactive and focused on maintaining health. This requires determining what care is needed;

having clear roles and tasks on a care team to ensure that the patient gets the care; making sure that everyone taking care of a patient has centralized, up-to-date information; and making follow-up a part of standard procedure. Patients with complex or multiple problems may need more intensive management (care or case management) to optimize clinical care and self-management. Health literacy and cultural sensitivity are two important emerging concepts in health care, and systems must respond effectively to the diverse cultural and linguistic needs of their patients as they perform these functions.

The PCMH described previously is one example of an effort to become proactive and team-based in caring for patients with chronic disease. This transformation is in response to health care systems that have tended to be disjointed, variable in processes across practice settings, and poorly designed for clear communication between primary care and specialty providers.[24] Medical homes attempt to better coordinate care across health, behavioral, community, and long-term services. Health care systems taking on financial risk for the overall costs of care through ACOs are developing complex care management programs to improve care, and thereby control costs, for the highest-need, highest-cost patients. Complex care management extends beyond medical issues, attempting to address how patients' psychosocial circumstances affect their ability to follow treatment recommendations and achieve a healthy lifestyle.[25] The goals are to maintain or improve functional status, increase the capacity to self-manage conditions, eliminate unnecessary clinical testing, and reduce the need for acute care services.

Decision Support

An important problem in health care is the significant gap between optimal evidence-based medical practice and the care delivered. Clinical decision support provides timely information, usually at the point of care, to help inform decisions about a patient's care backed by evidence and guidelines. Examples include order sets created for particular conditions or types of patients, practice guidelines accessible at the point of care, databases that can provide information relevant to particular patients, reminders for preventive screening, and alerts about potentially dangerous situations such as medication interactions. Health care organizations can creatively integrate these functions into the day-to-day practice of providers in an accessible and easy-to-use manner. Providers should receive ongoing education to stay up to date on the latest evidence, and guidelines should also be discussed with patients so that they can understand the principles behind their care. Clinical decision support can potentially lower costs, improve efficiency, and reduce patient inconvenience.[26]

In the past many clinical decision support systems were stand-alone and not well integrated with other electronic health records (EHRs), or into clinical workflow. With the passage of the Health Information Technology for Economic and Clinical Health (HITECH) Act of 2009, which provides the Department of Health and Human Services with the authority to establish programs to improve health care quality, safety, and efficiency through the promotion of health information technology, much work has been done to integrate decision support tools into EHRs.[27] EHRs with integrated decision support and chronic care management tools help providers manage patient information and monitor health outcomes. Early adopters of this technology have found that it supports the PCMH and CCM models by allowing redistribution of patient care tasks to nonphysician support personnel. Integrated laboratory and pharmacy information systems can further bolster decision support functions, promote coordinated care, and reduce errors and duplication.[26]

Advances in this arena have not been without obstacles. Significant investments of time and resources are required to transition practice settings to EHRs and configure clinical decision support tools to meet the needs and clinical workflows of practice environments. Usability amid busy clinical schedules is key to successful adoption and functionality. Ultimately, these systems must prove return on investment through better clinical management of chronic disease and cost savings to maintain financial support from health care system leadership, insurers, and grant-based sources. Findings thus far point toward evidence that incorporating health information technology in chronic disease management efforts can yield improved quality of care and significant cost savings.[28]

Clinical Information Systems

Effective chronic disease management is virtually impossible without information systems that guarantee ready access to key data on individual patients, as well as populations served by a health care system. A comprehensive clinical information system, or registry, can enhance care by providing timely reminders for needed services such as laboratory tests and immunizations, with the summarized data helping to track and plan care and outreach. At the population level the registry can identify groups of patients overdue for services or who might benefit from outreach and can facilitate performance monitoring and quality improvement efforts. Most disease registries are used to support care management for groups of patients with one or more chronic diseases and are the foundation for successful integration of all the CCM elements. Similar to decision support tools, patient registries are increasingly being integrated into EHRs to allow for more streamlined disease management and communication among care teams. Some registries with more advanced features may even include clinical decision support functionality that can prompt users with care recommendations.

Also supported by the HITECH Act, the establishment of electronic health information exchanges is a promising area for further development and implementation of computerized disease registries. Health information exchanges share clinical and administrative data across the boundaries of health care institutions, health data repositories, and states.

Many stakeholder groups (e.g., health care systems, insurers, patients) realize that if such data are shared, health care processes would improve with respect to safety, quality, cost, and other indicators. As it relates to chronic disease, a health information exchange offers the ability to effectively identify and manage patients across health care settings, not only for the individual patient who may have multiple chronic conditions managed by a variety of providers and settings but also to guide prevention and management initiatives for a population of interest.[26]

Sharing such data from a cultural and technical standpoint is not easy. Competing priorities, financial concerns, issues related to data ownership, and privacy and security are among some of the most difficult barriers to overcome. Regional health information organizations and other groups that facilitate health information exchange must combat the issue of supporting interfacing from different providers' health IT systems. The few currently operating registries have limited real-time data-feeding capabilities or have little integration into clinicians' workflows at the point of care.[26] Nonetheless, implementation of computerized disease registries by health information exchange organizations poses a promising opportunity to better manage chronic diseases.

Self-Management Support

All patients with chronic illness make decisions and engage in behaviors that affect their health. Disease control and outcomes depend to a significant degree on the effectiveness of this self-management. The greatest contributor to premature death from preventable chronic illness is patient behavior.[29] The degree to which patients are informed and active in their care is therefore critical.

Effective self-management support by heath care systems requires not only counseling patients on what to do in their care but also acknowledging their central role and fostering a sense of responsibility for their own health. It includes the use of proven programs that provide basic information, emotional support, and strategies for living with chronic disease. Using a collaborative approach and evidence-based techniques that emphasize patient activation or empowerment, providers and patients can work together to enhance these skills. Care teams must also be sensitive to the role that families, caregivers, and communities play in these activities.

One of the most widely recognized and studied self-management initiatives is the Stanford Chronic Disease Self-Management Program. Developed at Stanford University in the early 1990s in collaboration with the National Council on Aging and CDC, this community-based program provides in-person and online courses in which individuals with chronic diseases, such as heart disease, hypertension, cancer, stroke, arthritis, and diabetes, learn and practice problem-solving, coping, and communication skills to deal with their condition. They discover lifestyle strategies for good health, including diet, exercise, medications, managing pain and fatigue, living with disability, social support for change, and overcoming depression. The Stanford Chronic Disease Self-Management Program has been studied extensively, with results showing significant, measurable improvements in the health, quality of life, and communication with providers for people living with chronic conditions. The program also appears to have saved enough through reductions in health care expenditures to pay for itself within the first year. Studies have indicated fewer outpatient and emergency department visits and fewer hospitalizations, and a health care cost savings of approximately $590 per participant.[30,31]

Patient activation, or engagement—that is, the knowledge, skills, and confidence persons have in managing their own health and health care[32]—is now recognized as a crucial element to successful management of chronic disease. Multiple studies show that an individual's level of activation is predictive of most health behaviors, including preventive behaviors (e.g., obtaining screenings and immunizations), healthy behaviors (e.g., healthy diet and regular exercise), self-management behaviors (e.g., medication management), and health information seeking.[33] Highly activated individuals also have better health outcomes and lower rates of costly utilization, such as emergency department use and hospitalizations, than do less engaged persons. Furthermore, evidence shows that providing support and appropriate interventions can increase activation levels in patients. These interventions focus on helping patients gain new skills and encouraging a sense of ownership over their health. Health care systems are also increasingly applying patient activation measures to help inform population risk stratification and distribution of appropriate levels of support as well as to measure the performance and effectiveness of interventions.[32]

The Community

Health care systems can enhance care for patients, make strides in population health improvement, and avoid duplication of efforts by reaching out to form powerful alliances and partnerships with state and local agencies, nonprofit organizations, and schools, businesses, and other community stakeholders to share resources and collaborate on chronic disease initiatives. Local and state health policies, insurance benefits, and other health-related regulations also play a critical role in chronic disease care. Health care systems can make a difference for their patients by advocating on their behalf at the policy level.[34]

This collaboration signals a recognition that factors beyond the walls of clinical care must be recognized and addressed to effect positive change in chronic disease management and that individuals, social support systems, community resources, health care systems, and public policy leaders must be engaged and working together. (The role of clinical–community linkages in chronic disease prevention and management is explored later in this chapter.)

These six components of the CCM are interdependent and build upon one another. For instance, community resources can support patients with self-management skills.

For chronic disease registries to be successful, redesigning delivery systems is necessary so that a designated team member can manage the registry and perform indicated patient outreach, order placement, and data management. Clinical practice guidelines are the evidence upon which physician reminder systems and performance feedback are based. Chronic Care Model elements are unlikely to be introduced or maintained without an organizational environment featuring innovative leadership and favorable reimbursement structures.[23]

Support for the Chronic Care Model

Accumulated evidence appears to support the CCM as an integrated framework to guide practice redesign that leads to improved patient care and better health outcomes for a variety of chronic diseases.[31,35,36] Although work remains to be done in areas such as cost-effectiveness, the CCM, or adaptations of the model, has become a standard for health care delivery and performance measurement as it relates to chronic disease care. This includes several state programs in the United States, national certification agencies for chronic disease programs, and new models of primary care proposed by the American Academy of Family Physicians and American College of Physicians, as well as by the UK National Health Service, the World Health Organization, and several Canadian provinces.[34]

At the national level, and prompted by increased support from the ACA, the US Department of Health and Human Services developed the Strategic Framework on Multiple Chronic Conditions, building on elements of the CCM. This framework aims to convert the CCM into a set of specific, actionable, national-level strategies to "provide a foundation for realizing the vision of optimum health and quality of life for individuals with multiple chronic conditions" who frequently suffer suboptimal health outcomes and incur significant health care expenses.[37] The framework comprises four overarching goals:

1. Foster health care and public health system changes to improve the health of individuals with multiple chronic conditions.
2. Maximize the use of proven self-care management and other services by individuals with multiple chronic conditions.
3. Provide better tools and information to health care, public health, and social services workers who deliver care to individuals with multiple chronic conditions.
4. Facilitate research to fill knowledge gaps about, and interventions and systems to benefit, individuals with multiple chronic conditions.

Each of these goals includes several key objectives and strategies that the health care system, in conjunction with stakeholders and partners, should use to guide its efforts. Although this framework addresses individuals with multiple chronic conditions, many of the strategies also apply to persons with only one chronic disease as well as those with no chronic conditions.[37]

Level 2: Chronic Disease Screening Approaches

Moving along the prevention spectrum to more upstream approaches, chronic disease screening is a cornerstone of secondary prevention activities performed by health care systems. Screening aims to reduce the impact of chronic disease by detecting and treating it early to halt or slow its progress and by encouraging personal behaviors to restore wellness and prevent long-term problems.

Primary care clinics, as the ideal site of a patient's medical home, are an effective and efficient setting to provide evidence-based chronic disease screening. However, it can be challenging to optimally carry out recommended practices because of the competing care demands on primary care providers and support staff. One study found that the time required to provide all recommended preventive services to a typical family practice is 7.4 hours per working day, which would leave little time for any other patient care activities.[38] Patients with multiple chronic conditions or other complexities to their health care needs can experience even larger gaps between recommended screening practices and receipt of these services because of the many other issues that must be addressed during clinical encounters. The challenge for health care systems is to develop strategies for improving rates of evidence-based recommended chronic disease screening that can be incorporated into workflows without undue provider burden or compromised quality and efficiency of care.

The PCMH model, now implemented broadly across a variety of practice settings, emphasizes the core primary care function of providing clinical preventive services, including chronic disease screening, within its comprehensive approach to care over a patient's life course. Increased use of recommended preventive services is considered a key indicator for evaluating the success of the PCMH.[39] Early evaluations have shown consistent evidence of a positive association between implementation of the PCMH and cancer screening, for example.[40] Findings also suggest that the effects of the PCMH model on cancer screening rates vary depending on the socioeconomic context of the practice, with greater effects occurring in lower socioeconomic contexts.[41] Thus, the PCMH model could also contribute to reductions in disparities in screening rates across socioeconomic contexts. The model may be especially effective in lower-socioeconomic-status areas by overcoming some of the challenges that drive disparities through improved access to care, care coordination, and health literacy. Although this research focused on cancer screening, one might hypothesize that similar impact could be observed for other chronic disease screening.

Concurrent with the adoption of the PCMH is the integration of health information technology capacity that can support chronic disease screening activities. Outlined earlier, the use of patient registries can identify those who are overdue for recommended screening services, for which a designated member of the care team can perform outreach. Evidence-based reminders at the point of care, triggered by patient characteristics, and prevention-focused hubs within the EHR are two methods of clinical decision support tools that allow for increased delivery of screening services. Online "patient wellness portals" have also been created that focus on wellness, prevention, and longitudinal health, alerting patients when they are due for screening. A significantly greater proportion of patients who used these portals received all recommended preventive services compared with controls.[42]

As the health demands of populations grow, there is more interest in how health care systems can use the skills and competencies of other allied health professionals outside the walls of the examination room to increase access to care and decrease burden on physician workload. One such profession is pharmacists, who are increasingly performing activities around health promotion and disease prevention in addition to their medication-dispensing roles. The nature and frequency of contact between patients and pharmacists provides significant opportunities for chronic disease screening and healthy lifestyle counseling, as well as assisting patients with monitoring and management of their chronic condition(s). Community pharmacists can play a key role in population-based screening programs or initiatives targeting populations with certain risk behaviors. Close collaboration with other primary care and public health professionals is essential to avoid duplication of work and to ensure continuity of patient care. To realize the potential of pharmacists and other allied health professionals as a resource for chronic disease screening and prevention efforts, they must be allowed the time, training, and regulatory and policy support to perform these functions within the health care system.[43]

A notable signal of increased investment in chronic disease screening is the ACA mandates that eliminate consumer cost-sharing (e.g., co-payments and deductibles) for selected preventive services in marketplace plans and many other individual health plans. States are also encouraged to extend preventive health services in their Medicaid programs, paid for in large part by increased federal payments for Medicaid. This elimination of cost-sharing helps overcome the financial barriers that deter people from getting the screenings and preventive services that are recommended for them.[44]

Level 3: Chronic Disease Prevention and Health Promotion

The third level of chronic disease prevention activities targets primary prevention of chronic diseases and the promotion of wellness, which can deter the development of chronic diseases from the outset. The economic argument for investing in this prevention is compelling. It is estimated that 25% of all direct medical costs are attributable to a small number of excess risk factors such as smoking, obesity, physical inactivity, and poor nutrition; however, less than 1% of health care dollars are spent on scientifically proven, effective prevention strategies.[45] A report by Trust for America's Health estimated that investments in community-based initiatives that address such factors can yield an overall $5.60 return in health cost savings for every $1 spent on prevention.[46]

Individual- and population-level improvements in chronic disease prevention require primary prevention actions targeting the multiple determinants of health, including medical care, health behaviors, and the social and physical environment.[11] Although health care organizations' core responsibility is to improve population health through the delivery of clinical services, they can also work beyond this core mission to address other determinants of health. Unfortunately, health care systems have traditionally had little success in tackling such factors. Without concerted efforts to link clinical services with social-environmental and political efforts, success will continue to be elusive in health care system efforts to prevent disease and improve the overall health of the population. Acknowledging that no single entity can be held accountable for achieving improved outcomes, Kindig and Isham proposed a "community health business model," forming a new generation of partnerships among health care systems, government, schools, businesses, and community organizations.[47] In this model these entities are tasked with making substantial changes in how they approach health, allocate resources, and work together collectively on disease prevention and population health efforts.

An overarching theme within this call for partnership is the important foundation of primary care as a location and vehicle for both delivering preventive services and catalyzing engagement with the community and public health.[48] The fields of primary care and public health in the United States have, for the past century, tended to function independently of each other despite both having chronic disease prevention objectives. To foster collaboration, the Institute of Medicine released a report in 2012 titled "Primary Care and Public Health: Exploring Integration to Improve Population Health," which reviewed promising models of primary care and public health integration. From this report came a set of principles deemed essential for successful integration of primary care and public health: (1) a shared goal of population health improvement; (2) community engagement in defining and addressing population health needs; (3) aligned leadership; (4) sustainability, including shared infrastructure; and (5) sharing and collaborative use of data and analysis.[49,50]

Examples of this integration include a joint referral system for services provided by a community health center and local public health department and the use of trained health department representatives within primary care offices in medically underserved areas to promote clinical preventive services and chronic disease management targeted by the health department.[48] These partnerships must overcome the obstacles of varied training backgrounds and perspectives; the isolation in which each sector operates, which contributes to a general lack of awareness of each other's activities and resources; and funding limitations. The ACA contains certain provisions aimed at alleviating this last hurdle, encouraging combined efforts and leveraging resources between public health and health care systems to achieve common goals.[51]

The CCM explored earlier was geared mainly toward clinically oriented systems and is difficult to apply for broader prevention and health promotion practices such as these. In 2003 Barr and colleagues proposed the Expanded Chronic Care Model (ECCM),[52] which includes elements of the population health promotion field so that broadly based prevention efforts, recognition of the social determinants of health, and enhanced community participation could also be integrated into the work of health system teams as they seek to address chronic disease issues. The ECCM includes three additional components in terms of community resources and policies: building healthy public policy, creating supportive environments, and strengthening community action. These interrelated components and relationships are shown in Figure 5-5.

The ECCM represents the shift from health care systems focused on illness and disability to community-oriented services that focus on primary prevention. Working on both the prevention and the treatment ends of the continuum from such a broad perspective offers the best potential for improved health outcomes in the long term.[52] This change is a vital element of responsible, accountable, and population-focused health care management in today's climate of health care reform and innovation.

One example of evolving mechanisms for community-based chronic disease prevention efforts is the integration of community health workers into clinical care teams. Known by a variety of names (community health adviser, outreach worker, *promotoras/ promotores de salud* [health promoters], patient navigator, and lay health adviser) these

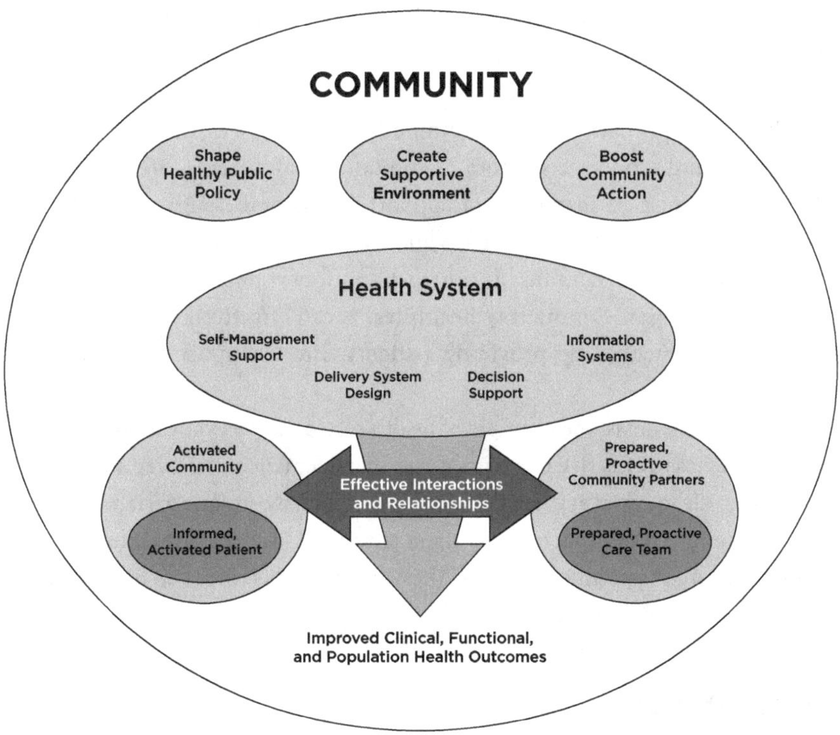

Source: Barr et al.[52] Adapted with permission of Longwoods Publishing.

Figure 5-5. The Expanded Chronic Care Model

are frontline public health workers who are trusted members of or possess an unusually close understanding of the community served. This relationship enables community health workers to be liaisons between health and social services and the community. This role both facilitates access to services and improves the quality and cultural competence of service delivery. Community health workers also build individual and community capacity by increasing health knowledge and self-sufficiency through activities such as outreach, community education, informal counseling, social support, and advocacy.[53]

In addition, community health workers can educate health care providers and administrators about the community's health needs and the cultural relevancy of interventions. Using their unique position, skills, and knowledge base, community health workers can help reduce system costs for chronic disease management. Mechanisms for these savings include linking patients to community resources, helping avoid unnecessary hospitalizations and other forms of more expensive care through improved and proactive disease management, and having an impact on the upstream determinants of disease.[53]

Using an even more robust concept for community–clinical linkages, Vermont's Blueprint for Health is an example of the ECCM in action. This statewide public–private initiative incorporates community health teams as a key aspect of the state's model to transform care delivery, improve health outcomes, and enable everyone in the state to receive seamless, well-coordinated care. These teams, supported by medical homes, comprise locally based, multidisciplinary members (e.g., nurse coordinators, community health workers, behavioral health counselors, dietitians, social workers) who provide a link between primary care and community-based services, connecting patients to medical, social, and economic support. Community health teams offer individual care coordination and disease management support, behavioral health counseling, health and wellness coaching, health system navigation, and teaching of self-management skills. In addition, they perform community outreach to support public health initiatives such as screening campaigns. Community health teams can effectively expand the capacity of primary care practices by providing patients direct support and individualized follow-up.

The Blueprint model is one example of health care delivery innovation incorporating various approaches to effective chronic disease management and prevention highlighted in this chapter. Although every health care system will have unique variables to consider when crafting effective approaches to address chronic disease according to their populations, resources, and operational climate, the Vermont experience can help inform these efforts at a local as well as national scale.[54]

MOVING FORWARD

It is now evident that health care systems will need creative and collaborative strategies to address chronic disease prevention and management at all levels of the prevention spectrum—from primary, to secondary, to tertiary prevention—if they are to make any noticeable impact on the concerning trends of chronic diseases in their populations. With proven frameworks as a guide, bolstered by health care reform incentives and innovative new models of care delivery, health care systems now have a robust toolkit for crafting strong prevention and care management systems to tackle chronic diseases, which can lead to significant cost savings and improved population health outcomes.

DISCUSSION QUESTIONS

1. Why should health care systems be concerned about chronic disease? What will happen if health care systems neglect to manage and prevent chronic disease in their populations?
2. Provide examples of successful health care reform initiatives that were supported by the ACA. What challenges and/or barriers do health care systems continue to face in moving health care reform forward?
3. What role should health care systems play in the prevention of chronic disease (as opposed to treatment of chronic disease)? Which external partners do health care systems need to engage in prevention initiatives to successfully affect community and population health?

REFERENCES

1. Boersma P, Black LI, Ward BW. Prevalence of multiple chronic conditions among US adults, 2018. *Prev Chronic Dis.* 2020;17:200130.
2. Agency for Healthcare Research and Quality. Advancing patient-centered care for people living with multiple chronic conditions. 2014. Updated December 2022. Available at: https://www.ahrq.gov/patient-safety/settings/long-term-care/resource/multichronic/mcc.html. Accessed January 10, 2023.
3. Anderson G. *Chronic Care: Making the Case for Ongoing Care.* Princeton, NJ: Robert Wood Johnson Foundation; 2010.
4. Parekh AK, Goodman RA, Gordon C, Koh HK; The HHS Interagency Workgroup on Multiple Chronic Conditions. Managing multiple chronic conditions: a strategic framework for improving health outcomes and quality of life. *Public Health Rep.* 2011;126(4):460–471.
5. Michener JL, Briss P. Health systems approaches to preventing chronic disease: new partners, new tools, and new strategies. *Prev Chronic Dis.* 2019;16:190248.
6. Marks S, Levin D; Amatihealth. Population health methodology, step 2: stratification. Blogpost, 2015. Available at: http://amatihealth.com/blog/2015/6/3/population-health-methodology-step-2-stratification. Accessed March 30, 2016.
7. Nash DB. The population health mandate: a broader approach to care delivery. The Boardroom Press. The Governance Institute. 2012. Available at: http://www.populationhealthcolloquium.com/readings/Pop_Health_Mandate_NASH_2012.pdf. Accessed January 10, 2023.

8. Kindig D, Stoddart G. What is population health? *Am J Public Health*. 2003;93(3):380–383.
9. Abrams MK, Nuzum R, Zezza MA, et al. The Affordable Care Act's payment and delivery system reforms: a progress report at five years. The Commonwealth Fund. May 7, 2015. Available at: https://www.commonwealthfund.org/publications/issue-briefs/2015/may/affordable-care-acts-payment-and-delivery-system-reforms. Accessed January 10, 2023.
10. Bauer UE, Briss PA, Goodman RA, Bowman BA. Prevention of chronic disease in the 21st century: elimination of the leading preventable causes of premature death and disability in the USA. *Lancet*. 2014;384(9937):45–52.
11. Remington PL, Catlin BB, Gennuso KP. The County Health Rankings: rationale and methods. *Popul Health Metr*. 2015;13:11.
12. Centers for Medicare and Medicaid Services. State Innovation Models Initiative: general information. Updated September 14, 2022. Available at: https://innovation.cms.gov/innovation-models/state-innovations. Accessed January 10, 2023.
13. Health Care Transformation Taskforce. The Center for Medicare and Medicaid Innovation: paving the way for value-based payment reform. September 2020. Available at: https://hcttf.org/wp-content/uploads/2020/10/HCTTF-Assessment_Impact-of-CMMI.pdf. Accessed January 10, 2023.
14. Centers for Medicare and Medicaid Services. Medicare Shared Savings Program. Shared Savings Program fast facts—as of January 1, 2022. Available at: https://www.cms.gov/files/document/2022-shared-savings-program-fast-facts.pdf. Accessed January 10, 2023.
15. Centers for Medicare and Medicaid Services. Affordable Care Act's Shared Savings Program continues to improve quality of care while saving Medicare money during the COVID-19 pandemic. CMS.gov Newsroom. August 25, 2021. Available at: https://www.cms.gov/newsroom/press-releases/affordable-care-acts-shared-savings-program-continues-improve-quality-care-while-saving-medicare. Accessed January 10, 2023.
16. Health Care Transformation Taskforce. Accountable care organizations: a gateway to a value-based delivery system. September 2020. Available at: https://hcttf.org/wp-content/uploads/2020/10/HCTTF-Assessment_-Impact-of-ACOs.pdf. Accessed January 10, 2023.
17. Health Care Transformation Taskforce. Impact of the Bundled Payment for Care Improvement Advanced Initiative. Available at: https://hcttf.org/wp-content/uploads/2021/04/HCTTF-Assessment_Impact-of-BPCIA_updated042021.pdf. Accessed January 10, 2023.
18. Nielsen M, Gibson A, Buelt L, Grundy P, Grumbach K. The patient-centered medical home's impact on cost and quality: annual review of evidence, 2013–2014. Patient-Centered Primary Care Collaborative, Milbank Memorial Fund. 2015. Available at: http://www.milbank.org/uploads/documents/reports/PCPCC_2015_Evidence_Report.pdf. Accessed January 10, 2023.
19. Center for Medicare and Medicaid Innovation. 2020 report to Congress. 2021. Available at: https://innovation.cms.gov/data-and-reports/2021/rtc-2020. Accessed January 10, 2023.
20. Centers for Medicare and Medicaid Services. Strategic direction. Available at: https://innovation.cms.gov/strategic-direction. Accessed January 10, 2023.
21. Wagner E. Chronic disease management: what will it take to improve care for chronic illness? *Eff Clin Pract*. 1998;1(1):2–4.
22. Fiandt K. The Chronic Care Model: description and application for practice. *Top Adv Prac Nurs eJ*. 2006;6(4).

23. Bodenheimer T, Wagner EH, Grumbach K. Improving primary care for patients with chronic illness. *JAMA*. 2002;288(15):1909–1914.
24. Agency for Healthcare Research and Quality. Care coordination. June 2014. Updated August 2018. Available at: http://www.ahrq.gov/professionals/prevention-chronic-care/improve/coordination/index.html. Accessed January 10, 2023.
25. Goodell S, Bodenheimer T, Berry-Millett R. *Care Management of Patients With Complex Health Care Needs*. Princeton, NJ: Robert Wood Johnson Foundation; 2009.
26. Agency for Healthcare Research and Quality. Clinical decision support. 2015. Available at: https://www.ahrq.gov/cpi/about/otherwebsites/clinical-decision-support/index.html. Accessed January 10, 2023.
27. Agency for Healthcare Research and Quality. Health information exchange. 2016. Archived. Available at: https://healthit.ahrq.gov/key-topics/health-information-exchange#projects. Accessed January 10, 2023.
28. Agency for Healthcare Research and Quality. Decisionmaker brief: chronic disease management. 2008. AHRQ publication 08-0084. Available at: https://digital.ahrq.gov/sites/default/files/docs/page/08-0084_cdm_0.pdf. Accessed January 10, 2023.
29. Nash DB, Reifsnyder J, Fabius RJ, Skoufalos A, Clarke JL. *Population Health: Creating a Culture of Wellness*. Burlington, MA: Jones and Bartlett Publishers; 2015:1–15.
30. National Council on Aging. Chronic disease self-management. 2015. Available at: https://www.ncoa.org/wp-content/uploads/Chronic-Disease-Fact-Sheet_Final-Sept-2015.pdf. Accessed April 10, 2016.
31. Ory MG, Ahn S, Jiang L, et al. Successes of a national study of the chronic disease self-management program. *Med Care*. 2013;51(11):992–998.
32. Hibbard J, Gilbert H. *Supporting People to Manage Their Health: An Introduction to Patient Activation*. London, UK: The King's Fund; 2014.
33. Greene J, Hibbard JH, Sacks R, Overton V, Parrotta CD. When patient activation levels change, health outcomes and costs change, too. *Health Aff (Millwood)*. 2015;34(3):431–437.
34. The Chronic Care Model. Center for Accelerating Care Transformation (ACT Center). Available at: https://www.act-center.org/application/files/1616/3511/6445/Model_Chronic_Care.pdf. Accessed January 10, 2023.
35. Coleman K, Austin BT, Brach C, Wagner EH. Evidence on the Chronic Care Model in the new millennium. *Health Aff (Millwood)*. 2009;28(1):75–85.
36. Stock S, Pitcavage JM, Simic D, et al. Chronic Care Model strategies in the United States and Germany deliver patient-centered, high-quality diabetes care. *Health Aff (Millwood)*. 2014;33(9):1540–1548.
37. US Department of Health and Human Services. Multiple chronic conditions: a strategic framework: optimum health and quality of life for individuals with multiple chronic conditions. December 2010. Available at: https://www.hhs.gov/sites/default/files/ash/initiatives/mcc/mcc_framework.pdf. Accessed January 10, 2023.
38. Yarnall KSH, Pollak KI, Østbye T, Krause KM, Michener JL. Primary care: is there enough time for prevention? *Am J Public Health*. 2003;93(4):635–641.
39. Rosenthal M, Abrams M, Bitton A; Patient-Centered Medical Home Evaluators' Collaborative. Data brief: recommended core measures for evaluating the patient-centered medical

home: cost, utilization, and clinical quality. The Commonwealth Fund. May 2012. Available at: http://www.commonwealthfund.org/~/media/files/publications/data-brief/2012/1601_rosenthal_recommended_core_measures_pcmh_v2.pdf. Accessed January 10, 2023.

40. Jackson GL, Powers BJ, Chatterjee R, et al. Improving patient care: the patient centered medical home: a systematic review. *Ann Intern Med.* 2013;158(3):169–178.
41. Markovitz AR, Alexander JA, Lantz PM, Paustian ML. Patient-centered medical home implementation and use of preventive services. The role of practice socioeconomic context. *JAMA Intern Med.* 2015;175(4):598–606.
42. Nagykaldi Z, Aspy CB, Chou A, Mold JW. Impact of a wellness portal on the delivery of patient-centered preventive care. *J Am Board Fam Med.* 2012;25(2):158–167.
43. George J, Zairina E. The potential role of pharmacists in chronic disease screening. *Int J Pharm Pract.* 2016;24(1):3–5.
44. Shearer G. Prevention provisions in the Affordable Care Act. APHA Issue Brief. October 2010. Available at: https://www.apha.org/~/media/files/pdf/topics/aca/prevention_aca_final.ashx. Accessed January 10, 2023.
45. Koh H. Statement to the Committee on Health, Education, Labor and Pensions, United States Senate. The state of chronic disease prevention. October 12, 2011. Available at: https://www.govinfo.gov/content/pkg/CHRG-112shrg87561/pdf/CHRG-112shrg87561.pdf. Accessed January 10, 2023.
46. Levi J, Segal LM, Juliano C. Prevention for a healthier America: investments in disease prevention yield significant savings, stronger communities. Trust for America's Health. 2009. Available at: http://resource.nlm.nih.gov/101511510. Accessed January 10, 2023.
47. Kindig D, Isham G. Population health improvement: a community health business model that engages partners in all sectors. *Front Health Serv Manage.* 2014;30(4):3–20.
48. Koo D, Felix K, Dankwa-Mullan I, Miller T, Waalen J. A call for action on primary care and public health integration. *Am J Public Health.* 2012;102(S3):S307–S309.
49. Institute of Medicine. *Living Well With Chronic Illness: A Call for Public Health Action.* Washington, DC: National Academies Press; 2012.
50. Institute of Medicine. *Primary Care and Public Health: Exploring Integration to Improve Population Health.* Washington, DC: National Academies Press; 2012. Available at: https://doi.org/10.17226/13381. Accessed January 10, 2023.
51. Elliott L, Mcbride TD, Allen P, et al. Health care system collaboration to address chronic diseases: a nationwide snapshot from state public health practitioners. *Prev Chronic Dis.* 2014;11:E152.
52. Barr V, Robinson S, Marin-Link B, et al. The expanded Chronic Care Model: an integration of concepts and strategies from population health promotion and the Chronic Care Model. *Hosp Q.* 2003;7(1):73–82.
53. Brownstein JN, Hirsch GR, Rosenthal EL, Rush CH. Community health workers "101" for primary care providers and other stakeholders in health care systems. *J Ambul Care Manage.* 2011;34(3):210–220.
54. Bielaszka-DuVernay C. Vermont's blueprint for medical homes, community health teams, and better health at lower cost. *Health Aff (Millwood).* 2011;30(3):383–386.

II. UPSTREAM RISK FACTORS

6

The Social Determinants of Chronic Disease

Carlyn M. Hood-Ronick, MPA, MPH, Parvathy Pillai, MD, MPH,
and Paula M. Lantz, PhD, MS

LEARNING OBJECTIVES

After completing this chapter, readers should be able to

1. Describe the multilevel (macro/structural, neighborhood/community, individual) factors that drive health differences.
2. Apply a framework to chronic diseases that includes pathways by which multilevel factors lead to positive, negative, and disparate health outcomes.
3. Explore how more proximate metrics, such as food, housing, and education, affect health and are ultimately shaped by public policy.
4. Identify challenges and future areas of research related to the interconnected nature of social and structural determinants of health.

INTRODUCTION

Places where people live, learn, work, pray, and play affect a wide range of health risks and outcomes.[1] The conditions of these places and how they are shaped through social, political, and economic forces are known as the social determinants of health. These determinants include an array of upstream or macro-level structural, system and neighborhood/community-level factors that drive differences in individual socioeconomic status (SES)—including income, employment, and education—that in turn create differences in individuals' exposure to the multitude of factors that matter for health. In sum, the social determinants of health represent a complex array of factors at the macro, mezzo, and micro levels of society that shape individuals' health-related opportunities, resources, and advantages and also their risks, exposures, and disadvantages in synergistic ways over the life course.[2]

While there are varying definitions and models of the social determinants of health, the key overarching theme is that health and health inequities are socially produced by myriad cultural, social, economic, and political factors that extend far beyond the reach of medicine and the health care system. Research suggests that these factors—collectively defined as "social"—drive approximately half of all individual health outcomes[3] and are especially important for understanding and addressing social and racial/ethnic disparities in chronic disease.[4] As such, it is important to recognize these factors and their powerful and sustained influence on chronic disease risk, disease, premature death, and mortality in the population.

This chapter addresses the social determinants of health, with a focus on the factors that play a major role in chronic disease risk and development and on the pathways by which such factors lead to positive, negative, and disparate health outcomes. It will be helpful to review these concepts within the framework used throughout this text, considering the causes of more proximate determinants, the pathways by which social factors influence health, and what positions subpopulations and particular groups at higher risk (Figure 6-1).

A key point to emphasize is that while the social drivers of health are visible in individual circumstances, risk factors, exposures, and behaviors, they operate at and must be addressed at levels above and beyond the individual. For example, it is well documented that achieving optimum health and minimizing the risk of chronic disease occurs through such health-promoting behaviors as eating well, staying physically active, avoiding smoking and excessive alcohol consumption, and receiving appropriate clinical preventive services.[5] However, the ability to trust and adhere to behavioral recommendations is influenced not only by individual knowledge and psychosocial factors but also by family and cultural contexts, community/neighborhood environments and resources, and structural/system-level factors including food systems, transportation

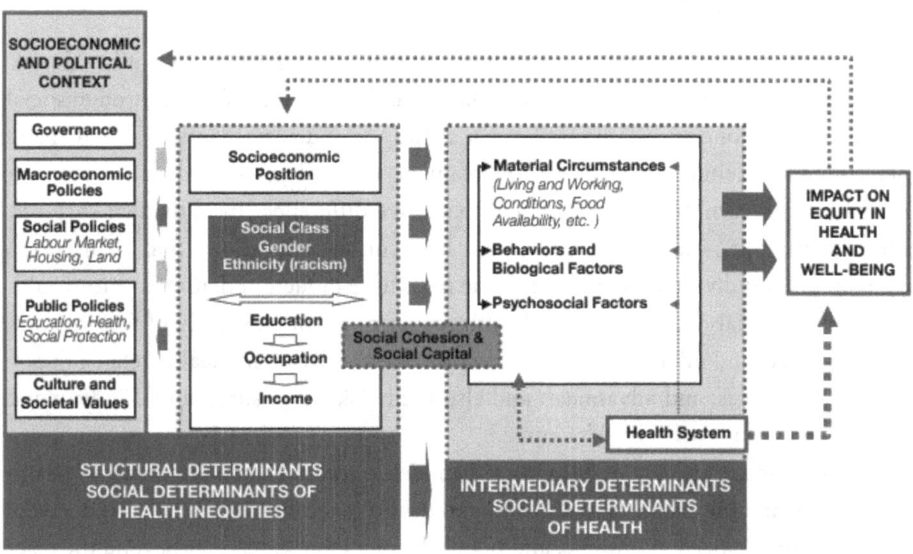

Source: Solar and Irwin.[2] Reprinted with permission of WHO.

Figure 6-1. World Health Organization Conceptual Framework

systems, education quality, public safety, and a wide array of public policies that sometimes reinforce rather than mitigate socioeconomic and racial inequities.

UPSTREAM DRIVERS AND DOWNSTREAM CONSEQUENCES

Conceptual Model

The World Health Organization (WHO) has developed a conceptual model of the social determinants of health that attempts to elucidate how macro-level social, economic, and political systems and structures produce significant stratification in society by factors such as income, education, occupation, wealth, race/ethnicity, and gender.[2]

It is the upstream structural determinants of health—including macroeconomic forces, public policies, and cultural factors—that drive the socioeconomic stratification (what social epidemiologist Nancy Krieger calls "structured chance") in society that in turn shapes both neighborhood and individual risk factors, exposures, disadvantages versus resources, power, and advantages.[6] Individuals can have important social needs such as food, income, housing, and health insurance, but these needs are not the social determinants of health. Again, the social drivers of health and health disparities are primarily upstream at the macro and mezzo (neighborhood/community) levels, which conspire to create individual social needs and ultimately downstream health outcomes.

Figure 6-2 summarizes how the WHO model can be used to understand a specific health behavior—physical inactivity—emphasizing that it is the macro-level systems,

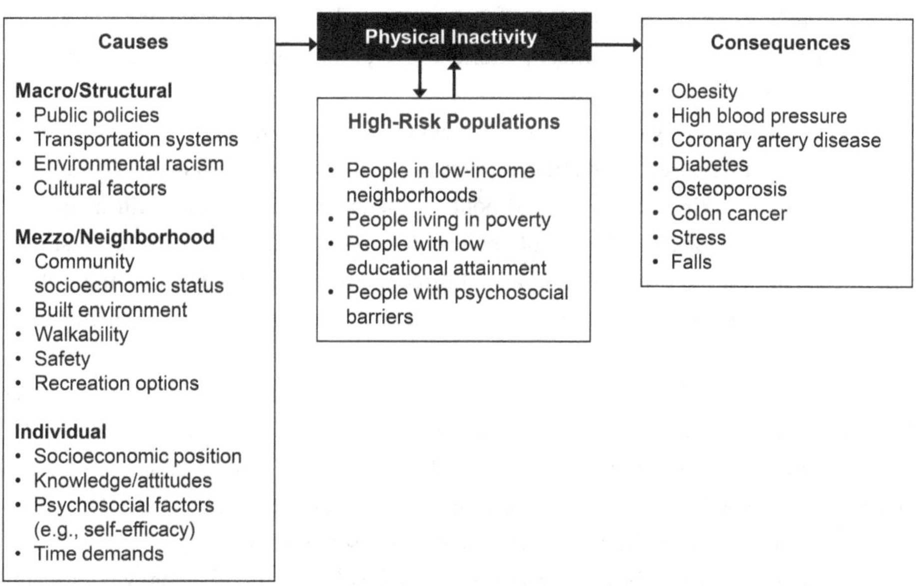

Figure 6-2. Physical Inactivity: Causes, Consequences, and High-Risk Populations

structures, and policies that drive the myriad ways in which an individual might understand, have access to, time for, and/or ability to afford the resources necessary to support being physically active. These macro- and mezzo-level forces affect the downstream outcomes such as one's material conditions, health behaviors (like being physically active), psychosocial factors, access to health care services, and ultimately the increased risk of disease, disability, and premature death. Importantly, the social factors that provide health-promoting benefits, resources, and advantages for some versus health risks, exposures, and disadvantages for others occur and accumulate over the entire life course.

Macro-Level/Structural Factors and Racism

WHO defines the structural, upstream socioeconomic and political contexts as "the system of values, policies and institutions by which society manages economic, political and social affairs through interactions within and among the state, civil society and private sector."[2] These powerful factors drive the ways in which a society allocates resources and develops policy to address issues, including those related to social inequality.

Several scholars and policy advocates have emphasized the need to focus on the structural, upstream determinants of social inequality in efforts to research or develop policy that addresses population health outcomes and inequities.[7] The primary or fundamental social determinants of health are the systems, institutions, and policies that create, codify, reaffirm, and sometimes reform the more proximate determinants of health and health inequity. This includes what has come to be labeled as the "commercial determinants of health" or the ways in which private markets/marketing for products such as tobacco, alcohol, and highly processed foods and associated regulatory and policy systems operate to generate profit in ways that affect patterns of risk, illness, injury, disability, and death within and across populations.[8]

There is also a growing focus on the role that public policy at the local, state, and federal levels plays in addressing and creating, reinforcing, and sustaining systems and conditions that produce the social, economic, and political inequality that drives health inequality. This includes a key focus on the role of public policy in systemic and structural racism. As Jones[9] explains, racism primarily operates at three levels in societies: (1) racism by which systems of culture/ideology/entrenched norms and structures such as laws, regulations, and institutional practices differentially provide access to resources, goods, services, and opportunities by race; (2) personally mediated racism between individuals, which includes both intentional and unintentional prejudice (differential assumptions about the worth, motives, and abilities of others by race) and discrimination (differential actions toward others by race); and (3) internalized racism or the acceptance of negative societal messages about one's own worth, abilities, opportunities, and deservedness.[9]

Braveman et al.[10] describe how design elements deeply embedded in many US systems and structures are racist (prejudicial and/or discriminatory) and damage health through many causal pathways, including material deprivation, economic and social disadvantage, increased negative exposures, and stress processes. Some examples include political disempowerment and disenfranchisement, residential segregation, and the concentration of advantage and disadvantage in neighborhoods; discriminatory lending policies and their historical negative impact on Black homeownership, economic mobility, and wealth accumulation; environmental racism; and the significant racial differences in every aspect of the criminal justice system. As Jones has articulated, "Race is a social construct, a social classification based on phenotype, that governs the distribution of risks and opportunities in our race-conscious society."[9] As such, it is racism at all levels, not race, that drives and explains persistent racial disparities in virtually every social and health outcome in the United States.

A growing amount of research regarding self-reported experiences of discrimination on the basis of race, ethnicity, and social class demonstrates significant associations with a number of health outcomes.[11,12] The research literature is most developed in the case of perceived racial/ethnic discrimination and mental health disorders (i.e., depression, anxiety disorders) and the physical health outcomes of hypertension and low birth weight.[13–15] Strong associations between perceived discrimination and some health outcomes have been observed in longitudinal studies after adjusting for psychosocial and other potential confounders.[16] Nonetheless, as described later in the Moving Forward section of this chapter, causal inference is a significant challenge, along with measurement challenges and the difficulty of observing institutional or structural discrimination.[11,15,16]

Mezzo-Level/Neighborhood Factors

Neighborhood factors and conditions can provide both health benefits/advantages and health risks/disadvantages and are driven in large part by the systemic and structural factors described in the foregoing. Macintyre et al.[17] identified five main features of neighborhoods that are related to health: (1) the physical infrastructure and environment shared by residents, including water, air, and street and sidewalk conditions; (2) the level of risk in the environments in which people work, play, and rest; (3) the quality of public and private services provided to residents, such as garbage removal, police protection, and social services; (4) sociocultural features of neighborhoods, including norms, values, social cohesion, social networks, and civic engagement; and (5) the reputation of a neighborhood, which signals how it is perceived by residents and nonresidents and involves shared community morale.[17]

A growing body of neighborhood effects research has shown that neighborhood context plays a critically important role in producing disparities in major health risk behaviors and their related outcomes.[18] For example, many features of the built environment and urban design (including land-use patterns, sidewalks, transportation systems, and street connectivity) are associated with physical activity and other features of mobility important to health.[18] (For detailed information on this concept, see Chapter 9 on physical activity.) Similarly, neighborhood characteristics such as the absence of grocery stores and the types of food available are associated with dietary patterns and obesity rates across communities. One US study found that features of urban food deserts, such as distance between stores and high prices, were associated with obesity and that price was the main driver of this relationship.[19] (For more detailed information on these concepts, see Chapter 8 on diet and nutrition and Chapter 11 on obesity.)

A recent literature review of 53 longitudinal studies of the effects of long-term neighborhood deprivation on health suggests that the effects of living in a low-socioeconomic neighborhood accumulate over the life course when exposure is sustained.[20] Neighborhood context was found to have an effect above and beyond individual SES for a number of health outcomes, including smoking, body mass index, chronic conditions, functional symptoms, disability, allostatic load, and all-cause mortality.

Another critically important part of material conditions is the physical environment, including air and water quality. Recent literature has documented that neighborhoods or communities with high levels of poverty and unemployment are significantly more likely to experience air pollution, water pollution, and other environmental hazards.[21] The unequal and disproportionate exposure of poor, minority, and marginalized populations to environmental hazards has been labeled environmental injustice and is viewed as a contributing factor to socioeconomic and racial/ethnic health status inequities.[22]

In the past 50 years there has been a significant increase in research attempting to link neighborhood socioeconomic, cultural, institutional, and physical conditions with health outcomes and using the conditions as an explanation for persistent social inequalities in health.[18] Neighborhood effects research, however, is challenging both conceptually and methodologically. It is difficult to control for neighborhood selection processes and to take into account cumulative exposures, lagged effects, and the dynamic nature of neighborhood contexts.[23]

Micro-Level/Individual Factors

The documented links between individual SES and health are consistent across time and geography and a variety of outcomes.[24] This includes chronic disease, as most health risks and exposures related to cancer, cardiovascular disease, and other chronic illnesses are patterned by SES. For example, individuals with low educational attainment and low income are more likely to smoke,[25] less likely to engage in physical activity, and less physically fit than their higher-income peers,[26] and they are less likely to consume fiber and fresh fruits and vegetables.[27] Research has clearly demonstrated that education promotes knowledge and life skills, which increase access to information and resources that promote health.[28] In addition, education builds occupational opportunities and earning potential, which in turn can lead to better nutrition, housing, schooling, and recreation.[28]

Research that attempts to distinguish the effects of education and income suggests that education is more strongly related to the onset of illness and chronic conditions, and income is more predictive of health trajectories and mortality after illness onset.[29]

The ways in which upstream social drivers of health influence the intermediary or more downstream determinants of health and create health inequities within populations are multiple and interrelated.[30] As described, these intermediary or more proximate determinants can be categorized as (1) pathways that work through material living conditions, (2) health-promoting and health risk behaviors, (3) psychosocial risk factors, and (4) access to and receipt of high-quality health care services. In addition, as emphasized earlier, these exposures and risk factors work at both the individual and contextual levels, including at the neighborhood and policy levels.

By applying what is known about the social determinants of health, improvements in individual and population health can be realized along with advancements in health equity.[31,32] This is especially important for the field of public health as we focus on prevention and control of chronic disease. Some key takeaways from a large and growing body of research regarding the social determinants of health include the following:

- The social determinants of health affect everyone, as they drive all the ways—positive and negative—in which social, economic, commercial, and political factors affect the health of populations, communities, and individuals.
- The social determinants of health are factors that primarily operate at the macro/structural and mezzo levels of society.
- While identifying and meeting individual social and material needs (e.g., food insecurity, housing insecurity, poverty, lack of transportation, exposure to violence) is necessary for individual health and well-being, this does not constitute addressing the social determinants of health. Only focusing on individual needs is downstream from the actual structural and system drivers of poor health outcomes and inequality.
- Policy and system reform and new, innovative interventions are needed at all levels to address outcomes, including chronic disease incidence, mortality, and inequities (discussed in more detail later in this chapter).

PUBLIC HEALTH IMPACT

The burden of chronic disease is large and growing in every country and is a serious global public health problem. Chronic diseases are among the most prevalent and costly health conditions in the United States. Nearly half of all Americans (approximately 45%, or 133 million) suffer from at least one chronic disease, and these illnesses account for 75% of aggregate health care spending.[33]

The structural factors laid out above affect several key intermediate influences that in turn lead to the greatest chronic disease burden and resulting public health impact: poverty, education attainment (and resulting ability to pay for food, housing, and health care) and health behaviors. This section of the chapter highlights the specific way these factors lead to poor outcomes and can have a large and multigenerational impact on the public's health.

Poverty and Education

There is ample evidence within and across societies that SES is highly correlated with the material conditions needed for individual and community well-being, including financial resources, food, shelter, transportation, health care, and safe environments.[30,34] Adults with low levels of income and education and their children have high rates of nearly every major health risk factor or health-damaging process, creating health inequities over the entire life course. Having higher levels of education and income affords individuals not only with the material conditions that are essential for health (e.g., security in income, healthy food, clothing, clean and safe shelter, and health care) but also with a number of other resources that are fundamental to the production of health.[35] These include knowledge (through education), power, prestige, access to health-promoting technology, and beneficial social relationships. Also included are the resources to be mobile and to select neighborhood, school, and employment contexts that bring individual benefits and that also build social capital.[36]

Importantly, there is growing evidence that income security is extremely important for the health and well-being of infants and children over the life course. The results of numerous studies suggest that children's development and health is greatly affected by the social environments in which they are raised and that exposure to childhood abuse, trauma, neglect, and poverty is linked to a number of chronic conditions in adulthood through multiple physiological pathways.[37]

People living in poverty may struggle to pay their rent, buy food, bear the costs of transportation, purchase education-related supplies for their children, pay for health care, and provide other material necessities for well-being (food, quality housing) and often have to make difficult trade-offs.[38] Food insecurity is a serious problem in low-income families, even in high-income countries. Adults who experience food insecurity have higher rates of physical and mental health problems and lower self-reported health than the rest of the population.[39] Individuals and families with few financial resources are also more likely to experience homelessness and/or housing instability and unhealthy and unsafe housing conditions.[40] Housing is an important material condition for health, and one of the most researched. Based on the existing research evidence, Taylor summarizes that housing has several methods by which it can support/hurt health outcomes and health care costs: (1) housing stability; (2) home quality and safety problems; (3) housing affordability; and (4) neighborhood conditions.[41]

Along with food and housing, health care remains a challenge for individuals who cannot afford it. A plethora of research demonstrates that people with few socioeconomic resources underuse health care services relative to their needs, are more likely to delay or forgo diagnostic and treatment services because of financial concerns, and are less likely to receive evidence-based clinical preventive services, including immunizations, teeth cleaning, cancer screening, and behavioral counseling.[42] In an assessment of the Affordable Care Act (ACA) at its tenth anniversary, Lantz and Rosenbaum concluded that there is significant evidence that the ACA has reduced social disparities in key health care outcomes, including insurance coverage, health care access, and the use of primary care.[43] In addition, research evidence suggests that the part of the ACA that has had the greatest impact on reducing socioeconomic and racial disparities in health outcomes, including in preterm births and mortality, is the Medicaid expansion.[44,45]

Health Behaviors

The majority of health-related behavioral risk factors are patterned by income and educational attainment.[46] An inverse relationship between individual SES and health risk behaviors (i.e., as SES increases, the prevalence of risky behavior decreases) has been observed for a wide variety of behaviors, including but not limited to tobacco use, illicit drug use, obesity, physical inactivity, sexual risk-taking, driving while intoxicated, and not wearing a helmet on a bicycle or motorcycle.

For example, although there are some differences in the epidemiology of tobacco use across countries, a prominent pattern is higher rates of cigarette smoking and other forms of tobacco use among people of lower socioeconomic position.[47] The socioeconomic background of individuals and the contexts in which they live, work, and age play a major role in creating the underlying disparities in the risk factors and exposures and are challenging to modify.[36] As information regarding the health risks of tobacco use has been disseminated and as policies, technologies, and resources for smoking prevention and cessation have been implemented and supported, socioeconomic disparities in tobacco use have widened.[48] This is an important illustration of how the deployment of resources (e.g., money, knowledge, expertise, access to technology, and positive policy attention) is a critical component of how SES influences, maintains, and sometimes exacerbates health disparities beyond simply the differential prevalence of risk behavior across social strata.[36,47]

Public Health Impacts of the COVID-19 Pandemic

The COVID-19 pandemic not only highlighted but also exacerbated inequities by socioeconomic strata across the country and globe. Ability to adhere to public health official guidance to prevent contraction of the virus has not been possible for all populations, including those who rely on frontline work to earn a living; families, individuals, and groups living in crowded spaces or houseless scenarios; and individuals unable to consistently handwash because of a lack of water. (The descriptive epidemiology portion of this chapter provides more detail on this issue.)

The field of public health itself will likely take new form as the work that has historically been underfunded and scarcely staffed to accomplish public health priorities evolves and changes post-pandemic. Many public health workers have been or were redeployed to COVID-19-related duties during the pandemic response, deprioritizing or suspending other critical public health issues by as much as 40% in the chronic disease realm.[49] And many others—often the most experienced with similar pandemic-related issues like H1N1, Zika, or Ebola—are burnt out or retiring.[49] The impact on chronic disease in years to come could be great.

PATHOPHYSIOLOGY

The social determinants of health influence individual health outcomes by structuring exposures and risks across the life course, especially as they relate to the material conditions of health. However, socioeconomic and racial inequality and disadvantage also influence health through stress and other psychosocial factors through complex physiologic pathways. Multiple regions of the brain are thought to play a role in recognizing and responding to stress, which in turn regulate hormone production through various pathways. These pathways include the hypothalamic-pituitary-adrenal (HPA) axis and the sympathetic nervous system. Activation of the HPA axis as part of the stress response results in the production of glucocorticoids, including cortisol. Cortisol, a steroid hormone, regulates multiple other physiological processes, among them those involving the metabolic, cardiovascular, and immune systems. Activation of the sympathetic nervous system results in the production of catecholamines, including epinephrine and norepinephrine, which also have a wide range of systemic effects, including increasing heart rate and blood pressure.[50]

The interaction of these multiple systems is critical in adapting to stressors, a process termed allostasis. However, over time these adaptations can have adverse effects, described as the allostatic load. It has been postulated that chronic stress, especially those experiences early in life, can result in pathophysiologic changes and adverse health outcomes through multiple hypothesized mechanisms, including those involving altered neuroplasticity, insulin resistance, immunosuppression, and epigenetic modifications.[50,51]

DESCRIPTIVE EPIDEMIOLOGY

It has been well recognized across multiple health conditions that populations experiencing inequities across social determinants, in turn the result of structural determinants, have faced worse health outcomes than populations who have not be subjected to such inequities.[52,53] As a variety of studies have shown, housing, for example, acts as a social determinant resulting in stark health differences between those identifying as homeless and those housed: individuals without housing are more likely to have depression, anxiety, hypertension, cardiovascular disease, asthma, and/or tuberculosis.[54,55]

Although the social determinants on health and their impact did not suddenly emerge because of COVID-19, the pandemic has nonetheless shone a spotlight on their importance.[52] Increasingly recognized associations between chronic disease conditions and COVID-19 include the following: increased risk of severe COVID-19 infection for those with underlying chronic diseases; decreased health care utilization secondary to the pandemic, resulting in decreased chronic disease prevention and care; and potential long-term impacts of COVID-19.[56]

High-Risk Populations

Greater exposure due to occupational and housing circumstances, less access to current health information, less access to quality health care services, and greater risk for comorbid conditions have been described as challenges that place certain communities, including low-income, non-US-born, and communities of color, at higher risk for adverse COVID-19 disease and adverse health outcomes.[53] However, it is important to recognize that these populations and those that face intersecting challenges, such as racial/ethnic minority status and low educational attainment level,[57] experience elevated risk for COVID-19 not because of intrinsic factors, but rather because of structural inequities that have led to differential exposure to upstream and downstream protective factors and risk factors that drive health over the life course.

Multiple studies have examined race/ethnicity-related inequities in COVID-19, with Karmakar and colleagues noting that racial/ethnic disparities seen in descriptive statistics represent underlying disparities in macro- and mezzo-level determinants of health, including structural racism.[58] In the United States, rates of COVID-19 infection have been shown to be higher among non-Hispanic American Indian/Alaska Native, non-Hispanic Black, and Hispanic populations relative to non-Hispanic White populations. These trends remained consistent even when examining multiple methods for grouping race and ethnicity.[59] As seen in Table 6-1, as of March 2022 marked racial/ethnic

Table 6-1. Risk for COVID-19 Infection, Hospitalization, and Death by Race/Ethnicity

Rate ratios compared to White, Non-Hispanic persons	American Indian or Alaska Native, Non-Hispanic persons	Asian, Non-Hispanic persons	Black or African American, Non-Hispanic persons	Hispanic or Latino persons
Cases[1]	1.6x	0.7x	1.1x	1.5x
Hospitalization[2]	3.1x	0.8x	2.4x	2.3x
Death[3]	2.1x	0.8x	1.7x	1.8x

Race and ethnicity are risk markers for other underlying conditions that affect health, including socioeconomic status, access to health care, and exposure to the virus related to occupation, e.g., frontline, essential, and critical infrastructure workers.

Source: Reprinted from CDC.[60]

inequities exist not only across age-adjusted COVID-19 case rates but also for age-adjusted COVID-19-related hospitalizations and age-adjusted death rate for COVID-19.[61] Additional racial/ethnic inequities have also been demonstrated with regard to COVID-19 outpatient treatment and vaccination.[58,62]

Geographic Distribution and Time Trends

While the US Centers for Disease Control and Prevention's Social Vulnerability Index (SVI) includes community-level data on race/ethnicity, its use has allowed for the examination of the role of additional community-level social factors in the COVID-19 pandemic. The SVI ranks census tract-level data on 15 population-based social indicators grouped into four categories: (1) SES; (2) household composition and disability; (3) racial/ethnic minority status and English proficiency; and (4) housing type and transportation.[63] Higher SVI, indicating greater social vulnerability, has been associated with increased COVID-19 incidence and mortality, overall and across all four subcategories.[56] In addition, when COVID-19 vaccination coverage was examined by overall SVI, first-dose vaccine coverage was greater in low-social-vulnerability counties compared with high-social-vulnerability counties, with similar findings seen across the SES, household composition and disability, racial/ethnic minority status, and English proficiency SVI subcategories.[61]

In summer 2020, counties with higher SVIs were noted to more likely become COVID-19 hotspots (i.e., counties with rapidly increasing COVID-19 incidence) and had a higher incidence of COVID-19 after becoming a hotspot.[63] Examining the subcomponents of the SVI, counties with a high percentage of racial/ethnic minority residents, high-density housing structures, and crowded housing conditions were at greater risk of becoming a COVID-19 hotspot, particularly in less urban areas.[63] Furthermore, racial/ethnic inequities have been noted throughout the course of the pandemic and have been shown to widen during pandemic surges.[64,65] How multiple different components of social vulnerability—including but not limited to race/ethnicity—interplay with COVID-19 disease, treatment, and outcomes serves as a critical and timely reminder of the need to ensure that health professionals, public health providers, and policymakers understand and proactively influence these macro- and mezzo-level factors to improve the health of our communities.

It should be noted that the links between SES and health have been well documented and are consistent across time, well beyond the onset of COVID-19. Having higher levels of education and income not only affords individuals the material conditions essential for health (e.g., security in income, healthy food, clothing, clean and safe shelter, health care) but also provides them a number of other resources that are fundamental to the production of health,[66,67] such as knowledge (through education), power, prestige, access to health-promoting technology, and beneficial social relationships.

Additional advantages include the resources to be mobile and to select neighborhood, school, and employment contexts that bring individual benefits and build social capital.[67]

IMPLICATIONS FOR POLICY AND PRACTICE

The upstream structural and systemic drivers of the more proximate social determinants of health—such as poverty, low educational attainment, low-paying jobs, or unemployment—are inextricably related to broad social and economic policies and the political context of communities, states, and the nation. A comprehensive analysis of the root causes of inequities in the social determinants and potential policy responses is beyond the scope of this chapter. However, the following section describes four main implications of the social determinants of chronic disease for public policy and public health/clinical practice:

- The prevention and control of chronic illness requires interventions beyond changing individual health behaviors and increasing access to medical care.
- The social determinants of health are not a checklist of patient or individual social and economic needs. Upstream policy reform is needed to shift and create more equitable distributions of advantages, resources, and the material conditions for health.
- Complex population health problems such a diabetes, cardiovascular disease, cancer, and other chronic diseases need a wide array of policies and other interventions at multiple levels.
- Early childhood interventions are crucial.

Each of these broad implications is discussed in further detail next.

Further Interventions to Prevent and Control Chronic Illness

The prevention and control of chronic illness requires interventions beyond changing individual health behaviors and increasing access to medical care. Despite increasing awareness about the social determinants of health, many people still believe that health is largely improved by reducing unhealthy behaviors and increasing access to health care.[68] In fact, the United States is the only developed country that spends more on the diagnosis and treatment of health issues than on providing social care programs.[69] In 2010 Frieden developed the Health Impact Pyramid (Figure 6-3), a five-tier pyramid showing varying health interventions that occur at different levels of society and gauging the potential impact of the interventions.[70] This model shows the increasing reach of population-based interventions focused on the upstream social determinants of health compared with a focus on individual counseling, personal education, or even clinical interventions.[68] (For additional discussion of the Health Impact Pyramid, see Chapter 1.)

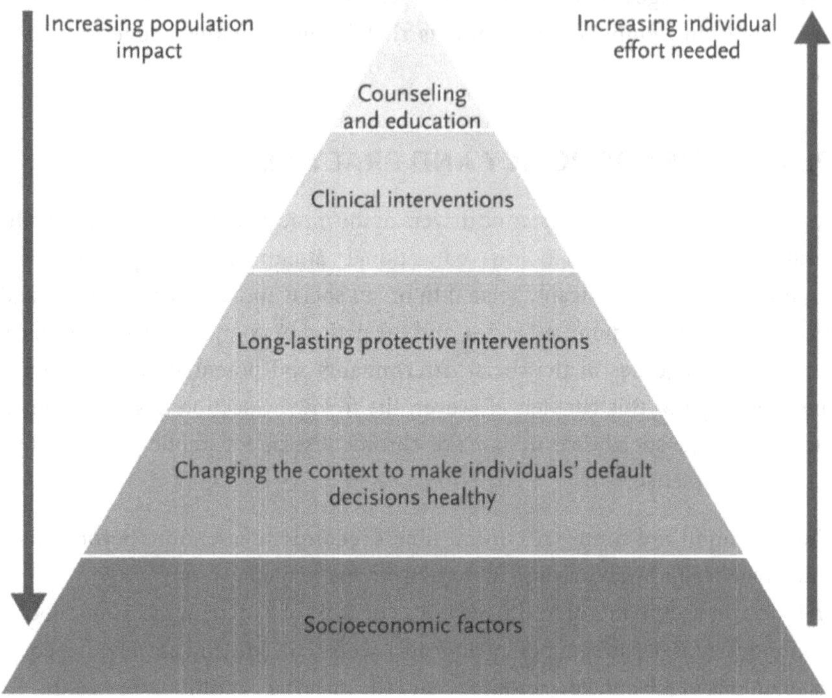

Source: Reprinted from Frieden.[70]

Figure 6-3. The Health Impact Pyramid

Achieving health improvement not only requires promoting healthy behaviors and access to high-quality medical care but also demands a focus on the broader set of factors that lie outside an individual and beyond the traditional spheres of both medical care and public health.[70]

Healthy People 2030—the current population health blueprint and strategic plan for the nation—presents a set of "leading health indicators" that, for the first time, include a number of evidence-based social indicators that are fundamental to improvements in population health and health equity.[71] In addition to the standard population health indicators (e.g., rates of infant death, drug overdose death, suicide, tobacco use, cancer screening, health insurance), the leading health indicators for the United States now include exposure to unhealthy air, household food insecurity and hunger, adult employment rates, and fourth-grade reading levels. An additional list of social indicators that should be considered as leading population health indicators was recommended by a National Academy of Medicine committee, including the Neighborhood Divestment Index, measures of residential segregation, the Heat Vulnerability Index, the prevalence of adverse childhood experiences, and voter registration rates.[72]

Policy Reform for Equitable Distributions

Policy reform is needed to shift and create more equitable distributions of advantage, resources, and the material conditions for health. The social determinants of health model emphasizes that the downstream distribution of the key, proximate material conditions is largely driven by upstream macro/structural/systemic political, economic, and social forces. As such, interventions at the individual level are necessary but are insufficient for addressing and changing the upstream forces that create the population distributions of risks/exposures/disadvantages versus resources/benefits/advantages in the first place.

A fundamental principle in epidemiology is that an individual's risk of illness cannot be separated from the risk distribution within the population to which he or she belongs.[73] Key to this core insight is that there is a difference between sick individuals and sick populations. In the latter case, a disease or health condition becomes more prevalent in a population or subpopulation primarily because of an increase in the number of people at some risk rather than high risk. This has important implications for prevention and control. If the primary strategy is to identify those individuals at high risk for a condition or disease, the incidence and prevalence will not be altered as much as if prevention efforts attempt to shift the distribution of all risk within the population. For example, in many countries attempts to address high rates of diabetes mellitus are primarily focused on identifying and targeting intervention for people at high risk because of body mass index or hemoglobin A1c levels. While this approach can indeed benefit people at high risk, this type of strategy is quite inefficient if the overall goal is to reduce the incidence, prevalence, and racial/ethnic inequities of diabetes within the population. Population-level strategies that attempt to address systemic, structural, and environmental barriers related to healthy food security, physical activity, safe communities, health care access, and so on will shift the risk distribution of the entire population and thus be more efficient and effective in terms of the overall health of the population. Simulation models and empirical analyses have demonstrated that low-cost population-level interventions often have better cost–benefit ratios than interventions tailored to individuals at highest risk.[74]

While public policy can have a positive impact on individual health risks and risk distributions within communities and societies, it also can be a structural factor that contributes to or produces social inequalities that have a negative impact on health. That is, public policy is often the *cause* of the structural or macro-level forces that create health inequities within society. For example, the significant racial disparities in wealth in the United States stem in large part from social structures and public policies, including redlining that has systematically hindered African Americans from access to mortgages and thus home ownership. As another example of how public policy can fuel social and health disparities, land use planning and zoning policies have exacerbated the concentration of environmental hazards in low-income and racial minority neighborhoods, contributing to environmental racism and its impact on health.

Braveman et al. posit that reducing the long-standing and stark racial/ethnic inequities in health risks and outcomes in the United States requires dismantling the structural and systemic racism that is built into myriad systems, laws, and policies.[10] They suggest prioritizing systems/structures that are the key proximate determinants of health; these include economic security, housing security, educational opportunities, and treatment by the criminal justice system. A multipronged set of strategies will be required for such dramatic reform, including enforcing existing antidiscrimination laws; introducing and passing new legislation at the local, state, and federal levels; using the power of broad-based advocacy coalitions; ensuring affirmative action; reducing earlier damage through "healing-centered" and "truth and reconciliation approaches"; and changing White attitudes.[10]

Complex Interventions for Complex Problems

Complex problems such a diabetes, cardiovascular disease, cancer, and other chronic diseases need a wide array of policies and other interventions at multiple levels. The causes of high rates and social inequities in chronic disease in populations are complex and multifaceted. As such, a simple yet fundamental point to emphasize is that chronic disease prevention and control, like any other complex issue in society, requires a wide array of interventions and policy changes aimed at structural/system reform, neighborhood environments, family factors, and individual behavioral and psychosocial processes. There is no magic intervention bullet or stand-alone policy reform that itself will make a significant impact.

A useful example of the need for multilevel interventions is that of tobacco use prevention and control. Smoking rates in the United States have dropped significantly over the past several decades because of a combination of effective interventions aimed at tobacco use initiation among youth (primary prevention) and cessation (secondary prevention).[75] This includes policy changes such as significant increases in the price of tobacco through taxation, regulatory changes in tobacco marketing and packaging, well-designed mass media campaigns and school-based educational interventions, the passage of smoke-free laws in public places and most worksites, and clinical interventions such as clinician-based interventions and nicotine-replacement products. As a result of this wide range of interventions and the synergies among them, adult smoking rates plummeted from 37.4% of adults in 1970 to 12.5% in 2020.[76] However, additional progress is necessary and will also require a coordinated set of public policy changes and interventions. Socioeconomic and racial/ethnic disparities in tobacco use remain and have actually increased over time, as many of the social determinants of this important health risk behavior have been left unchecked. Thus, many low-SES urban neighborhoods face increased exposure to tobacco advertising yet continue to have differential access to health care environments and health insurance that promotes evidence-based smoking cessation interventions.

It is important to recognize that challenging ethical issues sometimes arise in public policies related to chronic disease prevention and control. For example, smoking bans in public housing and limitations on what Supplemental Nutrition Assistance Program benefits can purchase may indeed have a positive impact on health behaviors, yet these policies also impose limits and restrictions on people by virtue of their income status and their reliance (often temporary) on resources in the public safety net.

The Importance of Early Childhood Interventions

Early childhood interventions are crucial. At a fundamental level, early childhood education has strong and consistent evidence for positively influencing health over the life course, as noted earlier in this chapter. WHO's Commission on Social Determinants of Health has identified early childhood education as a priority area, urging governments to put resources into the area.[30] Children who attend high-quality early learning programs see gains later in life, including improved graduation rates and earnings, as well as decreased rates of crime and teen pregnancy.[77] In addition, randomized controlled preschool intervention trials have shown that early childhood education is associated with improved adult health status, lower behavioral risk factors, and lower criminal activity.[78,79] Other educational policies and programs that have been proven to affect health outcomes can be seen in Table 6-2.

MOVING FORWARD

The myriad levels and interconnected nature by which different social and structural factors affect health make it difficult to determine the fundamental root cause of a specific outcome or the concrete impact of a particular intervention. Chronic disease and social epidemiologists should be extremely careful about causal inference. Causality and reverse-causality in the relationship between socioeconomic position and health are especially challenging to sort out in most population-based research studies. Nonetheless, the bulk of existing evidence strongly suggests that although causality works in both directions, the dominant direction is that the socioeconomic position of individuals and the social conditions in which they live precede and are the fundamental causes of subsequent health outcomes and health inequities across sociodemographic groups in society.[1,29]

One priority for research in the field necessitates strengthening the basis for causal inference between upstream structural determinants of health and downstream mediating or moderating factors and health outcomes. As it is impossible to randomly assign people or communities to socioeconomic conditions, the vast majority of scholarship in this area suffers from research designs with significant threats to internal validity. Selection processes, endogeneity concerns, omitted variable bias, lack of temporal ordering of exposures and outcomes, long lag periods, measurement issues, and bidirectional

Table 6-2. Education-Related Policies and Programs With Scientific Evidence of Health Impact

Program or Policy	Details
Career academies	Establish small learning communities in high schools focused on fields such as health care, finance, technology, communications, or public service.
[Chicago] Child Parent Centers	Provide preschool education and comprehensive support to low-income families, including small classes, student meals, and home visits with referrals for social service support as needed.
Dropout prevention programs	Provide services such as remedial education, vocational training, case management, and life skills training to help students complete high school.
Dropout prevention programs for teen mothers	Provide teen mothers with services such as remedial education, vocational training, case management, health care, and transportation assistance to support high school completion.
Early Head Start	Provide childcare, parent education, physical health, mental health services, and other family supports to pregnant women with low incomes and children aged 0–3 years.
Families and Schools Together	Convene small groups of families for facilitated weekly meetings that include a family meal, structured activities, parent support time, and parent-child play therapy.
Full-day kindergarten	Offer kindergarten programs for children aged 4–6 years 5 days/week for at least 5 hours/day.
Health career recruitment for minority students	Recruit and train minority students for careers in health fields via information about health careers, classes, practicum experiences, advising about college or medical school admissions, etc.
Incredible Years	Support young children who exhibit or are at risk for behavioral problems with interpersonal relationship training and parents and teachers who are trained to meet their needs.
Knowledge Is Power Program in middle schools	Emphasize high expectations for all students, parent and student commitment, empowered principals, and regular student assessments that inform continuous improvement in a lengthened school year.
Mentoring programs for high school graduation	Establish programs that connect at-risk students with trained adult volunteers who provide ongoing guidance for academic and personal challenges
No-excuses charter school model	Focus heavily on reading and math achievement, enforce high behavioral expectations through a formal discipline system, lengthen instructional time, and increase feedback on teacher performance.
Preschool education programs	Provide center-based programs that support cognitive and social-emotional growth among children who are not old enough to enter formal schooling.
Preschool programs with family support services	Provide center-based programs that support cognitive and social-emotional growth among young children from low-income families, usually with supports such as home visiting or parental skills training.
Reach Out and Read	Partner with doctors, nurse practitioners, and other medical professionals to incorporate literacy support into regular well-child visits, especially in lower-income communities.

(Continued)

Table 6-2. (Continued)

Program or Policy	Details
School-based social and emotional instruction	Implement focused efforts to help children recognize and manage emotions, set and reach goals, appreciate others' perspectives, and maintain relationships; also called social and emotional learning.
School-based violence and bullying prevention programs	Address students' disruptive and antisocial behavior by teaching self-awareness, emotional self-control, self-esteem, social problem-solving, conflict resolution, teamwork, social skills, etc.
School breakfast programs	Provide free, nutritious breakfasts for eligible school-aged children in public and private schools, as well as residential childcare settings.
School-wide Positive Behavioral Interventions and Supports (SWPBIS; Tier 1)	Teach positively stated behavior expectations to all students, often reinforced with prizes or privileges and supported with coaching and data; SWPBIS is Tier 1 of Positive Behavioral Interventions and Supports.
Summer learning programs	Provide academic instruction to students during the summer, often along with enrichment activities such as art or outdoor activities.
Targeted programs to increase college enrollment	Help students prepare academically for college, complete applications, and enroll, especially first-generation applicants and students from low-income families.
Targeted truancy interventions	Support interventions that provide chronically truant students with resources to improve self-esteem, social skills, etc., as well as familial and school-related factors that can contribute to poor attendance.
Technology-enhanced classroom instruction	Incorporate technology into classroom instruction via computer-assisted instruction programs, computer-managed learning programs, use of interactive whiteboards, etc.
Universal pre-kindergarten	Provide pre-kindergarten (pre-K) education to all 4-year-olds, regardless of family income.

relationships are just some of the challenges that researchers face when trying to establish causation between the potential benefits of social and economic policies and programs, and health outcomes. The increased use of longitudinal studies, natural experiments, regression discontinuity designs, sophisticated simulation modeling, and other research designs that are better able to identify causal relationships is needed. In all cases researchers need to be extremely careful not to overinterpret significant associations as causal relationships.

Structural racism, in particular, remains a challenge to measure, given that most relevant research today relies on self-reported exposures of racism. In fact, in 2020 the top four medical journals saw a dramatic increase in the number of articles that included the word *racism*, but fewer than 10% contained any measures of structural racism.[80] Hardeman et al. explore new measurement approaches which capture the multifaceted nature of structural racism as a system and the use of intersectionality to assess how structural racism exposure interacts with individual-level characteristics to shape health.[80] In addition, more research on the pathology of the social determinants of health is needed, including increased understanding of the cumulative impact of stressors on health, the role of social determinants of health in epigenetics, and the multiple biological pathways by which social determinants of health "get under one's skin."[81]

Finally, there is a need at the community, program, and policy level to establish an evidence base for programs and policies addressing the social determinants of health and to develop a better understanding of the relative impacts of various programs on health outcomes. This will allow for maximum efficiency and effectiveness when allocating resources and guiding social policy. This research could further be extended to determine the role government, payers, and others can play in effectively moving beyond social needs to address the social and structural determinants of health.

DISCUSSION QUESTIONS

1. What is the difference between social needs and the social determinants of health?
2. What are the ways in which race and health interact to result in disparate chronic disease outcomes?
3. In what ways and why did COVID-19 disproportionally affect the health of communities of color?

REFERENCES

1. Braveman P, Egerter S, Williams DR. The social determinants of health: coming of age. *Annu Rev Public Health*. 2011b;32:381–398.
2. Solar O, Irwin A. A Conceptual Framework for Action on the Social Determinants of Health. Social Determinants of Health discussion paper 2 (Policy and Practice). Geneva, Switzerland: World Health Organization; 2010. Available at: https://apps.who.int/iris/bitstream/handle/10665/44489/?sequence=1. Accessed January 25, 2023.
3. Hood CM, Gennuso KP, Swain GR, Catlin BB. County health rankings: relationships between determinant factors and health outcomes. *Am J Prev Med*. 2016;50(2):129–135.
4. Cockerham W, Hamby BW, Oates BR. The social determinants of chronic disease. *Am J Prev Med*. 2017; 52(1 suppl 1):S5–S12.
5. Centers for Disease Control and Prevention. Core functions of public health and how they relate to the 10 essential services. 2016. Archived. Available at: https://www.cdc.gov/nceh/ehs/10-essential-services/index.html. Accessed January 11, 2023.
6. Krieger N. Who and what is a "population"? historical debates, current controversies, and implications for understanding "population health" and rectifying health inequities. *Milbank Q*. 2012;90(4):634–681.

7. Zambrana RE, Williams DR. The intellectual roots of current knowledge on racism and health: relevance to policy and the national equity discourse. *Health Aff (Millwood).* 2022 Feb;41(2):163–170. doi:10.1377/hlthaff.2021.01439
8. Lee K, Freudenberg N, Zenone M, et al. Measuring the commercial determinants of health and disease: a proposed framework. *Int J Health Serv.* 2022;52(1):115–128. doi:10.1177/00207314211044992
9. Jones CP. Invited commentary: "race," racism, and the practice of epidemiology. *Am J Epidemiol.* 2001;154(4):299–304.
10. Braveman PA, Arkin E, Proctor D, Kauh T, Holm N. Systemic and structural racism: definitions, examples, health damages, and approaches to dismantling. *Health Aff.* 2022;41(2): 171–178.
11. Williams DR. Miles to go before we sleep: racial inequities in health. *J Health Soc Behav.* 2012;53(3):279–295.
12. Bleich SN, Jarlenski MP, Bell CN, LaVeist TA. Health inequalities: trends, progress, and policy. *Ann Rev Public Health.* 2012;33:7–40.
13. Gee G, Ford C. Structural racism and health inequities: old issues, new directions. *Du Bois Rev.* 2011;8(1):115–132.
14. Dolezsar CM, McGrath JJ, Herzig AJ, Miller SB. Perceived racial discrimination and hypertension: a comprehensive systematic review. *Health Psychol.* 2014;33(1):20–34.
15. Priest N, Paradies Y, Trenerry B, Truong M, Karlsen S, Kelly Y. A systematic review of studies examining the relationship between reported racism and health and wellbeing for children and young people. *Soc Sci Med.* 2013;95:115–127.
16. Lewis TT, Cogburn CD, Williams DR. Self-reported experiences of discrimination and health: scientific advances, ongoing controversies, and emerging issues. *Annu Rev Clin Psychol.* 2015;11:407–440.
17. Macintyre S, Ellaway A, Cummnins S. Place effects on health: how can we conceptualise, operationalize and measure them? *Soc Sci Med.* 2002;55(1):125–139.
18. Diez-Roux A, Mair C. Neighborhoods and health. *Ann N Y Acad Sci.* 2010;1186:125–145.
19. Ghosh-Dastidar B, Cohen D, Hunter G, et al. Distance to store, food prices, and obesity in urban food deserts. *Am J Prev Med.* 2014;47(5):587–595.
20. Jivraj S, Murray ET, Norman P, Nicholas O. The impact of life course exposures to neighbourhood deprivation on health and well-being: a review of the long-term neighbourhood effects literature. *Eur J Public Health.* 2020;30(5):922–928.
21. Kruize H, Droomers M, van Kamp I, Ruijsbroek A. What causes environmental inequalities and related health effects? an analysis of evolving concepts. *Int J Environ Res Public Health.* 2014;11(6):5807–5827.
22. Brender JD, Maantay JA, Chakraborty J. Residential proximity to environmental hazards and adverse health outcomes. *Am J Public Health.* 2011;101(suppl 1):S37–S52.
23. Diez-Roux A. Neighborhoods and health: where are we and where do we go from here? *Rev Epidemiol Sante Publique.* 2007;55(1):13–21.
24. Marmot M, Goldblatt P, Allen J, et al. Fair society, healthy lives: the Marmot review. Institute of Health Equity. 2010. Available at: https://www.instituteofhealthequity.org/resources-reports/fair-society-healthy-lives-the-marmot-review. Accessed January 11, 2023.

25. Centers for Disease Control and Prevention. Current cigarette smoking among adults in the United States. 2020. Updated March 17, 2022. Available at: https://www.cdc.gov/tobacco/data_statistics/fact_sheets/adult_data/cig_smoking/index.htm. Accessed January 11, 2023.
26. Jin Y, Jones-Smith JC. Associations between family income and children's physical fitness and obesity in California, 2010–2012. *Prev Chronic Dis*. 2015;12:E17.
27. Darmon N, Drewnowski A. Does social class predict diet quality? *Am J Clin Nutr*. 2008;87(5): 1107–1117.
28. Adler NE, Newman K. Socioeconomic disparities in health: pathways and policies. *Health Aff (Millwood)*. 2002;21(2):260–276.
29. Herd P, Goesling B, House JS. Socioeconomic position and health: the differential effects of education versus income on the onset versus progression of health problems. *J Health Soc Behav*. 2007;48(3):223–238.
30. World Health Organization. Closing the gap in a generation: health equity through action on the social determinants of health. Final report of the Commission on the Social Determinants of Health. August 27, 2008. Available at: https://www.who.int/publications/i/item/WHO-IER-CSDH-08.1. Accessed January 11, 2023.
31. Williams DR, Costa MV, Odunlami AO, Mohammed SA. Moving upstream: how interventions that address the social determinants of health can improve health and reduce disparities. *J Public Health Manag Pract*. 2008;14(suppl):S8–S17.
32. Marmot M; Commission on Social Determinants of Health. Achieving health equity: from root causes to fair outcomes. *Lancet*. 2007;370(9593):1153–1163.
33. Raghupathi W, Raghupathi V. An empirical study of chronic diseases in the United States: a visual analytics approach. *Int J Environ Res Public Health*. 2018;15(3):431. doi:10.3390/ijerph15030431
34. Adler NE. Health disparities: taking on the challenge. *Perspect Psychol Sci*. 2013;8(6):679–681.
35. Link BG, Phelan JC. Social conditions as fundamental causes of disease. *J Health Soc Behav*. 1995;35(extra issue):80–94.
36. Phelan JC, Link BG, Tehranifar P. Social conditions as fundamental causes of health inequalities: theory, evidence and policy implications. *J Health Soc Behav*. 2010;51(suppl 1):S28–S40.
37. Furumoto-Dawson A, Gehlert S, Sohmer D, Olopade O, Sacks T. Early-life conditions and mechanisms of population health vulnerabilities. *Health Aff (Millwood)*. 2007;26(5):1238–1248.
38. Edin KJ, Shaefer HL. *$2.00 a Day: Living on Almost Nothing in America*. New York, NY: Houghton Mifflin Harcourt Publishing; 2015.
39. Stuff JE, Casey PH, Szeto KL, et al. Household food insecurity is associated with adult health status. *J Nutr*. 2004;134(9):2330–2335.
40. Braveman P, Dekker M, Egerter S, Sadegh-Nobari T, Pollack C. Housing and health. Exploring the Social Determinants of Health Series. Issue Brief 7. Robert Wood Johnson Foundation. May 2011. Available at: https://www.dhss.delaware.gov/dhss/dph/mh/files/housingandhealth.pdf. Accessed January 11, 2023.
41. Taylor LA. Housing and health: an overview of the literature. Health Affairs Health Policy Brief. June 7, 2018. doi:10.1377/hpb20180313.396577
42. Regenstein M, Lantz PM. Socioeconomic status and health care. In: Wright JD, ed. *International Encyclopedia of the Social and Behavioral Sciences*. Oxford, UK: Elsevier; 2015:937–941.

43. Lantz PM, Rosenbaum S. The potential and realized impact of the Affordable Care Act on health equity. *J Health Politics, Policy Law*. 2020;45(5):831–845.
44. Miller S, Alterkruse S, Johnson N, Wherry LR. Medicaid mortality: new evidence from linked survey and administrative data. NBER Working Paper 26081. Cambridge, MA: National Bureau of Economic Research; 2019.
45. Brown CC, Moore JE, Felix HC, et al. Association of state Medicaid expansion status with low birth weight and preterm birth. *JAMA*. 2019;321(16):1598–1609.
46. Pampel FC, Krueger PM, Denney JT. Socioeconomic disparities and health behaviors. *Annu Rev Sociol*. 2010;36:349–370.
47. Garrett BE, Dube SR, Babb S, McAfee T. Addressing the social determinants of health to reduce tobacco-related disparities. *Nicotine Tob Res*. 2015;17(8):892–897.
48. Ding D, Do A, Schmidt HM, Bauman AE. A widening gap? changes in multiple lifestyle risk behaviours by socioeconomic status in New South Wales, Australia, 2002–2012. *PLoS One*. 2015;10(8):e0135338.
49. Kintzenger KW, Stone KW, Jagger MA, Horney JA. The impact of the COVID-19 response on the provision of other public health services in the US: a cross sectional study. *PLos One*. October 14, 2021. Available at: https://journals.plos.org/plosone/article?id=10.1371/journal.pone.0255844. Accessed January 11, 2023.
50. Egerter S, Braveman P, Barclay C. Stress and health. Exploring the Social Determinants of Health Series. Issue Brief 3. Robert Wood Johnson Foundation. 2011. Available at: https://www.rwjf.org/content/dam/farm/reports/issue_briefs/2011/rwjf70441. Accessed January 11, 2023.
51. McEwen BS. Brain on stress: how the social environment gets under the skin [published correction appears in *Proc Natl Acad Sci*. 2013 Jan 22;110(4):1561]. *Proc Natl Acad Sci*. 2012; 109(suppl 2):17180–17185. doi:10.1073/pnas.1121254109
52. Abrams EM, Szefler SJ. COVID-19 and the impact of social determinants of health. *Lancet Respir Med*. 2020;8(7):659–661. doi:10.1016/S2213-2600(20)30234-4
53. Thakur N, Lovinsky-Desir S, Bime C, Wisnivesky JP, Celedón JC. The structural and social determinants of the racial/ethnic disparities in the US COVID-19 pandemic. what's our role? *Am J Respir Crit Care Med*. 2020;202(7):943–949. doi:10.1164/rccm.202005-1523PP
54. Bensken WP, Krieger NI, Berg KA, Einstadter D., Dalton J, Perzynski AT. Health status and chronic disease burden of the homeless population: an analysis of two decades of multi-institutional electronic medical Records. *J Health Care Poor Underserved*. 2021;32(3): 1619–1634. Available at: https://doi.org/10.1353/hpu.2021.0153. Accessed January 11, 2023.
55. Harper S, Ali M, Rosenoff E. Individuals experiencing homelessness are likely to have medical conditions associated with severe illness from COVID-19 issue brief. Office of the Assistant Secretary for Planning and Evaluation; US Dept Health and Human Services. June 24, 2020. Available at: https://aspe.hhs.gov/reports/individuals-experiencing-homelessness-are-likely-have-medical-conditions-associated-severe-illness-0. Accessed January 11, 2023.
56. Hacker KA, Briss PA, Richardson L, Wright J, Petersen R. COVID-19 and chronic disease: the impact now and in the future. *Prev Chronic Dis*. 2021;18:E62. doi:10.5888/pcd18.210086
57. Feldman JM, Bassett MT. Variation in COVID-19 mortality in the US by race and ethnicity and educational attainment. *JAMA Netw Open*. 2021;4(11):e2135967. doi:10.1001/jamanetworkopen.2021.35967

58. Karmakar M, Lantz PM, Tipirneni R. Association of social and demographic factors with COVID-19 incidence and death rates in the US. *JAMA Netw Open*. 2021;4(1):e2036462. doi:10.1001/jamanetworkopen.2020.36462
59. Yoon P, Hall J, Fuld J, et al. Alternative methods for grouping race and ethnicity to monitor COVID-19 outcomes and vaccination coverage. *MMWR Morb Mortal Wkly Rep*. 2021;70(32): 1075–1080. doi:10.15585/mmwr.mm7032a2
60. Centers for Disease Control and Prevention. Risk for COVID-19 infection, hospitalization, and death by race/ethnicity. Available at: https://stacks.cdc.gov/view/cdc/105453. Accessed January 25, 2023.
61. Hughes MM, Wang A, Grossman MK, et al. County-level COVID-19 vaccination coverage and social vulnerability—United States, December 14, 2020–March 1, 2021. *MMWR Morb Mortal Wkly Rep*. 2021;70(12):431–436. doi:10.15585/mmwr.mm7012e1
62. Wiltz JL, Feehan AK, Molinari NM, et al. Racial and ethnic disparities in receipt of medications for treatment of COVID-19—United States, March 2020–August 2021. *MMWR Morb Mortal Wkly Rep*. 2022;71(3):96–102. doi:10.15585/mmwr.mm7103e1
63. Dasgupta S, Bowen VB, Leidner A, et al. Association between social vulnerability and a county's risk for becoming a COVID-19 hotspot—United States, June 1–July 25, 2020. *MMWR Morb Mortal Wkly Rep*. 2020;69(42):1535–1541. doi:10.15585/mmwr.mm6942a3
64. Hill L, Artiga S. COVID-19 cases and deaths by race/ethnicity: current data and changes over time. Kaiser Family Foundation. August 22, 2022. Available at: https://www.kff.org/coronavirus-covid-19/issue-brief/covid-19-cases-and-deaths-by-race-ethnicity-current-data-and-changes-over-time. Accessed January 11, 2023.
65. Taylor CA, Whitaker M, Anglin O, et al. COVID-19-associated hospitalizations among adults during SARS-CoV-2 Delta and Omicron variant predominance, by race/ethnicity and vaccination status—COVID-NET, 14 States, July 2021–January 2022. *MMWR Morb Mortal Wkly Rep*. 2022;71(12):466–473. doi:10.15585/mmwr.mm7112e2
66. Link BG, Phelan JC. Social conditions as fundamental causes of disease. *J Health Soc Behav*. 1995;35(extra issue):80–94.
67. Phelan JC, Link BG, Tehranifar P. Social conditions as fundamental causes of health inequalities: theory, evidence and policy implications. *J Health Soc Behav*. 2010;51(suppl 1):S28–S40.
68. Robert SA, Booske BC, Rigby E, Rohan AM. Public views on determinants of health, interventions to improve health, and priorities for government. *WMJ*. 2008;107(3):124–130.
69. Squires D, Anderson C. US health care from a global perspective: spending, use of services, prices, and health in 13 countries. The Commonwealth Fund. October 2015. Available at: http://www.commonwealthfund.org/publications/issue-briefs/2015/oct/us-health-care-from-a-global-perspective. Accessed January 11, 2023.
70. Frieden T. A framework for public health action: the Health Impact Pyramid. *Am J Public Health*. 2010;100(4):590–595.
71. Healthy People 2030. Available at: https://health.gov/healthypeople/objectives-and-data/leading-health-indicators. Accessed January 11, 2023.
72. National Academy of Medicine Committee on Social Indicators. Healthy People 2030's leading health indicators should track health effects of climate change, residential segregation, civic engagement. National Academies of Science, Engineering, and Medicine. January 22,

2020. Available at: https://www.nationalacademies.org/news/2020/01/healthy-people-2030s-leading-health-indicators-should-track-health-effects-of-climate-change-residential-segregation-civic-engagement. Accessed January 11, 2023.

73. Rose G. Sick individuals and sick populations. *Int J Epidemiol.* 1985;14:32–38.
74. Ahern J, Jones MR, Bakshis E, Galea S. Revisiting Rose: comparing the benefits and costs of population-wide and targeted interventions. *Milbank Q.* 2008; 86(4):581–600
75. Levy DT, Tam J, Kuo C, Fong GT, Chaloupka F. The impact of implementing tobacco control policies: the 2017 Tobacco Control Policy Scorecard. *J Pub H Mgmt Prac.* 2018;24(5):448–457.
76. Centers for Disease Control and Prevention. Burden of cigarette use in the US. 2020. Updated August 3, 2022. Available at: https://www.cdc.gov/tobacco/campaign/tips/resources/data/cigarette-smoking-in-united-states.html. Accessed January 11, 2023.
77. Ahmad FZ, Hamm K. The school-readiness gap and preschool benefits for children of color. Center for American Progress. November 12, 2013. Available at: https://www.americanprogress.org/issues/education/report/2013/11/12/79252/the-school-readiness-gap-and-preschool-benefits-for-children-of-color. Accessed January 11, 2023.
78. Muennig P, Robertson D, Johnson G, Campbell F, Pungello EP, Neidell M. The effect of an early education program on adult health: the Carolina Abecedarian Project randomized controlled trial. *Am J Public Health.* 2011;101(3):512–516. doi:10.2105/AJPH.2010.200063
79. Muennig P, Schweinhart L, Montie J, Neidell M. Effects of a prekindergarten educational intervention on adult health: 37-year follow-up results of a randomized controlled trial. *Am J Public Health.* 2009;99(8):1431–1437.
80. Hardeman RR, Homan PA, Chantarat T, Davis BA, Brown TH. Improving the measurement of structural racism to achieve antiracist health policy. *Health Aff (Millwood).* 2022;41(2):179–186. doi:10.1377/hlthaff.2021.01489
81. Seeman T, Epel E, Gruenewald T, Karlamangla A, Mcewen BS. Socio-economic differentials in peripheral biology: cumulative allostatic load. *Ann N Y Acad Sci.* 2010;1186(1):223–239.

7

Tobacco Use

Adrienne L. Johnson, PhD, Margaret B. Nolan, MD, MS, Vicki Huntington, BA, Melissa Doud, BBM, and Madison N. Alvarez, BS

LEARNING OBJECTIVES

After completing this chapter, readers should be able to

1. Understand the burden of tobacco use on the American public.
2. Describe the most evidence-based treatments for tobacco dependence.
3. Identify various populations that are particularly at risk for the harms of tobacco use and explain the factors that increase these risks.

INTRODUCTION

Combustible cigarette smoking is the leading preventable cause of death and disease in the United States, accounting for one in five deaths annually and costing more than $300 billion per year in direct and indirect costs.[1,2] Decades of research have elucidated the causes, consequences, and groups at high risk of tobacco use (Figure 7-1).[1,2] This chapter summarizes this information as well as identifies effective interventions to reduce tobacco use in children and adults and eliminate exposure to secondhand smoke. Importantly, we aim to differentiate between traditional tobacco and commercial tobacco.

Traditional tobacco is and has been used in ceremonial ways by American Indians for thousands of years. Its use differs by tribe, with Alaska Natives generally not using traditional tobacco at all. The tobacco plant is considered a sacred gift and used for medicinal and spiritual purposes. Traditional tobacco is planted, nurtured, and harvested, then processed to remove the harsh chemicals found in the plant. It is then sometimes smoked in a pipe, but not inhaled. Once harvested, processed, and dried, it can be used for ceremonial purposes to communicate with the spirit world. It is believed to remove negative energy, to cleanse and protect people and bring them good feelings, and to be offered as a gift to others who need help or guidance. Understanding the different practices around traditional tobacco will build a strong foundation when working with sovereign Native communities, who are essential partners in addressing the harm of commercial tobacco use.

Commercial tobacco is filled with chemicals and toxins known to cause harm to individuals when used the way it is intended. These manufactured items are created by big

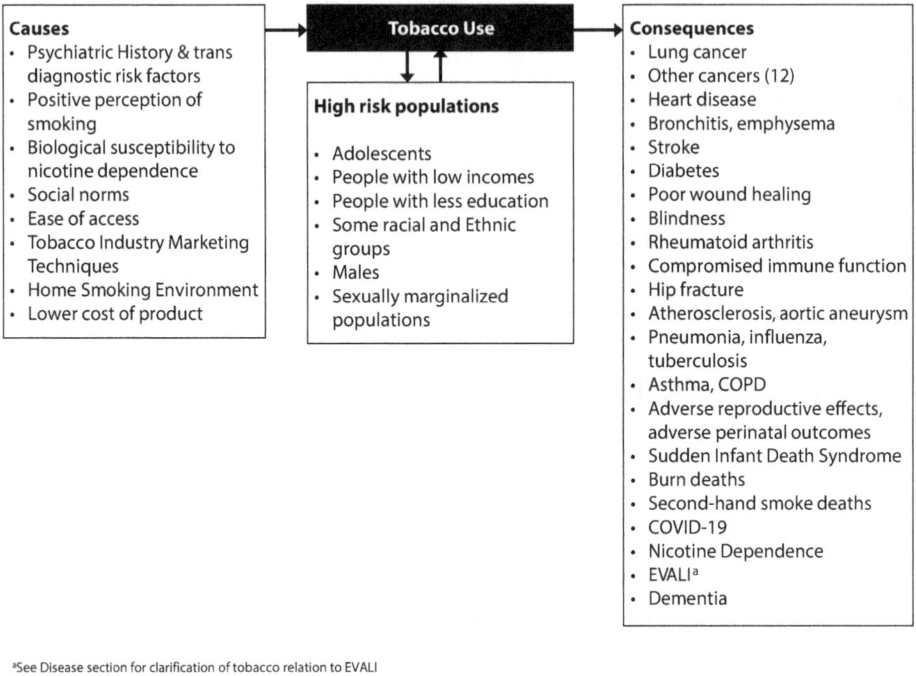

Note: COPD = chronic obstructive pulmonary disease; EVALI = e-cigarette, or vaping product, use associated lung injury.
[a]See Disease section later in this chapter for clarification of tobacco relationship to EVALI.

Figure 7-1. Causes, Consequences, and High-Risk Populations for Tobacco Use

tobacco companies for recreational use. They are specifically designed to be attractive, addictive, and sold for profit. When discussing tobacco in a public health context, remember that the health risks of commercial tobacco cannot be generalized to traditional tobacco. Whenever you read the word *tobacco* throughout the rest of this chapter, understand that it refers to commercial tobacco only, unless we explicitly mention traditional use. Learning to differentiate commercial and traditional tobacco will enable us to build strong relationships that will carry into the future.

Pathophysiology

Cigarette smoking harms nearly every organ of the body, causing a wide array of diseases (Figure 7-2a).[1] For example

- Cardiovascular diseases, including coronary heart disease, atherosclerosis, abdominal aortic aneurysm, and cerebrovascular disease.
- A variety of cancers, including lip, mouth, pharynx, esophagus, stomach, pancreas, liver, colon, larynx, trachea, lung, cervix, kidney, bladder, and acute myeloid leukemia.
- Respiratory problems, including chronic obstructive pulmonary disease, pneumonia, active tuberculosis, reduced lung function in infants, impaired lung growth during

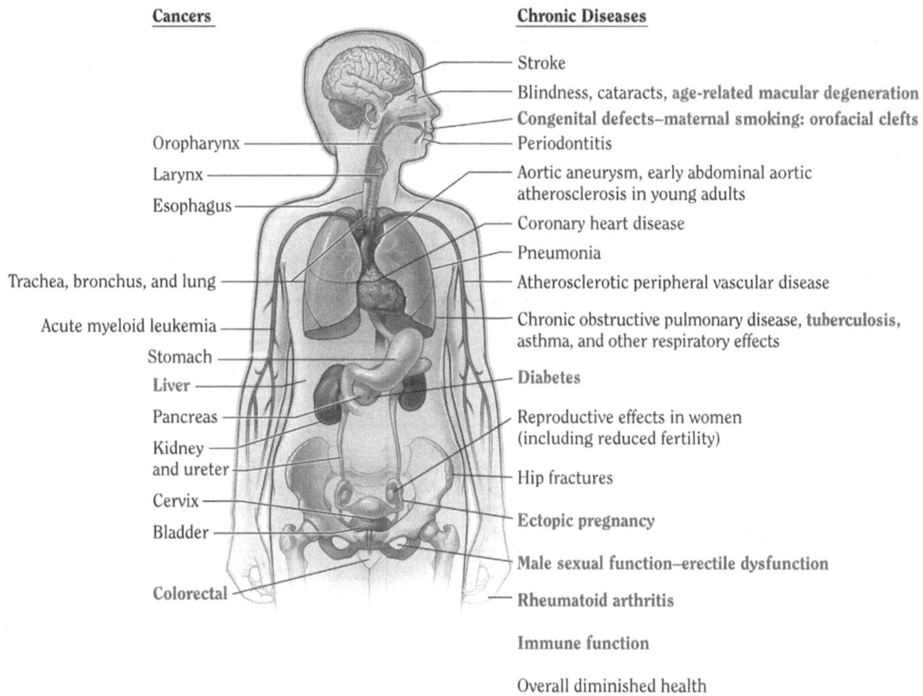

Source: Adapted from USDHHS.[1]

Figure 7-2a. The Health Effects of Cigarette Smoking on the Human Body

childhood and adolescence, lung function decline in adolescents and young adults, respiratory symptoms in children and adolescents, asthma-related symptoms in childhood and adolescence, premature onset and accelerated age-related decline in lung function among adults, major respiratory symptoms in adults (coughing, phlegm, wheezing, shortness of breath), and poor asthma control.

- Reproductive disorders, including reduced fertility, fetal death, stillbirth, low birthweight, and pregnancy complications.
- Dementia and cognitive decline, via effects on stroke and vascular dementia risk, as well as independent increased risk of Alzheimer's disease.[3]
- Other diseases, such as diabetes, rheumatoid arthritis, periodontitis, congenital defects such as orofacial clefts, sudden infant death syndrome (SIDS), blindness, cataracts, age-related macular degeneration, adverse surgical outcomes related to wound healing and respiratory complications, low bone density in postmenopausal women, hip fractures, altered immune function, peptic ulcer disease in persons who are *Helicobacter pylori*–positive, and overall diminished health.

The relative risk of these adverse health outcomes by age and smoking status can be seen in Table 7-1.[1]

Table 7-1. Relative Risk of Adverse Health Outcomes by Age and Smoking Status

Variables	Current Smokers, Age, y				Former Smokers, Age, y			
	35–54	55–64	65–74	≥75	35–54	55–64	65–74	≥75
Men								
Lung cancer	14.3	19	28.3	22.5	4.4	4.6	7.8	6.5
Other cancers	1.7	1.9	2.4	2.2	1.4	1.3	1.5	1.5
Coronary heart disease	3.9	3	2.8	2	1.8	1.5	1.6	1.3
Other heart disease	NA	NA	2.2	1.7	NA	NA	1.3	1.2
Cerebrovascular disease	NA	NA	2.2	1.5	NA	NA	1.2	1.1
Other vascular diseases	NA	NA	7.2	4.9	NA	NA	2.2	1.7
Diabetes mellitus	NA	NA	1.5	1	NA	NA	1.5	1.1
Other cardiovascular diseases	2.4	2.5	NA	NA	1.1	1.5	NA	NA
Influenza, pneumonia, tuberculosis	NA	NA	2.6	1.6	NA	NA	1.6	1.4
Chronic obstructive pulmonary disease	NA	NA	29.7	23	NA	NA	8.1	6.6
Influenza, pneumonia, tuberculosis, chronic obstructive pulmonary disease	4.5	15.2	NA	NA	2.2	4	NA	NA
All causes	2.6	3	3	2.4	1.3	1.5	1.6	1.4
Women								
Lung cancer	13.3	19	23.6	23.1	2.6	5	6.8	6.4
Other cancers	1.3	2.1	2.1	1.9	1.2	1.3	1.3	1.3
Coronary heart disease	5	3.2	3.3	2.2	2.2	1.2	1.6	1.4
Other heart disease	NA	NA	1.8	1.8	NA	NA	1.3	1.3
Cerebrovascular disease	NA	NA	2.3	1.7	NA	NA	1.2	1.1
Other vascular diseases	NA	NA	6.8	5.8	NA	NA	2.3	2
Diabetes mellitus	NA	NA	1.5	1.1	NA	NA	1.3	1.1
Other cardiovascular diseases	2.4	2	NA	NA	1	1.1	NA	NA
Influenza, pneumonia, tuberculosis	NA	NA	1.8	2.1	NA	NA	1.3	1.2
Chronic obstructive pulmonary disease	NA	NA	38.9	21	NA	NA	15.7	7.1
Influenza, pneumonia, tuberculosis, chronic obstructive pulmonary disease	6.4	9	NA	NA	1.8	4.8	NA	NA
All causes	1.8	2.6	2.9	2.5	1.2	1.3	1.5	1.4

Source: Adapted from USDHHS.[1]

Note: NA = not applicable. For detailed footnotes, see Table 12.3 in USDHHS.[1] Relative risks are rounded to the tenth decimal.

The Surgeon General[1] has also concluded that secondhand smoke (a mixture of sidestream smoke given off by a smoldering cigarette and the mainstream smoke exhaled by the person smoking) causes lung cancer, stroke, coronary heart disease, odor annoyance, and nasal irritation in adults and reduced birthweight, reduced lung function, lower respiratory infections (pneumonia, bronchitis), middle-ear disease (acute and recurrent otitis media and chronic middle-ear effusion), respiratory symptoms (cough, phlegm, wheeze, breathlessness), more severe asthma, and SIDS in children.

Smokeless tobacco, such as snuff or snus, causes several forms of cancer and oral diseases. Data on novel tobacco products such as electronic nicotine delivery devices, including e-cigarettes, are much more limited, but concerns have been raised about some of the chemicals used to generate the aerosol, exposure to metals leached from the device, the toxicity of certain flavorings when they are inhaled, and exposure to nicotine. Recent evidence suggests that regular use of e-cigarettes in adults increases the risk of developing respiratory disease (chronic obstructive pulmonary disease, asthma, emphysema, and chronic bronchitis). This is especially true for adults who co-use combustible cigarettes and e-cigarettes.[4]

Tobacco Products

Multiple types of tobacco products are available and in use today. Following is a brief description of these various products and their relative public health significance.

Combustible Cigarettes

Combustible cigarettes remain the most commonly used form of tobacco by US adults, used by 80% of American adults who use tobacco products.[5] It is the second most commonly used form of tobacco by adolescents (1.5%) in the United States (behind electronic cigarettes).[6] Combustible cigarettes are primarily sold in a pack (containing 20 cigarettes), although the sale of single cigarettes (loosies) in urban, low-socioeconomic-status (low SES), younger, and certain marginalized racial and ethnic groups is common.[7] Despite the illegality of these single cigarette sales, this practice is a way to circumvent public health efforts to decrease cigarette use (i.e., price increases) and may be associated with certain health inequities linked with smoking (see Public Health Impact section in this chapter).

Smokeless Tobacco

Smokeless tobacco is defined as any finely cut, ground, powdered, or leaf tobacco that is intended to be placed in the oral cavity. Use of smokeless tobacco causes addiction as well as precancerous oral lesions; cancer of the oral cavity, esophagus, and pancreas; and adverse reproductive effects, including low birthweight, preterm birth, and stillbirth.

Data suggest that some smokeless tobacco products also cause heart disease, stroke, and diabetes.[8] Given the great diversity of smokeless tobacco products, the level of risk can vary by product characteristics, ingredients, how the products are used, and interaction with other tobacco products (through dual or poly-tobacco use). For example, smokeless tobacco products vary in their concentration of nicotine, tobacco-specific nitrosamines, polyaromatic hydrocarbons, toxic metals, and other toxicants. Nitrosamines are formed primarily during tobacco processing, curing, fermentation, and storage. Polyaromatic hydrocarbons are formed during the fire-curing process. A variety of toxic metals have been found in smokeless tobacco products; this is caused by levels of these metals in the soil where the tobacco is grown and from the use of fertilizers. Alkaline agents added to the product increase the absorption of nicotine by the user.

Dual or poly-tobacco use can increase risk because of delayed cessation of cigarette smoking and increased toxicant exposure. Reduced benefit from cessation of cigarette smoking occurs among those who switch to smokeless tobacco rather than quit tobacco use completely. There is also concern that smokeless tobacco use by youth could increase their use of combusted tobacco products.[8]

Cigars

Cigars consist of tobacco wrapped in a tobacco leaf or in a substance that contains tobacco.[9] Cigarettes, by contrast, are wrapped in paper or another substance without tobacco in it. The three main types of cigars in the United States are large cigars, cigarillos, and little cigars.[5,6] Cigars contain the same harmful ingredients as cigarettes, and result in many of the same negative health effects, including multiple types of cancer, gum disease, heart disease, emphysema, and chronic bronchitis.[10]

Cigar use is higher among youth who use other tobacco products or addictive substances.[9] Cessation rates of cigarettes among youth who co-use cigarettes and other tobacco products do not vary compared with those who solely use cigarettes, but there is a lower prevalence of quitting all tobacco products versus quitting cigarettes only.[2] This highlights that cigar use can continue even in the presence of a cigarette quit attempt.

Pipes

Current pipe smoking, independent of other tobacco product use, is associated with increased risk of mortality from multiple forms of cancer, coronary heart disease, and cerebrovascular disease when compared with individuals who never used tobacco.[11] Although pipe smoke contains the same toxic chemicals and main addictive ingredient (nicotine) as cigarette smoke, patterns and prevalence of use can result in lower levels of risk for disease.[11] However, pipe smokers who previously smoked cigarettes are more likely to inhale,[1] which increases their risk of associated diseases.

Hookah or Water Pipe

Hookah products are unique in that the tobacco pipe pulls smoke through water prior to inhalation by the user. Similar to e-cigarettes, there are myriad forms of hookah products that differ in terms of size, materials used, and flavoring of products. Currently 0.8% of middle and high school students use hookah and 1.1% of US adults use a pipe/hookah/ water pipe.[5,6] Hookah products contain several compounds and byproducts found in combustible cigarettes, but at dramatically higher levels.[12] The existence of these toxicants in water pipe tobacco smoke, including carcinogens and heavy metals, may place users at risk for many of the same diseases faced by cigarette smokers, including lung and esophageal cancer, respiratory illness, cardiovascular disease, and low birthweight.[12] Concerns have also been raised about the high levels of carbon monoxide produced and the potential for acute carbon monoxide poisoning.[12] Given that water pipe tobacco smoking sessions last significantly longer than smoking a cigarette, smoking water pipe tobacco could potentially be even more dangerous than smoking a cigarette.[12]

Electronic Cigarettes

First introduced in the United States around 2007, electronic cigarettes, or e-cigarettes, are another novel tobacco product whose use has rapidly increased. Because of the newness and rapid evolution of the products, the potential benefits or risks of these products are not yet fully understood. At present there is significant variability in the concentration of chemicals among products. There is also variability between labeled content and concentration and the actual content and concentration, including nicotine levels.[13]

Studies show that e-liquid tobacco products contain nicotine, propylene glycol, glycerin, tobacco-specific nitrosamines, tobacco alkaloids, carbonyls, ethylene glycol, diacetyl, and acetyl propionyl.[13] Chemicals such as nicotine, carbonyls, tobacco-specific nitrosamines, heavy metals, and volatile organic compounds have also been identified in e-cigarette aerosols.[13] Carcinogen levels in e-cigarettes vary widely across the products, and some chemicals, such as formaldehyde, have been found at levels at, or greater than, those found in cigarettes under certain conditions.[13] (See the Public Health section of this chapter for more information on impacts of e-cigarettes.)

Flavored e-cigarettes raise particular concerns because of the potential dangers of these chemical flavorings when inhaled and the preferred nature of flavored aerosols among youth. In 2020 (and again in 2021) the US Food and Drug Administration (FDA) passed a ruling that banned the sale of flavorings in an attempt to address the public health crisis of e-cigarette use among youth. However, a 2021 report by the Campaign for Tobacco Free Kids found that three months after the 2021 deadline for removal of flavored e-cigarette products, over 100 flavors were found in online retailers and that flavored products were still widely available in stores across the country.[14] E-cigarette use rates have decreased since 2019,[15] but e-cigarettes remain the number one form of nicotine or tobacco product among middle and high school students (7.6%) and second most common among adults (3.7%).[5,6]

The long-term health effects of e-cigarettes are unknown, although completely switching from combusted cigarettes to e-cigarettes would likely reduce the risk of tobacco-related disease for individuals unable to quit use of combusted products. Nicotine causes addiction, and some data suggest that nicotine can adversely affect the adolescent brain.[13] Nicotine is also known to cause adverse reproductive outcomes.[1,16] Although levels of many toxicants are lower than the amounts found in combusted products, some of the chemicals in e-cigarettes have been linked to cancer and other adverse outcomes, so use by youth or former tobacco users should be discouraged. There are anecdotal reports of e-cigarettes helping some cigarette smokers completely switch from cigarettes to e-cigarettes, but data from research are mixed on whether e-cigarettes can help smokers quit, and none have as yet been approved as cessation aids.[2]

PUBLIC HEALTH IMPACT

As the tobacco industry continually evolves with the development of new products, the use of new marketing strategies, and targeting to populations and communities already dealing with the social determinants of health, the public health impact is felt broadly by all communities. These adjustments by the industry provide greater challenges to public health professionals who are also dealing with the intersects of tobacco prevention and control and other public health issues such as COVID-19 and environmental and behavioral health conditions.

Social and Health Equity Impacts of Tobacco

Historical Perspectives of Tobacco's Impact

It took centuries for public health to reach agreement on whether tobacco even caused any negative health effects, and if it did, whether it was worthy of concern. Some of this delay resulted from the necessarily slow progress of health science and the requirements of the scientific process, but both those processes were also stymied by the extent to which early scientific studies were obscured in public messaging by industry-funded counter-research.

Most early tobacco industry messaging focused on smoking's supposed health benefits. By the 1930s cigarette advertising featured a slew of dubious (later determined to be outright fabricated) health claims. These ranged from arguments that the newest product was somehow healthier than others on the market to claiming outright that smoking improved health. Kool, for example, pushed its cigarettes to nose and throat specialists to give to patients "suffering from colds and kindred disorders."[1]

By the 1950s the evidence linking smoking and lung cancer was clear. While scientists worked to make the negative health consequences of tobacco known, the tobacco industry concentrated on casting as much doubt on that evidence as possible. Executives of major tobacco companies met with the advertising firm Hill & Knowlton in December 1953 to organize a unified counter-information campaign and establish an industry-funded research organization. The strategies created at that meeting, including "denying the harms of its products, discrediting the scientific evidence that showed these harms, funding research that was intended to divert attention from cigarettes, and marketing new products with implied lower risks" would be used for decades.[1]

Public perceptions of the risks of tobacco have changed dramatically since the generation of widespread scientific consensus on the health risks of tobacco in the 1950s and 1960s and the rise of the modern tobacco-control movement.[2] In the early days of the movement smoking was often framed as a matter of habit, something people chose despite or because they did not know better. This understanding, which primarily put responsibility on the individual, determined the type of public health policies chosen to address tobacco use, which were heavily focused on public education.[1]

Social Determinants of Tobacco-Related Health and Illness

Now, with access to scientific understandings of the psychological impacts of tobacco, individual tobacco use is understood to be driven by addiction, rather than solely by habit.[2] Still, the addictiveness of tobacco alone does not explain the high rates of youth e-cigarette initiation or why smoking-related disease persists despite expanded access to addiction treatment. Therefore, the social determinants of health and, even more recently, health equity models have gained prominence as frameworks for understanding the full impact of tobacco on public health.

For example, when researchers wanted to study why so few people who smoke are successfully able to quit, despite a majority wanting to, they found the issue was deeper than a matter of willpower or addiction.[2] Instead, one of the primary causes of low quit rates at the time was that almost no health insurance policies covered smoking cessation services or pharmacotherapy. Many who wanted to quit tobacco use were being prevented by a systemic failure of health policy to allow them access to the basic treatment they needed.[2] In the same way, much of the public health impact of tobacco is a direct consequence of social and political systems that shape population trends in smoking initiation and cessation.

The full health burden of tobacco as a social determinant of health cannot be measured just through the prevalence of disease directly caused by tobacco exposure. Because tobacco use causes such a broad range of negative health effects and because those health effects can be spread through second- and thirdhand exposure, it must be addressed simultaneously as a consequence of social determinants of health and itself as a social determinant of many other negative public health outcomes. For example, many employers have expressed that they are less willing to hire candidates who smoke than those who do not, given the increased costs associated with use of insurance and sick leave by employees who smoke.[1] However, in the United States, where health insurance is uniquely tied to employment, an inability to get hired is itself a major social determinant that shapes nearly every aspect of a person's health.

Heath Equity and Tobacco

Public policy regulating tobacco sales is one social determinant that commonly produces tobacco health disparities, particularly when that policy is not equitably enforced across different communities. Many of these prevention policies have been far more effectively codified and enforced in White and high-income communities, which have greater access to the wealth and social capital needed to regulate tobacco sales. This disparity in enforcement leaves communities of color even more disproportionately vulnerable to targeting by the tobacco industry, and ultimately, race-based disparities in tobacco-related disease have worsened over time.[17]

In addition, commercial tobacco worsens non-health social and economic inequalities in numerous ways that by themselves become self-reinforcing social determinants of health inequality. While this cycle of health inequality is incredibly difficult to break, the interconnectedness of these shared determinants of social and health inequalities pose an opportunity for partnerships between public health, the tobacco-control advocacy organizations, and community-based coalitions to leverage a larger pool of resources to address these shared challenges.[17]

Global Tobacco Equity

The first treaty ever negotiated under the World Health Organization was the Framework Convention on Tobacco Control (FCTC), which quickly became "one of the most rapidly and widely embraced treaties in the United Nations' (UN) history."[1] The adoption of the FCTC demonstrated for the first time that the international community could work together effectively to improve public health.

Although there are 176 parties to the FCTC, the United States is one of only a handful of countries that are not members.[18] The United States signed the treaty when it was first written, but the US Senate has never held a vote to ratify its provisions into federal law; as a result, the United States retains the largely symbolic status of FCTC signatory.[1] Despite not being party to the FCTC, the United States. still dominates issues of global tobacco use.

American tobacco companies account for a growing portion of tobacco sales outside the United States. For example, just as the United States. passed its Tobacco Control Act in 2009, US-based Philip Morris split itself into two separate companies, Altria and Philip Morris International (PMI), to cover domestic and foreign markets, respectively.[1] PMI now sells 27% of all cigarettes purchased outside the United States and China (which has its own state-run monopoly), and its most popular brand, Marlboro, sells more than any other cigarette brand in the world.[18] PMI has invested much of its wealth in litigation against countries attempting to regulate its products. To date PMI has sued 13 (primarily low-income) countries in the World Trade Organization or in their local courts for enforcing FCTC provisions within their borders.[18]

Across the industry, companies have turned toward countries with few public health resources to compensate for declining sales in wealthier, more regulated countries. Cigarette sales, for example, dropped by 30% in high-income countries between 2008 and 2018 but increased by 8% in low-income countries over the same period.[18] In this way American institutions still hold significant sway over international tobacco regulation and the state of tobacco-related illness globally, despite the United States not being party to the FCTC.

Economics: Health Care and Lost Productivity

A clear link exists between the diminished health of people who smoke and increased absenteeism from work, along with increased health care utilization and cost. In the United States smoking tobacco caused an economic burden of annual public and private health care costs totaling $226.7 billion in 2014. Of this amount, annual federal and state government smoking-caused Medicaid payments equaled $68.3 billion and federal Medicare expenditures equaled $57.4 billion. In addition, the federal government continues to incur tobacco-caused health care costs of $20.5 billion annually, including health care for veterans through the Department of Veterans Affairs. Secondhand smoke exposure causes health care costs of $6.99 billion annually. Note that health care costs such as dental care or infant and maternal services incurred from other tobacco use are not included in these costs.[1*]

Each year smoking is estimated to cause productivity losses of $181 billion. which is calculated by costs from productive work lives shortened by smoking-caused death. Other costs that are incurred but not included in this figure are those from smoking-caused disability during work lives, smoking-caused sick days, or smoking-caused productivity declines when in the workforce.[1]

---

*The federal government reimburses the states, on average (weighted), for 58% of their Medicaid expenditures.[19] National health care costs are in 2014 dollars. Health care costs are updated to 2009 dollars.[20]

Disease

In addition to all the smoking-related diseases listed in Figure 7-1 and as noted earlier, recent research has shown the emergence of two other conditions affected by tobacco use.

EVALI

E-cigarette, or vaping product, use-associated lung injury (EVALI) is a lung condition that can develop with the use of e-cigarette (vaping) products. In 2019 the Centers for Disease Control and Prevention (CDC) started investigating a dramatic rise in hospitalizations connected to the use of vaping products. The patients presented with many respiratory symptoms such as a cough, shortness of breath, and chest pain, but they also had all used vaping products within the previous three months. CDC had tracked over 2,800 hospitalizations caused by EVALI along with 68 deaths by February 2020, but since September of 2020 there has been a significant drop in cases. It was determined that vitamin E acetate, a chemical added to some THC vaping products, was one of the main (but not only) causes, along with other chemicals found in nicotine and THC from vaping products. These chemicals caused damage to the person's lungs. Of note, 15% of EVALI patients were less than 18 years old, and EVALI emerged right at the same time as the "vaping epidemic" declared by the Surgeon General in 2016.[13,21]

COVID-19

As the COVID-19 pandemic reached its peak, it soon became clear that people who used tobacco seemed to be getting sicker, were having more difficult recoveries, and were dying more often than nonsmokers when they caught the illness. How tobacco use weakens the lungs, heart, and immune system in ways that increase vulnerability is now better understood,[22] but a solution to the impact of tobacco use on COVID-19 morbidity and mortality is still needed. Likewise, because of disparities in COVID-19 deaths,[23] which may reflect previously discussed disparities in tobacco use, diverse public health sectors must collaborate to address the health equity impacts of these intersecting illnesses.

There is still very little known about the longevity of COVID-19 vaccine immunity, treatments for severe COVID-19, and the nature of long-term impacts of COVID-19 infection—that is, of "long" or "long-haul" COVID-19—especially among individuals with comorbidities, including tobacco-related lung diseases, and from marginalized communities. Even as public health agencies begin to move away from the emergency stage of their COVID-19 responses, the need to address the intersections of COVID-19 and tobacco-related disease remains an urgent and immediate priority.

A longer-term challenge requires further research to address the intersection of tobacco use and other infectious diseases, particularly endemic illnesses like influenza, common colds, and mononucleosis. The COVID-19 pandemic has also demonstrated how addressing chronic disease determinants like tobacco is fundamental to the construction of health systems prepared to weather future epidemics of both familiar and novel pathogens.

Environmental Impact

Tobacco use not only impacts the health of individuals but also negatively affects the environment from the moment of its production to its end as litter and the resulting problem of waste management. Cigarette smoke causes environmental pollution by releasing toxic air pollutants into the air. Carbon dioxide, methane, and many other chemicals are found in secondhand smoke, which causes air pollution and poses a health risk to individuals around those who smoke. Cigarette butts and e-cigarette waste also litter the environment by polluting waterways, air, and soil with toxic chemicals. Approximately 766,571 metric tons of cigarette butts make their way into the environment every year, making cigarettes the most frequently littered item in the United States.[24] In 2019 cigarette butts were the most littered item on US beaches and in US waterways, with 900,178 pieces collected.[25] Preliminary studies show that compounds such as nicotine, pesticide residues, and metal seep from cigarette butts into water ecosystems and become acutely toxic to fish and microorganisms.[26,27]

The environmental impact comes not only from cigarettes but from disposable single-use e-cigarette products as well. How to safely handle this waste remains unclear, since it contains metal, circuitry, single-use plastic cartridges, batteries, and toxic chemicals in e-liquids.[28,29] Partially used liquid cartridges and refills contain nicotine salts and heavy metals such as lead and mercury, which can leak into soil and waterways or be ingested by wildlife.[30] Fires in garbage trucks and waste management plants have been caused by lithium-ion batteries in e-cigarettes that have been exposed to extreme heat and exploded.[31] The Drug Enforcement Agency started accepting e-cigarette devices and cartridges during its annual National Prescription Take Back Day in 2019, but the agency is not able to take devices that contain lithium-ion batteries.[32] Since the United States has no industry guidelines for recycling e-cigarettes, there are no policy requirements in place to hold manufacturers accountable.

The growing and manufacturing of tobacco products are also elements contributing to environmental problems. Deforestation is being caused by the growing of tobacco, as it decreases the ability of the land to support the growth of any other crops or vegetation.[33,34] Tobacco production depletes more water and wood and has more pesticides applied to it than most other crops, which further affects the water supplies and soil quality.

DESCRIPTIVE EPIDEMIOLOGY

High-Risk Populations

Cigarette Smoking

In 2020 an estimated 30.8 million American adults (12.5%) reported currently smoking cigarettes. At the time of the National Health Interview Survey (NHIS), they reported having ever smoked 100 cigarettes and having smoked every day or some days. Smoking prevalence was higher for men (14.1%) than for women (11.0%; Table 7-2). By age, prevalence was highest among those age 45 to 64 years (14.9%). Smoking prevalence was 8.0% among Asians, 8.0% among Hispanics, 14.4% among African Americans, 13.3% among Whites, and 27.1% among American Indians/Alaska Natives.[5] Formal educational attainment is strongly associated with smoking prevalence and cessation rates. In 2020 smoking prevalence was highest among people with a general equivalency diploma (GED; 32.0%), those with 9 to 11 years of education (21.5%), and only a high school diploma (17.6%); and lowest for persons with an undergraduate (5.6%) or graduate (3.5%) degree. In 2020 smoking prevalence was highest among persons with an annual household income less than $35,000 (20.2%), lower for those with an annual household income $35,000 to $74,999 (14.1%), and lowest for those with an annual household income greater than $100,000 (6.2%). In 2020 current smoking was also higher among persons who identified as gay, lesbian, or bisexual (16.1%), compared with those who identified as straight (12.3%).[5] (See Table 7-2.)

In 2020 more than three out of every five adults who were ever cigarette smokers had quit smoking. In 2017 the percentage of ever-smokers age 18 years and older who had quit was 61.7% overall, with 61.9% for men and 61.5% for women. It was 63.9% for non-Hispanic Whites, 61.5% for Hispanics, 64.3% for Asians, and 46.1% for non-Hispanic Blacks. In 2017 the percentage of ever-smokers who had quit was lowest among the group with a GED certificate (42.4%) and highest among persons with a graduate degree (82.8%). It was also higher among those at or above the poverty level (64.5%) than below it (42.2%).[2]

Each day in the United States about 1,600 youth smoke their first cigarette and nearly 200 youth start smoking every day. Tobacco use generally begins in early adolescence, and among those who smoke cigarettes daily, almost 90% first tried a cigarette before age 18 years. Essentially no initiation occurs after age 26 years.[16] In 2020, 4.6% of high school students and 1.6% of middle school students reported currently smoking cigarettes (had smoked in the past 30 days), which represents a significant decrease over the past decade. Note that CDC surveillance data from 2021 were collected via virtual surveys in addition to school surveys as a result of the COVID-19 pandemic. Although results may not be directly comparable for this reason, cigarette smoking was reported to be even lower: 1.0% among middle school students, 1.9% among high school students. In previous

Table 7-2. Percentage of Adults Aged 18 Years and Older Who Reported Tobacco Product Use "Every Day" or "Some Days" by Tobacco Product and Selected Characteristics: National Health Interview Survey, United States, 2020

Characteristic	Any Tobacco Product	Any Combustible Product	Cigarettes	Cigars	Pipes	E-cigarettes	Smokeless Tobacco Products	≥2 Tobacco Products
Overall	19.0	15.2	12.5	3.5	1.1	3.7	2.3	3.3
Sex								
Male	24.5	18.8	14.1	6.3	1.5	4.6	4.5	5.2
Female	13.9	11.7	11.0	0.8	0.7	2.8	0.3	1.5
Age, y								
18–24	17.6	10.9	7.4	4.1	2.1	9.4	2.4	5.7
25–44	22.9	18.0	14.1	5.0	1.7	5.2	2.8	4.9
45–64	20.4	16.9	14.9	2.8	0.6	2.2	2.5	2.3
≥65	11.8	10.4	9.0	1.8	0.3	0.6	1.2	1.0
Race/ethnicity								
White, non-Hispanic	21.1	16.3	13.3	3.8	0.9	4.2	3.2	3.6
Black, non-Hispanic	19.4	18.0	14.4	4.6	1.6	1.6	0.8	2.9
Asian, non-Hispanic	11.5	8.7	8.0	0.9	0.4	3.4	0.4	1.4
American Indian/Alaska Native, non-Hispanic	34.9	29.3	27.1	NA	NA	NA	6.8	10.9
Hispanic	11.7	9.8	8.0	2.2	0.9	2.8	0.4	2.2
Other, non-Hispanic	29.1	21.0	19.5	NA	NA	7.8	3.7	9.2
US census region								
Northeast	16.6	13.4	10.4	3.1	0.8	3.0	1.6	2.1
Midwest	22.0	18.2	15.2	3.7	1.3	4.1	2.6	4.1
South	21.1	16.9	14.1	4.1	1.1	3.6	2.7	3.7
West	15.0	11.1	9.0	2.5	1.1	4.0	1.9	2.8
Metropolitan statistical area								
Urban	17.7	14.2	11.4	3.4	1.1	3.7	1.7	3.0
Rural	27.3	21.3	19.0	3.7	1.0	3.9	5.9	5.0
Education (adults ≥25 y)								
0–12 y (no diploma)	24.8	22.7	21.5	3.1	0.7	1.4	2.4	3.6
General Educational Diploma (GED)	40.5	34.5	32.0	5.9	1.6	5.4	3.8	6.8
High school diploma	24.2	19.6	17.6	3.1	0.9	3.5	3.3	3.8
Some college, no diploma	21.7	17.3	14.4	4.0	0.8	4.1	2.6	3.5
Associate degree (academic or technical/vocational)	19.4	15.3	12.7	3.6	1.0	3.7	2.6	3.3

(Continued)

Table 7-2. (Continued)

Characteristic	Any Tobacco Product	Any Combustible Product	Cigarettes	Cigars	Pipes	E-cigarettes	Smokeless Tobacco Products	≥2 Tobacco Products
Education (adults ≥25 y)								
Undergraduate degree (bachelor's)	1.7	9.0	5.6	3.3	1.0	2.4	1.3	1.7
Graduate degree (master's professional, or doctoral)	8.6	6.9	3.5	3.0	0.9	1.5	0.8	1.1
Marital status								
Married/living with partner	17.5	13.8	10.9	3.6	0.8	3.1	2.6	2.9
Divorced/separated	21.6	18.9	17.3	2.3	0.8	2.6	1.6	2.6
Single/never married/not living with a partner	21.4	16.3	13.0	4.0	2.1	6.2	2.2	4.8
Annual household income, $								
<35,000	25.2	22.1	20.2	3.0	1.5	3.7	1.9	4.1
35,000–74,999	20.3	16.4	14.1	3.6	0.9	3.9	2.3	3.6
75,000–99,999	18.4	13.2	10.5	3.3	1.0	4.5	3.1	3.4
≥100,000	13.7	9.9	6.2	3.8	1.0	3.2	2.3	2.3
Sexual orientation								
Heterosexual/straight	18.8	15.0	12.3	3.5	1.0	3.5	2.4	3.2
Lesbian, gay, or bisexual	25.1	18.9	16.1	4.3	2.6	8.7	0.8	6.2
Health insurance coverage								
Private insurance	16.4	12.3	9.2	3.5	0.9	3.8	2.4	2.8
Medicaid	28.6	24.6	22.7	3.0	1.9	4.4	2.4	5.0
Medicare only (≥65 y)	12.5	11.3	10.2	1.6	0.1	0.7	1.1	1.0
Other public insurance	21.3	17.7	14.8	4.2	1.0	2.7	2.4	3.1
Uninsured	27.3	23.3	21.2	4.8	1.6	5.1	2.5	6.0
Disability								
Yes	25.4	21.6	19.8	3.4	1.2	3.5	2.9	4.8
No	18.4	14.6	11.8	3.5	1.1	3.7	2.3	3.2
Regularly having feelings of anxiety								
Yes	29.6	24.1	21.4	4.1	1.8	7.1	2.0	5.6
No	17.7	14.0	11.3	3.4	1.0	3.3	2.3	3.0
Regularly having feelings of depression								
Yes	35.6	29.6	26.9	3.7	2.8	8.3	2.6	6.7
No	18.3	14.5	11.8	3.5	1.0	3.5	2.3	3.1

Source: Adapted from Cornelius et al.[5]

Note: For detailed footnotes, see USDHHS.[1]

years boys were more likely to smoke cigarettes than girls, but in 2021 the prevalence of cigarette smoking was similar for high school boys (2.0%) and girls (1.8%). Among middle school students, prevalence of cigarette smoking was also comparable between boys (0.9%) and girls (1.2%).[6] Current youth cigarette use (middle and high school students combined) suggests cigarette use is higher among White, non-Hispanic youth (1.8%), lower among Hispanic youth (1.5%), and lowest among Black, non-Hispanic youth (1.0%).[6]

Use of Other Tobacco Products

In recent years the marketplace for tobacco products has become increasingly diverse, with the introduction of new tobacco products, such as e-cigarettes, and the reemergence of traditional products, such as certain types of cigars. In 2020 an estimated 19.0% (47.1 million) adults used any type of tobacco product; the large majority reported using cigarettes (12.5%, 30.8 million), but 3.7% (9.1 million) reporting e-cigarette use, 3.5% (8.6 million) cigars, 2.3% (5.7 million) smokeless tobacco, and 1.1% (2.6 million) pipes. Approximately 3.3% (8 million) of current adult tobacco product users reported using two or more tobacco products. E-cigarette use was highest among adults age 18 to 24 years old (9.4%), with over half (56.0%) of these young adults reporting that they had never smoked cigarettes.[5]

Since 2014 e-cigarettes have been the most commonly used tobacco product among youths. According to the most recent data from 2021, current e-cigarette use was reported by 11.3% of high school students and 2.8% of middle school students.[6] This represents a significant decrease from 2019, when current e-cigarette use was 27.5% among high school students and 10.5% among middle school students.[15] Other current tobacco product use (past 30-day use) among youth includes cigars (0.6% among middle school students, 2.1% among high school students), smokeless tobacco (0.6% of middle school students, 1.2% of high school students), hookah (0.4% of middle school students, 1.2% of high school students), nicotine pouches (0.3% of middle school students, 1.1% of high school students) and heated tobacco products, which heat tobacco leaves rather than vaporize a nicotine liquid (0.4% of middle school students, 0.8% of high school students).[6] Among current youth who use each tobacco product, the prevalence of frequent use (on ≥20 days of the preceding 30 days) ranged from 17.2% for nicotine pouches to 39.4% for e-cigarettes.[6]

Geographic Distribution

In 2021, as shown in Figure 7-2b, adult smoking prevalence varied substantially by state, ranging from 7.8% in Utah to 23.8% in West Virginia.[35] In 2020 cigarette smoking prevalence among youth ranged from 1.2% in California to 15.7% in Wyoming. In 2018

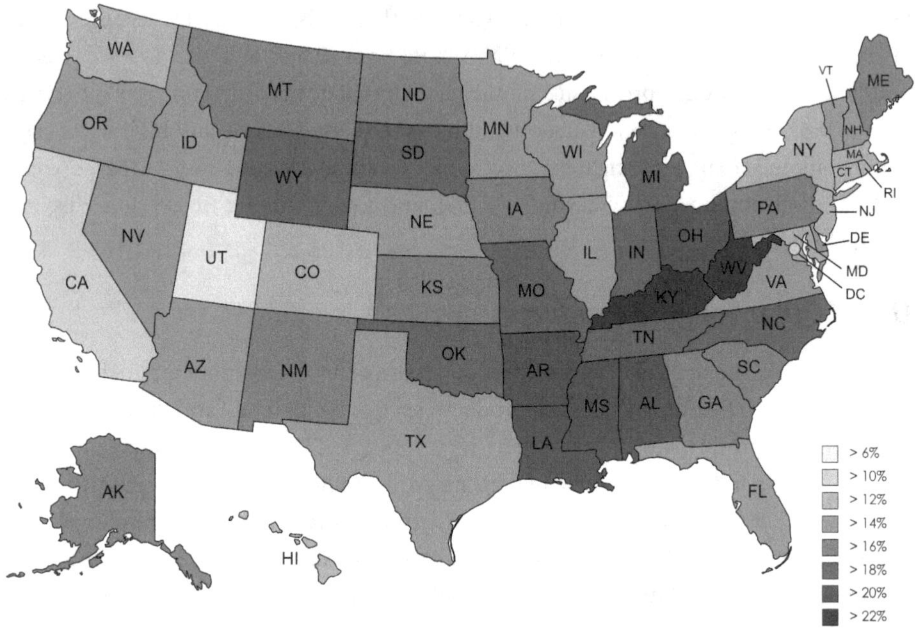

Source: Based on World Population Review.[35]

Figure 7-2b. Geographic Distribution of Tobacco Use in the United States, 2022

current smokeless tobacco use was highest in Wyoming (8.8%) and West Virginia (8.3%) and lowest in New Jersey (1.4%) and the District of Columbia (1.7%).[9]

Time Trends

Adults

In the early part of the 20th century the predominant forms of tobacco used by Americans were chewing tobacco, pipes, and cigars.[1] The first half of the 20th century saw a dramatic increase in annual per capita consumption of cigarettes to a peak of 4,345 in 1963, corresponding to more than half a pack a day per person in the United States. Except for an increase from 1971 through 1973, consumption has steadily declined since then.

Cigarette smoking prevalence among adults has declined dramatically from 42.4% in 1965 to 14.0% in 2019 (Figure 7-3a).[36–38] Before 1964, the prevalence of smoking among men had already begun to decline, whereas smoking among women was on the rise.[1] Although men historically had much higher smoking prevalence than women, the gap narrowed over time as more women started smoking and a greater decline in smoking prevalence was observed among men. Since about 1985 declines in smoking

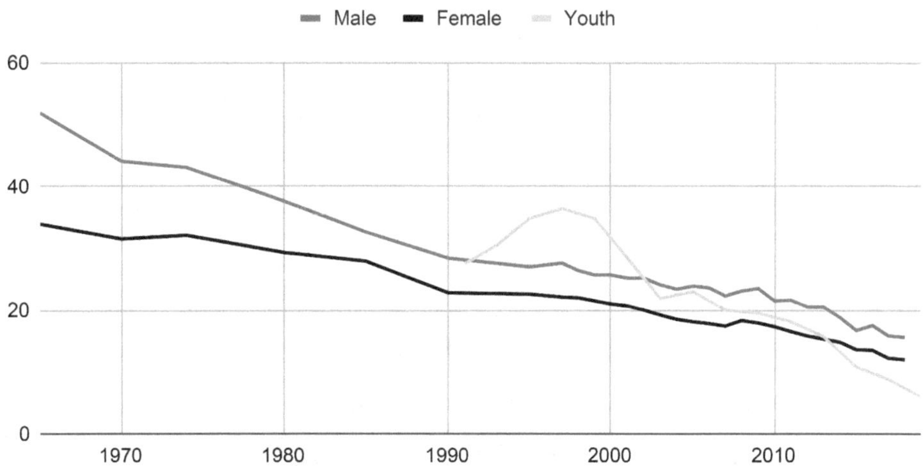

Source: Based on CDC.[37,38]

Figure 7-3a. Trends in Cigarette Use Among Youth and Adults by Sex, 1965–2019

prevalence are occurring at a comparable rate for women and men.[1] Although some differences in the rate of smoking prevalence declines have been observed by race/ethnicity, prevalence has nonetheless declined substantially in Black/African Americans, Whites, and Hispanics from 1965 to 2019. Smoking prevalence has declined fastest for persons with 16 or more years of education and slowest for persons with 9 to 11 years of education.[1]

E-cigarette use among adults has remained relatively stable despite a small increase in 2017 and 2018; prevalence of e-cigarette use among adults was 4.5% in 2016 and back to 4.5% again by 2019.[39] Of these, 36.9% also currently smoked cigarettes, and 39.5% formerly smoked cigarettes.[36]

Youth

From 2011 to 2021, current (past 30-day) cigarette smoking decreased dramatically among middle and high school students, from 4.3% in 2011 to 1.0% in 2020 among middle school students and from 15.8% in 2011 to 1.9% in 2021 among high school students (Figure 7-3b).[6,37,38] Over this same time period an initial increase in e-cigarette use was observed for these same age groups between 2017 and 2019, followed by a decrease from 10.5% of middle school students reporting current e-cigarette use in 2019 to 2.8% in 2021, and 27.5% of high school students currently using e-cigarettes in 2019 to 11.3% in 2021. Use of cigars and smokeless tobacco also went down from 2011 to 2021, from 11.6% of high school students reporting cigar use and 7.9% reporting smokeless tobacco use in 2011 down to 2.1% of high school students using cigars and 1.2% using smokeless tobacco in 2021 (Figure 7-3b).[6,40]

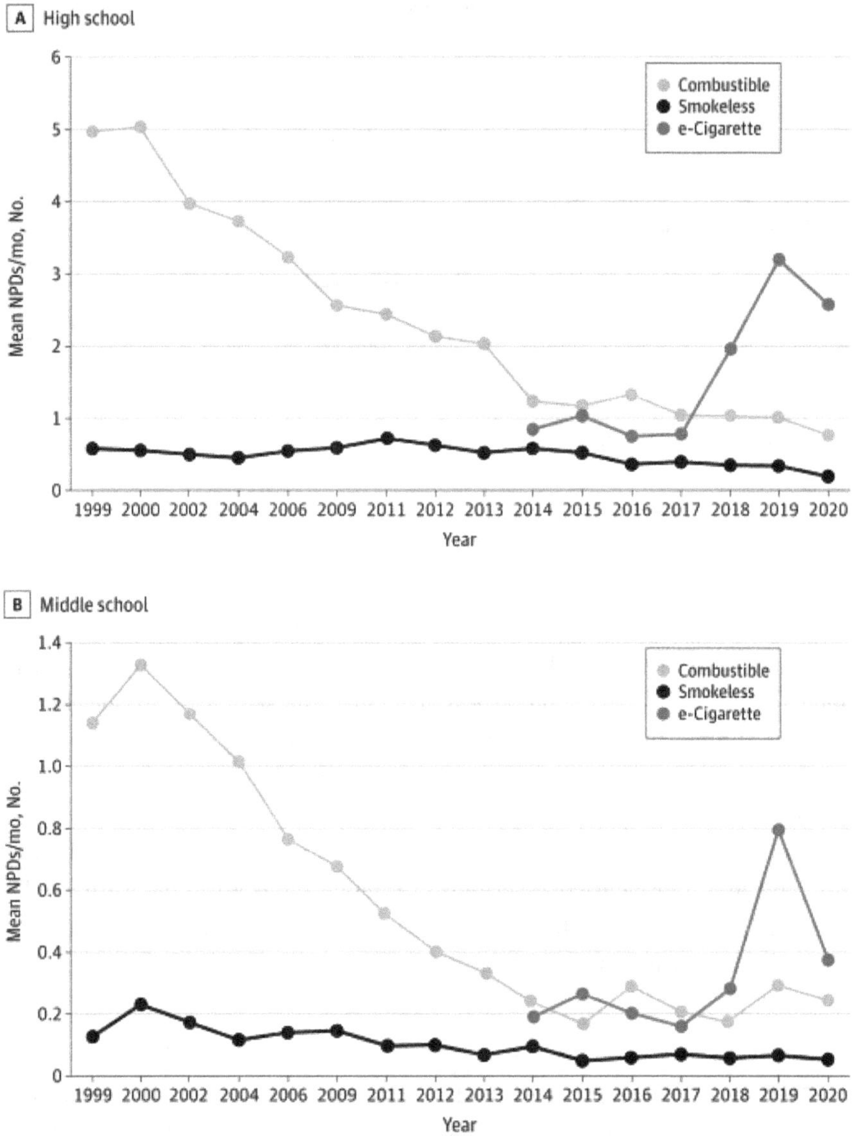

Source: Sun et al.[40] Reprinted under the terms of the CC BY license (https://creativecommons.org/licenses/by/4.0).
Note: NPD = nicotine product days.

Figure 7-3b. Trends in Nicotine Product Use Among US Adolescents, 1999–2020

CAUSES

Modifiable Risk Factors

There is no one factor that causes smoking initiation and maintenance. Although many factors are important for both smoking initiation and maintenance, certain factors have been identified to be particularly relevant to increasing risk (Figure 7-1). It is generally believed that the social and environmental influences are more likely to influence trying and experimenting with tobacco, and intrapersonal factors are more likely to predict frequent use, when development of nicotine dependence plays a larger role.[16] However, it is important to note the considerable variation in the trajectories of tobacco initiation and uptake of regular use and the factors that drive the development of tobacco-use behavior in youth and young adults.

Smoking Initiation

The average age of smoking onset has steadily increased from adolescence to young adulthood.[41] However, it is important to note that no one factor causes initiation. Further, the ever-changing landscape of nicotine and tobacco products highlights that combustible cigarettes are not the only form of use—e-cigarettes, for example, are an alternative. There are a multitude of interpersonal, environmental, intrapersonal, and biological factors that affect both the initiation and the maintenance of smoking (Table 7-3).

Interpersonal and Environmental Factors

Table 7-3 not only identifies important interpersonal and environmental factors that influence smoking initiation and maintenance but also provides salient yet clear examples of these factors.

Table 7-3. Environmental and Interpersonal Risk Factors for Smoking Initiation

Factor	Examples
Home smoking environment	• Parent, partner, or other housemate use of tobacco products
Community and cultural tobacco-use norms	• Having close friends who smoke or who use e-cigarettes • Overestimation of smoking prevalence among peers increases initiation
Relationship with parents and family	• Weaker relationship increases likelihood of initiation
Smoking in media	• Smoking or vaping in movies or television (smoking now part of audience rating)
Tobacco industry marketing techniques	• Sexualizing smoking behaviors • Discounts or coupons on cigarettes • Use of flavored products (including mentholated products) • Targeting advertisements to marginalized populations
Density of retail outlets selling tobacco	• Distance between convenience stores and gas stations
Level of enforcement of local police regarding sale of tobacco	• Frequency of ticketing for selling to a person aged < 21 y • Ticket amount and inclusion of jail time
Local policies regulating tobacco use	• Indoor smoking bans

Intrapersonal Factors

There are factors within an individual that can increase likelihood of smoking initiation. One such factor is psychiatric history, which is also linked to smoking maintenance. A history of psychiatric diagnosis is associated with almost two to five times higher likelihood of smoking initiation, depending on the psychiatric disorder.[42] There has also been substantial research examining the transdiagnostic risk factors and smoking initiation. Important transdiagnostic factors to consider in the initiation and maintenance of smoking (and other tobacco use behaviors) include anhedonia, anxiety sensitivity, distress tolerance, emotion regulation, and negative affect.[16,43]

Other individual risk factors for tobacco use include perception that smoking is more common than is actually true, low self-efficacy for refusal, low self-image, weak commitment to school and religion, belief that smoking can control weight and moods, and having a positive image of people who smoke.[16] Furthermore, as highlighted in the epidemiology section, certain groups are at greater risk for future use of cigarettes because of demographic factors, including their gender, race, age, socioeconomic status, and education.[16] All these factors, while uniquely important, are inherently affected by environmental factors and interpersonal experiences.

Biological Factors

Extant research highlights the impact of genetic factors on smoking initiation and maintenance.[16] While genetic factors are not modifiable among individuals, they do interact with other environmental and interpersonal factors to affect risk of smoking initiation and subsequent maintenance.[16] In addition to heritable biological factors, one notable factor associated with initiation is nicotine dependence. Nicotine dependence is the predominant reason for the continuation and maintenance of tobacco use. However, recent research suggests that for some adolescents, symptoms of nicotine dependence can develop early in the process of smoking initiation and at relatively low levels of use. Symptoms of nicotine dependence have been shown in people who use combustible and e-cigarettes prior to using even 100 cigarettes in a lifetime.[13,16] Emerging evidence suggests that the adolescent brain may be particularly vulnerable to the addictive properties of nicotine, including through alterations in structure and function that may influence lifelong susceptibility to addiction.[16]

Smoking Maintenance

Similar factors affect smoking maintenance, or cessation failures, and smoking initiation. Most notably, the impact of nicotine dependence is associated with the difficulty of many groups to successfully quit smoking. Research previously suggested individuals who smoke attempt to quit smoking at least 7 times before successfully stopping, but newer analyses suggest that 30 or more quit attempts are likely.[2] In this section we briefly highlight factors associated with cessation failure or smoking maintenance.

Interpersonal and Environmental Factors

All the factors listed in Table 7-3 remain as true for smoking maintenance as they do for initiation. The added problem is that once individuals want to quit smoking, they have already developed a certain level of nicotine dependence and must overcome this barrier.[44]

Intrapersonal Factors

Similarly, many factors that influence smoking initiation also influence maintenance. Individuals with particular difficulty quitting (highlighted in the High Risk Populations section) include those with low SES, low education, non-Hispanic Black race, psychiatric history, and lesbian, gay, or bisexual sexual orientation.[2,36] While decades of research have shown that persons with psychiatric disorders have greater difficulty quitting,[2] more recent analyses highlight that this may affect short-term cessation success, but not long-term cessation success.[45] This may point to the role of transdiagnostic risk factors in cessation success.[43,45]

Biological Factors

The most important biological factor associated with smoking and tobacco-use maintenance is nicotine dependence.[44] While certain groups have a greater predisposition to nicotine dependence (e.g., adolescents), the impact of nicotine dependence is observable across all populations. According to the US Surgeon General, the factors that influence developing nicotine dependence include

1. the effects of the product itself, including the addictive constituents, their pharmacokinetics and pharmacodynamics, and the design of the product that delivers the addictive constituents;
2. the response of the host, including genetic susceptibility and physiological response; and
3. the environmental setting that determines the availability of, accessibility to, and norms for use of the product.[44]

Population Attributable Risk

Table 7-4 represents the smoking attributable mortality (SAM) within the United States. Smoking causes 480,000 deaths annually and is the leading preventable cause of death and disability in the United States.[1] The relative risks (RR) from smoking are shown in Table 7-1. It is important to note that the risk for many smoking-related diseases decreases substantially after quitting.[2]

Table 7-4. Annual Deaths and Estimates of Smoking-Attributable Mortality for Adults

Disease	Men, Attributable Fraction			Women, Attributable Fraction			Total, Attributable Fraction		
	No. Deaths	SAM	%	No. Deaths	SAM	%	No. Deaths	SAM	%
Cancers									
Lung cancer	88,730	74,300	83.74	69,800	56,359	80.74	158,530	130,659	82.42
Other cancers	102,940	26,000	25.26	75,540	10,000	13.24	178,480	36,000	20.17
Total cancers	191,670	100,300	52.33	145,340	63,400	43.62	337,010	163,700	48.50
Cardiovascular and metabolic disease									
Coronary heart disease	218,870	61,800	28.24	193,720	37,500	19.36	412,590	99,300	24.07
Other heart diseases	75,670	13,400	17.71	96,200	12,100	12.58	171,870	25,500	14.84
Cerebrovascular disease	53,610	8,200	15.30	81,300	7,100	8.73	134,920	15,300	11.34
Other vascular disease	14,480	6,000	41.43	15,510	5,500	35.47	29,990	11,500	38.35
Diabetes mellitus	35,200	6,200	17.61	35,600	2,800	7.86	70,810	9,000	12.10
Total cardiovascular and metabolic diseases	397,840	95,600	24.03	422,330	65,000	15.39	820,170	160,600	19.58
Pulmonary disease									
Pneumonia, influenza, tuberculosis	25,300	7,800	30.83	30,290	4,700	15.52	55,590	12,500	22.49
Chronic obstructive pulmonary disease	61,430	50,400	82.04	66,300	50,200	75.71	127,740	100,600	78.76
Total pulmonary diseases	86,730	58,200	67.10	96,590	54,900	56.84	183,320	113,100	61.70
Total cancers, cardiovascular and metabolic diseases, pulmonary diseases	676,240	254,100	37.58	664,260	183,300	27.59	1,340,500	437,400	32.63

(Continued)

Table 7-4. (Continued)

Disease	Men, Attributable Fraction			Women, Attributable Fraction			Total, Attributable Fraction		
	No. Deaths	SAM	%	No. Deaths	SAM	%	No. Deaths	SAM	%
Perinatal conditions and sudden infant death syndrome									
Perinatal conditions	5,970	346	5.80	4,620	267	5.78	10,590	613	5.79
Sudden infant death syndrome	1,370	236	17.26	950	164	17.26	2,320	400	17.26
Total perinatal conditions	7,340	582	7.93	5,570	431	7.74	12,900	1,013	7.85
Residential fires		336			284			620	
Secondhand smoke									
Lung cancer	88,730	4,370	4.93	69,800	2,960	4.24	158,530	7,330	4.63
Coronary heart disease	218,800	19,150	8.75	193,720	14,800	7.64	412,590	33,950	8.23
Total secondhand smoke	307,600	23,530	7.65	263,520	17,760	6.74	571,120	41,280	7.23
Total attributable deaths		278,540			201,770			480,320	

Note: SAM = smoking attributable mortality.

EVIDENCE-BASED TREATMENT

Prevention

Comprehensive tobacco prevention programs may include mass media campaigns, price increases on tobacco products, regulatory initiatives such as those that ban advertising to youths, restrictions on youth access to tobacco, establishment of smoke-free public and workplace environments, and statewide, community-wide, and school-based programs and policies. These programs are effective in reducing the initiation, prevalence, and intensity of smoking among youth and young adults.[1,2,16]

Price Increase

There is a robust body of evidence on the effectiveness of price increases in reducing youth initiation.[2] Price increases are also one of the most effective interventions to increase cessation. Studies show that a 10% increase in cigarette price will result in a 3% to 5% reduction in overall cigarettes consumed.[2] Similarly, a 10% price increase in e-cigarettes reduced sales by 12% to 19% (higher sales reduction in reusable e-cigarettes).[46] More recent analyses highlight that higher combustible cigarette prices are associated with higher per capita sales of reusable e-cigarettes, suggesting that e-cigarettes may be used as a substitution for combustible cigarettes and that price increases should be applied across all forms of tobacco and nicotine delivery products.[47] In short, increases in cigarette prices decrease the prevalence of smoking and also the average number of cigarettes people smoke.[2] Further, cigarette price increases the motivation to quit, number of quit attempts, and rates of successful smoking cessation among people who smoke.[2]

Important to note is that youth and young adults are two to three times more responsive than adults to changes in cigarette prices.[16] This suggests that price increases may be a particularly helpful preventive measure to stop the initiation of tobacco produce use. However, price increases may not be as impactful in all populations (e.g., non-Hispanic African Americans),[2] resulting in greater health disparities.

School-Based Tobacco Prevention Programs

The Surgeon General has concluded that school-based programs with evidence of effectiveness, containing specific components, can produce at least short-term effects but noted that these programs produce larger and more sustained effects when they are implemented in combination with other initiatives, such as mass media public education campaigns, family programs, and state and community programs. Data suggest that the most effective programs are those that are interactive, address social influences, include components on intentions not to use tobacco, use peer leaders, add community components, and include life skills practice. Programs that showed evidence of longer-term effectiveness contained at least 15 sessions, including some up to at least ninth grade.[16]

Public Health Education

Public education campaigns change social norms about tobacco use, increase awareness of the health hazards of smoking and exposure to secondhand smoke, educate about tobacco industry actions, provide motivations for people to quit, inform people who use tobacco about resources available to help them quit, and support policy efforts. The first national, federally funded, anti-smoking campaign, TIPS From Former Smokers, demonstrated a significant increase in cessation attempts, sustained cessation, and call to quitlines. The 2020 Surgeon General's Report states that there is sufficient evidence to infer mass media campaigns increase quit rates and calls to quitlines.[2]

Advertising Bans

The 1998 Master Settlement Agreement (MSA) limits the advertising, marketing, and promotion of the four largest tobacco companies in the United States. While this has led to an overall decrease in the smoking rate, recent research highlights that tobacco industries have shifted their focus to the retail environment.[2] The 2020 Surgeon General's Report states that the current evidence for reducing retail point-of-sale advertising and retail density is suggestive but not sufficient in terms of impact on smoking cessation.[2] However, this report also notes that this should not deter us from continuing to work to ban advertisements and conducting more research on these effects so as to develop a more substantial research base.

Age Limit for Smoking

In December 2019 the US president signed into legislation an amendment to the Federal Food, Drug, and Cosmetic Act, which raised the minimum age for tobacco sales from 18 to 21 years. Notably, this law banned all tobacco product (including e-cigarettes) to anyone under 21 years. This effectively caused the remaining 31 states and territories that had not already imposed local or statewide ordinances to raise the smoking age to 21. Analyses of states that had previously enacted this law show a significant reduction in cigarette sales and menthol market share, which is of particular importance because these products are more commonly used by adolescents and young adults.[48]

Smoke-Free Policies

Smoke-free policies not only protect nonsmokers from secondhand smoke exposure but also reduce the prevalence of tobacco use, increase quit attempts, and prevent initiation among adolescents and young adults. Smoke-free laws are linked to a 3.4% decrease in tobacco-use prevalence and 6.4% higher cessation rates.[2] As of October 2019, the United States had 61% of its land area protected by a smoke-free law or policy.[2] When limiting smoking in public or private housing areas, it is important to provide low-cost or free cessation treatment options to prevent increasing health inequities among those who cannot otherwise access these treatments (see Treatment section below).

Screening

One of the most important screening strategies for health care professionals is to ask about a patient's tobacco use. Such information should be ascertained on every visit and documented in the medical record.[49] Routine screening for tobacco use is critical for ensuring that all people who use tobacco receive effective treatment every time they are seen by a health care professional.

Biochemical measures are available to assess whether a person is smoking cigarettes, is exposed to secondhand smoke, or uses e-cigarettes. These measures are generally used in research or surveillance studies but are not recommended for use as part of routine clinical care of patients who use tobacco. While screening is a key component of the clinical guidelines for tobacco-use dependence, it is not sufficient to alter smoking behavior and needs to be coupled with other treatment measures. Clinicians should be aware that certain subgroups of participants (i.e., pregnant women, patients with cardiac disease, patients with respiratory illness) may underreport smoking and that the use of multiple-choice questions as opposed to a yes-or-no question can increase disclosure among pregnant women by as much as 40%.[49]

Treatment

In addition to prevention and screening interventions to promote smoking cessation or prevent initiation, multiple evidence-based treatments exist to facilitate successful smoking cessation. These include pharmacotherapeutic interventions, counseling interventions, quitline interventions, mobile phone-based interventions, and internet-based interventions. These treatments have been shown to double or triple cessation success.[49] Further, while medications and counseling are each effective independently, the strongest effect on cessation success is the combination of these two treatments.[2]

Notably, while the reduction of out-of-pocket costs of treatments may not be an intervention in and of itself, there is strong evidence to support it. Of the 68% of adults who smoke and want to quit, 55% tried to quit in the past year, but only 31% of those who tried to quit used evidence-based treatment when doing so.[2] One of the greatest barriers to use of evidence-based treatment is the cost. Therefore, the 2020 Surgeon General's Report states that the evidence supports promotion of comprehensive, barrier-free evidence-based cessation insurance coverage.[2] The Affordable Care Act, passed in 2010, stated that insurers should provide coverage for treatment of at least two quit attempts per year, which includes counseling and all seven of the FDA-approved smoking cessation medications (discussed next).[2] Tobacco-use treatment for adults is extremely cost-effective, more so than other commonly covered preventive interventions, such as mammography, treatment for mild-to-moderate hypertension, and treatment for hypercholesterolemia.[49]

Medications

A total of seven first-line medications are FDA-approved for smoking cessation. The primary rationale for use of medications during a cessation attempt is to help alleviate symptoms of nicotine withdrawal.[2,49] While there is strong research to support the effectiveness of these medications, certain populations have insufficient evidence to support the use of these medications during cessation (i.e., pregnant women, adolescents, light smokers, people who use smokeless tobacco).[49] These medications can be separated by whether they are nicotine replacement therapies (5) or other oral medications (2). Furthermore, the previous boxed warning on both Varenicline and Bupropion were removed in December 2016 after a large trial showed no increased risk of neuropsychiatric symptoms compared with other cessation medications.[2]

Nicotine Replacement Therapies

All five forms of nicotine replacement therapy (NRT)—transdermal nicotine patch, nicotine gum, nicotine lozenge, nicotine nasal spray, and nicotine inhaler—work by delivering concentrations lower than those found a conventional cigarettes. The nasal spray and inhaler both require prescriptions for use, while the patch, gum, and lozenge are available over the counter. However, prescriptions may be required for all NRT products to ensure insurance coverage. All NRTs show similar rates of efficacy but are particularly helpful for people with high levels of nicotine dependence (vs. those with lower dependence levels). They are available in different dosages, with higher dosages corresponding to the nicotine consumption amount prior to quitting and nicotine dependence levels. These medications are used daily (some multiple times per day, as needed) for durations ranging from eight weeks to six months.[2] Dosage charts are readily available to assist clinicians.[2]

Varenicline

Varenicline is intended to be used 1 week prior to the quit date and used for 12 weeks (some patients may use it for an additional 12 weeks). This medication requires a prescription for use, and clinicians must use caution when prescribing to patients with severe renal impairment, as well as to women who are pregnant or breastfeeding, and to adolescents.[2]

Bupropion

Bupropion is intended to be used 1 to 2 weeks prior to the quit date and used for 7 to 12 weeks on average (some patients may use it for up to six months). This medication requires a prescription and is contraindicated for persons with a seizure disorder, concomitant bupropion therapy, or life history of bulimia or anorexia nervosa. It is also contraindicated for persons who have used MAO inhibitors in the last 14 days or are going through simultaneous abrupt cessation of alcohol or sedatives/benzodiazepines. Clinicians should use precaution before prescribing this medication to patients with hepatic impairments and concomitant therapy with medications/conditions known to lower seizure threshold (in addition to women who are pregnant/breastfeeding and adolescents).[2]

Counseling

The 2008 PHS Clinical Practice Guideline[49] reported the following findings: brief clinician advice to quit is effective (30% increase in cessation rates), and more intensive counseling is even more effective (doubles the cessation rate). Counseling can be delivered as individual, group, or telephone counseling. Medications approved by FDA increase cessation by twofold to threefold.[49] These findings are consistent with other published recommendations.[2] According to the 2020 Surgeon General's Report, although there are anecdotal reports about people who smoke using e-cigarettes to quit smoking and an increasing number of randomized controlled trials suggest they are effective cessation aids,[50] there are not sufficient data to support this as a cessation method at this time. Thus to date no e-cigarette has been approved as an effective cessation aid.[2]

Cessation counseling or coaching provides practical advice about quitting and provides social support to those who use tobacco as they try to quit. Using counseling and medication together or combining medications results in higher cessation rates.[49] A major problem, however, is that physicians are not providing the most effective treatments, few people are using them if they are provided,[2] and many people trying to quit smoking use fewer doses of the medications and use medication for a shorter period than recommended, which may contribute to lower success rates.[49]

The PHS Clinical Practice Guideline concluded that effective tobacco-use treatments should be offered to every patient who uses tobacco, recommending a brief intervention of three minutes, called the Five A's[49]:

- Ask every patient at every visit if he or she uses tobacco and document the patient's status in the medical chart (e.g., as a vital sign).
- Advise all patients who use tobacco to quit.
- Assess patients' interest in quitting.
- Assist people who smoke in quitting by helping them set a quit date, recommending or prescribing FDA-approved medications unless contraindicated, and providing or referring patients to more intensive individual, group, or telephone counseling.
- Arrange for follow-up (by telephone or by scheduling a return appointment) to assess progress and encourage those who relapse to try again.

Intensive treatment strategies that have the most evidence of success include behavior therapy, cognitive behavioral therapy, and motivational interviewing (for people who smoke but are not yet willing to quit).[2,49] These therapies have each shown significant success in improving cessation attempts, particularly when combined with cessation medications.[2] There is also growing research on the benefit of acceptance and commitment therapy, which draws from cognitive behavioral therapy but focuses on accepting rather than altering cognitions and offers contingency management and monetary incentives for quitting.[2] In addition, there is growing research on delivering these more intensive counseling interventions via alternate modalities such as the internet or mobile phone applications.[2]

Mobile Health Cessation Interventions

Mobile phone, internet, mobile application, or mobile text-based cessation interventions use interactive features to deliver evidence-based information, strategies, and behavioral support. Typically, participants receive text messages that support their quit attempt. However, with the growing capabilities of mobile phones, interventions can incorporate online content and other mobile health (mHealth) tools. Content may be adapted for specific populations and messages may be tailored for individuals. These interventions may be automated, and they may include text responses provided on demand to participants encountering urges to smoke. These interventions can also be coordinated with additional interventions, such as quitline-based cessation services or provision of medications. Perhaps most important is that these interventions allow many individuals access to evidence-based interventions they would otherwise not have because of cost, location, and unavailability of providers.[51] The 2020 Surgeon General's Report stated that short-text-message cessation services and web-based mHealth services independently improve cessation success, but there is inadequate research to infer that smartphone applications for smoking cessation are independently effective.[2]

Quitline Interventions

Telephone cessation quitlines increase quitting success and are recommended by multiple guiding agencies.[1,2,49] Telephone quitlines provide practical advice to people who smoke who are interested in quitting about how to deal with withdrawal symptoms and other challenges of quitting. Quitlines increase access to treatment because they are free; generally available days, evenings, and weekends, they do not require transportation or child-care arrangements. They also provide individually tailored help.[2] In addition, the semi-anonymous nature of the phone counseling encourages candid discussion, and the use of structured protocols promotes consistent quality control. Some quitlines also provide free nicotine replacement therapy.[1]

MOVING FORWARD

Continued research on the effect of various public health actions on reducing tobacco use is important in adapting interventions to maintain and increase effectiveness. The subsections that follow highlight key issues focusing on these areas:

- E-cigarette (vaping)–related issues
  - Regulation of ever-evolving noncombustible nicotine/tobacco products;
  - Utility of e-cigarettes in cessation of combustible cigarettes;
  - Effective cessation of e-cigarettes; and
  - Impact of e-cigarettes on health.
- Marijuana regulation and integration with the tobacco industry.
- Improved tobacco-use treatment interventions and finding ways to increase access to treatment.
- Assessing tobacco use and developing effective interventions for reducing tobacco use in disparate populations.

Regulatory Status of E-Cigarettes

A historical challenge of tobacco control that has become a major concern in recent years is the emergence of novel products specifically designed to avoid regulation, particularly the 2009 Tobacco Control Act, which gave the FDA power to require manufacturers of new tobacco products to submit premarket tobacco product applications (PMTAs) to determine whether the products would be allowed to enter the market.

This premarket review authority was not exercised over e-cigarettes until a September 2020 court order required it. Because these products had already been on the market for some time, they were given one year to submit a PMTA and could continue to be sold until FDA issued an authorization or a marketing denial order. Following the September 2021 application, FDA issued marketing denial orders for over a million e-cigarettes and a few approvals as well, but many applications are still awaiting review.[14] In the meantime, unauthorized products remain on the market and easily accessible to minors.

The retroactive PMTA approval of e-cigarettes is a prime example of the way in which the current federal tobacco regulatory framework leaves public health playing a desperate game of whack-a-mole, forever struggling to push back whatever new product has hooked their communities. As the industry continues to design new and more addictive products, the tobacco-control movement must rapidly address each new product to avoid backsliding on the past gains in reducing tobacco addiction and disease.

Synthetic Nicotine

One novel product that poses regulatory challenges is synthetic nicotine. Synthetic nicotine is manufactured in a laboratory rather than extracted from the tobacco plant itself. Manufacturers argue that synthetic nicotine is not a true "tobacco" product and therefore not subject to the Tobacco Control Act or most other state and local tobacco laws.[1] Currently there is no good way to determine whether products claiming to contain only synthetic nicotine are truly tobacco-free or simply claiming to be.

Puff Bar, by far the most popular e-cigarette brand among children, disappeared from the market for months only to return rebranded as a synthetic nicotine. Puff Bar, the manufacturer, has claimed that its products are not made of tobacco and used this claim to expand its many child-friendly flavors, such as "Kookie Krunch" and "Banana Fried Cream Cakes," over the market as its equivalent nonsynthetic competitors are removed from the shelves.[14]

Many e-cigarette manufacturers are using the regulatory loopholes around synthetic nicotine to stay in business after receiving PMTA marketing denial orders from FDA. Some manufacturers state very clearly that they are switching their denied products to synthetic nicotine only to avoid FDA regulation, while others passively market their product as "tobacco-free" to assert their belief that they are not subject to current tobacco laws. Many brands still awaiting PMTA review are offering both synthetic and tobacco-derived versions of the same product, ready to switch exclusively to synthetics the moment their tobacco-derived products receive FDA marketing denials.[14]

On April 14, 2022, new legislation came into effect that gave FDA the power to regulate products containing nicotine from any source. Manufacturers of synthetic nicotine were given until May 14, 2022, to submit PMTAs for FDA review. As of the writing of this chapter, it is unclear what enforcement of this new legislation will look like or whether it will be enough to change the direction of the epidemic of youth e-cigarette use.[52]

Disposable E-Cigarettes

Another emerging product that poses regulatory challenges is the disposable e-cigarette. Disposable e-cigarettes contain cartridges prefilled with e-liquid and are designed to be thrown away entirely after a certain number of uses. This is in contrast to traditional refillable e-cigarettes where people who vape keep the vaporizer device and refill the e-liquid only as needed. Disposable e-cigarettes tend to be incredibly cheap, with some available for less than $5. They can also contain higher concentrations of nicotine than refillable products, even Juul.[14]

Although flavored refillable e-cigarettes have been functionally banned through the PMTA process since February 2020, flavored disposable products have not. As such, sales of disposable e-cigarettes have grown by at least 258% since 2020.[14] This growth in popularity is primarily driven by youth who use e-cigarettes, a majority of whom now prefer disposables, Puff Bar in particular.[6]

E-Cigarettes as a Harm Reduction Technique

The use of e-cigarettes for cessation of combustible cigarettes remains a contentious subject in the US public health community.[53] A major concern is use among youth, as over two million middle and high school students reported currently using e-cigarettes in 2020.[6] However, e-cigarettes may also aid in cessation of combustible cigarettes.[54] Neither FDA nor the US Preventive Services Task Force has approved the use of e-cigarettes as cessation devices in the United States.[2] However, many people who smoke combustible cigarettes report using e-cigarettes to reduce their smoking or quit combustibles entirely,[55] and an increasing number of randomized controlled trials suggest they are effective cessation aids.[50] Unfortunately, a substantial proportion of people who use e-cigarettes continue to use combustible cigarettes.[56] The impact of e-cigarette use for sustained cessation of combustible cigarettes remains unclear, and more research is needed.

Similarly, while the effectiveness of e-cigarettes for smoking cessation is not fully understood, ample research suggests that e-cigarettes are less harmful than combustible cigarettes.[50] However, the long-term impact of e-cigarettes is unclear, particularly with the rapid evolution of these products and the difficulty regulating the chemical components. Moreover, there is a dearth of research examining effective and efficacious ways to successfully quit using e-cigarettes. In summary, ample work remains to be done in the area of e-cigarettes.

Marijuana Regulation and Integration With the Tobacco Industry

The wave of cannabis (marijuana) legalization across the United States also poses challenges for tobacco control. Secondhand smoke exposure from smoking marijuana is of particular concern. Without proper regulation of production and additives, marijuana smoke can contain added toxic chemicals like ammonia and hydrogen cyanide in concentrations up to 20 times higher than in the smoke of combustible tobacco cigarettes.[57] Many of the policies passed to prevent secondhand tobacco smoke exposure—including banning use in public spaces, workplaces, multiunit housing, and while driving—are challenged by gaps that do not account for increasingly common smoke from nontobacco products like marijuana.[57]

Because federal law regulates marijuana as a completely illegal Schedule 1 drug, there are currently no mechanisms to address these challenges at a national level.[57] Instead, state- and local-level tobacco-control movements must work to address these challenges as effectively as possible within their segmented communities, even as a nationwide marijuana industry grows.

Improving Treatment Efficacy and Access

Although current evidence-based treatments for tobacco cessation double or triple cessation success,[49] less than one-third of individuals trying to quit utilize these methods.[2] As discussed earlier, one of the main barriers to use is cost,[2] but additional barriers to treatment access exist (e.g., misperception of perceived treatment effectiveness, limited prescription by providers, distance from treatment providers, language barriers). Greater efforts are needed to ensure that existing treatments are made available for all people who smoke regardless of demographic characteristics.

There is, in addition, a call for improvement of the effectiveness of existing psychosocial treatments for smoking cessation.[58] Although there have been improvements in reaching more people who smoke, improvements attributable, in large part, to the advancement of digital interventions and health care system changes, more work is needed to identify psychosocial content and mechanisms to increase effectiveness of all cessation interventions.[58] On the prevention side, greater emphasis on policies to prevent the initiation of smoking among populations commonly targeted by the tobacco industry (e.g., African Americans) needs to be made, and the policies need to be enforced (i.e., enforcing the ban on mentholated cigarettes).

Assessing Tobacco Use and Developing Effective Interventions

There is clear evidence that the tobacco industry has a long-standing history of targeting multiple groups, among them African Americans, Native Americans, active and veteran military service members, lower-SES populations, and the psychologically distressed, to ensure increased likelihood of use and failure with cessation.[2] The reduction in tobacco use in the United States is considered a public health triumph,[2] but it is only half achieved. Perhaps most important, large disparities in tobacco use across groups defined by race, ethnicity, educational level, sexual orientation and identity, and SES and across regions of the country have emerged over the past 55 years. The diversification of product use and the increasing pattern of dual or poly-tobacco product use among both youth and adults have undermined progress in reducing overall tobacco use.

A research agenda that adapts to the changing tobacco-control landscape to continually identify the important emerging research needs, informs new tobacco-control interventions, and determines ways to quickly translate relevant research findings into action is critical. Careful evaluations of specific interventions, timely evaluation of new and innovative strategies, and macro-level analyses of the impact of interventions on tobacco use, health outcomes, and health care and productivity costs will be useful to inform future interventions. In particular, focusing on those populations that continue to smoke heavily or find it extremely difficult to quit is a worthy goal of the public health and research communities. Their targeted efforts aim to ensure that the predatory tactics of the tobacco industry are countered and that in so doing they can help improve the health of these marginalized communities.

Reducing tobacco use is a shared responsibility of federal, state, and local governments, the public health community, the health care system, the private sector, and individual communities. If each sector did its part to fully implement the proven strategies discussed in this chapter, one could expect faster progress in reducing tobacco use. A concerted effort is needed, analogous to the efforts to eliminate the morbidity and mortality resulting from polio or smallpox. The leading preventable cause of death in the world deserves no less.

DISCUSSION QUESTIONS

1. Why might the rate of utilizing evidence-based treatment be so low, despite its proven efficacy in helping people quit?
2. Provide several examples of how the tobacco industry has worked to keep the sale of tobacco products high. What groups has this industry's marketing strategies targeted?
3. Should e-cigarettes be used as a cessation method? What are the potential benefits of governing agencies approving e-cigarettes for cessation treatment and what are potential drawbacks?

REFERENCES

1. US Department of Health and Human Services. The health consequences of smoking—50 years of progress: a report of the surgeon general. 2014. Updated May 21, 2021. Archived. Available at: https://www.cdc.gov/tobacco/sgr/50th-anniversary/index.htm. Accessed January 11, 2023.
2. US Department of Health and Human Services. *Smoking Cessation: A Report of the Surgeon General.* Rockville, MD: US Dept of Health and Human Services, Center for Disease Control and Prevention, National Center for Chronic Disease Prevention and Health Promotion, Office on Smoking and Health; 2020.
3. Zhong G, Wang Y, Zhang Y, Guo JJ, Zhao Y. Smoking is associated with an increased risk of dementia: a meta-analysis of prospective cohort studies with investigation of potential effect modifiers. *PLoS One.* 2015;10(3):e0118333. doi:10.1371/journal.pone.0118333
4. Bhatta DN, Glantz SA. Association of e-cigarette use with respiratory disease among adults: a longitudinal analysis. *Am J Prev Med.* 2020;58(2):182–190. doi:10.1016/j.amepre.2019.07.028
5. Cornelius ME, Loretan CG, Wang TW, Jamal A, Homa DM. Tobacco product use among adults—United States, 2020. *MMWR Morb Mortal Wkly Rep.* 2022;71(11):397–405. doi:10.15585/mmwr.mm7111a1
6. Gentzke AS, Wang TW, Cornelius M, et al. Tobacco product use and associated factors among middle and high school students—National Youth Tobacco Survey, United States, 2021. *MMWR Surveill Summ.* 2022;71(5):1–29. doi:10.15585/mmwr.ss7105a1

7. Azagba S, Shan L, Manzione LC, Latham K, Rogers C, Qeadan F. Single cigarette purchasers among adult US smokers. *Prev Med Rep*. 2020;17:101055. doi:10.1016/j.pmedr.2020.101055
8. National Cancer Institute. Smokeless tobacco and public health; a global perspective. 2020. Updated July 14, 2022. https://cancercontrol.cancer.gov/brp/tcrb/smokeless-tobacco. Accessed January 11, 2023.
9. Centers for Disease Control and Prevention. Smokeless tobacco product use in the United States. 2022. Available at: https://www.cdc.gov/tobacco/data_statistics/fact_sheets/smokeless/use_us/index.htm. Accessed January 11, 2023.
10. Centers for Disease Control and Prevention. Smoking and tobacco use: cigars. Updated November 10, 2022. Available at: https://www.cdc.gov/tobacco/data_statistics/fact_sheets/tobacco_industry/cigars/index.htm#. Accessed January 11, 2023.
11. Henley SJ, Thun MJ, Chao A, Calle EE. Association between exclusive pipe smoking and mortality from cancer and other diseases. *J Natl Cancer Inst*. 2004;96(11):853–861.
12. Qasim H, Alarabi AB, Alzoubi KH, Karim ZA, Alshbool FZ, Khasawneh FT. The effects of hookah/waterpipe smoking on general health and the cardiovascular system. *Environ Health Prev Med*. 2019;24(1):58. doi:10.1186/s12199-019-0811-y
13. US Department of Health and Human Services. *E-Cigarette Use Among Youth and Young Adults: A Report of the Surgeon General*. 2016. Atlanta, GA: US Dept of Health and Human Services, Centers for Disease Control and Prevention, National Center for Chronic Disease Prevention and Health Promotion, Office on Smoking and Health; 2016. Available at: https://e-cigarettes.surgeongeneral.gov/documents/2016_SGR_Full_Report_non-508.pdf. Accessed January 11, 2023.
14. Campaign for Tobacco-Free Kids. An e-cigarette market update. 2021. Available at: https://www.tobaccofreekids.org/assets/content/press_office/2021/ecigreport.pdf. Accessed January 11, 2023.
15. Cullen KA, Gentzke AS, Sawdey MD, et al. E-cigarette use among youth in the United States, 2019. *JAMA*. 2019;322(21):2095–2103. doi:10.1001/jama.2019.18387
16. National Center for Chronic Disease Prevention and Health Promotion, US Office on Smoking and Health. *Preventing Tobacco Use Among Youth and Young Adults*. Atlanta, GA: Centers for Disease Control and Prevention; 2012. Available at: https://www.ncbi.nlm.nih.gov/books/NBK99237. Accessed January 11, 2023.
17. Center for Public Health Systems Science. *Best Practices User Guide: Health Equity in Tobacco Prevention and Control*. Atlanta, GA: US Dept of Health and Human Services, Centers for Disease Control and Prevention, National Center for Chronic Disease Prevention and Health Promotion, Office on Smoking and Health; 2015. Available at: https://www.cdc.gov/tobacco/stateandcommunity/best-practices-health-equity/pdfs/bp-health-equity.pdf. Accessed January 11, 2023.
18. Evans-Reeves K, Gilmore A, Zatonsky M. Addiction at any cost: Philip Morris International uncovered. 2020. Available at: https://exposetobacco.org/wp-content/uploads/STOP_Report_Addiction-At-Any-Cost.pdf. Accessed January 11, 2023.
19. Federal Register. Federal financial participation is state expenditures, federal matching shares for Medicaid, the Children's Health Insurance Program and Aid to the Needy, Aged, Blind or Disabled Persons. 2021;86(225):67479–67480. Available at: https://www.govinfo.gov/content/pkg/FR-2021-11-26/pdf/2021-25798.pdf. Accessed January 11, 2023.

20. Society of Actuaries. Economic effects of environmental tobacco smoke. 2021. Available at: https://www.soa.org/resources/research-reports/2000-2006/research-economic-effect. Accessed January 11, 2023.
21. Centers for Disease Control and Prevention. Outbreak of lung injury associated with the use of e-cigarette, or vaping, products. 2021. Archived. Available at: https://www.cdc.gov/tobacco/basic_information/e-cigarettes/severe-lung-disease.html. Accessed January 12, 2023.
22. Patanavanich R, Glantz SA. Smoking is associated with worse outcomes of COVID-19 particularly among younger adults: a systematic review and meta-analysis. *BMC Public Health.* 2021;21(1):1554. doi:10.1186/s12889-021-11579-x
23. Holmes L Jr., Enwere M, Williams J, et al. Black-White risk differentials in COVID-19 (SARS-COV2) transmission, mortality and case fatality in the United States: translational epidemiologic perspective and challenges. *Int J Environ Res Public Health.* 2020;17(12):4322. doi:10.3390/ijerph17124322
24. Stigler-Granados P, Fulton L, Nunez Patlan E, Terzyk M, Novotny TE. Global health perspectives on cigarette butts and the environment. *Int J Environ Res Public Health.* 2019;16(10):1858. doi:10.3390/ijerph16101858
25. Ocean Conservancy, International Coastal Cleanup. Together, We Are Team Ocean: 2020 report. 2020. Available at: https://oceanconservancy.org/wp-content/uploads/2020/10/FINAL_2020ICC_Report.pdf. Accessed January 12, 2023.
26. Micevska T, Warne MS, Pablo F, Patra R. Variation in, and causes of, toxicity of cigarette butts to a cladoceran and microtox. *Arch Environ Contam Toxicol.* 2006;50(2):205–212. doi:10.1007/s00244-004-0132-y
27. Register K. Cigarette butts as litter-toxic as well as ugly. *Underwater Naturalist.* 2000;25(2):23–29.
28. Krause MJ, Townsend TG. Hazardous waste status of discarded electronic cigarettes. *Waste Manag.* 2015;39:57–62. doi:10.1016/j.wasman.2015.02.005
29. SIMS Lifecycle Services. A closer look: lithium-ion batteries in e-waste. 2019. Available at: https://www.simslifecycle.com/2019/05/21/a-closer-look-lithium-ion-batteries-in-e-waste. Accessed January 23, 2023.
30. Hendlin YH. Alert: public health implications of electronic cigarette waste. *Am J Public Health.* 2018;108(11):1489–1490. doi:10.2105/AJPH.2018.304699
31. Forster M. What happens when you throw away e-cigarettes. November 18, 2018. Available at: https://missionlocal.org/2018/11/what-happens-when-you-throw-away-an-e-cigarette. Accessed January 12, 2023.
32. Drug Enforcement Administration. DEA to accept electronic vaping devices and cartridges as part of National Prescription Drug Take Back Day. 2019. Available at: https://www.dea.gov/press-releases/2019/10/18/dea-accept-electronic-vaping-devices-and-cartridges-part-national. Accessed January 12, 2023.
33. Geist HJ. Global assessment of deforestation related to tobacco farming. *Tob Control.* 1999;8(1):18–28. doi:10.1136/tc.8.1.18
34. Drope J, Schluger NW, Cahn Z, et al. Growing. In: Drope J, Schluger NW, eds. *The Tobacco Atlas.* 6th ed. Atlanta, GA: American Cancer Society; 2018:14–15. Available at: https://theunion.org/sites/default/files/2020-12/TobaccoAtlas_6thEdition_LoRes.pdf. Accessed January 12, 2023.

35. World Population Review. Smoking rates by state. 2022. Available at: https://worldpopulationreview.com/state-rankings/smoking-rates-by-state. Accessed January 12, 2023.
36. Cornelius ME, Wang TW, Jamal A, Loretan CG, Neff LJ. Tobacco product use among adults — United States, 2019. *MMWR Morb Mortal Wkly Rep.* 2020;69(46):1736–1742. doi:10.15585/mmwr.mm6946a4
37. Centers for Disease Control and Prevention. Trends in the prevalence of tobacco use national YRBS: 1991–2019. Available at: https://www.cdc.gov/healthyyouth/data/yrbs/factsheets/2019_tobacco_trend_yrbs.htm. 2020. Accessed January 25, 2023.
38. Centers for Disease Control and Prevention. Adult cigarette smoking rate trend by sex, race, and age. Available at: https://www.lung.org/research/trends-in-lung-disease/tobacco-trends-brief/data-tables/ad-cig-smoke-rate-sex-race-age. Accessed January 25, 2023.
39. Obisesan OH, Osei AD, Uddin SMI, et al. Trends in e-cigarette use in adults in the United States, 2016–2018. *JAMA Intern Med.* 1 2020;180(10):1394–1398. doi:10.1001/jamainternmed.2020.2817
40. Sun R, Mendez D, Warner KE. Trends in nicotine product use among US adolescents, 1999–2020. *JAMA Netw Open.* 2021;4(8):e2118788. doi:10.1001/jamanetworkopen.2021.18788
41. Barrington-Trimis JL, Braymiller JL, Unger JB, et al. Trends in the age of cigarette smoking initiation among young adults in the US from 2002 to 2018. *JAMA Netw Open.* 2020;3(10):e2019022. doi:10.1001/jamanetworkopen.2020.19022
42. Rohde P, Lewinsohn PM, Brown RA, Gau JM, Kahler CW. Psychiatric disorders, familial factors and cigarette smoking, I: associations with smoking initiation. *Nicotine Tob Res.* 2003;5(1):85–98.
43. Leventhal AM, Zvolensky MJ. Anxiety, depression, and cigarette smoking: a transdiagnostic vulnerability framework to understanding emotion-smoking comorbidity. *Psychol Bull.* 2015;141(1):176–212. doi:10.1037/bul0000003
44. US Department of Health and Human Services. How tobacco smoke causes disease: the biology and behavioral basis for smoking-attributable disease: a report of the surgeon general. 2010.
45. Johnson AL, Kaye J, Baker TB, Fiore MC, Cook JW, Piper ME. Psychiatric comorbidities in a comparative effectiveness smoking cessation trial: relations with cessation success, treatment response, and relapse risk factors. *Drug Alcohol Depend.* 2020;207:107796. doi:10.1016/j.drugalcdep.2019.107796
46. Huang J, Tauras J, Chaloupka FJ. The impact of price and tobacco control policies on the demand for electronic nicotine delivery systems. *Tob Control.* 2014;23(suppl 3):iii41–iii47. doi:10.1136/tobaccocontrol-2013-051515
47. Yao T, Sung HY, Huang J, Chu L, St Helen G, Max W. The impact of e-cigarette and cigarette prices on e-cigarette and cigarette sales in California. *Prev Med Rep.* 2020;20:101244. doi:10.1016/j.pmedr.2020.101244
48. Glover-Kudon R, Gammon DG, Rogers T, et al. Cigarette and cigar sales in Hawaii before and after implementation of a Tobacco 21 law. *Tob Control.* Jan 2021;30(1):98–102. doi:10.1136/tobaccocontrol-2019-055248
49. Fiore MC, Jaen CR, Baker TB, et al. Treating tobacco use and dependence: 2008 update. Rockville, MD: US Dept of Health and Human Services; 2008.

50. Hartmann-Boyce J, McRobbie H, Lindson N, et al. Electronic cigarettes for smoking cessation. *Cochrane Database Syst Rev.* 2020;10:CD010216. doi:10.1002/14651858.CD010216.pub4
51. Whittaker R, McRobbie H, Bullen C, Rodgers A, Gu Y. Mobile phone-based interventions for smoking cessation. *Cochrane Database Syst Rev.* 2016;4:CD006611. doi:10.1002/14651858.CD006611.pub4
52. US Food and Drug Administration. Requirements for products made with non-tobacco nicotine take effect April 14. 2022. 2022. Available at: https://www.fda.gov/tobacco-products/ctp-newsroom/requirements-products-made-non-tobacco-nicotine-take-effect-april-14. Accessed January 12, 2023.
53. Balfour DJK, Benowitz NL, Colby SM, et al. Balancing consideration of the risks and benefits of e-cigarettes. *Am J Public Health.* 2021;111(9):1661–1672. doi:10.2105/AJPH.2021.306416
54. National Academies of Science, Engineering, and Medicine. Report to Congress 2018. 2018. Available at: https://www.nationalacademies.org/annual-report. Accessed January 12, 2023.
55. Patel D, Davis KC, Cox S, et al. Reasons for current e-cigarette use among US adults. *Prev Med.* 2016;93:14–20. doi:10.1016/j.ypmed.2016.09.011
56. Owusu D, Huang J, Weaver SR, et al. Patterns and trends of dual use of e-cigarettes and cigarettes among US adults, 2015–2018. *Prev Med Rep.* 2019;16:101009. doi:10.1016/j.pmedr.2019.101009
57. Cork K; Tobacco Control Legal Consortium. Toking, smoking, and public health: lessons from tobacco control for marijuana regulation. 2018. Available at: https://publichealthlawcenter.org/sites/default/files/resources/Toking-Smoking-Public-Health-2018.pdf. Accessed January 12, 2023.
58. Baker TB, McCarthy DM. Smoking treatment: a report card on progress and challenges. *Annu Rev Clin Psychol.* 2021;17:1–30.

8

Diet and Nutrition

Juliana F. W. Cohen, ScD, ScM, Yara Gholmie, PhD, RD,
and Deborah Olarte, PhD, RD

LEARNING OBJECTIVES

After completing this chapter, readers should be able to

1. Understand the impact our food system has on public health and food availability.
2. Identify modifiable risk factors and different scale evidence-based interventions to improve diet, promote health, reduce risk of chronic disease, and meet nutrient needs.
3. Describe interventions and policy approaches to improve the diets of differing populations.

INTRODUCTION

Healthy dietary behaviors are a cornerstone of well-being, including physical and mental health, throughout the life span. Foods are also deeply connected to our cultures, lifestyles, and emotions. Dietary choices are complex and are influenced by multiple determinants, including biological (e.g., taste), economic (e.g., cost), physical (e.g., access), social (e.g., culture), and psychological (e.g., stress) factors, as well as attitudes and knowledge about food.

Poor nutrition is one of the leading causes of chronic disease worldwide, including increased risk of obesity, type 2 diabetes, cardiovascular disease (CVD), hypertension, poor oral health, osteoporosis, iron deficiency anemia, and many cancers. An unhealthy diet is a major modifiable risk factor for these noncommunicable diseases, which can have a significant impact on the global burden of chronic disease.

Public health nutrition must take a population-based approach to protect the human right to food by simultaneously addressing food security, health promotion, and disease prevention. The challenge for public health is to provide leadership across the public, nonprofit, and business sectors that will result in norms and environments where the healthiest food choices are also the most affordable and readily accessible to all segments of society. Public health must also partner with these sectors to enact change. The purpose of this chapter is to describe and discuss the downstream consequences of poor nutrition, the upstream modifiable risk factors that cause poor nutrition, the high-risk

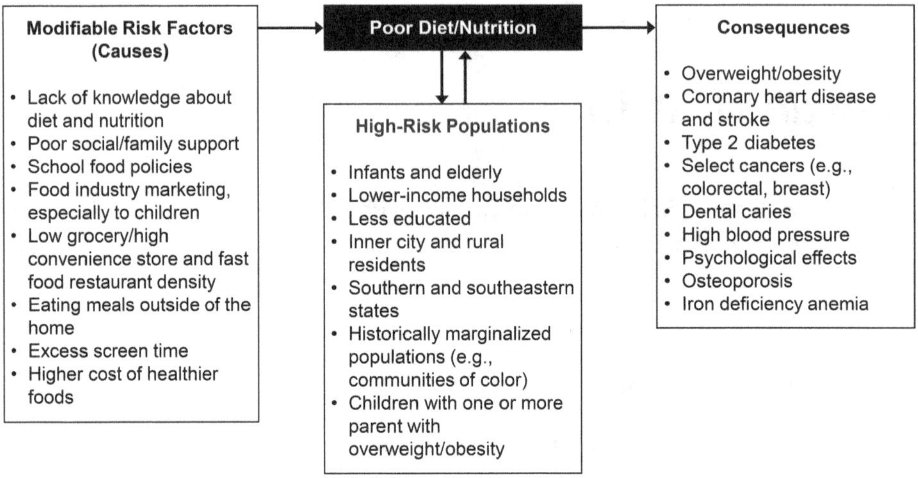

Figure 8-1. Causes, Consequences, and High-Risk Populations for Poor Nutrition

populations for poor nutrition, and the associated conditions and diseases related to poor nutrition (Figure 8-1).

PATHOPHYSIOLOGY

Good nutrition can be preventive against certain diseases and lower risks for adverse health outcomes. Conversely, poor nutrition—whether an excess or insufficient number of calories and nutrients—is a risk factor for many diseases. Given the amount and complexity of dietary research, only some of the most important relationships are described in the next paragraphs to illustrate ways that nutrition affects chronic disease biology.

Fruits and Vegetables

Only about 1 in 10 adults eats the recommended amount of fruit and vegetables. However, an adequate intake of fruits and vegetables has long been associated with a lower risk of many chronic diet-related diseases, including some cancers, type 2 diabetes, CVD, and obesity.[1] The protection comes from a variety of nutrients found in fruits and vegetables, including dietary fiber, vitamin C, vitamin E, folic acid, and potassium. Phytochemicals, particularly carotenoids found in yellow, orange, and red fruits and vegetables and dark, leafy green vegetables may reduce inflammation and oxidative stress.

One mechanism for the association between fruits and vegetables and reduced risk of CVD may be through antioxidants such as vitamins C, E, beta-carotene, and flavonoids.[2] They may act by reducing oxidized cholesterol levels in the body, thereby protecting arteries from damage by slowing or inhibiting the development of atherosclerotic plaques made up of low-density lipoprotein (LDL) particles. Diets that are rich in fruits and vegetables, such as a vegan, vegetarian, or Mediterranean diets, may be associated with lower levels of LDL cholesterol. A second protective mechanism for CVD may be through a reduction of serum cholesterol caused by soluble fiber found in fruits and vegetables.[1] For each incremental increase in fiber consumption, fiber may help to reduce both coronary events and coronary deaths. Natural substances in fruits and vegetables may also be responsible for a decreased risk of some cancers. Green cruciferous vegetables (e.g., broccoli, brussels sprouts, collards, and kale) have been shown to decrease total cancer risk.[1] Antioxidants are theorized to protect cell membranes and DNA from oxidative damage.

Fruits and vegetables are thought to influence body weight through a variety of mechanisms. Their high content of water and fiber and low fat content result in low energy density. Such foods have been associated with greater post-meal satiety. Nevertheless, studies examining an association between increased fruit and vegetable consumption and weight control are inconsistent. This may be attributable at least in part to the inherent complexity, multiple contributing factors, and long-term nature of dietary research.

Dietary Fiber and Whole Grains

Fruits and vegetables and whole grains (e.g., wheat and brown rice) are recommended as sources of dietary fiber. To be considered whole, a grain must have all components of the grain included (i.e., endosperm, germ, and bran). There are two types of fiber: soluble and insoluble fiber. Examples of fibrous foods include whole grains, fruits, vegetables, and nuts. They speed transit time and increase stool bulk, thereby decreasing exposure to and concentration of carcinogens in the gut. Soluble fiber has been shown to lower blood cholesterol levels, likely by binding bile acids, thereby preventing reabsorption. Furthermore, dietary fiber appears to be inversely associated with blood insulin levels, which may have benefits for the prevention of insulin resistance and type 2 diabetes.

Production of short-chain fatty acids occurs as dietary fiber is fermented in the colon. These short-chain fatty acids are absorbed, can be used for energy, and may protect against cancer by promoting differentiation, inducing apoptosis, or inhibiting secondary bile acid production. Many case-control studies have demonstrated a lower risk of cancer with high consumption of dietary fiber, yet large prospective studies have been largely inconsistent.[3]

Dietary Fat and Red Meat

Different types of fats affect bodies in different ways. Trans fats and saturated fats can have adverse effects on health, whereas unsaturated fats (e.g., monounsaturated and polyunsaturated fats [PUFAs]), are associated with health benefits.[4] Research has shown that reducing saturated fat intake is associated with reductions in CVD risk, and according to the American Heart Association, replacement of saturated fat with unsaturated fats lowers LDL cholesterol. Omega-3 PUFAs may be particularly beneficial and are present in fish oils, nuts and seeds, and plant oils (e.g., flaxseed oil and canola oil). In addition to providing energy for the body, omega-3 PUFAs also make up the membranes that surround the cells within the body, with high levels in the retina and brain. Omega-3 PUFAs may reduce the risk of CVD by lowering triglyceride levels and circulating markers of inflammation, thus potentially protecting against heart disease and atherosclerosis. However, clinical trials are not definitive. Furthermore, some studies have shown that an increased intake of PUFAs may reduce risk of breast cancer and colorectal cancer.

Red meat (e.g., beef, pork, lamb), when consumed in limited quantities, can be a rich source of protein, B vitamins, vitamin A, iron, folate, zinc, and selenium. In addition, the folate in red meat is of higher bioavailability than that provided in plant-based sources, which may explain the greater prevalence of iron deficiency anemia in populations that do not consume adequate amounts of red meat. However, the World Health Organization's International Agency for Research on Cancer recently classified processed meat (e.g., meat that has been salted, cured, fermented, or smoked) as carcinogenic to humans, and red meat was classified as probably carcinogenic to humans. High intake of red meat has been associated with some cancers, principally colorectal cancer. The possible mechanisms include the polycyclic hydrocarbons and mutagenic amines that can be generated by cooking at high temperatures; the nitrites and other similar compounds found in salted, smoked, and processed meats that can be converted to toxic N-nitroso compounds within the colonic wall; and the high level of iron, which can lead to the formation of mutagenic free radicals in the gut wall.

Milk and Dairy Products

Dairy intake can offer benefits to a balanced diet. Milk and dairy products from cows (e.g., cheese, yogurt) are rich sources of protein, calcium, potassium, vitamin B12, riboflavin, magnesium, phosphorous, and when fortified, vitamin D. The Dietary Guidelines for Americans recommends that all adults consume up to three servings of low-fat or nonfat milk, or equivalent milk products such as low-fat yogurt, each day. However, consumption can be precluded in many populations by lactose or milk protein intolerance. It is estimated that 80 million Americans have lactose intolerance or lactose malabsorption (alternative, lactose-free dairy options are available but with varying nutrient quality). Additionally, although milk contains beneficial fatty acids, vitamins, minerals, and bioactive compounds, evidence is more mixed on the impact on overall nutrition.[5] Among adults, research suggests that high daily consumption is not associated with reductions of fractures, body mass index (BMI), diabetes, or CVD. Some research suggests high dairy consumption is associated with an increased risk of some types of cancers (e.g., prostate cancer), while potentially reducing the risk colorectal cancer. The impact of high dairy consumption among children is also unclear, although it may be beneficial among children who have poorer overall diet quality.

Sugar-Sweetened Beverages

Sugar-sweetened beverages include soft drinks, fruit drinks, sweetened waters, teas and coffees, and energy drinks that are sweetened by high-fructose corn syrup or sucrose. They do not include beverages with naturally occurring sugars and/or artificial sweeteners. Sugar-sweetened beverages account for the highest amount of added sugar consumption and top source of calories in the United States, easily out-numbering the consumption percentages of added sugar from desserts, candy, and ready-to-eat cereals. On average, sugar-sweetened beverages account for 8% of total energy intake in young adults and nearly 7% in children. Overconsumption of energy-dense, nutrient-poor beverages has been associated with type 2 diabetes, obesity, dental caries, and cardiovascular risks.[6] Research shows that for every daily serving of a sugar-sweetened beverage, the risk of developing type 2 diabetes increases by 20%.[7] The low cost, convenience, variety of options, lack of satiety, and aggressive and widespread marketing campaigns all contribute to the high intake of sugar-sweetened beverages. Research suggests that interventions aimed at decreasing sugar-sweetened beverage consumption and replacing it with water are successful in children but less successful among adults.[7]

The Microbiome

The microbiome—a living ecosystem of microorganisms that inhabit the human body—serves an important role in human health.[8] Colonization occurs during the earliest years of life and a long-term, well-rounded diet is believed to have the greatest influence on gut microbiome diversity. However, we are still unaware of how the variation of microbes in the gut over time affects health, wellness, or the onset of disease. Disruption in the microbiome is correlated with the onset of disease such as cancer and obesity. Given the association between the microbiome and diet-related diseases, there is increasing research into the relationship between diet and microbiome and how they influence each other, including research on genetics, epigenetics, and microbiome health, and modification as a method of disease reduction. Gene sequencing is becoming more widespread, and our knowledge of colonization is growing. Once the complexities of the genetics–diet–microbiome–disease relationship are better understood, genetics may become a tool for nutritional advice and the microbiome may become a modifiable risk factor to improve health and wellness and fight chronic disease.

PUBLIC HEALTH BURDEN

As noted in Figure 8-1, the consequences of poor nutrition are numerable and severe. Poor diet quality is the leading risk factor associated with death in the United States. High blood pressure, high cholesterol, low fruit and vegetable intake, high BMI, and alcohol consumption are leading contributors to chronic noncommunicable, diet-related diseases in developed countries. Noncommunicable, diet-related diseases include type 2 diabetes, cancer, and CVD. Across the globe, poor nutrition accounts for approximately 11 million deaths and 255 million disability-adjusted life years annually.[9]

In the United States the food system plays a large role in the type and availability of foods people have access to eat. Lack of access to proper nutrition and food insecurity increase consumption of nonnutritive, hyperpalatable foods that can cause noncommunicable, diet-related diseases. In 2020 about 10.5% of US households were food insecure and 3.9% (5.1 million) of US households experienced very low food security.

Local food availability also affects disease rates. More than 23 million Americans live in food deserts—areas that have limited access to supermarkets, grocery stores, and other sources of affordable and healthy foods, exacerbating the lack of access to proper nutrition. People who live more than a mile away from a supermarket are 25% less likely to eat a healthy diet compared with those with a supermarket nearby. Specifically, rural communities are at high risk of poor diet and struggle to access fresh food. In many inner-city neighborhoods, supermarkets have relocated to more affluent neighborhoods, causing a reduction in healthy dietary options within those less affluent communities. This has particularly affected historically marginalized communities, such as those with a greater percentage of racial and/or ethnic minorities, increasing disparities in poor dietary intakes and corresponding disease risks.[10,11]

PUBLIC HEALTH IMPACT

Outlined in Table 8-1 are the consequences of noncommunicable, diet-related diseases such as CVD, type 2 diabetes, and colon cancer. Most Americans consume more than the recommended amounts of solid fat and added sugars, refined grains, sodium, and saturated fat, while eating fewer fruits and vegetables, whole grains, and dairy products.[12–14] As a result, more than half of adults have one or more chronic diet-related diseases. However, good nutrition paired with an active lifestyle can help Americans achieve and maintain health.

DESCRIPTIVE EPIDEMIOLOGY

High-Risk Populations and Health Disparities

A healthy dietary pattern is necessary to reduce the prevalence of noncommunicable diet-related diseases. However, the US population is at high risk of developing diet-related chronic disease; Americans' energy-dense diets include saturated fats, red meat, and sugar-sweetened beverages and few vegetables, fruits, and whole grains. Surveillance of nutritional intake is difficult, especially within the current public health and health care

Table 8-1. The Complications and Consequences of Noncommunicable, Diet-Related Diseases

Factor	Complications and Consequences
Coronary heart disease	• Buildup of plaque on the arterial walls of the heart • Chest pain (angina) among other symptoms (e.g., shortness of breath, weakness, pain in arms/shoulders) • Heart attack
Type 2 diabetes	• Heart disease • Chronic kidney disease • Nerve damage • Vision/hearing loss
Colon cancer	• Blood in stool • Change in bowel habits (i.e., diarrhea or constipation, urinary incontinence [post cancer treatment]) • Unintentional weight loss • Bowel obstruction
High blood pressure	• Heart disease • Heart attack • Stroke • Chronic kidney disease
Osteoporosis	• Weakened bones • Bone fractures
Falls	• Bone fractures • Limited mobility
Psychological effects	• Anxiety and stress • Poor body image • Poor self-esteem

Source: Based on WHO, CD, and Academy of Nutrition and Dietetics.[12-14]

infrastructure, and relies on national surveys or epidemiological studies, such as the National Health and Nutrition Examination Survey (NHANES) and the Behavioral Risk Factor Surveillance System. These efforts reveal disparities in dietary quality among demographic groups.

Age and Life Course

For infants, the Academy of Nutrition and Dietetics recommends breastfeeding for the first six months of life with the addition of complementary foods starting at six months to one year. Children ages two to five on average have a high diet quality. However, youth gravitate toward heavily marketed, energy-dense foods and drinks. Poor dietary habits established at an early age are often carried into adulthood and can be difficult to change. On any given day almost two-thirds of adolescents consume at least one sugar-sweetened beverage.[15] In children and adolescents, taste preferences, family support for healthy foods, and food availability are strongly correlated with a healthy, balanced diet.

Healthy dietary patterns and regular physical activity at every life stage are associated with a lower risk of mortality. Eating a well-rounded diet of fruits, vegetables, legumes, nuts, whole grains, and fish and unsaturated vegetable oils and limiting red and processed meats and high-fat dairy are essential for health. Aging involves many psychosocial, economic, and physiological changes. Nutritional requirements change, and the pleasure of eating may wane. Many older adults struggle to meet dietary recommendations because of factors such as disability, caregiver limitations, or living arrangements. Older adults require more calcium and vitamin D to maintain bone health and vitamin B12, fiber, and potassium. In this population, a regular multivitamin may be recommended. However, according to the Healthy Eating Index–2015 (HEI), older Americans (i.e., ≥65) have the highest diet quality.

Race and Ethnicity

Diet contributes to disparities and chronic diet-related diseases experienced by many racial and ethnic populations. These differences are largely attributable to a variety of interlinked cultural preferences and socioeconomic, environmental, educational, and psychosocial factors, as well as structural inequities in access to healthier foods. For instance, on average those populations who are Black face overall greater chronic health conditions, are least likely to achieve healthy diets, and generally have a higher BMI compared with those populations who are White.[16] In comparison, Hispanic populations have a higher-than-average HEI score, as more than 25% of Hispanic adults consume recommended amounts of proteins, fruits, greens, and beans.[16] Among Black and Hispanic populations, there is also greater access to fast food from quick-service restaurants.[17,18] Asian populations in the United States have been documented to consume more fruits and vegetables in general than other populations.[19] Research has found that low percentages of American Indians consume the recommended number of fruits and vegetables.[20]

Income

The relationship between income and diet quality holds along a gradient of income levels. As the affluence of a community decreases, access to healthy food also decreases. Energy-dense diets with poor nutritional value are more likely to be consumed by persons of lower economic means. Healthier foods are generally more expensive and take time to prepare. In addition, compared with populations living in more affluent communities, lower-income populations have greater access and live in greater proximity to fast-food restaurants, which typically offer foods that cost less than healthier whole grain, fruit, or vegetable options. Research suggests that this effect can, in part, be mitigated by federal safety net programs through the US Department of Agriculture (USDA), such as the Supplemental Nutrition Assistance Program (SNAP) and Women, Infants and Children (WIC), which are available to low-income individuals and families. According to the US Department of Agriculture Economic Research Service, these programs provide assistance in supplementing families' food budgets to ensure that low-income families can purchase healthy foods.[21]

Education

Education and income are highly interrelated, and both have been shown to strongly correlate with nutrition and chronic disease. An inverse relationship exists between educational attainment and unhealthy weight gain; individuals who attain college degrees are less likely to become obese. Additionally, higher consumption of fruits, vegetables, and foods with vitamins A and C, calcium, and potassium have been associated with higher levels of education.[16,22] Maternal education is positively related to the nutritional content of meals prepared at home, with college-educated primary food providers spending the most per capita on fruits and vegetables.[23]

Food Insecurity

Food insecurity can be defined as limited or unstable access to healthy foods and can have major impacts on physical and mental health. Food insecurity can be temporary or long term and can range from marginal food security (i.e., one or two indications of problems accessing food) to low food security (i.e., indication of reduced quality, variety, or desirability in the diet), to very low food security (i.e., multiple indications of disrupted eating patterns and reduced food intake). Food insecurity has been linked to poor diet, obesity, and hunger, although these relationships are complex and may be modified by participation in food benefit programs such as SNAP and WIC. Low-cost, highly palatable but nutritionally poor foods may be consumed more in low-income areas. Those who are from historically marginalized populations are more likely to be food insecure, highlighting the role of structural inequities in food insecurity. This relationship was further highlighted during the COVID-19 pandemic, with the prevalence of food insecurity among households with children under the age of 18 rising from 13.6% in 2019 to 14.8% in 2020.[24,25] The greatest increases were observed among those who were racial and/or ethnic minorities; for example, in 2020 during the pandemic Hispanic children were more than twice as likely, and Black children almost three times more likely, to live in a food-insecure household compared with White children.[25]

Geographic Distribution

Within the United States there exist important and long-standing regional differences in food consumption patterns. Generally, fruit and vegetable consumption is lower, and saturated fat consumption higher, in regions that also have high rates of obesity, such as the South and lower Midwest. Populations in many southern states maintain diets high in saturated fats (e.g., fried foods, processed meats) and sugary drinks. By state, Vermont had the highest percentage of adults who achieved the recommended daily vegetable consumption (16%) in 2019, while Kentucky had the lowest (5.6%).[26]

Climate change is also negatively affecting the food system and therefore public health.[27] The current practice of reducing the variety of crops grown and increasing the quantity of specific crops (e.g., corn, soy) is depleting the nutrients in the soil and could also be reducing food quality. Natural disasters (e.g., droughts, increased fires, tornadoes, hurricanes) also impair the ability to grow food and deplete crop yields. For example, with less water as a result of drought, farmers have increasing difficulty growing crops and, consequently, providing fewer fruits and vegetables for consumption. As climate change continues to affect the planet, noncommunicable, diet-related diseases will continue to pose a great risk to public health.

Industrial Development and Immigration

As climate change continues to affect the land, more and more nutritionally vulnerable, food-insecure people are being forced to leave their homes. Because many immigrants enter Western countries as food insecure and experience language barriers, their ability to access their healthier native foods becomes difficult. Research shows that as immigrants establish themselves in a new country, their dietary habits and patterns shift toward that of the new country (e.g., a Western country such as the United States) and their BMI increases. Thus, in transitional groups, it is important to preserve their healthy diets and prevent the uptake of highly advertised, inexpensive, low-nutrient foods, especially by children.

Time Trends

Since NHANES was first administered in 1971, there have been many changes in food consumption patterns.[28] Food marketing has influenced what and how we eat, thus influencing and contributing to the rise of chronic diet-related diseases. The rise of fast food and ready-to-eat meals in grocery stores has caused average energy intake to increase for all populations, likely contributing to the increased prevalence of obesity over time. Portion sizes have also increased both inside and outside the home, and portions for sugar-sweetened beverages and snacks have grown markedly. In fact, snacks account for the greatest caloric intake.

Examining unhealthy weight gain, researchers have shown that between 1999 and 2018 the prevalence of obesity has risen from 30.5% to 42.4% in adults. In children and adolescents aged 2 to 19, the prevalence of obesity has increased from 13.9% in 1999 to 19.3% in 2018. Historically marginalized populations experience some of the highest rates of obesity. Generally, Western developed countries have experienced a "double burden" of undernutrition (i.e., decreased nutrients from a regular, healthy dietary intake) and overnutrition (i.e., increased energy intake from high-calorie, low-nutrient foods) simultaneously. (For more information on obesity, see Chapter 11.)

CAUSES

Modifiable Risk Factors

Diet choice, like any complex human behavior, is determined by multiple factors working independently and concurrently. Time, location, psychology, social relationships, culture, and environmental contexts (e.g., family, school, community, structural inequities) are factors that affect diet choices. Understanding the multiple layers of these interacting factors can help us to assess forces, direct efforts, and interactions within and among individuals; families, peers, and social groups; institutions and communities; businesses, nonprofits, and government programs; and larger forces of society and culture.[29]

Individual-Level Factors

Individuals' personal preference for certain foods, including taste, texture, and appearance, can vary considerably.[30] Food preference can override nutritional knowledge and drive resistance to the adoption of a healthy diet. In the absence of economic barriers and poor availability, personal preference is the best predictor of food choice. But what about consumption? It is important to note that hunger is not a necessary stimulus for food consumption; the sight and proximity of food have been found to stimulate food intake independent of hunger. In fact, food "convenience" ranks high among the factors influencing purchases. Individuals recognize that food cravings, which typically involve the desire to eat energy-dense, high-fat foods, influence their diet. Cravings and their subsequent indulgence lead to increased unhealthy food intake and consequently weight gain.

Emotional state and stress are important determinants of diet and eating patterns. Higher stress levels have been found to significantly decrease the amount of fruits and vegetables consumed. The demands of individual lifestyles can affect the ability to eat a healthy diet as well. Self-esteem and body dissatisfaction are also associated with disordered eating patterns. Other potential predictors include perceived barriers, strength of intention, attitudes and beliefs, and autonomous motivation to consume a healthy diet.

Yet, sufficient evidence shows that advertising, nutrition education, and repeated exposures to new foods, as well as introduction of healthy foods early in life, can alter population taste preferences.

Social Environment

One aspect of the family environment is the "family health climate." Families provide considerable influence on dietary habits, through learned behavior, parent or peer modeling, household food purchasing, and regularity of family meals. Beliefs regarding what or how much is eaten are influenced by those with whom we eat and the social acceptability of eating patterns. As more family members work long hours outside the home, the number of family meals can become limited and replaced by unhealthy snacking, missed meals, or fast food. Adolescents in particular resort to low-cost, energy-dense foods when there is little parental oversight. Furthermore, child and adolescent eating patterns are particularly influenced by their friends in the absence of parents, and foods recommended among peers are typically savory snacks, sugary drinks, and fast-food options. Thus family meals are important to healthy eating, and strong parental modeling and enforcement of home rules for healthy eating are promising strategies to improve nutrition.

Physical Environment

Food prices have a significant effect on the food choices of individuals, specifically those at lower socioeconomic levels. There is a perception of less-healthy foods being cheaper than healthy foods, yet access to heathy food options is affected by the current built environment. As mentioned earlier, areas of lower socioeconomic status, minority communities, and rural areas typically have fewer options for food purchasing and increasingly rely on fast food from quick-service restaurants and convenience stores. In such areas shopping may be limited to convenience stores tending to stock foods high in solid fats, salt, and sugar, with little produce, whole grains, or lean meat for sale. When healthy food choices are not available, individuals may settle for foods that are energy dense and have low nutritional value. Having healthy food easily accessible and affordable in large supermarkets or a mix of markets with a variety of competitively priced nutritious foods allows people to make healthy food choices.

Schools also influence the eating behaviors of children. Many schools provide students with access to two meals each school day. Students' access to meals comes through federal school meal programs (i.e., the National School Lunch Program and the School Breakfast Program). These programs meet federal standards, as they are administered by USDA. The nutritional standards were revised in 2012 to include more fruits, vegetables, and whole grains and to decrease the amount of sodium and trans fat. Other programs offer financial support to provide children and youth with nutritious snacks and meals.

These programs particularly reach children from low-income areas and include the National School Lunch Program's Afterschool Snack Service, the At-Risk Snack and Meals component of the Child and Adult Care Food Program, and the Summer Food Service Program. Research suggests that students who participate in these programs consume more whole grains, milk, fruits, and vegetables during mealtimes and have better overall diet quality than children who do not participate.

As children transition to adulthood, they move from school to work environments. Foods obtained in and around the workplace are generally high in calories, sodium, solid fat, added sugars, and refined grains. Workplace modifications can have real impacts on dietary habits, particularly for low-income workers. One way to improve diets is to increase the availability of healthier food and beverage options at food service venues, including cafeterias, concession stands, snack bars, and vending machines. Another way is to implement workplace health programs. Improving workplace social networks can also result in significant improvement to dietary choices.

Macro-Level Environment

On the broadest level, economics, mass media, and public policy modulate the complexities of food choice. Food companies are the second-largest advertiser on television, spending billions of dollars and competing vigorously to persuade consumers to select their products. In the United States more than 80% of food advertising promotes fast food, sugary drinks, candy, and unhealthy snacks. Children exposed to advertisements for unhealthy foods consume more of these products as a result. In 2017–2018, the average daily intake of added sugars was 17 teaspoons for children and young adults.[31] Modifications to existing policies or introduction of a new policy can greatly affect access to healthy foods, and these changes should align with the most recent Dietary Guidelines for Americans. Many strategies can contribute to healthy environments, including food or menu nutritional labeling practices, food labeling policy, food quality regulation, restrictions against using food benefits to purchase unhealthy foods (or incentives to purchase healthy ones), simplification of benefits, modification of benefit cycles, nutrition education, and improvement of built food environments.

Population-Attributable Risk

Diet is a modifiable factor that contributes to the primary and secondary prevention of most noncommunicable diseases and the leading causes of disability and mortality affecting Americans.[32] However, estimating the population-attributable risk attributable to diet is difficult. Poor nutrition is associated with many chronic diseases throughout the life course. Estimates for population-attributable risk may determine specific components of food or broad dietary measures associated with all-cause mortality or specific diseases.

Many Americans have one or more chronic diet-related health conditions, and the prominent contributors are unhealthy dietary patterns and a lack of physical activity. According to the 2020–2025 Dietary Guidelines for Americans, the US population consumes on average more than 13% of total calories from added sugars (~270 calories) per day compared with recommendations to limit added sugars to no more than 10% of calories.[33] Similarly, only one in four Americans (23%) is meeting the recommendation of energy intake from saturated fat of less than 10%.[33] Current intake of fruits, vegetables, and whole grains is also lower than recommended intake.[33] More than 70% of US adults are overweight or obese[34]; this important public health problem is a driver for prevalent diet-related chronic disease such as heart disease, stroke, type 2 diabetes, hypertension, liver disease, certain types of cancer, dental caries, and/or metabolic syndrome.

EVIDENCE-BASED INTERVENTIONS

Prevention

Since 1980 USDA and the US Department of Health and Human Services have updated the Dietary Guidelines for Americans (https://www.dietaryguidelines.gov) in line with new public health science every five years. The guidelines have provided evidence-based advice on what to consume to promote health, reduce risk of chronic disease, and meet nutrient needs.[32] The guidelines were developed so that policymakers and nutrition and health professionals could help Americans develop healthy dietary patterns at every life stage from infancy through older adulthood. Federal food and nutrition education programs such as WIC, child nutrition programs, and SNAP use the guidelines as the foundation for their programs. Other target audiences include educators and the food industry.

The Dietary Guidelines for Americans emphasize customizable recommendations of essential elements within which individuals make tailored and affordable choices that meet their personal, cultural, and traditional preferences. The 2020 guidelines were the first to provide guidance for healthy dietary patterns by life stage, from birth through older adulthood, including women who are pregnant and lactating. Key suggestions were to (1) follow a healthy eating pattern across the life span; (2) customize and enjoy nutrient-dense food and beverage choices to reflect personal preferences, cultural traditions, and budgetary considerations; (3) focus on meeting food group needs with nutrient-dense foods and beverages and stay within calorie limits; and (4) limit foods and beverages high in added sugars, saturated fat, and sodium and limit alcoholic beverages.

The Dietary Guidelines for Americans form the basis of MyPlate, an interactive food guide developed by USDA. It was introduced in 2011 to replace MyPyramid (MyPlate). Intended as a graphic display to help all Americans know what to eat, MyPlate is USDA's interactive food guide. At the website (https://www.supertracker.usda.gov), people can enter their age, sex, weight, height, and level of physical activity to calculate personalized diet and

Table 8-2. MyPlate Plan

Age Group	Calorie Level									
Ages 12–23 Mos.	700	800	900	1000						
Ages 2–3 Yrs.	1000	1200	1400							
Ages 4–8 Yrs.	1200	1400	1600	1800	2000					
Ages 9–13 Yrs.	1400	1600	1800	2000	2200	2400	2600	2800	3000	3200
Ages 14+ Yrs.	1600	1800	2000	2200	2400	2600	2800	3000	3200	

Source: Reprinted from FDA.[35]

exercise recommendations based on the guidelines. The output details the grains, vegetables, fruits, milk, meat and beans, oils, discretionary calories, and physical activity the individual needs on a daily basis.[35] A pictorial representation of MyPlate is shown in Table 8-2.

Screening

National Surveys

Screening is a key component of assessing the health and nutritional status of children and adults. One of the largest dietary assessments among the US population is conducted by NHANES, the National Health and Nutrition Examination Survey. These surveys are cross-sectional and longitudinal and combine interviews and physical examinations. NHANES incorporates measures of diet; physical activity; biological measures such as weight, anemia, CVD risk factors, and diabetes; school food; school health policies and programs; and youth media. The survey's dietary intake interview component, What We Eat in America (WWEIA), collects US food consumption data. This involves obtaining two 24-hour dietary recalls for each participant, one through an initial in-person interview and the second over the phone within 3 to 10 days. USDA's dietary data collection instrument, the Automated Multiple-Pass Method, a computerized method for collecting 24-hour dietary recalls in person or by telephone, is used to collect WWEIA data. Data gathered include types and amounts of foods consumed as well as information on the food nutrients and energy.

Other surveys and data collection systems with state-specific data include the Behavioral Risk Factor Surveillance Survey, Pediatric Nutrition Surveillance, the Youth Risk Factor Behavioral Surveillance System, School Health Policies and Practices Study, and the National Survey of Children's Health. Similarly, state-specific data about participation in USDA nutrition assistance programs are available annually and can be calculated at the county level. A growing number of states, counties, and cities are conducting their own surveys and developing new approaches, such as geographic information systems, to map and evaluate factors contributing to dietary, physical activity, and obesity risks.

Dietary Assessment Measures

Several methods have been developed to assess overall dietary quality, and these primarily rely on self-report. Food frequency questionnaires are the most popular form of assessing dietary quality in public health practice. These questionnaires ask about the average intake of foods and dishes in a defined food list over a given time period. This dietary assessment method tends to be easy to administer and has a low respondent burden. However, it also has limitations; it is circumscribed by the foods included on the questionnaire, does not capture day-to-day variation, requires respondents to have literacy skills, and relies on respondents' memory (and therefore may not be a questionnaire suitable for children). The Diet History Questionnaire is a food frequency questionnaire that is freely available and can be used with adults aged 19 and older. The most recent version consists of 135 food and beverage line items and 26 dietary supplement questions; it can be used by researchers, clinicians, or educators to assess food and dietary supplement intakes.

Another method of assessing diet is 24-hour recall, where individuals are interviewed about their food and beverage consumption during the past 24 hours. Strengths of this method include that it does not require literacy and can be useful for estimating intakes in culturally diverse populations with a range of foods. This method also has limitations, however; these include typically requiring a trained interviewer, needing multiple days of assessments to determine usual intake, and relying on memory (which can often make it an expensive and unsuitable questionnaire for children). To help address some of these limitations, the Automated Self-Administered 24-Hour dietary assessment tool, commonly referred to as ASA24, is a free, web-based tool that can be used in many different settings (epidemiologic, interventional, behavioral, or clinical research) and by anyone with access to a computer or a mobile device with internet connection.

Many other dietary instruments have been designed for the purpose of assessing the quantity and quality of dietary intake, among them brief food screeners and food diaries, all with varying strengths and limitations. One such instrument developed by USDA is the HEI, or Healthy Eating Index. The HEI assesses 12 aspects of dietary consumption and provides a validated tool for public health practitioners to track population characteristics and help modulate interventions. It is a summary measure of overall diet quality. Such tools have helped reveal associations between population characteristics and nutrition.

Examples of Evidence-Based Interventions

Economic concerns and a growing awareness of the role of social determinants are accelerating the pressure to use social marketing, environmental change, and policy as affordable and effective large-scale approaches for populations.

Large-Scale Initiatives

Historically, the drive to use large-scale approaches for healthy nutrition promotion started with the National Cancer Institute–Kellogg's Campaign in the early 1980s. The then controversial partnership between government and industry used a marketing approach that included mass media advertising, information on cereal boxes, in-store merchandising, and other commercial techniques to reach the general adult market and health professionals. The campaign increased consumer awareness of diet–cancer relationships and extended beyond the Kellogg's brand to a wide range of bran products.

The largest and longest-running partnership for nutrition and chronic disease prevention is the Fruits & Veggies—More Matters campaign. The program was originally created by the California Department of Health Services in 1988 and was initially called the National 5 A Day Program. The Dietary Guidelines for Americans, released in January 2005, changed fruit and vegetable recommendations to more than five servings of fruits and vegetables. Previous dietary guidelines recommended a range of five to nine servings of fruits and vegetables a day. As with 5 A Day, state agencies are licensed by CDC, or the Produce for Better Health Foundation, to serve as health authorities, implement interventions, and ensure conformity among public and nonprofit partners.

More recently, the Salad Bars to Schools program was initiated by the Chef Ann Foundation, National Fruit and Vegetable Alliance, and Whole Foods Market in support of the Let's Move initiative of former first lady Michelle Obama. As of 2021 almost 6,000 schools across the nation have salad bars delivered by the program. With more variety of choices delivered through self-serve salad bars, children eat more fruits and vegetables each day at school.

Site-Based Interventions

Worksites

The rising cost of health care benefits, together with lost work productivity attributable to obesity and other chronic diseases, is driving employers to apply worksite modifications and workplace health programs.[36] Worksites are in a unique position to promote health to their employees, who typically spend more than one-third of their day on the job. Effective workplace health programs and policies can lead to a decrease of health risks and improve the quality of life for the approximately 138 million workers in the United States. Examples of initiatives include behavioral nudges, point-of-choice messages (e.g., signage near a food bay to encourage healthy food choices), healthy options on cafeteria menus and in vending machines, employee recognition programs, management training, and health objectives as management goals. Additional examples and resources for environmental interventions are available at the CDC Workplace Health Promotion website, including lactation support for breastfeeding mothers and healthier foods at meetings (https://www.cdc.gov/workplacehealthpromotion).

Preschool Interventions

Changes targeting early care and education providers, especially in child-care settings, have the potential to reach large numbers of children who spend prolonged periods of time with providers each day. Providers have existing infrastructure for meeting the nutritional and activity needs of children, which may be enhanced to more effectively improve nutrition. Licensing and accreditation standards that shape the early care and education setting offer additional points for intervention. Implementing wellness policies and training caregivers in best practices for nutrition can promote healthy weight and good nutrition for young children in child-care settings.

One such intervention, Eat Well Play Hard in Child Care Settings (EWPHCCS) (https://www.health.ny.gov/prevention/nutrition/cacfp/ewphccs.htm), is a multicomponent intervention that focuses on improving the nutrition and physical activity behaviors of preschool-age children and their parents/caregivers. EWPHCCS uses educational approaches and skill-building activities to encourage healthy behavior change. This intervention targets families with children ages three to five years, participating in or eligible for SNAP and children enrolled in child-care centers participating in the Child and Adult Care Food Program. Studies have shown that children in centers that received the EWPHCCS program increased daily at-home consumption of vegetables and child-initiated vegetable snacking, increased their daily at-home use of 1% milk or fat-free milk, and experienced increased parental offering of vegetables.[37]

Faith Organizations

Comprehensive interventions supported by respected spiritual leaders using approaches such as peer support, motivational interviewing, community coalitions, health fairs, grocery store promotions, cooking classes, healthy options at church meals, and printed materials as part of established religious infrastructures have been shown to be effective, especially among historically marginalized communities. Some of the more influential dietary interventions have included serving vegetables or fruits in church and presenting verbal or printed messages from spiritual leaders.[38] Fit Body and Soul, a faith-based diabetes prevention program, demonstrated improvements in participants' weight status after 12 program sessions; 48% of participants lost at least 5% of baseline body weight.[38]

Schools

Schools offer a venue to reach virtually all children and youth through education, skill-building, environmental change, and social support. Most large interventions in schools that focus on strong nutrition policies (e.g., limiting the sale of snack foods in vending machines, ensuring sufficient time to eat lunch) or providing more choices that are healthy, convenient, and taste good have a positive effective on dietary consumption.[39]

Schools can provide more healthy options by using cost-effective food procurement strategies, such as purchasing USDA commodity foods, participating in the USDA Department of Defense Fresh Fruit and Vegetable Program, buying locally grown and produced foods, and incorporating produce grown in school gardens. There is also evidence that multicomponent obesity prevention programs at schools can improve student nutrition and weight. For example, programs utilizing both school- and community-level interventions, such as Shape Up Somerville and CATCH, the Coordinated Approach to Child Health, have demonstrated positive outcomes.[40,41]

INTERVENTIONS FOCUSING ON SPECIFIC POPULATIONS

Emerging Community Approaches

Increasing access to a diverse array of nutritious foods is needed to ensure population improvements in nutrition, particularly in historically marginalized communities (e.g., lower-income communities, communities of color). Increasingly, advocates and public health departments are working to bring more affordable and healthy options to communities, such as through community gardens, farmers markets, and farm-to-institution networks. In addition, expanding healthy food options at grocery and convenience stores, as well as schools, restaurants, and fast-food entities, is necessary. Furthermore, policies at the local and state level can expand on or fill in gaps in policies at the federal level to ensure communities have equitable access to healthy foods.

Federal Safety Net Programs

The Food and Nutrition Service (https://www.fns.usda.gov/programs) within USDA administers 15 federal nutrition assistance programs that are designed to reduce the risk of food insecurity and obesity among children and lower-income households and individuals. In collaboration with state and tribal governments, these federal safety net programs serve one in four Americans over the course of a year.

SNAP, the nutrition program formerly known as the Food Stamp Program, is an entitlement program considered the centerpiece of the US food security safety net. It uses Electronic Benefit Transfer cards to provide households with incomes less than 130% of the federal poverty level with a monthly cash allotment for food. The value of the food benefit is based on the cost of USDA's Thrifty Food Plan. Complex means testing to determine eligibility is typically administered through state and local social services departments. Means testing includes questions about household income, the number of qualifying household members, specific types of expenses possibly incurred by the household, documentation of US citizenship or residency, and regular recertification. In 2020, over 41 million people received SNAP benefits in an average month. All foods, except hot, ready-to-eat items, qualify for SNAP. While SNAP addresses food insecurity, research has generally not found improvements in diet quality among SNAP participations.[42] The obesity prevention and nutrition education side of SNAP (SNAP-Ed) is reimbursed as an optional administrative activity that requires detailed documentation of in-kind state share funds from nonfederal sources. Budgets and activities require annual federal approval of a SNAP-Ed state plan. Although the amount per state depends on the matching funds a state can identify, all states now offer some SNAP-Ed. In the United States SNAP-Ed and WIC, the Special Supplemental Nutrition Program for Women, Infants, and Children, are the two largest sources of nutrition education funding. Research examining the effectiveness of SNAP-Ed programs on improvements in dietary quality have been mixed.[43]

WIC supports nutritionally at-risk pregnant, breastfeeding, and non-breastfeeding postpartum women, and their children up to age five. WIC provides federal grants to states for nutrient-rich supplemental foods, health care referrals, and nutrition education. Over half of infants in the United States participate in WIC. The program's foods include whole grains, fruits, vegetables, dried/canned beans and peas, eggs, milk, cheese, peanut butter, and iron-fortified cereals. Given these healthier foods available through WIC, participants have on average healthier dietary consumption compared with similar eligible nonparticipants.[44]

The National School Lunch Program is USDA's largest program for America's schoolchildren. On average, nearly 30 million children in the United. receive a school meal daily. Children can be eligible for free school meals if they come from a household with an income less than 130% of the federal poverty level or reduced-price meals if they come from a household within 130% to 185%. Children from households with incomes greater than 185% of the federal poverty level can purchase full-price meals, with the price varying by school district. School districts are reimbursed by the federal government based the number of free, reduced-price, or full-price meals served. Schools or school districts with high poverty rates among their students (based on means-tested programs such as SNAP) can also participate in federal school meal provisions, such as the Community Eligibility Provision, which enables all students to receive free school meals. School meal standards are based on the 2010 Healthy Hunger-Free Kids Act, which requires school meals to provide whole grains, fruits, vegetables, milk, and a meat/meat alternative while also placing limits on calories, sodium, and saturated fats. Research has found that school meal consumption is associated with healthier dietary intakes.[45]

Additional federal nutrition assistance programs include the School Breakfast Program, Child and Adult Care Food Program, Summer Food Service Program, and Afterschool Snacks. These programs are updated by Congress through Child Nutrition and WIC reauthorization, which typically occurs every five years. Also, SNAP and other more agriculturally based programs, such as the Fresh Fruit and Vegetable Snack Program, the WIC Farmer's Market Nutrition Program, the Senior Farmer's Market Nutrition Program, and some commodity and emergency food programs, are reauthorized every five years in a statute commonly known as the Farm Bill.

Marketing to Children

Food marketing to children is widespread across the globe, and the products most heavily marketed are energy dense and nutrient poor. Multiple persuasive marketing methods are used to alter children's food preferences and consumption, with the most prominent techniques and platforms including television/movies, digital games, endorsers, print advertising, packaging, and the internet. Research has found these marketing strategies strongly influence children's food preferences, requests, purchases, and dietary behaviors. Further research is needed to understand newly emerging marketing techniques (e.g., embedded in online games and in film), which policies most effectively limit children's exposure to marketing, and the long-term impact this type of marketing has on diets and excess weight gain.[46] Public health, medical, and advocacy groups, as well as health agencies like the World Health Organization and the National Academy of Medicine, have therefore recommended policies that restrict unhealthy food marketing to children. Despite the strong evidence, the United States continues to have only voluntary regulations.

Eliminating Disparities

Disparities in health and disease burden among historically marginalized communities, especially those that are racial and ethnic minorities, are increasingly gaining attention as a public health priority. Initiatives and policies to improve nutrition are particularly important to addressing disparities, as diet is a key contributor. At the individual level, targeted, tailored, and culturally appropriate nutrition education, dietary counseling, and dietary programming should consider demographic characteristics, the environment, psychosocial factors, and literacy levels. Appropriate venues for programming should also be considered, including churches, local schools, and senior and community centers. In addition, racially and ethnically diverse staff can help to develop greater buy-in from participants. At the community level, improving access to affordable healthy options in schools and in local markets can help address barriers to healthier diets.

Policy Approaches

Although federal policies focus most directly on nutrition for women, children, and those with low incomes, the effects of poor nutrition on health have far-reaching effects on nearly everyone. Policies that shape the supply, production, distribution, and promotion of food can have a significant impact on population-level dietary behaviors.

Agricultural Policy

Food and agricultural policy helps determine which crops farmers will produce and the prices they will get, thereby influencing the food products that retailers, food services, and restaurants offer the public. Federal agriculture policy has supported particular crop production through funding for research, enhancement of infrastructure, and subsidies. In particular, long-standing policies have promoted the production of grains, corn, and soybeans, an approach that has important implications for the food supply because such crops are often converted to energy-dense food products laden with either simple sugars or saturated fats. These agricultural policies result in lower prices, which can influence purchasing decisions, leading purchasers to buy these less healthy foods. Federal agricultural policies (as well as federal safety net programs, including SNAP) are governed by the Farm Bill, which is updated approximately every five years.

School Nutrition Policies

Policy within the public school system also plays a key role in the diets of children throughout the United States. The Healthy, Hunger-Free Kids Act of 2010 updated the National School Lunch Program and School Breakfast Program nutrition standards, as well as nutrition standards for competitive foods (e.g., foods and beverages sold outside the school meal programs, such as in vending machines) to bring them in closer alignment with the concurrent Dietary Guidelines for Americans. The Healthy, Hunger-Free Kids Act also strengthened the requirements for local school wellness policies, including plans related to implementation, evaluation, and public reporting. Overall, these policies have had a positive impact on children's diets and have not adversely affected BMI.[39]

Nutrition Labeling

Access to clearer and/or more detailed nutrition information can help consumers make more informed purchasing decisions. To help address this, updates have been made to the nutrition information available when placing orders in restaurants, as well as to the Nutrition Facts label.

First, to address the lack of visible nutrition information when purchasing fast food and food away from home, given the high consumption of these products among Americans, the Affordable Care Act requires chain restaurants and vending machines with 20 or more locations to disclose calorie information at the point of purchase (e.g., menus and menu boards). Research examining the impact of this policy has found mixed results with regards to product reformulation or changes to purchasing decisions.[47] Second, in 2016 the US Food and Drug Administration issued regulations to update the Nutrition Facts label for the first time in over 20 years. These changes, which were implemented over time, included updates on serving sizes and calories (including a larger, bolder font), and for the first time, information on added sugars (in addition to total sugars). More research is needed to understand the impact of these recently implemented changes.

MOVING FORWARD

This chapter has introduced issues and trends in public health nutrition. It has illustrated that although vast areas of intervention research and theory should be explored, there are many proven effective public health solutions. The disparities in nutrition between socioeconomic, racial/ethnic, and geographic divides that lead to chronic disease are being exposed, along with concerns about vulnerable groups who live in environments that promote poor nutrition, especially in historically marginalized communities. Understanding the gaps and interconnections in policy and environmental information, built environment, community intervention, and surveillance systems increases clarity about opportunities for change. As the burden of poor nutrition has grown, so has the willingness to find solutions. These solutions have been increasingly brokered by broad-based partnerships, multilevel interventions, public policy, and collaborative efforts among policymakers, advocates, researchers, communities, and food producers.

Intervention resources and research to effectively promote healthier and sustainable dietary intakes are needed in proportion to the magnitude of existing disparities. Research has highlighted successful strategies but also identified key gaps in information that will be essential to inform nutrition initiatives and policy decisions at the local, state, and federal levels. Moving forward, the focus must be on advancing research and initiatives that positively influence individual factors that affect food choice and foster environments that make the healthy choice the easy choice for consumers. More is needed to better understand marketplace factors such as economic incentives and disincentives, effective nutrition education and media campaigns, and to recognize how organizations on the national, state, regional, and local levels can complement and gain synergy from each other's efforts. Efforts must also be customized to be both age-appropriate and culturally tailored. Vulnerable populations, such as children from lower-income households or who are racial/ethnic minorities, should be prioritized. According to the World Health Organization's Report on the Commission on Ending Childhood Obesity (https://www.who.int/publications/i/item/9789241510066), the most effective nutrition strategies should focus on school foods, food marketing to children, and price policies to promote healthier diets.

Given the scope of the food system, large-scale comprehensive initiatives will require interdisciplinary professionals and stakeholders to increase access to healthy food, generate resources, and deliver communication programs. Specialists will be needed in the fields of public health nutrition, health education, marketing, epidemiology, mass communications and public relations, health care and health insurance, public policy, and community organizing. Professionals from schools, business, design and the creative arts, culinary arts, retail merchandising, public health law, resource development, and applied research, evaluation, and administration will also be needed. Although some of the specialties may be available through public–private partnerships, public health agencies need dedicated resources for these functions. The challenges in nutrition are large, but the growing interest and innovation is equally large. As public health interventions become more multifaceted, wider-reaching, and creative, the prospect of a healthier global diet grows more promising.

DISCUSSION QUESTIONS

1. Which modifiable risk factors influence dietary choices and lifestyle behaviors?
2. What are the strengths and limitations of different ways to assess diets?
3. How does the food system affect our eating habits and patterns?
4. Which policy approaches might be the most effective at improving nutrition and reducing diet-related disparities?

REFERENCES

1. Aune D, Giovannucci E, Boffetta P, et al. Fruit and vegetable intake and the risk of cardiovascular disease, total cancer and all-cause mortality—a systematic review and dose-response meta-analysis of prospective studies. *Int J Epidemiol.* 2017;46(3):1029–1056.
2. Blekkenhorst LC, Sim M, Bondonno CP, et al. Cardiovascular health benefits of specific vegetable types: a narrative review. *Nutrients.* 2018;10(5):595.
3. Veronese N, Solmi M, Caruso MG, et al. Dietary fiber and health outcomes: an umbrella review of systematic reviews and meta-analyses. *Amer J Clin Nutr.* 2018;107(3):436–444.
4. Hooper L, Summerbell CD, Thompson R, et al. Reduced or modified dietary fat for preventing cardiovascular disease. *Cochrane Database Syst Rev.* 2011;(7):CD002137.
5. Willett WC, Ludwig DS. Milk and health. *N Engl J Med.* 2020;382(7):644–654.
6. Malik VS, Pan A, Willett WC, Hu FB. Sugar-sweetened beverages and weight gain in children and adults: a systematic review and meta-analysis. *Amer J Clin Nutr.* 2013;98(4):1084–1102.
7. Vargas-Garcia E, Evans C, Prestwich A, Sykes-Muskett B, Hooson J, Cade J. Interventions to reduce consumption of sugar-sweetened beverages or increase water intake: evidence from a systematic review and meta-analysis. *Obes Rev.* 2017;18(11):1350–1363.
8. Gilbert JA, Blaser MJ, Caporaso JG, Jansson JK, Lynch SV, Knight R. Current understanding of the human microbiome. *Nat Med.* 2018;24(4):392–400.
9. Afshin A, Sur PJ, Fay KA, et al. Health effects of dietary risks in 195 countries, 1990–2017: a systematic analysis for the Global Burden of Disease Study 2017. *Lancet.* 2019;393(10184):1958–1972.
10. Walker RE, Keane CR, Burke JG. Disparities and access to healthy food in the United States: a review of food deserts literature. *Health & Place.* 2010;16(5):876–884.
11. Larson NI, Story MT, Nelson MC. Neighborhood environments: disparities in access to healthy foods in the US. *Amer J Prev Med.* 2009;36(1):74–81.
12. World Health Organization. Noncommunicable diseases. September 16, 2022. Available at: https://www.who.int/news-room/fact-sheets/detail/noncommunicable-diseases. Accessed January 25, 2023.
13. National Center for Chronic Disease Prevention and Health Promotion, Centers for Disease Control and Prevention. About chronic diseases: poor nutrition. Updated September 8, 2022. Available at: https://www.cdc.gov/chronicdisease/resources/publications/factsheets/nutrition.htm. Accessed January 25, 2023.

14. Eat Right. Academy of Nutrition and Dietetics website. Available at: https://www.eatright.org. Accessed January 25, 2023.
15. Rosinger A, Herrick KA, Gahche JJ, Park S. Sugar-sweetened beverage consumption among US youth, 2011–2014. *NCHS Data Brief.* 2017(271):1–8.
16. Hiza HA, Casavale KO, Guenther PM, Davis CA. Diet quality of Americans differs by age, sex, race/ethnicity, income, and education level. *J Acad Nutr Diet.* 2013;113(2):297–306.
17. Block JP, Scribner RA, DeSalvo KB. Fast food, race/ethnicity, and income: a geographic analysis. *Amer J Prev Med.* 2004;27(3):211–217.
18. Sturm R. Disparities in the food environment surrounding US middle and high schools. *Public Health.* 2008;122(7):681–690.
19. Satia JA. Diet-related disparities: understanding the problem and accelerating solutions. *J Amer Diet Assoc.* 2009;109(4):610.
20. Berg CJ, Daley CM, Nazir N, et al. Physical activity and fruit and vegetable intake among American Indians. *J Community Health.* 2012;37(1):65–71.
21. US Department of Agriculture Economic Research Service. Documentation. Updated October 20. 2022. Available at: https://www.ers.usda.gov/data-products/food-access-research-atlas/documentation. Accessed January 26, 2023.
22. Kant AK, Graubard BI. Secular trends in the association of socio-economic position with self-reported dietary attributes and biomarkers in the US population: National Health and Nutrition Examination Survey (NHANES) 1971–1975 to NHANES 1999–2002. *Public Health Nutr.* 2007;10(2):158–167.
23. Blisard N, Stewart H, Jolliffe D. Low-income households' expenditures on fruits and vegetables. Agricultural Economic Report AER-833. US Dept of Agriculture. May 2004. Available at: https://www.ers.usda.gov/publications/pub-details/?pubid=41663. Accessed January 14, 2023.
24. US Department of Agriculture. Food security in the US—key statistics and graphics. 2021. Updated October 17, 2022. Available at: https://www.ers.usda.gov/topics/food-nutrition-assistance/food-security-in-the-u-s/key-statistics-graphics. Accessed January 14, 2023.
25. Coleman-Jensen A, Rabbitt MP, Gregory CA, Singh A. Household food security in the United States in 2019. Economic Research Report ERR-275. US Dept of Agriculture. Updated September 9, 2020. Available at: https://www.ers.usda.gov/publications/pub-details/?pubid=99281. Accessed January 14, 2023.
26. Lee SH, Moore LV, Park S, Harris DM, Blanck HM. Adults meeting fruit and vegetable intake recommendations—United States, 2019. *MMWR Morb Mort Wkly Rep.* 2022;71(1):1.
27. Fanzo JC, Downs SM. Climate change and nutrition-associated diseases. *Nat Rev Dis Primers.* 2021;7(1):1–2.
28. Kearney J. Food consumption trends and drivers. *Philos Trans Royal Soc B: Biol Sci.* 2010;365(1554):2793–2807.
29. McGuire S; Institute of Medicine. 2012. *Accelerating Progress in Obesity Prevention: Solving the Weight of the Nation.* Washington, DC: the National Academies Press; 2012.
30. Scaglioni S, De Cosmi V, Ciappolino V, Parazzini F, Brambilla P, Agostoni C. Factors influencing children's eating behaviours. *Nutrients.* 2018;10(6):706.
31. Centers for Disease Control and Prevention. Get the facts: added sugars. Updated November 28, 2021. Available at: https://www.cdc.gov/nutrition/data-statistics/added-sugars.html. Accessed January 14, 2023.

32. US Department of Health and Human Services; US Department of Agriculture. *Dietary Guidelines for Americans, 2015–2020*. 8th ed. Washington, DC: US Dept of Health and Human Services; 2015.
33. US Department of Health and Human Services; US Department of Agriculture. *Dietary Guidelines for Americans, 2020–2025*. 9th ed. December 2020. Available at: https://www.dietaryguidelines.gov/sites/default/files/2020-12/Dietary_Guidelines_for_Americans_2020-2025.pdf. Accessed January 14, 2023.
34. Fryar CD, Carroll MD, Ogden CL; Division of Health and Nutrition Examination Surveys. Prevalence of overweight, obesity, and severe obesity among children and adolescents aged 2–19 years: United States, 1963–1965 through 2015–2016. National Center for Health Statistics: Health E-Stats. September 2018. Available at: https://www.cdc.gov/nchs/data/hestat/obesity_child_15_16/obesity_child_15_16.pdf. Accessed January 14, 2023.
35. US Department of Agriculture. MyPlate plan. Available at: https://www.myplate.gov/myplate-plan. Accessed January 25, 2023.
36. Goetzel RZ, Hawkins K, Ozminkowski RJ, Wang S. The health and productivity cost burden of the "top 10" physical and mental health conditions affecting six large US employers in 1999. *J Occup Environ Med.* 2003;45(1):5–14.
37. New York State Department of Health. Eat Well Play Hard in Child Care Settings. December 2012. Updated May 2013. Available at: https://www.cdc.gov/nccdphp/dnpao/state-local-programs/pdf/ewphccs_practice-tested_template.pdf. Accessed January 14, 2023.
38. Dodani S, Fields J. Implementation of the Fit Body and Soul: a church-based life style program for diabetes prevention in high-risk African Americans. *Diabetes Educator.* 2010;36(3):465–472.
39. Cohen JF, Hecht AA, Hager ER, Turner L, Burkholder K, Schwartz MB. Strategies to improve school meal consumption: a systematic review. *Nutrients.* 2021;13(10):3520.
40. Economos CD, Hyatt RR, Must A, et al. Shape Up Somerville two-year results: a community-based environmental change intervention sustains weight reduction in children. *Prev Med.* 2013;57(4):322–327.
41. Nader PR, Stone EJ, Lytle LA, et al. Three-year maintenance of improved diet and physical activity: the CATCH cohort. *Arch Pediatr Adol Med.* 1999;153(7):695–704.
42. Andreyeva T, Tripp AS, Schwartz MB. Dietary quality of Americans by Supplemental Nutrition Assistance Program participation status: a systematic review. *Amer J Prev Med.* 2015;49(4):594–604.
43. Rivera RL, Maulding MK, Eicher-Miller HA. Effect of Supplemental Nutrition Assistance Program–Education (SNAP-Ed) on food security and dietary outcomes. *Nutr Rev.* 2019;77(12):903–921.
44. Schultz DJ, Shanks CB, Houghtaling B. The impact of the 2009 Special Supplemental Nutrition Program for Women, Infants, and Children food package revisions on participants: a systematic review. *J Acad Nutr Diet.* 2015;115(11):1832–1846.
45. Fox MK, Gearan E, Cabili C, et al. School nutrition and meal cost study: student participation, satisfaction, plate waste, and dietary intakes. Vol. 4. US Department of Agriculture, Food and Nutrition Service, Office of Policy Support. April 23, 2019. Available at: https://www.mathematica.org/publications/school-nutrition-and-meal-cost-study-final-report-volume-4-student-participation-satisfaction-plate. Accessed August 9, 2023.
46. Smith R, Kelly B, Yeatman H, Boyland E. Food marketing influences children's attitudes, preferences and consumption: a systematic critical review. *Nutrients.* 2019;11(4):875.
47. VanEpps EM, Roberto CA, Park S, Economos CD, Bleich SN. Restaurant menu labeling policy: review of evidence and controversies. *Curr Obes Rep.* 2016;5(1):72–80.

9

Physical Activity

Barbara E. Ainsworth, PhD, MPH, and Caroline A. Macera, PhD

LEARNING OBJECTIVES

After completing this chapter, readers should be able to

1. Recognize the public health approach in presenting physical activity as a health-enhancing behavior.
2. Acquire information needed to understand why physical inactivity is a public health concern.
3. Compare differences in the prevalence of physical activity by demographic factors and geographic areas.
4. Evaluate the impact of physical inactivity on health conditions.
5. Explain the public health approach to promoting physical activity.

INTRODUCTION

The importance of being physically active is shown repeatedly in countless studies of various populations. Physically active people have a longer life expectancy than physically inactive people, and are less likely to be diagnosed with chronic diseases such as diabetes, heart disease, and some cancers. In 1996, Physical Activity and Health: A Report of the Surgeon General summarized the many health benefits of physical activity (PA). The report suggested that the minimum level required to achieve health benefits was a daily expenditure of 150 kilocalories in moderate or vigorous activities (https://www.cdc.gov/nccdphp/sgr/index.htm). This recommendation is consistent with a 1995 consensus statement issued by the Centers for Disease Control and Prevention (CDC) and the American College of Sports Medicine recommending that every adult accumulate at least 30 minutes of moderate activity most days of the week.[1]

In 2008 an update to these recommendations was published as the Physical Activity Guidelines of Americans (hereafter cited as federal PA guidelines) that incorporated recommendations for a combination of 150 minutes per week of moderate-intensity PA or 75 minutes per week of vigorous-intensity PA and muscle-strengthening activities at least twice a week for all adults. Accumulating the equivalent amount of either moderate or vigorous activity was acceptable. Also, added health benefits occur by doubling

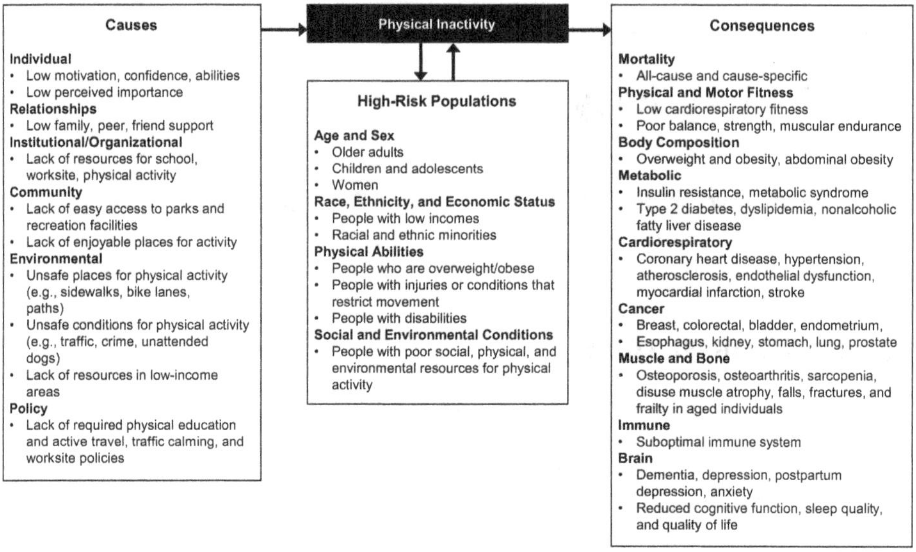

Figure 9-1. Physical Inactivity: Causes, High-Risk Populations, and Consequences

the duration of moderate- and vigorous-intensity PA. Children and adolescents should have 60 minutes per day of moderate- and vigorous-intensity PA, with muscle- and bone-strengthening activities performed at least three days a week. The guidelines highlighted the importance of minimizing sitting, referred to as "sedentary" time, regardless of the type and amount of PA obtained during the rest of the day (https://health.gov/sites/default/files/2019-09/paguide.pdf). The federal PA guidelines were updated and expanded in 2018 to include guidelines for preschool-age children, women during pregnancy and the postpartum period, and adults with chronic health conditions and disabilities and to make recommendations for safe PA (https://health.gov/sites/default/files/2019-09/Physical_Activity_Guidelines_2nd_edition.pdf). In 2020 the World Health Organization (WHO) published similar guidelines, the WHO Guidelines on Physical Activity and Sedentary Behaviour (https://www.who.int/publications/i/item/9789240015128). Figure 9-1 summarizes the causes of not engaging in PA at federally recommended levels (deemed physical inactivity) or prolonged sitting and reclining (classified as sedentary behaviors) and identifies not only the health consequences of such behaviors but also the populations at high risk for physical inactivity and sedentary behaviors. Note that physical inactivity, as subsequently described in this chapter, includes sedentary behaviors (for detailed definitions, see Table 9-1).

Pathophysiology

PA affects all body systems associated with energy production, metabolism, and bodily movement. Table 9-1 shows the acute and chronic changes in body systems and

Table 9-1. Public Health Burden: Acute and Chronic Changes Associated With Disease Risk Following Moderate Amounts of Physical Activity

System	Acute Changes	Chronic Changes
Cardiovascular	Increased • Heart rate • Stroke volume • Cardiac output • Systolic blood pressure • Oxygen consumption • Heart contractility • End diastolic filling • Sheer stress on vascular endothelium • Dilation of peripheral vessels to dissipate heat	Increased • Aerobic capacity • Maximal stroke volume • Maximal cardiac output • Coronary circulation • Mitochondrial density • Oxygen extraction in muscles • Endothelial function • Heart rate variability • Blood clot lysis • Heart size • Blood volume
		Reduced • Resting blood pressure • Resting heart rate • Heart rate and blood pressure at submaximal work • Blood and plasma viscosity • Cardiac output during submaximal work
Pulmonary	Increased • Breath rate and depth • Breath rate during submaximal activity • Oxygen diffusion • Dilatation of airways	Increased • Endurance of ventilatory muscles • Total lung capacity • Maximum voluntary ventilation • Maximum tidal volume • Oxygen extraction from circulating blood • Aerobic capacity
		Reduced • Submaximal breath rate
Neuromuscular	Increased • Rate of nerve impulses • Mobility • Oxygen utilization • Mitochondria • Anaerobic enzymes • Aerobic enzymes • Release of Interleuken-6 peptide from skeletal muscle • Release of myokines (e.g., cytokines and peptides) from skeletal tissue that influence metabolism in other organs	Increased • Size of motor nerves • Size of muscle fibers • Strength, power, endurance • Aerobic capacity • Functional independence • Fat and carbohydrate utilization • Muscle flexibility • Muscle mass

(Continued)

Table 9-1. (Continued)

System	Acute Changes	Chronic Changes
Skeletal, ligaments, tendons, joints	Increased • Osteocalcin production in bone and release in blood to stimulate glycogen breakdown • Mechanical loading	Increased • Bone mass and density • Tendon and ligament strength • Joint stability
Endocrine	Increased • Release of hormones from pituitary (most), adrenal, thyroid, parathyroid, kidney, ovaries, testes, pancreas (glucagon and insulin), endorphins • Release of glucose during activity • Release of adrenaline during rest	Increased • Insulin sensitivity • Psychological well-being Reduced • Insulin requirement during submaximal exercise
Metabolic	Increased • ATP demand • Glucose utilization • Glycogen breakdown • Fatty acid utilization • Insulin signaling	Increased • ATP-CP energy stores in muscles • Ratio of lipid-to-carbohydrate oxidation • Glucose and free fatty acid in adipose, muscle, or liver cells • Insulin sensitivity Reduced • Circulating triglyceride, LDL, VLDL • Body fat stores • Adipose cell volume • Fatty acid synthesis in liver
Immune	Increased • Lymphocyte activity and proliferation • Circulating neutrophils • Leukocyte distribution • Humoral immunity (IgA, IgG, IgM) • Pro-inflammatory cytokines following intense exercise	Increased • Lymphocyte levels with moderate-intensity physical exercise • Resistance to illness Decreased • Lymphocyte levels (only with long-term intensive training)

Source: Based on Booth et al.[2,3]
Note: ATP-CP = adenosine triphosphate-creatine phosphate; Ig = immunoglobulin; LDL = low-density lipoprotein; VLDL = very low-density lipoprotein.

associated disease risks following moderate amounts of PA.[2,3] The time required for PA (or physical inactivity) to produce changes in the body may range from one week (i.e., neuromuscular system) to several years (i.e., metabolic hormones, enzymes, and tissue changes). Many physiological responses to PA reflect a gene–environment interaction that influences responses to PA. About 40% to 50% of maximal aerobic capacity is attributable to genetics, and the remaining part results from the level of chronic voluntary PA. Aerobic capacity refers to the ability to carry out daily tasks with vigor and alertness, without undue fatigue, and with ample energy to enjoy leisure-time pursuits and to meet unforeseen emergencies. Aerobic capacity increases with moderate-to-vigorous PA (MVPA) at all ages, although absolute aerobic capacity decreases with increasing age. Higher aerobic capacity is associated with better health. This capacity decreases when there is chronic absence of movement (e.g., bed rest, physical inactivity). However, this decrease is secondary to reductions in cardiac output (the amount of oxygenated blood leaving the heart each minute) and the body's ability to deliver oxygen to muscle tissues. Consequently, low aerobic capacity is associated with increased chronic diseases and increased mortality rates. Alternatively, regular MVPA produces positive adaptations to enhance the delivery of oxygen and metabolites to and from tissues and organs.[2,3]

Regular PA can directly affect health-related fitness (changes in the body tissues as a result of PA) or may indirectly modify health-related fitness through other changes in health status. In either case PA causes tissue-specific changes that positively influence the function of nearly all bodily systems and processes and alters regulatory enzymes and hormones that reduce disease risks. For example, regular PA reduces cardiovascular disease (CVD) by increasing shear stress to vascular walls promoting endothelial cell remodeling, increasing high-density lipoprotein that reduces circulating atherogenic low-density lipoproteins, and increasing lipoprotein lipase that breaks down triglycerides. It also lowers systolic blood pressure and resting heart rate to reduce the work of the heart at rest. The absence of these mechanisms promotes vascular endothelium thickness, reduces blood flow to cardiac tissues, and increases the risk for CVD. Regular PA can reduce the threshold for angina pectoris during activities and also reduce the risks for sudden death among people with chronic heart disease. PA at levels recommended by the federal PA Guidelines is inversely associated with obesity and glucose-insulin intolerance and is positively associated with immune function, muscular strength, mobility, psychological well-being, and increased bone mass. By modifying these intermediate factors, regular PA can reduce the risks for diabetes mellitus, depression, injuries, osteoporosis, and some forms of cancer associated with immune deficiencies and excess body fat.[2,3]

Burden of Physical Inactivity

Physical inactivity is a result of many causal and correlational upstream factors among high-risk populations that increase the risks for various downstream health consequences (Figure 9-1). Multiple factors adversely affect one's decision to engage in PA, ranging from one's immediate environment to more indirect environmental factors in communities and policies that govern PA settings. Socioecological models have been used in public health to provide a framework to understand the multiple factors influencing behavior. These factors can deter one's decision to initiate and maintain regular PA. At the model's center are individual factors such as low motivation, physical abilities, confidence, and low perceived importance for PA. Interacting with individuals in their immediate environment are relationships with families, peers, and friends that can influence PA behaviors. Institutional and organizational factors are essential resources for places for PA. Schools failing to provide a physical education program or worksites limiting PA opportunities during the workday can lead to individuals' prolonged physical inactivity during the day. Community and environmental settings have an influential role in indirectly facilitating or inhibiting PA. Living in a community with few parks within walking distance from home, lack of safe and enjoyable places to walk and bicycle (e.g., no sidewalks or bike lanes), cities with high crime rates, and frequent unattended dogs are deterrents to PA outdoors. In addition, local, state, and community policies govern how institutions and organizations indirectly support PA. Communities provide PA opportunities, organize PA infrastructures, and spend resources on facilities for PA. Evidence shows that people engage in PA when policies support active living for transportation, recreation, schools, and occupations, and when exercise resources are near one's home environment.[4] Many of these factors interact in causal ways to support or deter choices for PA.

Certain people, termed high-risk populations, are more susceptible to the multiple factors increasing physical inactivity. At a population level these include older adults, children and adolescents, women, people with low incomes, and some racial and ethnic minorities (e.g., African Americans, Hispanics). Persons with overweight and obese status, injuries, and conditions that restrict movement (e.g., knee, hip arthritis) and persons with disabilities often find it challenging to engage in regular PA. Further, persons who live in environments with poor infrastructure or social support for PA have fewer opportunities for PA outside the home.

There are many disease risk-reducing and health-enhancing effects of regular, moderate PA that integrate body systems. Conversely, physical inactivity has powerful effects on increasing disease risks for adverse health consequences. The body makes specific adaptations to imposed demands of stresses placed on the body by PA or lack of stress placed by physical inactivity. The downstream adaptations to physical inactivity include increased risks for all-cause and cause-specific mortality, reductions in physical and motor fitness, and changes in body composition contributing to overweight and obesity. Alterations in skeletal muscle and bone tissues associated with physical inactivity contribute to osteoporosis, sarcopenia, disuse muscle atrophy, falls, fractures, and frailty in older persons. Physical inactivity is also causally related to developing metabolic diseases (e.g., metabolic syndrome, type 2 diabetes, nonalcoholic fatty liver disease), CVD, and several types of cancers. Regular PA is necessary for optimal brain development in young children, enhances the quality of life, and is a form of treatment for adults with dementia, anxiety, depression, and postpartum depression.[3] The benefits of regular PA depend on the frequency, intensity, and duration of the activities and the types and amounts of stress imposed on tissues, organs, and body systems. PAs that exert considerable stress on most systems are aerobic (i.e., MVPA), high-intensity interval, weight-bearing, and resistance activities. These include most sports and conditioning activities, weight training, brisk walking and bicycling, gardening, home repair, manual labor occupations, and vigorous house cleaning.

PUBLIC HEALTH IMPACT

Physical inactivity is a public health problem that affects the health and well-being of persons and has worldwide social and economic consequences if not urgently addressed. Physical inactivity is estimated to account for 6% to 10% of deaths globally[5] and 8.3% of US deaths.[6] An analysis of data from the National Health Information Survey has shown that adults who engaged in aerobic and muscle-strengthening PA consistent with the 2018 federal PA Guidelines between 1997 to 2014 reduced their risks of premature mortality by 40% to 60% compared with those who were inactive or insufficiently active. This reduction in risk includes deaths from all-causes, cause-specific conditions for CVD, all cancer types, type 2 diabetes, Alzheimer's disease, influenza and pneumonia, and kidney diseases.[7] Compared with levels of PA insufficient to meet PA recommendations, regular PA also can reduce the percentage burden of disease incidence for coronary heart disease (6.7%), type 2 diabetes (8.3%), breast cancer (10.8%), and colon cancer (11.0%).[5] The costs for chronic disease management have an enormous economic impact in the United States as well as globally. For example, estimates for the annual costs of diagnosed diabetes in the United States in 2017 was $327 billion in direct medical costs ($237 billion) and reduced productivity ($90 billion). People with diagnosed diabetes incurred average medical expenditures of $16,752 per year, of which about $9,601 was attributed to diabetes (https://www.diabetes.org/about-us/statistics/cost-diabetes). Overall, in 2013 physical inactivity in the United States resulted in expenditures of $29 billion (direct and indirect costs) on health care expenses and productivity losses. The proportion of the expenditures paid by the public sector (47.1%), private sector and third-party payers (40.1%), and households (12%) reflects a tremendous financial burden.[8] Physical inactivity among older adults exacerbates the risks for poor health, thereby increasing the economic burden and straining the public and private health care systems. Of particular concern is the public health burden of lonely and socially isolated older persons who have high physical inactivity levels and poor nutritional habits, placing them at increased risks for depression, anxiety, dementia, CVD, and stroke.[9]

DESCRIPTIVE EPIDEMIOLOGY

High-Risk Populations and Health Disparities

What we know about population levels of PA is obtained by large-scale systems using standardized questions designed to elicit this information regularly. These systems (usually called surveillance systems) can help monitor PA patterns among the general population and assist in developing and evaluating interventions. Although surveillance systems typically rely on self-report rather than objectively measured data and, thus, may overestimate actual PA, they are the best measures currently available to obtain information on a population level. Not only do self-report measures provide information on types of PA, they also form the basis for research identifying the long-term health effects. Furthermore, they have been used to develop the federal PA Guidelines (Physical Activity Guidelines for Americans: https://health.gov).

Current surveillance systems can assess whether people meet the federal PA Guidelines (including obtaining 150 minutes per week of moderate or vigorous activity in leisure time) and activities specifically designed to increase muscle mass twice a week. However, even though some of these systems also collect information on transportation- and occupation-related PA, leisure-time PA (LTPA) is activity performed during one's leisure time. It is the measure that has the most complete data over time. This type of PA is also strongly associated with overall health and all-cause mortality.

There are several separate surveillance systems in the United States to measure PA. They include

- State-level data: The Behavioral Risk Factor Surveillance System (BRFSS) is a telephone survey that provides ongoing data on major behavioral risk factors among American adults, emphasizing state-level surveillance (https://www.cdc.gov/brfss).
- National-level data: The National Health Interview Survey (NHIS) collects data on a broad range of health topics through personal household interviews,(modified to telephone interviews during the COVID-19 pandemic. The survey provides national-level estimates about the health of Americans used to track progress toward national health objectives (https://www.cdc.gov/nchs/nhis).

Two other important survey instruments are used:

- The National Health and Nutrition Examination Survey (NHANES) provides information about the health of Americans through a combination of personal interviews and direct physical examinations (modified during COVID-19). The survey examines a nationally representative sample of about 5,000 people each year (https://www.cdc.gov/nchs/nhanes).
- The Youth Risk Behavior Surveillance System (YRBSS) monitors priority health-risk behaviors that contribute markedly to the leading causes of death, disability, and social problems among adolescents in the United States. YRBSS includes a national school-based survey conducted by CDC and state, territorial, tribal, and local surveys. PA data are collected every two years and are used to monitor progress toward national objectives (https://www.cdc.gov/healthyyouth/data/yrbs).

Using national data for adults combining leisure-time aerobic MVPA and muscle-strengthening activities, the prevalence of meeting the federal PA guidelines is shown in Table 9-2 for adults by demographic.[10] In 2018 about 24% of adults adequately met the

Table 9-2. Percentage of Adults Aged 18 Years and Older by Selected Characteristics Who Met and Did Not Meet 2008 Federal Physical Activity Guidelines for Leisure-Time Aerobic and Muscle-Strengthening Activities: United States, 2018

Characteristic	Met Both Aerobic and Muscle-Strengthening Guidelines (% ± SE)	Did Not Meet Either Aerobic or Muscle-Strengthening Guidelines (% ± SE)
Overall	24.2 ± 0.4	42.2 ± 0.5
Age, y		
18–44	30.0 ± 0.6	36.5 ± 0.7
45–54	21.3 ± 0.8	44.2 ± 1.0
55–64	18.2 ± 0.7	45.2 ± 1.0
65–74	16.4 ± 0.7	49.6 ± 0.9
≥75	10.2 ± 0.7	62.9 ± 1.0
Sex		
Men	27.7 ± 0.6	38.2 ± 0.6
Women	20.9 ± 0.5	46.0 ± 0.6
Race		
White only	25.0 ± 0.4	41.1 ± 0.6
Black or African American only	20.1 ± 1.1	50.1 ± 1.3
Asian only	22.9 ± 1.4	41.6 ± 1.7
Hispanic origin		
Hispanic or Latino	21.6 ± 0.9	49.5 ± 1.3
Education		
No high school or GED	9.9 ± 0.8	63.7 ± 1.4
High school or GED	14.9 ± 0.7	52.5 ± 1.0
Some college or more	27.6 ± 0.5	37.1 ± 0.5
Poverty level, %		
<100	14.9 ± 0.8	56.5 ± 1.2
100–199	16.6 ± 0.8	52.7 ± 1.1
200–399	21.8 ± 0.7	45.8 ± 0.8
≥400	31.6 ± 0.6	32.0 ± 0.6
Geographic region		
Northeast	24.9 ± 0.9	41.0 ± 1.1
Midwest	24.1 ± 0.8	42.2 ± 1.0
South	21.6 ± 0.6	46.2 ± 0.9
West	27.8 ± 0.8	37.1 ± 1.0

Source: Adapted from CDC.[10]

Note: SE = standard error. Characteristics are age-adjusted to the 2000 US population.

guidelines necessary to achieve health benefits, but over 40% did not meet the aerobic or muscle-strengthening guidelines. From these data men appear to be more active than women, and younger adults are more active than older adults. Although the guidelines apply to all adults, including older adults, few meet the guidelines after age 75. As in previous years there continues to be a lower prevalence of meeting the federal PA guidelines among those who identify as Black or African American compared with White or Asian.

As for education, the dose–response effect previously reported appears again when comparing the prevalence of meeting the guidelines among those with no high school diploma (9.9%) with those who have some college or more (27.6%). Likewise, of those in the lowest poverty level (<100%), 14.9% met the federal guidelines compared with 31.6% for those with an income 400% or more of the poverty level.

A high-risk population not reflected in Table 9-2 is school-aged youth. Data from the YRBSS suggest that some notable changes have occurred in youth PA levels. For example, in 2019, while 44% participated in PA for at least 60 minutes on five or more days, only 23% were physically active for at least 60 minutes on seven days prior. In this instance, they defined PA as engaging in any PA that increased their heart rate and made them breathe hard. Attending physical education classes is another measure that is useful in documenting the opportunities available for youth PA. In 2019 about one-quarter of school-aged youth participated in physical education classes on all five days, while slightly more than half attended at least one class per week. That suggests that about half of these youth did not have any physical education class. For sedentary behaviors, in 1999 YRBSS added to the survey a question on watching television for three hours or more on a school day. The good news is that while 43% reported this behavior in 1999, by 2019 only 20% reported this behavior. However, when in 2003 YRBSS incorporated a question on playing video or computer games three hours or more per day on a school day, 22% reported this behavior, increasing to 46% by 2019.

Geographic Distribution

There continue to be differences in the prevalence of meeting the federal PA guidelines throughout the United States. Prevalence of meeting PA guidelines is lowest in the South (21.6%), followed by the Midwest (24.1%) and the Northeast (24.9%), with the highest in the West (27.8%). This pattern is pictured by the map (Figure 9-2a), showing the prevalence of meeting only the aerobic component of the guidelines obtained by the BRFSS in 2019.[11] A similar but opposite pattern appears when looking at those who reported no PA in the previous month (Figure 9-2b).[12] The areas with the highest levels of physical inactivity are in the South, and the lowest levels of physical inactivity are primarily in the West. These data reflect three years (2015–2018), so specific events, such as extreme heat or cold periods, are not solely responsible for the

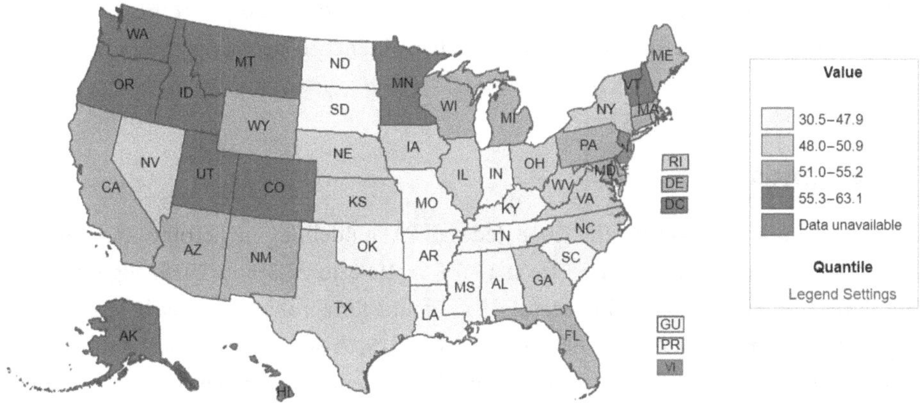

Source: Adapted from CDC.[11]

Note: Shown in quartiles. Data are age-adjusted to the 2000 US population.

Figure 9-2a. Percentage of US Adults Who Achieve at Least 150 Minutes of Moderate-Intensity Aerobic Physical Activity or 75 Minutes of Vigorous-Intensity Aerobic Activity (or an Equivalent Combination): Behavior Risk Factor Surveillance System, 2019

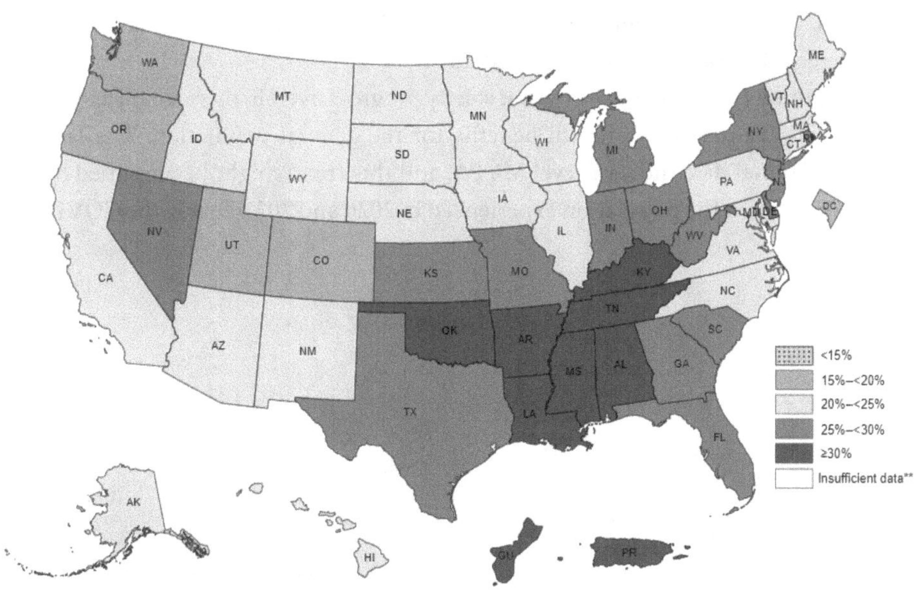

Source: Adapted from CDC.[12]

Note: Respondents were classified as physically inactive if they responded "no" to the following question: "During the past month, other than your regular job, did you participate in any physical activities or exercises such as running, calisthenics, golf, gardening, or walking for exercise?"

Figure 9-2b. Prevalence of Self-Reported Physical Inactivity Among US Adults by State and Territory: Behavior Risk Factor Surveillance System, 2015–2018

patterns seen here. Because these data are state-specific, state programs have many opportunities to focus on ways to assist their residents in becoming more physically active.

Time Trends

The prevalence of meeting the 2018 federal PA guidelines in aerobic and muscle-strengthening activities increased from 14.5% in 1998 to 23.3% in 2018 (Figure 9-3).[10] Similarly, those not meeting the federal PA guideline for aerobic and muscle-strengthening decreased from 56.3% in 1998 to 43.0% in 2018. A state-based study published in 2021 found that although the overall national prevalence did not change from 2011 to 2019, the prevalence of meeting the federal PA guidelines decreased in 12 states, increased in 11 states, and remained the same in 29 states.[13]

While MVPA is only one aspect of PA, it is worth noting that other measures such as sedentary behavior have not decreased. A nationally representative sample of individuals aged 12 years and older in the United States found that the prevalence of sitting and watching television or videos for at least two hours a day did not change between 2001 and 2016. Furthermore, they found that the prevalence of computer use during leisure time increased among adolescents and adults.[14]

While these figures suggest slow but steady progress overall, there is still a long way to go to ensure maximum health benefits for the general population. The last few years of national data indicate level MVPA, and this trend might be amplified by the lockdown most of the population experienced in 2020 and 2021 during the COVID-19 pandemic.

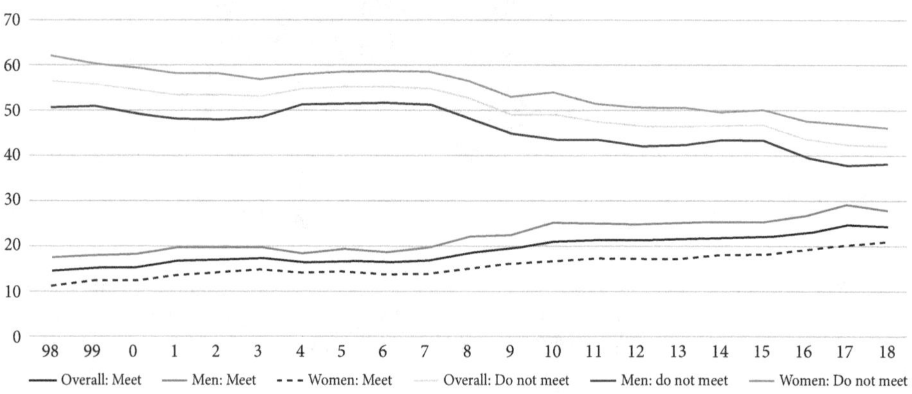

Source: Adapted from CDC.[10]

Figure 9-3. Participation in Leisure-Time Aerobic and Muscle-Strengthening Activities That Meet Federal Guidelines and Those That Do Not Meet Either Aerobic or Muscle-Strengthening Guidelines Among Adults Aged 18 Years and Older by Selected Characteristics, 1998–2018

CAUSES

Modifiable Risk Factors

Identifying factors associated with a physically active lifestyle—also called correlates and determinants of PA—is essential for developing effective interventions. The influence of factors differs by age groups, cultures, and a country's income level. PA factors include self-efficacy (i.e., confidence in one's ability to be physically active), previous PA, reported health, intention to exercise in adults, and family social support in adolescents.[15] Several investigators have applied a socioecological approach to correlates of PA behaviors. These include a variety of factors, among them individual (e.g., demographic, psychological, biological), interpersonal (e.g., social support, cultural norms, practices), environmental (e.g., social, built, natural environment), regional or related to national policy (e.g., transportation systems, urban planning, parks and recreation, national PA plans, advocacy organizations, the corporate sector), and global efforts (e.g., economic development, urbanization, advocacy efforts, social and cultural norms).[4]

Barriers to PA differ with gender, age, mobility, health status, socioeconomic status, residence, culture, and country. Common barriers are lack of time, fatigue and lack of energy, financial restrictions, health-related restrictions, low motivation, fear of injury, lack of skill, weather conditions, and high cost and shortage of facilities.[16] CDC offers advice on overcoming many of these barriers (https://www.cdc.gov/physicalactivity/basics/adding-pa/barriers.html). In particular, commuting long distances to work, sedentary jobs, watching television, and using computers during leisure are low-intensity activities that contribute to time spent physically inactive (https://sites.google.com/site/compendiumofphysicalactivities/home). More research is needed to understand and modify lifestyle behaviors associated with physically inactive lifestyles.

Among women, researchers cite lack of time, lack of enjoyment, self-consciousness about body size, shape, and physical ability, and urinary incontinence concerns as common barriers to being physically active.[17] Women who work full time and have home and family responsibilities report less PA than working women without family care responsibilities. Minority women report additional barriers, including hair concerns, safety and weather concerns, lack of role models, lack of social support, and monetary cost of recreational facilities.[18]

Living in rural areas is associated with lower levels of LTPA compared with living in urban areas.[19] However, this association is not consistent in different geographical locations. These differences may be attributable to differences in PA patterns not captured on sport- and recreation-focused questionnaires, where rural respondents would not cite house, yard, and farm work or animal care. It is also possible that rural respondents might not report a lack of environmental supports for LTPA such as sidewalks, parks, and stores near their homes for walking or for transportation. Consequently, more studies are needed to understand the PA patterns of rural dwellers.

For some individuals other health conditions may contribute to physical inactivity. Overweight status, chronic and infectious disease, injury, and physical disability may increase the energy cost of PA, making movement less enjoyable and possibly prohibiting one from being physically active. Often, because of existing health conditions or inaccessible facilities, physical inactivity may create a positive feedback response by which the condition may worsen with decreased PA.

An emerging view for understanding the determinants of PA is a systems approach that describes the complex dynamic influences (i.e., correlates/determinants) that interact together in ever-changing ways to drive desired outcomes. It is understood that in complex environments people have different needs that influence behavior, and the context of the socioecological settings that influence behavior constantly changes. An example of the complex nature of obesity, for example, is visually presented in the 2007 UK government Foresight report *Tackling Obesities,*[20] which provides a visual causal loop diagram of the determinants of PA and nutrition. Researchers have developed similar systems approaches to identify community PA and nutrition influences on obesity,[21] understand and promote global and national PA plans,[22] and help plan and implement citywide PA programs.[23]

Population-Attributable Risk

In an examination of deaths attributable to physical inactivity (≤150 minutes per week of MVPA), Carlson et al.[6] estimated 8.3% of all causes of mortality in the United States could be avoided if inactive and insufficiently active adults became more active. Population-attributable risk (PAR%) has been applied to understanding the proportion of physical inactivity in Canadian adolescents that could be avoided if neighborhoods were more suitable for PA. Nearly 15% to 23% of adolescents' physical inactivity (defined as engaging in <60 minutes per day, ≤4 days/week) could be avoided if neighborhoods were built with environmental features for moderate or high walkability, low cul-de-sac density, and moderate amounts of park space.[24] These PAR% estimates show that increased PA results in preventable premature mortality and that environmental support in neighborhoods positively influences adolescents' PA. It is possible to compute PAR% for other PA correlates/determinants with more information about relative risks and the prevalence of exposures.

EVIDENCE-BASED INTERVENTIONS, PROGRAMS, AND DOCUMENTS

Prevention

As with any public health problem, prevention works best when operating at many levels: personal, medical, worksite, school, and community. To guide prevention efforts and measure the improvement in the risk profiles of the US population, the government routinely develops national health objectives. The most recent document, Healthy People 2030, was published in 2020 and lists eight broad, global outcomes and 355 core, measurable objectives in five categories: health conditions, health behaviors, populations, settings and systems, and social determinants. The document also identifies 39 research objectives (2 related to PA) with high health or economic burden or significant disparities between groups. These objectives provide baseline prevalence data and set 10-year targets for each objective. Developing and modifying objectives for the next decade is an ongoing process. More information and opportunities for input are available at http://www.healthypeople.gov.

The US Preventive Services Task Force (USPSTF) provides recommendations and summarizes clinical and community practice strategies to improve PA among adults and children. *USPSTF Clinical Perspective* provides clinicians with updated screening and counseling information. This guide contains recommendations for prevention based on a review of evidence-based screenings and interventions to prevent 102 different illnesses and conditions. In 2017 and 2020, respectively, USPSTF added recommendations for PA and healthful diet behavioral counseling in adults without and with known risk factors for CVD. In 2018 the task force added a recommendation for a multicomponent behavioral intervention (including PA) for weight loss in adults to prevent obesity-related morbidity and mortality. USPSTF notes that linking primary care patients to community-based PA programs provides the best setting to enhance clinician counseling in primary care. The USPSTF website provides additional resources about recommendations in clinical settings (https://www.uspreventiveservicestaskforce.org/uspstf).

Released in 2001 and updated annually, *The Guide to Community Preventive Services* (hereafter The Community Guide) provides evidence-based recommendations for programs and policies designed to promote population health in community settings. The Community Guide contains intervention approaches for 21 behaviors and conditions. It is intended for public health professionals, legislators, policymakers, community-based organizations, providers of health care services, researchers, employers, and purchasers of health care services to promote public health. Recommended intervention approaches have "sufficient evidence" demonstrating the effectiveness of the interventions in research studies. Approaches with "insufficient evidence" need more research showing consistent and desired results. The Community Guide identifies 24 intervention approaches for PA categorized as campaigns and information and as behavioral and social, environmental, and policy interventions. Of these, 20 intervention approaches have strong or sufficient evidence, and 4 approaches have insufficient evidence. The Community Guide website provides supporting materials for each evidence-based approach (https://www.thecommunityguide.org/topic/physical-activity).

The National Physical Activity Plan (hereafter The Plan) is a comprehensive set of policies, programs, and initiatives designed to increase PA in all segments of the US population. Released in 2010 and expanded in 2016, The Plan aims to improve health, prevent disease and disability, and enhance quality of life by fostering a national culture that supports physically active lifestyles. The Plan contains nine societal sections, each with specific strategies to promote participation in PA: business and industry; community, recreation, fitness, and parks; education; faith-based settings; health care; mass media; public health; sport and; transportation, land use, and community design. The Plan website provides detailed information about specific strategies for each sector to increase PA participation in populations (https://paamovewithus.org/national-physical-activity-plan).

CDC's Division of Nutrition, Physical Activity, and Obesity provides resources and publications about PA as a health-enhancing behavior. It also posts data, statistics, and reports from PA surveillance, shares community strategies to increase PA, and suggests worksite PA programs. The website provides many resources for use in education and state and local public health settings (https://www.cdc.gov/physicalactivity/index.html).

The President's Council on Sports, Fitness & Nutrition is a federal advisory committee that promotes healthy eating and PA for Americans. The council has two membership categories: council members of accomplished athletes, coaches, and sports advocates, appointed by the president, who participate in events to promote healthy and active lifestyles, and a science board consisting of experts from academia who support initiatives identified by the executive director, such as contributing to the Healthy People midcourse review report on older adults. The council website provides additional information about meetings, initiatives, and activities (https://health.gov/our-work/nutrition-physical-activity/presidents-council).

Screening

Identifying insufficiently active people is essential to reduce the incidence of disease and disability associated with physical inactivity. Exercise is Medicine (EIM) is a global health initiative to make PA assessment and promotion a standard in clinical care and to connect patients with evidence-based PA resources. Managed by the American College of Sports Medicine, EIM has three goals for providers: first, to assess their patients' current PA levels according to the federal PA guidelines of 150 minutes per week of moderate-intensity PA; second, to provide brief advice and write an exercise prescription as needed; and third, to refer patients to PA resources such as qualified exercise professionals and evidence-based programs to help patients increase their PA. The EIM website provides physicians and health care providers resources for PA screening and referrals for patients (https://www.exerciseismedicine.org).

Treatment

Youth and adults who are insufficiently active at federal PA guideline levels have several resources to increase their PA, including EIM and The Community Guide. For adults,

The Community Guide recommends digital health interventions for adults 55 years and older, use of activity monitors for adults with overweight and obesity, worksite digital health and telephone interventions to increase healthy eating and PA, family-based interventions, and combined diet and PA promotion programs to prevent type 2 diabetes in people at increased risk for diabetes. For youth, The Community Guide recommends eight programs, including classroom-based PA breaks, lesson interventions involving PA, enhanced school-based physical education programs, and increased travel (i.e., walking or biking) to school for children and youth.

MOVING FORWARD

Researchers have studied the health effects of PA for nearly three-quarters of a century. From the 1950s to the 1960s their emphasis was on identifying the benefits of occupational MVPA and LTPA in reducing all-cause mortality and CHD mortality. Then the 1970s introduced laboratory studies to understand the mechanisms of PA in reducing mortality and disease risk. Exercise scientists also conducted studies to identify the dose of PA (frequency, intensity, type, and duration) sufficient to increase performance and aerobic capacity. By the 1980s and 1990s the emphasis shifted from performance and aerobic capacity benefits of exercise to understanding the myriad health benefits that we now know accompany even small increases in MVPA. Consensus conferences set a research agenda for PA, fitness, and health.[25] In the 2000s and beyond the focus has expanded to measuring and improving PA globally by using technology to measure PA, understanding how environmental and policy factors can increase opportunities for people to be physically active, and reducing sedentary behaviors. PA recommendations and federal guidelines identify types and doses of health-enhancing PA for people of all ages and health conditions. The Robert Wood Johnson Foundation (https://www.rwjf.org), the Women's Sports Foundation (https://www.womenssportsfoundation.org), and the National Fitness Foundation (http://fitness.foundation), among other foundations, have supported research and practice efforts to modify the environment, to understand how policies can promote PA, and to increase PA in women and older adults. Other organizations, like Girls on the Run (https://www.girlsontherun.org) and First Tee (https://firsttee.org), support research and practice to increase PA in youth. The National Institutes of Health funds research grants to advance the assessment of PA and conduct home and community PA interventions to improve the health of wheelchair users (https://prevention.nih.gov/research-priorities/physical-activity). Nevertheless, gaps remain in understanding how to integrate technology into PA surveillance and disseminate and translate research to public health practice, promoting PA and reducing sedentary behavior in underserved population sectors, as well as integrating the complexity of PA in research and interventions. The future directions for research are outlined next.

Integrating Technology With Questionnaires in Surveillance

In the past 30 years considerable progress has been made in assessing PA by using questionnaires and objective measures in the field. Most questionnaires address MVPA for walking, sports, conditioning, and recreational activities based on the federal PA guidelines. NHANES also assesses MVPA in household and worksite settings; walking and bicycling for transport; and sitting, watching media on a computer or smartphone, and using a computer outside of work (https://wwwn.cdc.gov/nchs/data/nhanes/2017-2018/questionnaires/PAQ_J.pdf). In 2003 NHANES started monitoring movement using accelerometers for seven days in a subsample of respondents. This has allowed monitoring time spent in sedentary behaviors, light-intensity PA, MVPA, and count steps taken per day. Assessment of movement with accelerometers also enables comparison of surveillance data obtained by questionnaire with objective measures in different population sectors.

It is challenging to assess self-report PA behaviors with sufficient accuracy to track long-term trends and measure the success of intervention studies. Low-cost and nonobtrusive uses of integrated technology can help researchers obtain objective measures of movement data. For example, it may be possible to monitor steps taken with smartphones. The Pew Research Center reports that 85% of US adults across a wide range of demographics own a smartphone (https://www.pewresearch.org/internet/fact-sheet/mobile). Generalizing the prevalence of PA estimates using accelerometers is difficult because of variability in surveillance system methodologies, including differences in cut points used to manage objective monitors and estimate time spent in MVPA.[26] For accelerometers to be useful for PA surveillance, public health professionals need to standardize accelerometer methodologies and cut points used to estimate PA intensity levels. Also, researchers should conduct feasibility studies using smartphones to obtain step data for PA surveillance. Researchers should conduct these studies in diverse groups, including ethnic minorities and older adults.

Translating and Disseminating Research Into Public Health Practice

Translation of PA intervention research into formats understood by the public and disseminated for use in public health practice can effectively reduce physical inactivity among targeted populations. Unfortunately, many research projects end with presentations at scientific conferences and publications in research journals. Instead, innovative, evidence-based PA interventions can be translated and disseminated to low-cost and accessible locations, such as community centers, churches, and recreation centers. PA intervention programs can be delivered effectively by community health advisers, exercise specialists, and volunteers without losing fidelity to the PA program. Collaboration with community stakeholders and exercise specialists can help identify effective channels and settings suitable for disseminating PA programs.

Foundations, centers, and institutes provide website access to evidence-based PA programs for children, adolescents, adults, and older adults. Examples of a few organizations that list evidence-based PA programs are National Cancer Institute evidence-based cancer control programs (https://www.cancer.gov), the National Council on Aging (https://www.ncoa.org), Healthy People 2030 evidence-based resources (https://health.gov/healthypeople), and the National Center on Health, Physical Activity and Disability (https://www.nchpad.org).

The more integrated these approaches are with everyday activities, the more successful they will be changing behavior. Even though behavior change is the ultimate goal, removing obstacles and providing effective ways to be physically active will help achieve this goal.

Promoting Physical Activity and Reducing Sedentary Behaviors

In 2021, according to the US Census Bureau, the United States had 71.6 million older adults aged 57 to 75, a cohort that represented 16.5% of the US population of 332 million people (https://www.census.gov/quickfacts/fact/table/US/PST045221). These baby boomers are the largest-ever cohort of adults approaching retirement age in the United States, with nearly 8,000 adults turning 60 years of age every day. By 2030 more than 21% of the US population (71 million) will be 65 years and older. Another 22 million will be 75 and older (https://www.census.gov/newsroom/press-releases/2018/cb18-41-population-projections.html). With age, the proportion of adults failing to meet either the aerobic or muscle-strengthening goals from the 2018 federal PA guidelines increases. Nearly 50% of adults aged 65 to 75 years and 63% of adults aged 75 years and older fail to meet either goal. Further, fewer than 16.4% of adults aged 65 and older meet the aerobic and muscle-strengthening goals. This lack of PA during older ages increases the risks for mortality, low physical and aerobic fitness, and loss of muscle strength and power, leading to muscle wasting (sarcopenia), poor balance, frailty, and risk for falls.

Researchers and practitioners have translated evidence-based PA programs for delivery in community settings for older adults. These programs effectively reduce physical inactivity if they are available and if older persons attend the programs. Three examples of community PA programs, discussed next, are available for download from websites:

- Active Living Every Day
- Fit & Strong
- FallProof! Comprehensive Balance and Mobility Program

Active Living Every Day is a 12-week evidence-based behavior change program designed to address the root causes of physical inactivity. The program uses facilitated group-based problem-solving methods to integrate PA into participants' everyday living. Program outcomes include increases in MVPA and total PA, with concomitant decreases in depressive symptoms and stress, and increases in satisfaction with body appearance and function, along with decreases in body mass index (https://www.ncoa.org/article/evidence-based-program-active-living-every-day).

Fit & Strong is an eight-week evidence-based group exercise program designed for persons with osteoarthritis, a common cause of disability among older adults and a significant barrier to participation in PA. In past research studies, program outcomes included improved joint pain, stiffness, and function, along with lower extremity strength and increased mobility. Additional positive results include improved mood and greater self-confidence to manage osteoarthritis with PA (https://www.ncoa.org/article/evidence-based-program-fit-strong).

The award-winning FallProof! Comprehensive Balance and Mobility Program aims to improve balance and mobility in older adults. FallProof! is a theory-driven, multidimensional, community-based program that targets intrinsic risk factors of impaired balance and gait and muscle weakness associated with fall risk. Certified instructors and standard program content ensure fidelity of the program.

While evidence-based programs are available for application in senior communities, older people need PA programs that are effective, convenient, and enjoyable to slow the decline in PA with aging. Researchers have an urgent task to understand more about the "efficacy" (i.e., Does it work in controlled research settings?) and "effectiveness" (i.e., Does it work in real-world settings?) of PA programs designed for older people. Also, sports and recreational programs should be encouraged to offer programs for older people to enable them to maintain physical function and prevent physiological decline and disability associated with aging.

Racial/Ethnic Minorities and Low Socioeconomic Status

Data from PA surveillance systems consistently show that African Americans, Hispanic women, and persons with low socioeconomic status, reflected by education and income, have the lowest prevalence of meeting federal PA guidelines. These populations also have a higher prevalence of sedentary inactivity than other groups (see Table 9-2). As shown in Figure 9-1, there are many adverse health consequences resulting from physical inactivity. Racial/ethnic minorities and persons with low socioeconomic status experience higher levels of chronic and behavioral health conditions such as hypertension, overweight and obesity, type 2 diabetes, and psychological stress than do non-Hispanic Whites and persons with higher socioeconomic status (https://www.commonwealthfund.org). PA has a powerful effect on preventing chronic health conditions and, indeed, helps manage the progression of chronic conditions. Increasing PA levels of racial/ethnic minorities and persons with lower socioeconomic status can help reduce the burden of chronic diseases in these populations.

More research is needed not only to show the efficacy and effectiveness of strategies to reduce the barriers to PA but also to increase the facilitators for PA in these underserved populations. Research can help us understand the causal factors associated with physical inactivity (see Figure 9-1). These causal factors are complex in that they interact in additive and multiplicative ways to increase the difficulty for long-term PA participation. For example, individuals faced with family demands, lack of peer support, and work requirements may perceive PA to be less important to their daily lives than these other issues, thus reducing their odds of initiating PA. Add to these factors sedentary worksites, parks and recreation centers far from home, and environments unsafe for recreational purposes or transportation, and the difficulties individuals face are compounded. To untangle a starting place for developing interventions to increase PA, more research is needed to understand how these barriers interact.

As noted by Bantham et al.,[27] a one-size-fits-all approach is insufficient to provide interventions and programs to eliminate barriers to PA for racial/ethnic minorities and persons with low socioeconomic status. Researchers and practitioners must address different barriers to PA and preferences for PA types with tailored approaches.

Children and Adolescents

PA is essential for children's and adolescents' physical and cognitive development. School physical education programs are an effective source of PA for children and adolescents. Students who receive regular physical education classes have higher grades and standardized test scores, better classroom behaviors, and lower absenteeism rates. However, only 3.7% of elementary school students and 25% of high school students receive regular physical education classes (https://www.cdc.gov/healthyschools/physicalactivity/physical-education.htm). Adopting federal PA guidelines to promote PA in and out of school settings provides a framework to address increasing physical inactivity among US children and adolescents. In a report of global trends in insufficient PA among adolescents, in 2016, an estimated 64% of boys and 80.7% of girls (overall prevalence 72%) were active at levels insufficient to meet the WHO PA guideline.[28] In addition to conducting recent research designed to test interventions to prevent declines in PA among adolescent girls, researchers and practitioners need to identify effective strategies to encourage this group. These strategies are crucial if girls and young women are to remain active during adolescence and balance activity levels with adequate nutrition required for growth and development.

Research and Interventions: Understanding the Complexity of Physical Activity

PA behaviors operate in a complex system where intrinsic and extrinsic factors, such as those identified in Figure 9-1, interact or are dependent on each other in ever-changing ways that influence interventions to increase PA. In traditional research, upstream causal and correlational factors for physical inactivity are often studied in isolation to identify a factor's influence on changes in PA. In a complex system, researchers must study the upstream factors collectively to understand how factors may become dependent on each other, interact in additive or multiplicative ways, and form relationships in ways influencing outcomes of increased PA. For example, the success of an intervention that builds a series of walking trails in a community must consider community residents' personal, social, and cultural factors that can influence trail walking. For example, in a community with many families, parents pushing strollers require paved rather than gravel trails. Accordingly, PA interventions must be adaptable to account for the unpredictability of emergent behaviors and properties in a complex system. They must account for competing factors that can influence behavior change. Also, in complex environments, people must be taught adaptative behaviors to adjust to ever-changing internal and external factors that influence their choices to be more active.

Future research into the complexity of PA systems can provide insight into new ways to promote health-enhancing PA behaviors in diverse populations. Research can focus on the complexity of factors influencing personal PA behavior change outcomes and address community systems that influence the acquisition and sustainability of resources and policies supporting active living.[22,23]

Policy and Environmental Approaches

Two public health approaches to increasing PA rely on policy and environmental strategies. Changes in public policy to promote PA often arise from grassroots community organizations designed to effect change at local, state, and national levels. Public health, education, and advocacy groups in recent years have coordinated their efforts to change policies for programs and facilities that promote regular PA in children and adults.

Advocates can focus policy changes on removing environmental barriers for nonmotorized travel (e.g., walking, using bicycles, scooters, or skateboards), de-emphasizing automation in labor-saving devices and systems, and building more accessible facilities to enhance movement. They can support policies that require physical education programs in schools, for example, or buildings to be designed with open, well-lit, safe, and accessible stairways in visible locations as an alternative to elevators and escalators. They also can influence how state and federal funds are used, whether to support PA initiatives at large or subsidize parks and recreational facilities to provide PA programs for people of all ages. For instance, Federal Highway Administration funding through the US Department of Transportation can be directed to support bicycle and pedestrian safety in specific areas. Projects may include building pedestrian and bicycle lanes on bridges, increasing walkway lighting, making trail maps, repairing sidewalks, and building and maintaining bicycle lanes separated from traffic (https://www.fhwa.dot.gov/environment/bicycle_pedestrian/funding/funding_opportunities.cfm).

Organization and community leaders can enact PA-friendly policies for worksites, schools, neighborhoods, and recreation centers. For example, community developers and city councils could be encouraged to install bicycle trails, walking trails, and sidewalks and to designate parkland and green spaces in and around new housing developments. Employers can provide safe and convenient exercise facilities and flexible work schedules to promote increased PA during the workday. Other examples of environmental opportunities for promoting PA include building bicycling paths and sidewalks along busy streets and providing access to shopping malls and schools as safe, heated, or air-conditioned walking and exercise spaces.

In the past 15 years much legislation and numerous statutes have been introduced to state and federal legislatures to increase not only the number of PA programs but also their availability and people's access to them. In reviewing the databases for PA provided by the National Conference of State Legislatures, one can see that nearly every state has introduced legislation to mandate state and local school boards to require school physical education programs focusing on activities that students can practice throughout their lifetime (https://www.ncsl.org). Similarly, some states have enacted legislation to increase access to open space for recreation, ensure bicycle and pedestrian safety, and assess aerobic capacity and percentage of body fat in school-age children. Funding for such legislation has come from various sources, such as deposits on recyclable soda cans for PA programs.

Given the public health impact of physical inactivity in terms of personal health, the economy, and societal integration, policy and environmental approaches provide an effective way to increase opportunities for PA for people of all ages.

DISCUSSION QUESTIONS

1. Characterize the federal PA guidelines and describe why are they meaningful to public health.
2. Identify the chronic changes of PA in body systems and recommend which chronic changes you think are most important for health and longevity.
3. Rank the top three upstream causes of physical inactivity listed in Figure 9-1, then explain how they can influence PA in populations at the highest risk for not meeting the aerobic and muscle-strengthening guidelines listed in Table 9-2.
4. Name the main PA surveillance systems and explain why they are useful for tracking the prevalence of PA and evaluating interventions.
5. Explain why policy and environmental supports for PA are public health approaches to promote PA.
6. Characterize reasons why physical inactivity is a public health problem.
7. Considering the suggestions presented in the Moving Forward section of this chapter, prioritize an order for action to fill the gaps for advancing PA in public health and defend your priorities.

REFERENCES

1. Pate RR, Pratt M, Blair SN, et al. Physical activity and public health: a recommendation from the Centers for Disease Control and Prevention and the American College of Sports Medicine. *JAMA*. 1995;273(5):402–407.
2. Booth FW, Thyfault JP, Ruegsegger GN, Toedebusch RG. Role of inactivity in chronic diseases: evolutionary insight and pathophysological mechanisms. *Physiol Rev*. 2017;97:1351–1402.
3. Booth F, Roberts CK, Laye M. Lack of exercise is a major cause of chronic diseases. *Compr Physiol*. 2012;2(2):1143–1211.
4. Sallis J, Cervero RB, Ascher W, Henderson KA, Kraft MK, Kerr J. An ecological approach to creating active living communities. *Annu Rev Public Health*. 2006;27:297–322.
5. Lee I-M, Shiroma EJ, Lobelo F, et al. Effect of physical inactivity on major non-communicable diseases worldwide: an analysis of burden of disease and life expectancy. *Lancet*. 2012; 380(9838):219–229.
6. Carlson S, Adams EK, Yang Z, Fulton JE. Percentage of deaths associated with inadequate physical activity in the United States. *Prev Chronic Dis*. 2018;15(March):1–11.
7. Zhao M, Veeranki SP, Magnussen CG, Xi B. Recommended physical activity and all cause and cause specific mortality in US adults: prospective cohort study. *BMJ*. 2020;370:1–10.
8. Ding D, Lawson KD, Kolbe-Alexander TL, et al. The economic burden of physical inactivity: a global analysis of major non-communicable diseases. *Lancet*. 2016;388:1311–1324.
9. Matos A, Barbosa F, Cunha C, Voss G, Correia F. Social isolation, physical inactivity and inadequate diet among European middle-aged and older adults. *BMC Pub Health*. 2021;21:1–12.
10. Centers for Disease Control and Prevention. Data finder. Available at: https://www.cdc.gov/nchs/hus/contents2019.htm. Accessed January 15, 2023.
11. Centers for Disease Control and Prevention. 2019 data. Available at: https://www.cdc.gov/brfss/annual_data/annual_2019.html. Accessed August 15, 2023.
12. Centers for Disease Control and Prevention. Adult physical inactivity prevalence maps by race/ethnicity 2015–2018. Available at: https://www.cdc.gov/physicalactivity/data/inactivity-prevalence-maps/2015-2018.html. Accessed August 15, 2023.
13. Ussery E, Omura JD, McCain K, Watson KB. Change in prevalence of meeting the aerobic physical activity guidelines among US adults, by states and territories—Behavioral Risk Factor Surveillance System, 2011 and 2019. *J Phys Act Health*. 2021;18:S84–S85.
14. Yang L, Cao C, Kantor ED, et al. Trends in sedentary behavior among the US population. *JAMA*. 2019;321(16):1587–1597.
15. Bauman A, Reis RS, Sallis JF, Wells JC, Loos RJF, Martin BW; Lancet Physical Activity Series Working Group. Correlates of physical activity: why are some people physically active and others not? *Lancet*. 2012;380(9838):258–271.
16. Pederson M, Hansen AF, Elmose-Østerlund KE. Motives and barriers related to physical activity and sport across social backgrounds: implications for health promotion. *Int J Environ Res Pub Health*. 2021;18:1–16.
17. Moreno JP, Johnston CA. Barriers to physical activity in women. *Amer J Lifestyle Med*. 2014;8(3):164–166.

18. Joseph R, Ainsworth BE, Keller C, Dodgson JE. Barriers to physical activity among African American women: an integrative review of the literature. *Women Health.* 2015;55(6):679–699.
19. Whitfield G, Carlson SA, Ussery EN, Fulton JE, Galuska DA, Petersen R. Trends in meeting physical activity guidelines among urban and rural dwelling adults—United States, 2008–2017. *MMWR Morb Mort Wkly Rep.* 2019;68(23):513–518.
20. Butland B, Jebb S, Kopelman P, et al. *Tackling Obesities: Future Choices—Project Report.* London, UK: Government Office for Science; 2007.
21. Allender S, Owen B, Kuhlberg J, et al. A community based systems diagram of obesity causes. *PLoS ONE.* 2015;10(7):1–12.
22. Rutter H, Cavill N, Bauman A, Bull F. Systems approaches to global and national physical activity plans. *Bull World Health Organ.* 2019;92(2):162–165.
23. Cavill N, Richardson D, Faghy M, Bussell C, Rutter H. Using system mapping to help plan and implement city-wide action to promote physical activity. *J Pub Health Res.* 2020;9:278–284.
24. Laxer RE, Janssen I. The proportion of youth's physical inactivity attributable to neighborhood built environment features. *Int J Health Geog.* 2013;12:1–13.
25. Bouchard C, Shephard RJ, Stephens T. *Physical Activity, Fitness, and Health.* Champlain, IL: Human Kinetics; 1994.
26. Pedišić Ž, Bauman A. Accelerometer-based measures in physical activity surveillance: current practices and issues. *Mr J Sports Med.* 2015;49(4):219–223.
27. Bantham A, Ross SET, Sebastião E, Hall G. Overcoming barriers to physical activity in underserved populations. *Prog Cardiov Dis.* 2021;64:64–71.
28. Guthold R, Stevens GA, Riley LM, Bull FC. Global trends in insufficient physical activity among adolescents: a pooled analysis of 298 population-based surveys with 1.6 million participants. *Lancet Child Adolesc Health.* 2020;4:23–35.

10

Alcohol Use

Alyssa Bruehlman, MD, Bri Deyo, MPH, Jordan Mills, DO, PhD,
and Randall Brown, MD, PhD

LEARNING OBJECTIVES

After completing this chapter, readers should be able to

1. Describe the prevalence of alcohol use in the United States and important trends in current use patterns.
2. Identify health conditions affected by acute alcohol intoxication and chronic alcohol use as well as the diagnosis of alcohol use disorder.
3. Demonstrate prevention and intervention strategies for unhealthy alcohol use at both the societal and the individual level.

INTRODUCTION

Human consumption of alcohol, including descriptions of both favorable and adverse effects, has been documented for millennia. In the present day, the distinction between low-risk and disordered alcohol use involves complex physiological, psychological, behavioral, social, and economic considerations.

For individuals who use alcohol, current guidelines recommend limiting daily consumption to two drinks or less for males or one drink or less for females.[1] One standard drink equivalent contains 14 grams of pure alcohol, which is equivalent to the alcohol found in 12 ounces of beer (5% alcohol by volume, or ABV), 5 ounces of wine (12% ABV), or 1.5 ounces of 80 proof distilled spirits (40% ABV), as shown in Figure 10-1.[2] The caloric density of alcohol (7 kcal/gram) is closer to dietary fat (9 kcal/gram) than carbohydrates (4 kcal/gram) or protein (4 kcal/gram), raising concern that regular alcohol use could contribute to obesity. Some prospective studies suggest that light-to-moderate alcohol use does not increase the risk for obesity, whereas heavy drinking is more consistently associated with weight gain.[3] The 2020 US Department of Agriculture (USDA) dietary guidelines recommend considering the caloric density of alcoholic beverages to stay within recommended daily limits.[1]

Alcohol can be safe when consumed in moderation in the healthy adult population and is often an integral component to family, social, and cultural gatherings or celebrations.

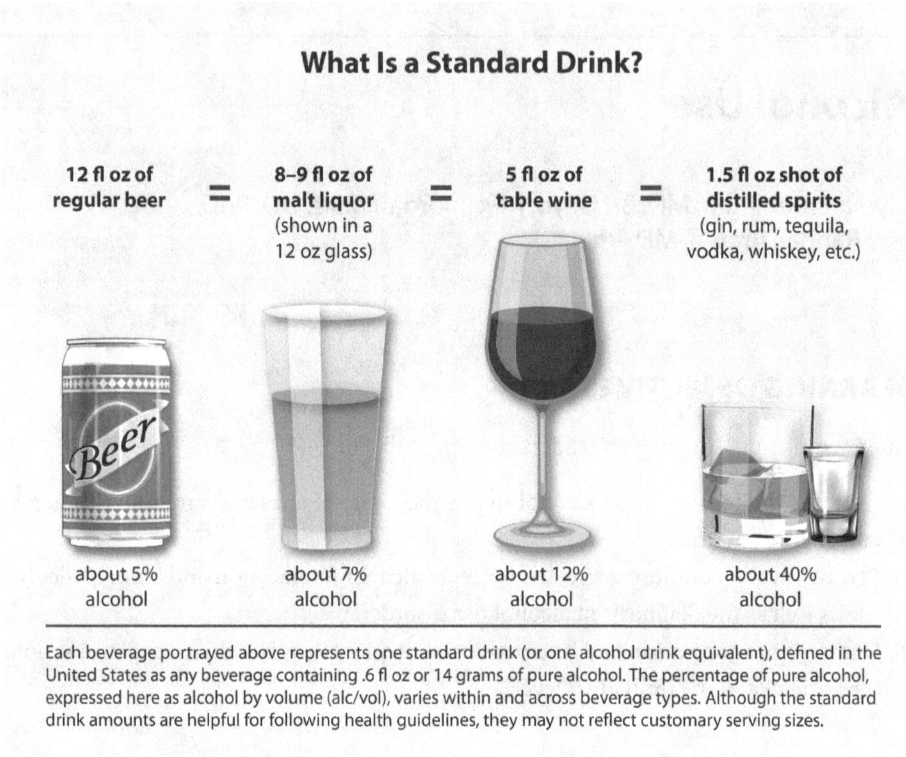

Source: Reprinted from NIAAA.[2]

Figure 10-1. Standard Drink Equivalents

Although moderate alcohol use is accepted in the United States, its objective physical health benefits are still an emerging area of research. A growing body of literature describes potential protective effects of low-level alcohol consumption against coronary heart disease, though this remains controversial, as discussed later in this chapter.

Negative health consequences related to alcohol use are of three broad types: (1) the acute consequences of alcohol intoxication such as motor vehicle crash injuries, violence, and alcohol poisoning; (2) chronic disease consequences, such as liver disease, cancer, and cardiomyopathy; and (3) the primary chronic disease of alcohol use disorder.

Alcohol affects every organ of the body. Most critical to heavy consumption are the effects of alcohol on the brain (Table 10-1).[4] It has been known for millennia that alcohol ingestion creates a pleasurable state of mind. Alcohol intoxication affects areas of the brain controlling judgment, motor function, and memory, resulting in adverse consequences, including injuries, violence, and alcohol-induced blackouts. Progressive drinking leads to confusion, incoordination, sedation, and even an alcohol overdose in which basic life-supporting functions of breathing and heart rate begin to shut down.[5]

Table 10-1. Effect of Blood Alcohol Concentration (BAC)

BAC (~no. drinks)	Typical Effects	Predictable Effects on Driving
0.02% (2)	• Some loss of judgment • Relaxation • Slight body warmth • Altered mood	• Decline in visual functions (rapid tracking of a moving target) • Decline in ability to perform 2 tasks at the same time (divided attention)
0.05% (3)	• Exaggerated behavior • May have loss of small-muscle control (e.g., focusing your eyes) • Impaired judgment • Usually good feeling • Lowered alertness • Release of inhibition	• Reduced coordination • Reduced ability to track moving objects • Difficulty steering • Reduced response to emergency driving situations
0.08% (4)	• Muscle coordination becomes poor (e.g., balance, speech, vision, reaction time, hearing) • Harder to detect danger • Judgment, self-control, reasoning, and memory are impaired	• Impaired concentration • Short-term memory loss • Impaired speed control • Reduced information-processing capability (e.g., signal detection, visual search) • Impaired perception
0.10% (5)	• Clear deterioration of reaction time and control • Slurred speech, poor coordination, and slowed thinking	• Reduced ability to maintain lane position and brake appropriately
0.15% (7)	• Far less muscle control than normal • Vomiting may occur (unless this level is reached slowly or a person has developed a tolerance for alcohol) • Major loss of balance	• Substantial impairment in vehicle control, attention to driving task, and in necessary visual and auditory information processing

Source: Adapted from NHTSA.[4]

With long-term daily exposure, the brain adapts to the presence of alcohol and eventually functions more normally in its presence. This physiologic change is known as tolerance. Repeated drinking causes an imbalance of central nervous system signaling chemicals called neurotransmitters. When alcohol consumption is discontinued or reduced suddenly, this maladaptive imbalance of neurotransmitters can lead to symptoms of alcohol withdrawal, including tremors, hallucinations, delirium, and seizures.[5]

Long-standing alcohol use can lead to a variety of chronic health disorders.[5] Liver disease (steatosis, hepatitis, cirrhosis, and liver failure) is a leading cause of death in people who drink heavily. Chronic alcohol consumption may also lead to conditions in other organ systems, including cardiovascular (dilated cardiomyopathy, arrhythmia, hypertension, stroke), gastrointestinal (nutrient malabsorption, gastritis, pancreatitis), and reproductive (testicular atrophy, fetal alcohol spectrum disorders). Heavy alcohol use is associated with increased risk of cancer of the head and neck, esophagus, breast, colon, and liver.[5] Chronic alcohol use may lead to a form of brain damage due to thiamine (vitamin B1) deficiency called Wernicke encephalopathy that presents as altered mental status, gait changes, and visual symptoms. These changes are reversible with replacement of high doses of thiamine in the medical setting; however, if not recognized and treated appropriately, they can cause irreversible memory problems (also called Korsakoff syndrome).[6]

Public health and medical organizations use varying terms to describe patterns of alcohol use (Table 10-2).[7–11] In 2013 the *Diagnostic and Statistical Manual of Mental Disorders*, Fifth Edition (*DSM-5*) established the diagnosis of "alcohol use disorder" in place of previously used terminology. Alcohol use disorder (AUD) is a clinical diagnosis defined by symptoms of (1) impaired control, including difficulty limiting consumption; (2) social problems, including adverse effects on relationships and responsibilities; (3) risky use despite harms and consequences; and (4) physical dependence, including tolerance and withdrawal symptoms.[11] AUD may be classified as mild, moderate, or severe depending on the number of diagnostic criteria met. The term *alcohol use disorder* replaces the former terms *alcohol abuse* and *alcohol dependence* from the previous edition of the *Diagnostic and Statistical Manual of Mental Disorders* (*DSM-4*) as well as more colloquial terms including *alcoholism* or *alcohol addiction*, which are still broadly used but lack diagnostic specificity and carry some degree of stigma. Notably, the development of alcohol use disorder is not solely attributable to excess alcohol use in isolation. It is instead dependent on a multitude of risk factors and has myriad physical and psychosocial consequences (Figure 10-2).[8,12,13]

Table 10-2. Terms and Definitions

Term	Source	Definition
Unhealthy use	USPSTF[7]	Spectrum of alcohol-related behaviors, from at-risk use to alcohol use disorder
At-risk use	NIAAA[8]	A pattern of alcohol use that falls outside recommended limits (see "heavy use")
Binge drinking	NIAAA[8]	Drinking that brings BAC to 0.08%
	SAMHSA, NSDUH[9]	On a single occasion ≥5 drinks for males or ≥4 drinks for females
Heavy use	NIAAA[7]	>4 drinks/d or 14 drinks/wk for males, >3 drinks/d or 7 drinks/wk for females
	SAMHSA, NSDUH[9]	≥5 binge drinking days in the last mo
Hazardous use	ASAM[10]	Alcohol use that increases risk of future negative consequences
Alcohol use disorder	*DSM-5*[11]	A pattern of maladaptive use resulting in physical and psychosocial consequences over a 12-mo period

Note: ASAM = American Society of Addiction Medicine; BAC = Blood Alcohol Concentration; *DSM-5* = *Diagnostic and Statistical Manual of Mental Disorders*, Fifth Edition; NIAAA = National Institute on Alcohol Abuse and Alcoholism; NSDUH = National Survey on Drug Use and Health; SAMHSA = Substance Abuse and Mental Health Services; USPSTF = United States Preventive Services Task Force.

ALCOHOL USE DISORDER		
UPSTREAM CONTRIBUTORS (CAUSES)	DOWNSTREAM CONSEQUENCES	HIGH-RISK POPULATIONS
• Normative heavy alcohol use among peers or family • Local drinking culture • Alcohol outlet density • Alcohol laws and policy • Poverty and economic disparity • Structural inequity • Situational and environmental stress • Limited access to physical and mental health services	Cognitive: • Disruptions in adolescent brain development • Impaired decision-making • Hangovers • Memory loss • Dementia Psychosocial: • Relational dysfunction • Domestic violence • Criminal activity • Victimization • Accidental injury • Suicide • Legal entanglement • Absenteeism • Sexual dysfunction Physical: • Unintended pregnancy • Adverse pregnancy outcomes • Physical trauma • Chronic cardiovascular, liver, or gastrointestinal disease • Cancer • Withdrawal complications • Death	• Early age of first alcohol use • Family history of alcohol use disorder • Co-occurring substance use disorder • Co-occurring mental health conditions • History of trauma

Source: Based on NIAAA,[8] CDC,[12] and CPSTF.[13]

Note: CDC = Centers for Disease Control; CPSTF = Community Preventive Services Task Force; NIAAA = National Institute on Alcohol Abuse and Alcoholism.

Figure 10-2. Alcohol Use Disorder: Causes, Consequences, and High-Risk Populations

PUBLIC HEALTH IMPACT

Alcohol consumption is a part of contemporary life for many. Results from the 2020 National Survey on Drug Use and Health indicate that 34.6% of people aged 12 to 20 years and 86.5% of people aged 21 years and older in the United States have used alcohol in their lifetime. Although most people drink moderately and without negative effects, alcohol use disorders and alcohol-related consequences are major health problems in the United States.[9] The survey data from 2020 indicate that 4.9% of people aged 12 to 20 years and 11.1% of people aged 21 years and older in the United States meet *DSM-5* criteria for alcohol use disorder.[9] The presence of an alcohol use disorder increases the relative risk of mortality 3.5 times for males and 4.6 times for females.[14] Alcohol-related deaths made up 3.0% of all deaths in the United States in 2020.[15]

Patterns of unhealthy alcohol use without underlying alcohol use disorder are also prevalent. In 2020 in the United States 44.4% of adults who used alcohol reported binge drinking and 12.8% reported heavy drinking.[9] Healthy People 2030, a government-led effort to promote health and well-being nationally, has chosen binge drinking as one of its eight leading health indicators that affect the death and disease burden in the United States.[16]

In economic terms, alcohol-related costs are estimated to have been $250 billion in 2010, the most recent year for which such estimates are available.[17] Of these costs, more than 72% are in the form of indirect costs, such as productivity losses attributable to premature mortality, excess morbidity, and crime, while only 11% are for medical treatment of alcohol use disorders.

DESCRIPTIVE EPIDEMIOLOGY

The prevalence of past-month alcohol use, as well as binge drinking and heavy drinking among specific demographics from the 2020 National Survey on Drug Use and Health, is shown in Table 10-3.[9]

High-Risk Populations and Health Disparities

Youth and Young Adults

The National Institute on Alcohol Abuse and Alcoholism (NIAAA) calls underage drinking a "serious health problem." Brain development continues well beyond teenage years, thus earlier onset of alcohol use confers greater risk of both immediate (e.g., physical injury, relational dysfunction, legal entanglement) and long-term adverse outcomes (alcohol use disorder and premature death).[18,19]

In 1984 the Minimum Legal Drinking Age Act restricted the legal purchase of alcohol nationwide until the age of 21 years. The Centers for Disease Control and Prevention (CDC) estimates that raising the minimum legal drinking age from 18 to 21 years nationally significantly reduced motor vehicle crashes, drinking among people aged 18 to 25 years, and other adverse outcomes related to alcohol consumption, including suicide and death.[20] These downstream risks of early-age alcohol use are the impetus behind pervasive national, state, and local efforts and funding to address alcohol use among youth.

Table 10-3. Prevalence of Alcohol Use in Past Month Among Various US Demographic Groups Aged 12 Years and Older: NSDUH, 2020

Characteristic	Any Alcohol Use, %	Binge Use, %	Heavy Use, %
Total	50.0	22.2	6.4
Age, y			
12–17	8.2	4.1	0.6
18–25	51.5	31.4	8.6
26–49	59.6	30.2	8.1
≥50	50.2	16.5	5.5
Sex			
Male	52.6	24.9	8.3
Female	47.6	19.7	4.6
Origin			
Hispanic/Latinx	42.6	23.7	5.4
Not Hispanic/Latinx	51.6	21.9	6.6
Race			
White	55.3	23.1	7.3
Black	44.8	20.8	5.4
AIAN	NA	NA	7.9
NHPI	NA	NA	2.4
Asian	33.4	12.1	2.2
≥2 races	42.0	20.6	6.9
Education			
<High school	29.9	18.7	5.7
High school graduate	45.9	24.1	8.0
Some college/associate degree	56.8	26.1	7.2
College graduate	68.1	23.8	6.4
Employment			
Full-time	64.4	30.2	8.7
Part-time	55.3	23.9	6.2
Unemployed	46.4	26.6	7.3
Other[a]	41.8	15.9	5.0

Source: Adapted from SAMHSA.[9]

Note: AIAN = American Indians and Alaska Natives; NA = not available; NHPI = Native Hawaiian/Other Pacific Islander; NSDUH = National Survey on Drug Use and Health; SAMHSA = Substance Abuse and Mental Health Services Administration. A dash indicates a low-precision prevalence.

[a]Includes students, full-time caregivers, retired people, disabled people, and those not in the labor force.

Pregnancy and Lactation

Alcohol can affect fetal brain development at all stages of pregnancy. Alcohol use during pregnancy is the leading cause of preventable birth defects as well as intellectual and neurodevelopmental disability. Infants exposed to alcohol prenatally are at risk of fetal alcohol spectrum disorders, which can include growth limitations, abnormal facial features, and intellectual and developmental disability.[21] Because the diagnosis of fetal alcohol spectrum disorder has lifelong impacts, CDC recommends that reproductive-age females limit their alcohol use to avoid unintentional fetal alcohol exposure before a pregnancy is known.

Alcohol is also expressed in breas tmilk. Current guidelines recommend either complete avoidance of alcohol use while lactating or monitoring the quantity of alcohol consumed and time between alcohol consumption and feeding or expressing breast milk. CDC recommends avoidance of more than one drink per day while lactating and waiting two hours after a single drink before nursing or pumping.[22]

Genetic Predisposition

Genetic factors contribute to alcohol use disorder susceptibility. Supportive evidence comes from studies involving identical versus fraternal twins.[23,24] Inherited risk can be elucidated by a family history of alcohol use disorder, though underlying shared environmental factors within families also contributes to this elevated risk. Genes involved in alcohol metabolism as well as stimulus–reward networks in the brain may particularly contribute to increased risk of developing AUD.[25] Genetic influences have been associated with specific phenotypes, including behavioral (e.g., impulsivity, disinhibition) and physiologic traits (e.g., flushing response to alcohol, high tolerance to alcohol).[26]

Psychiatric Comorbidities, Trauma, and Other Substance Use

Research has suggested a link between post-traumatic stress disorder and higher rates of alcohol and other substance use disorders, suggesting that people with a history of trauma are more likely to use alcohol or drugs to mitigate their symptoms.[27] The National Institute on Drug Abuse suggests three main pathways underlying the high prevalence of comorbid substance use disorders and mental health conditions: (1) both substance use and psychiatric illness have common risk factors; (2) people with mental health conditions may use alcohol and/or other substances as a form of symptom management; and (3) substance use leads to brain changes that may contribute to psychiatric illness.[28] Rather than being a linear causal pathway, the interplay between trauma, mental health disorders, and substance use can be cyclic and exponential, such that each individual risk factor contributes to heightened risk for the others. In addition, populations who experience chronic or repeated stress and trauma related to their racial, ethnic, socioeconomic, or gender and sexual identities may be at greater risk of alcohol and other substance use disorders.

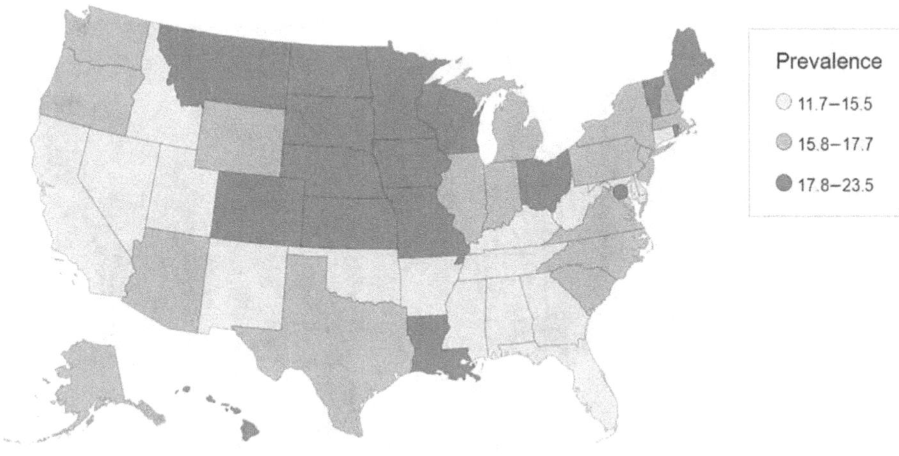

Source: Reprinted from CDC.[12]

Figure 10-3. Binge Drinking Prevalence Among US Adults by State in 2018

Geographic Distribution

Alcohol use patterns involve local and regional contexts. The Substance Abuse and Mental Health Services Administration (SAMHSA), along with CDC and NIAAA, publishes data to describe trends of alcohol use across the country.[9,12,29] Figure 10-3 portrays binge drinking prevalence by state from the CDC's 2018 Behavioral Risk Factor Surveillance System, with notably highest rates of binge drinking in the US Midwest.[12] Figure 10-4, made available by NIAAA, shows that most states did not meet goal metrics set by Healthy People 2020 for reducing alcohol consumption per capita.[29]

Rates of both past-month alcohol use and past-month heavy alcohol use are similar across geographic regions per age group. However, among those 21 years of age and older, the Northeast and Midwest regions show slightly higher than average rates for both consumption categories, while the South and West regions show slightly lower than average rates. When sorted by county type, rates are similar regardless of age group. However large metro and small metro counties show slightly higher than average rates for both consumption categories, while non-metro counties show slightly below average rates (see Tables 10-4a and 10-4b).[9]

Time Trends

American alcohol consumption in terms of volume per capita has been tracked since 1850, excluding the years of the Prohibition era, from 1920 to 1934.[29] NIAAA reports annually on gallons of ethanol consumed per capita including beer, wine, spirits, and all

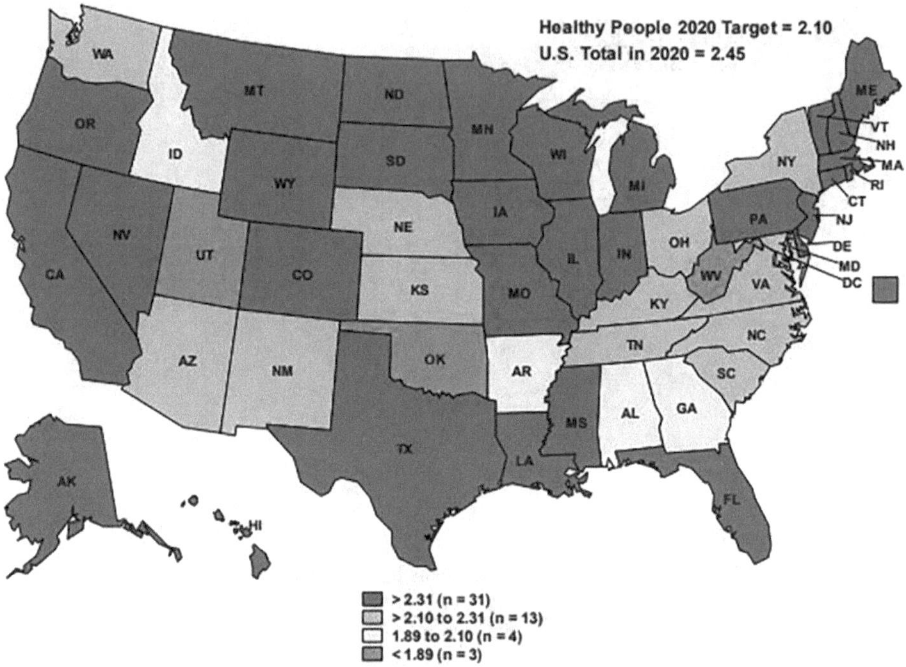

Source: Reprinted with permission of NIAAA.[29]

Figure 10-4. Per Capita Consumption of Gallons of Ethanol by State in 2020

Table 10-4a. Prevalence of Any Alcohol, Binge Alcohol Use, and Heavy Alcohol Use in the Past Month Among US Individuals Aged 12–20 Years and Older: NSDUH, 2020

	Any Alcohol Use, %	Binge Use, %	Heavy Use, %
Total	16.1	9.2	1.8
Region			
Northeast	15.7	9.7	2.3
Midwest	18.3	11.1	2.3
South	15.7	8.2	1.4
Southwest	15.2	8.7	1.6
County type			
Large metro	15.2	8.6	1.6
Small metro	16.5	9.2	1.8
Non-metro	18.9	11.6	2.5

Source: Adapted from SAMHSA.[9]

Note: NSDUH = National Survey on Drug Use and Health; SAMHSA = Substance Abuse and Mental Health Services Administration.

Table 10-4b. Prevalence of Any Alcohol, Binge Alcohol Use, and Heavy Alcohol Use in the Past Month Among US Individuals Aged 21 Years and Older: NSDUH, 2020

	Any Alcohol Use, %	Binge Use, %	Heavy Use, %
Total	55.3	24.3	7.1
Region			
Northeast	57.6	24.7	6.8
Midwest	57.6	26.0	8.7
South	52.5	23.3	6.6
Southwest	56.1	24.0	6.9
County type			
Large metro	58.7	25.4	7.1
Small metro	53.9	24.2	7.5
Non-metro	45.9	20.5	6.5

Source: Adapted from SAMHSA.[9]

Note: NSDUH = National Survey on Drug Use and Health; SAMHSA = Substance Abuse and Mental Health Services Administration.

alcoholic beverages. Available data show that volume of alcohol consumption per capita has remained relatively steady since 1850. In general, beer is the highest volume consumed by gallon, followed by spirits and then wine. For all alcoholic beverages, annual volume per capita has spanned from a low of 0.97 gallons in 1934 to a high of 2.76 gallons in 1981. The mean and median are similar at approximately 2.2 gallons of all alcoholic beverages per capita. Trends in consumption over the last 20 years have shown a general decrease in beer consumption and an increase in wine and spirit consumption (Figure 10-5)[29]; however, the mean and median of consumption per capita in each category are similarly matched: beer at approximately 1.1 gallons per capita, spirits at approximately 0.8 gallons per capita, wine at approximately 2.2 gallons per capita.[29] Despite the variations in measuring techniques and reporting methods throughout this sample from 1850 to the present, the similarities between the mean and median of all four categories suggest relative stability in volume of alcohol consumed over time.

From 2006 to 2018 the prevalence of people who reported at least one heavy drinking day in the past year remained stable for both males (mean 30.7%, median 30.9%) and females (mean 15.7%, median 14.5%).[30] Despite the stable prevalence of alcohol use, deaths attributed to alcohol have risen dramatically over the last two decades. According to the National Center for Health Statistics, deaths from alcohol poisonings were relatively consistent at 0.1 per 100,000 deaths from 1999 to 2006, then increased eightfold to 0.8 per 100,000 deaths from 2006 to 2020. Other alcohol-related causes of death rose steadily throughout the same time period, from 6.8 per 100,000 deaths in 1999 to 14.1 in 2020.[31]

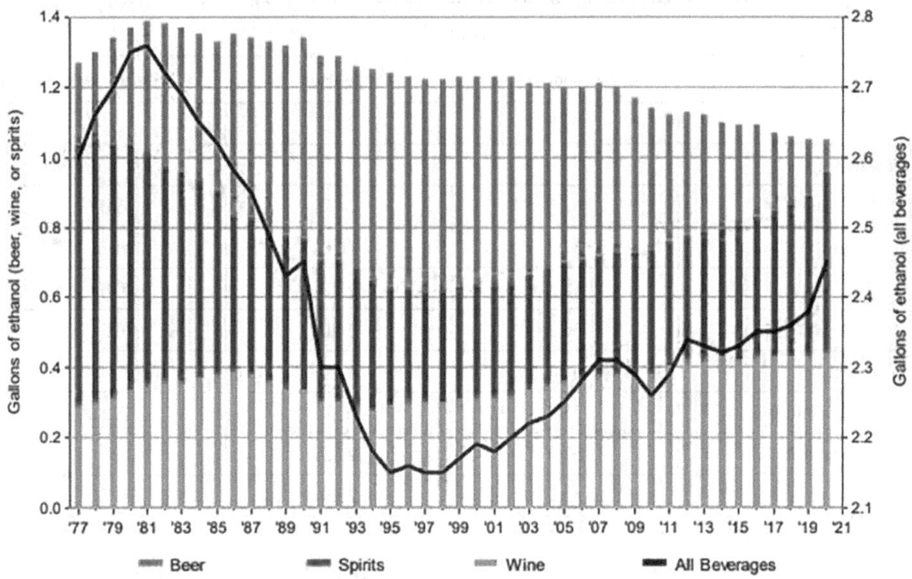

Source: Reprinted from NIAAA.[29]

Note: NIAAA = National Institute on Alcohol Abuse and Alcoholism.

Figure 10-5. Per Capita Ethanol Consumption by Beverage Type: 1977–2020

CAUSES

Modifiable Risk Factors

Although addiction is attributed in part to brain maladaptation, understanding the social determinants of health that contribute to alcohol use and its related harms is essential for prevention and treatment.[16] These include economic stability, education access and quality, health care access and quality, neighborhood and built environment, and social and community context (Table 10-5).[16,32,33]

While age is considered a nonmodifiable risk factor for many medical conditions, age of first drink and age of alcohol misuse onset are potential areas for modification and intervention. Early age at drinking onset poses an increased risk for lifetime alcohol-related problems. Almost half of individuals who develop signs of alcohol use disorder started drinking before 16 years of age.[34] Parent and other adult alcohol users influence the likelihood of heavy drinking in adolescence,[35–37] and an adolescent's choice between drinking and non-drinking peer groups can be correlated with home drinking environment.[38] The influence of alcohol advertising on young people is a subject of particular debate. Some ecological studies suggest little effect; however, longitudinal studies enrolling individual participants show associations between commercial and media exposure with alcohol use.[39,40]

Table 10-5. Social Determinants of Health Affecting Alcohol Consumption

Factor	Examples
Economic stability	• Limited employment opportunities • Income inequality • Taxes on alcohol sales • Happy hour specials
Education access and quality	• High school graduation/GED completion • Preventive education in schools
Health care access and quality	• Availability of mental health resources • Access to primary care • Insurance coverage
Neighborhood and built environment	• Local liquor stores • Restaurant and bar density • Housing availability
Social and community context	• Family or sibling use of alcohol • Celebrations involving alcohol • Targeted advertising on social media

Source: Based on USDHHS,[16] Swan et al.,[32] and Fone et al.[33]

Note: GED = General Educational Development Test; USDHHS = US Department of Health and Human Services.

How and where alcohol is sold also affects rates of excess consumption. A systematic review of studies of alcohol outlet density indicated greater prevalence of alcohol use disorders in neighborhoods with increased alcohol availability. Privatization rather than government control of retail alcohol sales also results in increased per capita alcohol consumption. Conversely, higher alcohol prices and taxes on alcohol sales are consistently related to reduced harms, including less youth drinking, fewer alcohol-related motor vehicle crashes, and decreased mortality from liver disease, as well as from all causes.[13]

Population-Attributable Risk

Alcohol consumption is associated with over 200 disease and injury conditions as well as increased mortality.[41] The World Health Organization releases yearly information on alcohol-attributable fractions (AAFs) through its Global Health Observatory dataset.[42] AAF is a measure of the population-attributable risk related to alcohol consumption (i.e., the proportion of a particular health outcome which can be attributed solely to alcohol use). Table 10-6 lists the AAF for various causes of death in the US population, though alcohol's impacts on mortality are broader than these conditions alone.[42]

While alcohol misuse is clearly associated with increased risks of cardiovascular disease,[43] the relationship between mild-to-moderate alcohol use and cardiovascular disease is complicated by data from large population studies in Europe[44] and Asia[45] showing a possible protective effect. A large meta-analysis of individual-participant data for nearly

Table 10-6. Alcohol-Attributable Fractions in the United States

Cause of Death	Alcohol-Attributable Fraction, %	
	Males	Females
All causes	7.5	2.1
Cancer	7.0	2.6
Road traffic	42.5	25.0
Liver cirrhosis	74.1	59.2

Source: Based on World Health Organization.[42]

600,000 people who use alcohol in 83 prospective studies showed a lower risk of myocardial infarction in people who use alcohol compared with those who do not. However, the data also showed increased risks of hypertensive disease, stroke, heart failure, aortic aneurysm, and death from coronary disease, excluding myocardial infarction, in those who use alcohol.[46]

Several biases have been suggested as confounders of the cardioprotective effect of mild- to-moderate alcohol use, including type of alcohol consumed,[47] genotype affecting alcohol metabolism,[48] and lifestyle factors like exercise and diet.[49] It has been suggested that if these biases were removed, the observed protective relationship may change to reflect a detrimental relationship.[50]

Other studies focus on intoxication-related public health outcomes such as violence or traffic fatalities. A 2000 study from Zador et al. estimated the relative risk (RR) of fatal motor vehicle crash at various blood alcohol concentrations (BAC). The relative risk of fatal motor vehicle accident was 2.6 to 4.6 at a BAC of 0.035% and jumped astronomically to RR 382 to 15,560 at a BAC of 0.22%. Drivers aged 16 to 20 years had an increased relative risk of fatal crashes at baseline even without alcohol involvement; however, their RR was increased substantially with any level of alcohol consumption, even at BACs less than 0.02% (the legal driving limit for that age group).[51]

EVIDENCE-BASED INTERVENTIONS

Prevention

Prevention measures aim to reduce negative alcohol-related consequences through strategies employed at the individual and community level, including policies regulating alcohol-related behavior as well as community and educational interventions. Most programs are focused on immediate goals, such as decreasing binge drinking among youth or preventing driving after drinking. If successful, however, these programs could affect longer-term health outcomes such as alcohol use disorder, liver disease, and mortality. Research has demonstrated that rates of consumption, intoxication, and driving after drinking are sensitive to the cost of alcohol, particularly among underage individuals

Intervention	CPSTF Finding
Dram Shop Liability	Recommended (strong evidence) March 2010
Electronic Screening and Brief Intervention (e-SBI)	Recommended (strong evidence) August 2012
Enhanced Enforcement of Laws Prohibiting Sales to Minors	Recommended (sufficient evidence) February 2006
Increasing Alcohol Taxes	Recommended (strong evidence) June 2007
Maintaining Limits on Days of Sale	Recommended (strong evidence) June 2008
Maintaining Limits on Hours of Sale	Recommended (sufficient evidence) February 2009
Overservice Law Enforcement Initiatives	Insufficient Evidence March 2010
Privatization of Retail Alcohol Sales	Recommended Against April 2011
Regulation of Alcohol Outlet Density	Recommended (sufficient evidence) February 2007
Responsible Beverage Service Training	Insufficient Evidence October 2010

Source: Reprinted with permission of Community Preventive Services Task Force.[13]

Figure 10-6. Summary of Intervention Approaches for Excessive Alcohol Consumption

and young adults. Happy hours, "all-you-can-drink" specials, and other commercial promotions encourage overconsumption by reducing prices. As of January 1, 2021, some 16 states have ordinances either prohibiting or restricting happy hours, and up to 24 states have restricted other drink specials.[52] Although nearly every state prohibits sales and service of alcohol to obviously intoxicated people, little is known about enforcement and adjudication of these laws and their public health impacts.[53] In the United States the Community Services Task Force has released a list of recommendations surrounding regulation of alcohol sales and availability as potential targets for ongoing prevention efforts (Figure 10-6).[13]

Screening

Early intervention programs focus on identifying people who use alcohol in unhealthy ways or experience adverse consequences of alcohol use. The US Preventive Services Task Force recommends routine screening for unhealthy alcohol use in the primary care setting in all adults including pregnant people. The task force notably concludes that current evidence is insufficient to make a firm recommendation about screening and brief interventions in adolescents.[54]

Many screening instruments are available. Both structured interviews and self-report instruments are rapid, inexpensive, and noninvasive ways to administer screening. A specific screening instrument should be selected based on staff experience and training, time constraints, and patient population.

NIAAA recommends screening for at-risk alcohol use with a single question about the number of heavy drinking days in the past year.[8] Additional assessment can follow depending on the individual's initial response (see Figure 10-7). This single-item question is both sensitive (0.73–0.88) and specific (0.74–1.0) for detecting unhealthy alcohol use.[54]

The Alcohol Use Disorders Identification Test (AUDIT; Table 10-7)[55] is a 10-question instrument assessing quantity and frequency of alcohol use, binge drinking behavior, symptoms of AUD, and alcohol-related problems. The AUDIT has been tested internationally in primary care settings and externally validated, including in female and minority populations as well as emerging promise in adolescents and young adults.[54] The first three questions of the AUDIT—assessing frequency of alcohol use, usual amount consumed, and number of binge drinking episodes within the past year—have been validated as an initial screen and termed the AUDIT-C. The AUDIT-C is generally more sensitive than specific (sn = 0.73–1.0, sp 0.28–0.91) while the full AUDIT questionnaire has variable sensitivity but is highly specific (sn = 0.38–0.73, sp = 0.89–0.97) for unhealthy alcohol use.[54]

Clinical laboratory tests can be used in conjunction with self-report and screening instruments to enhance objectivity. BAC detects the amount of alcohol within the bloodstream at a single point in time, typically reflecting alcohol use within the last 12 to 24 hours. In recent years tests to assist in the detection of chronic alcohol use have become more common in clinical practice. Carbohydrate-deficient transferrin can be elevated for weeks to months following sustained heavy use (~4 drinks/day); however, it can be elevated in other forms of liver disease as well as in pregnancy. Other direct markers of alcohol use include ethyl glucuronide and phosphatidylethanol. Ethyl glucuronide is excreted in urine for up to three days following alcohol use. Phosphatidylethanol serves as a blood test that can detect alcohol use within the last four weeks and has some correlation to amount consumed.[56]

Other laboratory tests are indirect biomarkers of alcohol use and can detect consequences of at-risk or chronic drinking. Elevations show up in markers of liver function, including serum alanine aminotransferase, aspartate aminotransferase, and gamma-glutamyl transferase, which are sensitive for alcohol-related liver injury. These tests are not particularly specific because other etiologies of liver damage can cause these lab values to be abnormal. Results may be more discriminating when interpreted in conjunction with complete blood cell count indices, including mean corpuscular volume, which increases

At-a-Glance Sample Workflow for Alcohol Screening, Brief Intervention, and Referral to Treatment (SBIRT)

This simplified model shows the general elements in an alcohol SBIRT workflow using an alcohol use disorder (AUD) symptom checklist as an assessment tool. Your health system may use different tools for screening and assessment.

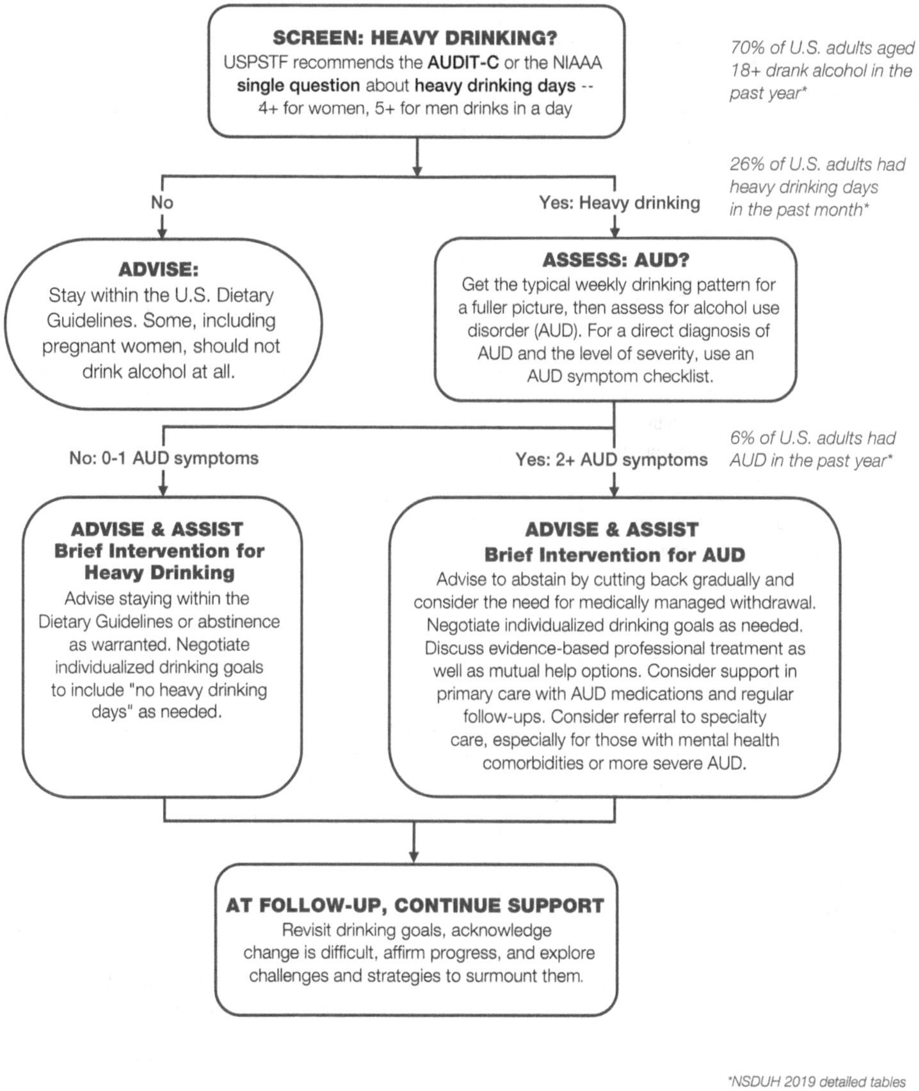

Source: Reprinted from NIAAA.[8]

Figure 10-7. Single-Question Screen for Heavy Drinking

Table 10-7. Alcohol Use Disorder Identification Test

AUDIT Question	0	1	2	3	4
1. How often do you have a drink containing alcohol?[a]	Never	<Monthly	2-4 times a month	2-3 times a week	≥4 times a week
2. How many drinks containing alcohol do you have on a typical day when you are drinking?[a]	1 or 2	3 or 4	5 or 6	7-9	≥10
3. How often do you have five or more drinks on one occasion?[a]	Never	<Monthly	Monthly	Weekly	Daily or almost daily
4. How often during the last year have you found that you were not able to stop drinking once you had started?	Never	<Monthly	Monthly	Weekly	Daily or almost daily
5. How often during the last year have you failed to do what was normally expected of you because of drinking?	Never	<Monthly	Monthly	Weekly	Daily or almost daily
6. How often during the last year have you needed a first drink in the morning to get yourself going after a heavy drinking session?	Never	<Monthly	Monthly	Weekly	Daily or almost daily
7. How often during the last year have you had a feeling of guilt or remorse after drinking?	Never	<Monthly	Monthly	Weekly	Daily or almost daily
8. How often during the last year have you been unable to remember what happened the night before because of your drinking?	Never	<Monthly	Monthly	Weekly	Daily or almost daily
9. Have you or someone else been injured because of your drinking?	No	NA	Yes, but not in the last year	NA	Yes, during the last year
10. Has a relative, friend, or doctor or other health care worker been concerned about your drinking or suggested you cut down?	No	NA	Yes, but not in the last year	NA	Yes, during the last year
TOTAL AUDIT SCORE: ___________ AUDIT scores between 8–15 are most appropriate for simple advice focused on the reduction of hazardous drinking. Scores between 16–19 suggest brief counseling and continued monitoring. Scores >20 warrant further diagnostic evaluation for alcohol use disorder.					

Source: Adapted from NIDA.[55]

Note: AUDIT = Alcohol Use Disorder Identification Test; NA = not applicable. To reflect drink serving sizes in the United States (14 g pure alcohol), the number of drinks in the third question was changed from 6 to 5.

[a]The first 3 questions of the AUDIT comprises the AUDIT-C, a 3-item alcohol screen scored on a scale of 0–12. A positive score for identifying alcohol misuse or active alcohol use disorders is 4 in males and 3 in females.

with excess alcohol intake because of the adverse nutritional and bone marrow–toxic effects of heavy alcohol use.[56]

Treatment

Brief Interventions

The term *brief intervention* is used to describe short one-on-one conversations with anyone who screens positive for harmful or at-risk drinking behavior. Brief interventions include counseling and information-sharing about alcohol use harms with an aim to moderate a person's drinking to safer levels and to reduce harmful practices, including binge drinking (see Figure 10-7).[8] Brief interventions are typically performed in the primary care or community setting, and notably not in a setting specific for alcohol use disorder treatment. Computerized or web-based interventions offer alternative means of implementing brief interventions, particularly in settings affected by time constraints or lack of resources or training in intervention techniques.[13] Brief interventions have shown benefit in reducing total alcohol use as well as reducing the number of excess drinking days.[54] Brief interventions do not preclude subsequent application of more intensive intervention or referral to additional services if indicated.

Despite evidence that brief interventions are useful and effective in the primary care setting,[54] they are not routinely or universally performed. A review of screening practices in US primary care from 2014 to 2016 showed that alcohol screening with a validated questionnaire occurred in only 2.6% of office visits, and counseling was documented in only 0.8% of visits. Screening was more likely if patients were seen by their primary care physician, had multiple medical comorbidities, or were new to the practice.[57]

Alcohol Use Disorder

Several settings are available for the treatment of alcohol use disorder. In many cases the beginning phase is detoxification, the set of interventions aimed at managing alcohol intoxication and subsequent withdrawal. Abstinence from alcohol may lead to acute alcohol withdrawal syndrome, the cluster of symptoms observed in people who stop drinking after continuous heavy consumption (Table 10-8).[58] Mild manifestations of alcohol withdrawal include tremulousness, anxiety, headache, nausea. More complicated withdrawal symptoms include hallucinations and seizures. Most concerning is delirium tremens, popularly known as the DTs, which typically begins 48 to 96 hours after the last drink and includes profound confusion, severe autonomic nervous system overactivity, and a serious risk of increased mortality. Risk factors for developing these more severe complications of alcohol withdrawal include previous withdrawal episodes, comorbid medical or surgical illness, age greater than 65 years, and previous complications of withdrawal, including seizures or delirium tremens. The preferred treatment for alcohol

Table 10-8. Alcohol Withdrawal Signs and Physical Symptoms

Severity Category	Symptom Description
Mild	Mild or moderate anxiety, sweating, and insomnia, but no tremor
Moderate	Moderate anxiety, sweating, insomnia, and mild tremor
Severe	Severe anxiety and moderate to severe tremor, but not confusion, hallucinations, or seizure
Complicated	Seizure or signs and symptoms indicative of delirium—such as an inability to fully comprehend instructions, clouding of the sensorium or confusion—or new onset of hallucinations

Source: Based on ASAM.[58]

Note: ASAM = American Society of Addiction Medicine. The timing of symptom onset may vary, and progression of symptoms and signs is not always linear from mild to moderate to severe. Risk factors for complicated withdrawal include previous history of alcohol withdrawal delirium or alcohol withdrawal seizure, numerous prior withdrawal episodes, comorbid medical or surgical illness, age >65 years, long duration of heavy and regular alcohol consumption, and physiological dependence on benzodiazepines or barbiturates

withdrawal includes benzodiazepines, a class of medications that dampen the sympathetic response while also preventing seizures. Additional medications can include gabapentinoids, antiseizure medications, phenobarbital, and alpha-adrenergic agents. Alcohol withdrawal is often managed and monitored in a dedicated detoxification facility or hospital. However, in appropriately selected patients, alcohol withdrawal may be managed in the outpatient setting with close monitoring.[58]

After detoxification most patients require ongoing engagement with medical and/or behavioral treatment for alcohol use disorder. Treatment options can include medication, psychotherapy, and peer support and may vary in terms of setting, intensity, duration, and philosophy. Alcohol treatment programs have three broad goals: (1) reducing or eliminating alcohol use, (2) improving life functioning, and (3) preventing or reducing relapse. The continuum of treatment settings from most to least intensive includes hospitalization, residential treatment (often 30- or 90-day programs), intensive outpatient treatment (3–5 hour sessions several days a week), and outpatient treatment (office-based visits per discretion of the provider). The American Society of Addiction Medicine Criteria is a nationally recognized set of guidelines aimed to match the care of patients with AUD to the most appropriate treatment setting for their level of need.[59]

There are three medications approved by the US Food and Drug Administration for management of alcohol use disorder: acamprosate, disulfiram, and naltrexone (Table 10-9). Additional evidence supports the off-label use of other medications, including topiramate and gabapentin in the appropriate clinical situations.[60]

Nonpharmacologic supports include substance use counseling, individual peer recovery coaches, and community-based support groups, among them Self-Management and Recovery Training (SMART) and 12-step programs like Alcoholics Anonymous. A Cochrane review in 2020 found high-quality evidence to support 12-step facilitation interventions over other behavioral treatments, including motivational interviewing

Table 10-9. US Food and Drug Administration-Approved Medications for Alcohol Use Disorder

Medication, Generic (brand name)	Method of Action	Contraindications, Cautions, Adverse Events
acamprosate (Campral)	Acts on the same neuroreceptors that alcohol does (gamma-aminobutyric acid).	• Greater benefit if abstinence prior to initiation • Mild gastrointestinal (GI) upset • Rarely worsening depression, insomnia, and suicide risk • Contraindicated in end-stage renal disease
disulfiram (Antabuse)	Causes aversive symptoms after ingestion of alcohol.	• Drowsiness • Nausea, vomiting • Visual symptoms • Liver damage • Best studied in highly structured treatment settings
naltrexone (Revia [oral]; Vivitrol [injectable])	Decreases the rewards or reinforcing effects of alcohol by blocking the opioid receptor.	• Cannot be using any opioid pain medications • Cannot be used in people with liver disease • Mild GI upset • Potential liver test elevations

Source: Based on Reus et al.[60] and Kelly.[61]

therapy and cognitive behavioral therapy, for increasing alcohol abstinence.[61] Peer recovery support services are usually free and available in person, via phone, or online.

MOVING FORWARD

Research on alcohol risk and use disorder vulnerabilities continues to flourish. The neural and developmental basis of alcohol use disorder is being further described with the help of advanced imaging techniques such as functional magnetic resonance imaging. Research into the influences of alcohol on neurotransmitter systems and intercellular networks are potential targets for the future of pharmacotherapy. Progress in understanding the genetics and epigenetics of alcohol use disorder may guide future diagnostics and therapeutics as well. We are also gaining a clearer understanding of alcohol's effects on cardiovascular disease risk.

Beyond basic science and translational research, there are ongoing efforts to assess effective behavioral interventions, including psychotherapy and peer support resources to enhance recovery. Current and future investigations seek to describe how psychosocial and environmental factors may further increase risk or confer protection. Research also needs to emphasize systems-level prevention and intervention strategies in diverse settings both medical (primary care clinics, emergency departments, substance use treatment centers) and public-facing (schools, community organizations, government programs). Furthermore, the role of technology and the internet, including social media and telehealth, is a rapidly developing area of study. These and other efforts will inform public health policymakers and practitioners in the present and the future.

DISCUSSION QUESTIONS

1. What trends surrounding alcohol use, including in relation to specific populations or health conditions, did you find surprising? Why do you think you were surprised?
2. How does alcohol's status as a legal substance for adult use and its acceptance in many social and cultural contexts complicate efforts to address its negative consequences?
3. How can the public health and medical fields collaborate on interventions to reduce alcohol use? List other stakeholders who should be involved in these efforts.

REFERENCES

1. US Department of Agriculture; US Department of Health and Human Services. *Dietary guidelines for Americans, 2020–2025*. 9th ed. December 2020. Available at: DietaryGuidelines.gov. Accessed January 16, 2023.
2. National Institute on Alcohol Abuse and Alcoholism. What is a standard drink? Available at: https://www.niaaa.nih.gov/alcohols-effects-health/overview-alcohol-consumption/what-standard-drink. Accessed March 31, 2023.
3. Traversy G, Chaput JP. Alcohol consumption and obesity: an update. *Curr Obes Rep*. 2015;4(1):122–130. doi:10.1007/s13679-014-0129-4
4. National Highway Traffic Safety Administration. Drunk driving. Available at: https://www.nhtsa.gov/risky-driving/drunk-driving. Accessed Mar 31, 2023.
5. National Institute on Alcohol Abuse and Alcoholism. Alcohol's effects on health. Available at: https://www.niaaa.nih.gov/alcohols-effects-health. Accessed January 16, 2023.
6. National Institute of Neurological Disorders and Stroke. Wernicke-Korsakoff syndrome information page. 2019. Available at: https://www.ninds.nih.gov/Disorders/All-Disorders/Wernicke-Korsakoff-Syndrome-Information-Page. Accessed January 16, 2023.
7. US Preventive Services Task Force. Screening and behavioral counseling interventions to reduce unhealthy alcohol use in adolescents and adults: US Preventive Services Task Force recommendation statement. *JAMA*. 2018;320(18):1899–1909. doi:10.1001/jama.2018.16789
8. National Institute on Alcohol Abuse and Alcoholism. Resources for clinicians, physicians, social workers, health care professionals, and members of community coalitions. Available at: https://www.niaaa.nih.gov/health-professionals-communities. Accessed March 19, 2023.
9. Substance Abuse and Mental Health Services Administration. 2020 National Survey on Drug Use and Health (NSDUH) annual national report. Available at: https://www.samhsa.gov/data/release/2020-national-survey-drug-use-and-health-nsduh-releases. Accessed January 16, 2023.
10. Alinsky RH, Hadland SE, Quigley J, Patrick SW, Committee on Substance Use and Prevention. Recommended terminology for substance use disorders in the care of children, adolescents, young adults, and families. *Pediatrics*. 2022;149(6):e2022057529. doi:10.1542/peds.2022-057529
11. American Psychiatric Association. *Diagnostic and Statistical Manual of Mental Disorders*. 5th ed. Arlington, VA: American Psychiatric Publishing; 2013.

12. Centers for Disease Control and Prevention. Alcohol and public health: data on excessive drinking. Updated November 28, 2022. Available at: https://www.cdc.gov/alcohol/data-stats.htm. Accessed January 16, 2023.
13. Community Preventive Services Task Force. CPSTF findings for excessive alcohol consumption. Updated April 16, 2019. Last reviewed February 28, 2022. Available at: https://www.thecommunityguide.org/content/task-force-findings-excessive-alcohol-consumption. Accessed January 16, 2023.
14. Roerecke M, Rehm J. Alcohol use disorders and mortality: a systematic review and meta-analysis. *Addiction*. 2013;108(9):1562–1578. doi:10.1111/add.12231
15. White AM, Castle IP, Powell PA, Hingson RW, Koob GF. Alcohol-related deaths during the COVID-19 pandemic [published online ahead of print, 2022 Mar 18]. *JAMA*. 2022;e224308. doi:10.1001/jama.2022.4308
16. US Department of Health and Human Services. Healthy People 2030. Available at: https://health.gov/healthypeople. Accessed January 30, 2023.
17. Sacks JJ, Gonzales KR, Bouchery EE, Tomedi LE, Brewer RD. 2010 National and state costs of excessive alcohol consumption. *Am J Prev Med*. 2015;49(5):e73–e79. doi:10.1016/j.amepre.2015.05.031
18. National Institute on Alcohol Abuse and Alcoholism. Underage drinking. 2019. Available at: https://www.niaaa.nih.gov/publications/brochures-and-fact-sheets/underage-drinking. Accessed January 16, 2023.
19. National Institute on Drug Abuse. Part 1: the connection between substance use disorders and mental illness. 2021. Available at: https://nida.nih.gov/publications/research-reports/common-comorbidities-substance-use-disorders/part-1-connection-between-substance-use-disorders-mental-illness. Accessed on January 16, 2023.
20. Centers for Disease Control and Prevention. Alcohol and public health: age 21 minimum legal drinking age. Updated December 7, 2022. Available at: https://www.cdc.gov/alcohol/fact-sheets/minimum-legal-drinking-age.htm. Accessed January 16, 2023.
21. Centers for Disease Control and Prevention. Fetal alcohol spectrum disorders (FASDs): basics. Updated November 4, 2022. Available at: https://www.cdc.gov/ncbddd/fasd/facts.html. Accessed January 16, 2023.
22. Centers for Disease Control and Prevention. Breastfeeding: alcohol. 2021. Updated October 4, 2022. Available at: https://www.cdc.gov/breastfeeding/breastfeeding-special-circumstances/vaccinations-medications-drugs/alcohol.html. Accessed January 16, 2023.
23. Kendler KS, Prescott CA, Neale MC, Pedersen NL. Temperance board registration for alcohol abuse in a national sample of Swedish male twins, born 1902 to 1949. *Arch Gen Psychiatry*. 1997;54(2):178–184. doi:10.1001/archpsyc.1997.01830140090015
24. Prescott CA, Aggen SH, Kendler KS. Sex differences in the sources of genetic liability to alcohol abuse and dependence in a population-based sample of US twins. *Alcohol Clin Exp Res*. 1999;23(7):1136–1144. doi:10.1111/j.1530-0277.1999.tb04270.x
25. Prom-Wormley EC, Ebejer J, Dick DM, Bowers MS. The genetic epidemiology of substance use disorder: a review. *Drug Alcohol Depend*. 2017;180:241–259. doi:10.1016/j.drugalcdep.2017.06.040
26. Schuckit MA. An overview of genetic influences in alcoholism. *J Subst Abuse Treat*. 2009;36(1):S5–S14.

27. Berenz EC, Coffey SF. Treatment of co-occurring posttraumatic stress disorder and substance use disorders. *Curr Psychiatry Rep*. 2012;14(5):469–477. doi:10.1007/s11920-012-0300-0
28. National Institute on Drug Abuse. Why is there comorbidity between substance use disorders and mental illnesses? NIDA. April 13, 2021. Available at: https://nida.nih.gov/publications/research-reports/common-comorbidities-substance-use-disorders/why-there-comorbidity-between-substance-use-disorders-mental-illnesses. Accessed January 16, 2023.
29. National Institute on Alcohol Abuse and Alcoholism. Surveillance Reports. NIAAA Surveillance Report 119. 2022. Available at: https://pubs.niaaa.nih.gov/publications/surveillance119/surveillance-report119.pdf. Accessed April 5, 2023.
30. Centers for Disease Control and Prevention. Early release of selected estimates based on data from the 2018 National Health Interview Survey. 2019. Available at: https://www.cdc.gov/nchs/nhis/releases/released201905.htm. Accessed on January 16, 2023.
31. Centers for Disease Control and Prevention; National Center for Health Statistics. Underlying cause of death, 1999–2020. CDC WONDER online database. 2021. Available at: http://wonder.cdc.gov/ucd-icd10.html. Accessed January 16, 2023.
32. Swan JE, Aldridge A, Joseph V, Tucker JA, Witkiewitz K. Individual and community social determinants of health and recovery from alcohol use disorder three years following treatment. *J Psychoactive Drugs*. 2021;53(5):394–403. doi:10.1080/02791072.2021.1986243
33. Fone DL, Farewell DM, White J, Lyons RA, Dunstan FD. Socioeconomic patterning of excess alcohol consumption and binge drinking: a cross-sectional study of multilevel associations with neighbourhood deprivation. *BMJ Open*. 2013;3(4):e002337. doi:10.1136/bmjopen-2012-002337
34. Hingson RW, Heeren T, Winter MR. Age at drinking onset and alcohol dependence: age at onset, duration, and severity. *Arch Pediatr Adolesc Med*. 2006;160(7):739–746. doi:10.1001/archpedi.160.7.739
35. Paschall MJ, Grube JW, Thomas S, Cannon C, Treffers R. Relationships between local enforcement, alcohol availability, drinking norms, and adolescent alcohol use in 50 California cities. *J Stud Alcohol Drugs*. 2012;73(4):657–665. doi:10.15288/jsad.2012.73.657
36. Haugland SH, Holmen TL, Ravndal E, Bratberg GH. Parental alcohol misuse and hazardous drinking among offspring in a general teenage population: gender-specific findings from the Young–HUNT 3 Study. *BMC Public Health*. 2013;13:1140. doi:10.1186/1471-2458-13-1140
37. Mares SH, Lichtwarck-Aschoff A, Engels RC. Intergenerational transmission of drinking motives and how they relate to young adults' alcohol use. *Alcohol Alcohol*. 2013;48(4):445–451. doi:10.1093/alcalc/agt025
38. Wang C, Hipp JR, Butts CT, Jose R, Lakon CM. Alcohol use among adolescent youth: the role of friendship networks and family factors in multiple school studies. *PLoS One*. 2015;10(3):e0119965. doi:10.1371/journal.pone.0119965
39. Hastings G, Anderson S, Cooke E, Gordon R. Alcohol marketing and young people's drinking: a review of the research. *J Public Health Policy*. 2005;26(3):296–311. doi:10.1057/palgrave.jphp.3200039
40. Anderson P, de Bruijn A, Angus K, Gordon R, Hastings G. Impact of alcohol advertising and media exposure on adolescent alcohol use: a systematic review of longitudinal studies. *Alcohol Alcohol*. 2009;44(3):229–243. doi:10.1093/alcalc/agn115

41. World Health Organization. Alcohol fact sheet. 2018. Updated May 9, 2022. Available at: https://www.who.int/news-room/fact-sheets/detail/alcohol. Accessed January 16, 2023.
42. World Health Organization. The global health observatory: alcohol-attributable fractions. Available at: https://www.who.int/data/gho/indicator-metadata-registry/imr-details/2332. Accessed January 16, 2023.
43. GBD 2016 Alcohol Collaborators. Alcohol use and burden for 195 countries and territories, 1990–2016: a systematic analysis for the Global Burden of Disease study 2016 [published correction appears in *Lancet.* 2018 Sep 29;392(10153):1116] [published correction appears in *Lancet.* 2019 Jun 22;393(10190):e44]. *Lancet.* 2018;392(10152):1015–1035. doi:10.1016/S0140-6736(18)31310-2
44. Ding C, O'Neill D, Bell S, Stamatakis E, Britton A. Association of alcohol consumption with morbidity and mortality in patients with cardiovascular disease: original data and meta-analysis of 48,423 men and women. *BMC Med.* 2021;19(1):167. doi:10.1186/s12916-021-02040-2
45. Saito E, Inoue M, Sawada N, et al. Impact of alcohol intake and drinking patterns on mortality from all causes and major causes of death in a Japanese population. *J Epidemiol.* 2018;28(3): 140–148. doi:10.2188/jea.JE20160200
46. Wood AM, Kaptoge S, Butterworth AS, et al. Risk thresholds for alcohol consumption: combined analysis of individual-participant data for 599 912 current drinkers in 83 prospective studies [published correction appears in *Lancet.* 2018 Jun 2;391(10136):2212]. *Lancet.* 2018; 391(10129):1513–1523. doi:10.1016/S0140-6736(18)30134-X
47. Jani BD, McQueenie R, Nicholl BI, et al. Association between patterns of alcohol consumption (beverage type, frequency and consumption with food) and risk of adverse health outcomes: a prospective cohort study. *BMC Med.* 2021;19(1):8. doi:10.1186/s12916-020-01878-2
48. Millwood IY, Walters RG, Mei XW, et al. Conventional and genetic evidence on alcohol and vascular disease aetiology: a prospective study of 500 000 men and women in China. *Lancet.* 2019;393(10183):1831–1842. doi:10.1016/S0140-6736(18)31772-0
49. Biddinger KJ, Emdin CA, Haas ME, et al. Association of habitual alcohol intake with risk of cardiovascular disease. *JAMA Netw Open.* 2022;5(3):e223849. doi:10.1001/jamanetworkopen.2022.3849
50. Schutte R, Smith L, Wannamethee G. Alcohol—the myth of cardiovascular protection. *Clin Nutr.* 2022;41(2):348–355. doi:10.1016/j.clnu.2021.12.009
51. Zador PL, Krawchuk SA, Voas RB. Alcohol-related relative risk of driver fatalities and driver involvement in fatal crashes in relation to driver age and gender: an update using 1996 data. *J Stud Alcohol.* 2000;61(3):387–395. doi:10.15288/jsa.2000.61.387
52. National Institute on Alcohol Abuse and Alcoholism. Alcohol beverages pricing: drink specials. Alcohol Policy Information System (APIS). 2021. Available at: https://alcoholpolicy.niaaa.nih.gov/apis-policy-topics/drink-specials/2. Accessed January 16, 2023.
53. Mosher J, Hauck A, Carmona C, et al. Laws prohibiting alcohol sales to intoxicated persons. National Highway Traffic Safety Administration. 2009. Available at: https://www.nhtsa.gov/sites/nhtsa.gov/files/811142.pdf. Accessed January 16, 2023.

54. US Preventive Services Task Force. Unhealthy alcohol use in adolescents and adults: screening and behavioral counseling interventions. November 13, 2018. Available at: https://www.uspreventiveservicestaskforce.org/uspstf/recommendation/unhealthy-alcohol-use-in-adolescents-and-adults-screening-and-behavioral-counseling-interventions. Accessed January 16, 2023.
55. National Institute on Drug Abuse. NIDA CTN common data elements: Instrument: AUDIT-C questionnaire. Available at: https://cde.nida.nih.gov/instrument/f229c68a-67ce-9a58-e040-bb89ad432be4. Accessed March 19, 2023.
56. Tawiah KD, Riley SB, Budelier MM. Biomarkers and clinical laboratory detection of acute and chronic ethanol use [published online ahead of print, 2022 Mar 22]. *Clin Chem.* 2022;68(5):635–645. doi:10.1093/clinchem/hvac004
57. Chatterton B, Agnoli A, Schwarz EB, Fenton JJ. Alcohol screening during US primary care visits, 2014–2016 [published online ahead of print, 2022 Jan 19]. *J Gen Intern Med.* 2022;37(15):3848–3852. doi:10.1007/s11606-021-07369-1
58. American Society of Addiction Medicine. The ASAM clinical practice guideline on alcohol withdrawal management [published correction appears in *J Addict Med.* 2020 Sep/Oct;14(5):e280]. *J Addict Med.* 2020;14(3S suppl 1):1–72. doi:10.1097/ADM.0000000000000668
59. American Society of Addiction Medicine. About the ASAM criteria. Available at: https://www.asam.org/asam-criteria/about-the-asam-criteria. Accessed January 6, 2023.
60. Reus VI, Fochtmann LJ, Bukstein O, et al. The American Psychiatric Association Practice Guideline for the Pharmacologic Treatment of Patients with Alcohol Use Disorder. APA. 2018. Available at: https://ajp.psychiatryonline.org/doi/10.1176/appi.ajp.2017.1750101. Accessed January 16, 2023.
61. Kelly JF, Humphreys K, Ferri M. Alcoholics Anonymous and other 12-step programs for alcohol use disorder. *Cochrane Database Syst Rev.* 2020;3(3):CD012880. doi:10.1002/14651858.CD012880.pub2

III. MIDSTREAM CHRONIC CONDITIONS

11

Obesity

Deborah A. Galuska, PhD, MPH, and Ellen W. Stowe, PhD, MPH

LEARNING OBJECTIVES

After completing this chapter, readers should be able to

1. Understand the association of age, sex, race/ethnicity, education, and income with obesity.
2. Describe how obesity is related to health outcomes, grouped in five major categories.
3. Understand the relationship of diet, physical activity, sleep, and prenatal exposures with obesity.
4. Describe the evidence for obesity-related interventions delivered in childcare, school, worksite, health care, and community settings.

INTRODUCTION

Obesity is a complex, common, and costly disease that contributes to poor health and quality of life. However, it has the potential to be prevented and managed. This chapter examines the epidemiology of obesity, its health and economic consequences, and the evidence on prevention and treatment strategies.

Obesity is both a disease and a risk factor for other diseases. As a disease, it is a result of excess accumulation of adipose tissue. This excess accumulation is caused by a complex interaction of genes; physiological and cognitive processes that affect food intake, energy metabolism, and energy expenditure; and the environment.[1,2]

As a risk factor for diseases, obesity is associated with many of the leading causes of morbidity and mortality in the United States, which are described in more detail in the next section. Multiple mechanisms are hypothesized to link obesity to health outcomes both because adipose tissue is physiologically active and because of its physical mass.[1–3] These mechanisms include the association of obesity with

- lipid, glucose, and steroid hormone metabolism;
- the activity of the sympathetic nervous system;
- the activity of the renin–angiotensin system;

- low levels of chronic inflammation; and
- mechanical stress on organs and joints.

Although obesity is defined as the accumulation of excess adipose tissue, in clinical and public health settings it is most often assessed by body mass index (BMI), a measure of weight that accounts for height and is estimated as weight in kilograms divided by height in meters squared (kg/m^2). Although BMI does not directly measure the amount of fat, it is easily assessed in clinical and large population settings and correlates reasonably well with more direct measures of body fat assessed through techniques such as skinfold thickness or dual X-ray absorptiometry.[4] For adults, an absolute value of BMI—a BMI greater than or equal to 30—is used to define obesity. The category of obesity can be subdivided into three classes: Class 1 is BMI 30.0 to 34.9; Class 2 is BMI 35.0 to 39.9; and Class 3 is BMI greater than or equal to 40 (this class is also called severe or extreme obesity).[4]

For children and adolescents aged 2 to 19 years, because of their growth patterns the classification of weight status is relative. BMI is compared to age- and sex-specific percentiles on the Centers for Disease Control and Prevention (CDC) growth charts, and obesity is defined as a BMI greater than or equal to the 95th percentile for age and sex.[5]

The burden of obesity and its sequelae in the United States is significant (Figure 11-1, Tables 11-1 and 11-2). Between 2017 and March 2020, 41.9% of adults (Table 11-1) and 19.7% of children and adolescents aged 2 to 19 years (Table 11-2) had obesity.[6]

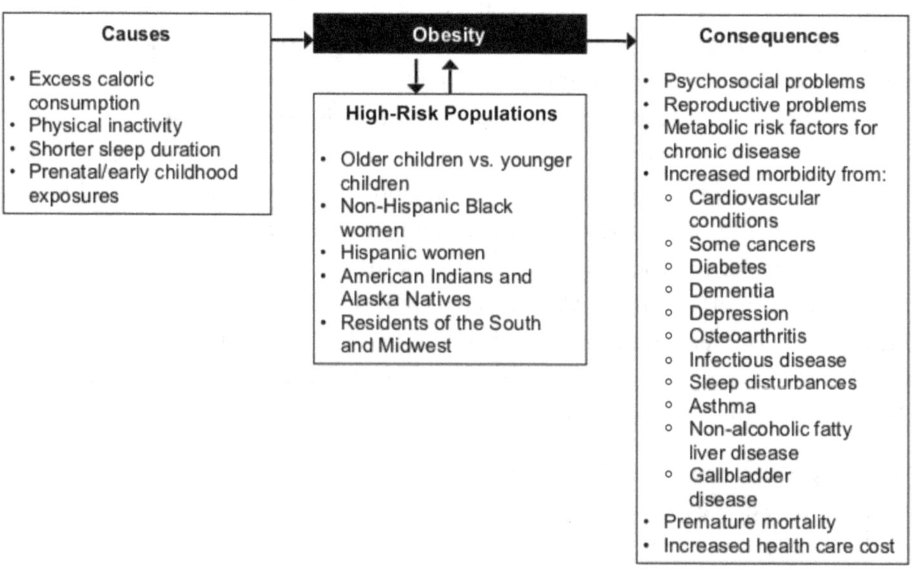

Figure 11-1. Obesity: Causes, Consequences, and High-Risk Populations

Table 11-1. Prevalence of Adults Aged 20 and Older With Obesity by Demographic Characteristics: United States, 2017–March 2020

Characteristic	Both Sexes	Men	Women
	Prevalence % (95% CI)	Prevalence % (95% CI)	Prevalence % (95% CI)
Total	41.9 (39.4-44.3)	41.8 (37.7-45.9)	41.8 (39.3-44.4)
Age, y			
20-39	39.8 (35.3-44.3)	39.9 (33.1-47.0)	39.6 (34.9-44.3)
40-59	44.3 (41.3-47.4)	45.9 (41.0-50.9)	42.8 (38.7-47.1)
≥60	41.5 (38.4-44.7)	38.4 (32.9-44.1)	44.2 (40.5-47.9)
Race and Hispanic origin			
Non-Hispanic White	41.4 (37.9-44.9)	43.1 (37.4-48.9)	39.6 (36.2-43.0)
Non-Hispanic Black	49.9 (47.2-52.6)	40.4 (36.3-44.6)	57.9 (54.0-61.7)
Non-Hispanic Asian	16.1 (13.6-18.9)	17.6 (13.7-22.2)	14.5 (11.4-18.1)
Hispanic	45.6 (42.9-48.2)	45.2 (41.7-48.8)	45.7 (42.4-49.1)
Family income relative to FPL			
≤130%	43.9 (41.7-46.1)	38.6 (33.6-43.8)	47.9 (44.0-51.7)
130%-350%	46.5 (43.6-49.4)	43.9 (40.5-47.3)	48.8 (44.5-53.0)
> 350%	39.0 (34.2-43.9)	42.4 (34.9-50.2)	35.1 (31.1-39.3)
Education			
< High school diploma	40.1 (36.5-43.8)	35.3 (30.4-40.6)	45.3 (41.0-49.7)
High school diploma or some college	46.4 (44.0-48.9)	45.9 (41.9-50.0)	46.8 (43.9-49.8)
> College degree	34.2 (30.1-38.5)	36.3 (29.0-44.1)	32.2 (28.5-36.1)

Source: Adapted from Stierman et al.[6]

Note: CI = confidence interval; FPL = federal poverty level. Obesity is defined as a body mass index of ≥30 kg/m^2.

PUBLIC HEALTH IMPACT

Obesity is associated with an increased risk of a multitude of deleterious health outcomes that can be grouped into five major categories: (1) psychosocial, (2) reproductive, (3) metabolic risk factors for chronic disease, (4) disease morbidity, and (5) mortality. The relationship of obesity to these outcomes has been extensively reviewed for both adults and children and is summarized in the next paragraphs.

Psychosocial Effects

Obesity can affect how people feel about themselves as well as how others in society feel about them. In general, obesity is associated with individual feelings of low self-esteem

Table 11-2. Prevalence of Children and Adolescents Aged 2–19 Years With Obesity by Demographic Characteristics: United States, 2017–March 2020

Characteristic	Both Sexes	Boys	Girls
	Prevalence % (95% CI)	Prevalence % (95% CI)	Prevalence % (95% CI)
Total	19.7 (17.9-21.6)	20.9 (18.9-22.9)	18.5 (16.3-21.0)
Age, y			
2-5	12.7 (10.8-14.8)	13.6 (10.8-16.8)	11.8 (9.3-14.8)
6-11	20.7 (17.9-23.7)	22.9 (19.5-26.5)	18.5 (15.2-22.1)
12-19	22.2 (19.7-24.8)	22.6 (19.7-25.7)	21.7 (18.1-25.7)
Race and Hispanic origin			
Non-Hispanic White	16.6 (13.7-19.8)	17.6 (14.8-20.7)	15.4 (11.2-20.5)
Non-Hispanic Black	24.8 (21.6-28.1)	18.8 (15.9-22.1)	30.8 (26.0-35.8)
Non-Hispanic Asian	9.0 (6.5-12.2)	13.1 (8.8-18.4)	[a]5.2 (2.3-9.9)
Hispanic	26.2 (22.4-30.2)	29.3 (23.1-36.0)	23.0 (19.6-26.6)
Family income relative to FPL			
≤130%	25.8 (22.8-29.1)	26.4 (22.4-30.8)	25.2 (22.3-28.3)
130%-150%	21.2 (18.5-24.0)	20.7 (17.6-24.1)	21.7 (18.3-25.3)
> 350%	11.5 (8.9-14.5)	15.1 (11.1-19.8)	8.2 (5.0-12.5)

Source: Adapted from Stierman et al.[6]

Note: CI = confidence interval; FPL = federal poverty level. Obesity is defined as a body mass index of greater than or equal to the age- and sex-specific 95th percentile of the 2000 CDC Growth Charts.

[a]Estimate does not meet National Center for Health Statistics standards of reliability.

for both adults and children.[7,8] In addition, individuals with obesity commonly report weight discrimination, which can occur across a variety of settings, including work and health care. Discrimination is more frequently reported by women and those who have a higher weight.[9] Obesity also may be correlated with lower levels of economic achievement, particularly for women.[10]

Reproductive Effects

Obesity can affect reproductive health from conception to delivery. Obesity is negatively associated with fertility in both men and women.[11] Women with obesity more often experience complications during pregnancy, including hypertension or preeclampsia and gestational diabetes, as well as complications during labor and delivery, including an increased risk of cesarean delivery.[12–14] Maternal obesity is also associated with increased adverse effects for the child such as preterm birth,[12,14] high birthweight,[12–14] fetal death,[12,13] and a range of congenital anomalies.[12]

Metabolic Risk Factors for Chronic Disease

The positive association between excess weight and metabolic risk factors for chronic disease, in particular cardiovascular disease (CVD) and type 2 diabetes, has been documented for both adults[15] and children.[16] These risk factors include elevated blood pressure, dyslipidemias, and insulin resistance. Obesity is also associated with low levels of chronic inflammation, which is hypothesized to affect a variety of chronic diseases, including CVD, type 2 diabetes, and cancer, by mechanisms such as its effect on insulin resistance and on cell mobility and differentiation.[17,18]

Disease Morbidity

Obesity is associated with greater morbidity from a number of chronic conditions, including some of the leading causes of death. Among adults, obesity or high-weight status increases the risk of cardiovascular conditions such as coronary heart disease,[15,19] ischemic stroke,[15,20] and type 2 diabetes.[15,19] Obesity and overweight together are associated with an increased risk of at least 13 cancers (adenocarcinoma of the esophagus, breast cancer in postmenopausal women, colon and rectum, endometrium, gallbladder, gastric cardia, kidney, liver, ovary, pancreas, thyroid, meningioma, and multiple myeloma).[21] In children, severe obesity is associated with having or developing type 2 diabetes.[22]

Obesity affects brain health. Obesity during midlife is associated with an increased risk of dementia or Alzheimer's disease.[23] However, this relationship is not evident for obesity in later life, where meta-analyses have found either no association[24] or a reduced risk of disease.[23] Obesity is also associated with an increased risk of depression in adults[25] and children.[26]

In addition, obesity affects bone and joint health. For example, obesity among adults is associated with osteoarthritis and its progression.[27] Children with obesity experience orthopedic problems such as Blount's disease (a growth disorder of the tibia that causes the bowing of legs) and slipped capital femoral epiphysis (a separation of the ball of the hip joint from the femur).[16]

Obesity is also associated with the severity of several infectious diseases. For example, among individuals with COVID-19 or influenza, obesity is associated with more severe outcomes such as hospitalization or mechanical ventilation.[28]

In addition to the conditions described, multiple other health outcomes are associated with obesity. For example, in both adults and children, obesity is associated with sleep apnea and other sleep disturbances,[16,29] asthma,[30,31] nonalcoholic liver disease,[16,32] and

Table 11-3. Relative Risks for the Association Between Obesity and Select Health Outcomes as Estimated by Meta-Analyses

Health Outcome	Adjusted Relative Risk (95% CI)[a]	Comparison
Cancer		
Breast, postmenopausal[37]	1.25 (1.07-1.46)	Obesity vs. normal weight[b]
Endometrial[37]	1.85 (1.30-2.65)	Obesity vs. normal weight[b]
Colon[37]	Women: 1.19 (1.04-1.36) Men: 1.57 (1.48-1.65)	Obesity vs. normal weight[b]
Renal[37]	Women: 1.72 (1.58-1.88) Men: 1.57 (1.38-1.77)	Obesity vs. normal weight[b]
Coronary heart disease[38]	Women: 1.61 (1.42-1.82) Men: 1.60 (1.43-1.79)	Obesity vs. normal weight[c]
Type 2 diabetes[39]	4.56 (3.69-5.64)	Obesity vs. normal weight[d]
Stroke, ischemic[20]	1.64 (1.36-1.99)	Obesity vs. normal weight[c]

Source: Based on Strazzullo et al,[20] Dobbins et al,[37] Mongraw-Chaffin et al,[38] and Yu et al.[39]

Note: CI = confidence interval; BMI = body mass index.

[a]Variables adjusted for varied by meta-analysis and studies within meta-analysis.

[b]Obesity (BMI ≥30); normal weight (BMI 18.4-24.9).

[c]Definition of obesity and normal weight varied by study within the meta-analysis.

[d]Non-Asian studies: obesity (BMI ≥ 30); normal weight (BMI 18.4-24.9); Asian studies: obesity (BMI ≥ 25); normal weight (BMI 18.5-23.0).

gallbladder disease.[16,33] Childhood obesity also appears to affect adult morbidity; it is associated with adult obesity[34] and cardiometabolic morbidity.[35,36] The association of childhood obesity with cardiometabolic morbidity may be mediated through adult obesity.[35] Table 11-3 documents the relative risks for the association of obesity with select health outcomes.[20,37,38,39]

Mortality

Among adults, obesity is associated with greater risk for all-cause mortality[40-43] and a number of cause-specific mortalities, including CVD[40,41] and some cancers.[40,42] One meta-analysis estimated that compared with persons with a BMI of 18.5 to 25.0, those with a BMI of 30 or higher had a relative risk of 1.22 for all-cause, 1.48 for CVD, and 1.07 for cancer mortality.[41] The association between obesity and mortality may weaken with age. A study using National Health and Nutrition Examination Survey data found no association among adults aged 70 years and older.[44] Obesity is also associated with reduced survival from diseases. For example, among adults with COVID-19, obesity increased the risk of mortality approximately 50% compared with those without obesity.[45] Among children, overweight or obesity is associated with increased overall mortality in adulthood.[39] Whether this association is independent of adult obesity remains unclear.

Economic Burden

In addition to its impact on health, obesity has a high economic burden. For example, one study estimated that in 2016 a high BMI among adults and children resulted in approximately $238.5 billion in US health care spending.[46] Another study found that obesity accounted for $173 billion of health care expenditures among adults and $1.32 billion among children in 2019 US dollars.[47] This same study estimated that adults with obesity had $1,861 excess costs per year compared with those without obesity and children had $116 excess costs.[47] Although the immediate costs of childhood obesity are relatively less than those for adults, childhood obesity, if maintained, can result in significant lifetime medical costs. One study estimated that a 10-year-old child with obesity has $12,660 to $19,630 excess lifetime cost when compared with a child with normal weight.[48] In addition to increased medical costs, obesity is also associated with increased costs in the workplace related to increased absenteeism and presenteeism.[49]

DESCRIPTIVE EPIDEMIOLOGY

High-Risk Populations

Data from the National Health and Nutrition Examination Survey demonstrate that obesity affects some demographic subgroups of the population more than others. Between 2017 and March 2020 adult obesity prevalence was 41.9% and the same among men and women (41.8%; Table 11-1).[6] Obesity prevalence did not differ by age overall or among women; however, men aged 40 to 59 years had a higher prevalence of obesity (45.9%) compared with men 60 years of age and older (38.4%). Racial/ethnic differences varied by sex. Among men, the prevalence of obesity was similar for Hispanic men (45.2%), non-Hispanic White men (43.1%), and non-Hispanic Black men (40.4%) and lower for non-Hispanic Asian men (17.6%). By contrast, among women, non-Hispanic Black women had the highest prevalence of obesity (57.9%), followed by Hispanic women (45.7%), non-Hispanic White women (39.6%), and non-Hispanic Asian women (14.5%). In 2018 the prevalence of obesity for American Indians and Alaska Natives was 48.1%, according to self-reported data.[50]

The prevalence of obesity differs among men and women by educational attainment.[6] Among men, those with a high school diploma or some college had the highest prevalence of obesity (45.9%), followed by men with a college degree or above (36.3%)

and men with less than a high school diploma (35.3%; Table 11-1). Among women, those with a high school diploma or some college had the highest obesity prevalence (46.8%), followed by women with less than a high school diploma (45.3%) and a college degree or above (32.2%). The prevalence of obesity also differs among men and women by income. Men with family income more than 130% through 350% of the federal poverty level (FPL) had the highest prevalence of obesity (43.9%), followed by men with family income more than 350% FPL (42.4%) and men with family income 130% or less FPL (38.6%; Table 11-1). Women with family income more than 130% through 350% FPL had the highest prevalence of obesity (48.8%), followed by women with family income 130% or less FPL (47.9%) and women with family income more than 350% FPL (35.1%).

Among children and adolescents aged 2 to 19 years between 2017 and March 2020, the prevalence of obesity was 19.7% and 20.9% for boys and 18.5% for girls (Table 11-2).[6] The prevalence in children aged 2 to 5 years (12.7%) was lower than that of those aged 6 to 11 years (20.7%) and 12 to 19 years (22.2%), a pattern consistent for boys and girls. Among boys, Hispanic boys had the highest prevalence of obesity (29.3%), followed by non-Hispanic Black boys (18.8%), non-Hispanic White boys (17.6%), and non-Hispanic Asian boys (13.1%). Among girls, non-Hispanic Black girls (30.8%) had the highest prevalence of obesity, followed by Hispanic girls (23.0%) and non-Hispanic White girls (15.4%). Non-Hispanic Asian girls (5.2%) had the lowest prevalence of obesity. In 2019 the obesity prevalence for American Indian and Alaska Native high school students was 21.3% according to self-reported data.[51]

In addition, among children and adolescents aged 2 to 19 years between 2017 and March 2020, obesity prevalence in children varied by family income.[6] Children with family income 130% or less FPL had the highest prevalence of obesity (25.8%), followed by children with family income 130% through 350% FPL (21.2%) and children with family income more than 350% FPL (11.5%). This pattern was consistent for boys and girls.

Geographic Distribution

In 2020 the state-specific prevalence of adult obesity based on self-report ranged from 24.2% in Colorado to 39.7% in Mississippi (Figure 11-2).[52] In general, the prevalence of obesity was lowest among states in the West and Northeast and highest among states in the Midwest and South. In 2019 similar geographic patterns were observed for adolescent obesity prevalence based on self-reported data.[51] Between 2013 and 2016 urbanization was associated with obesity. Adults living in large metropolitan statistical areas (MSAs) had a lower obesity prevalence compared with adults living in medium or small MSAs and non-MSAs.[53] For children and adolescents aged 2 to 19 years, obesity prevalence did not differ based on level of urbanization.[54]

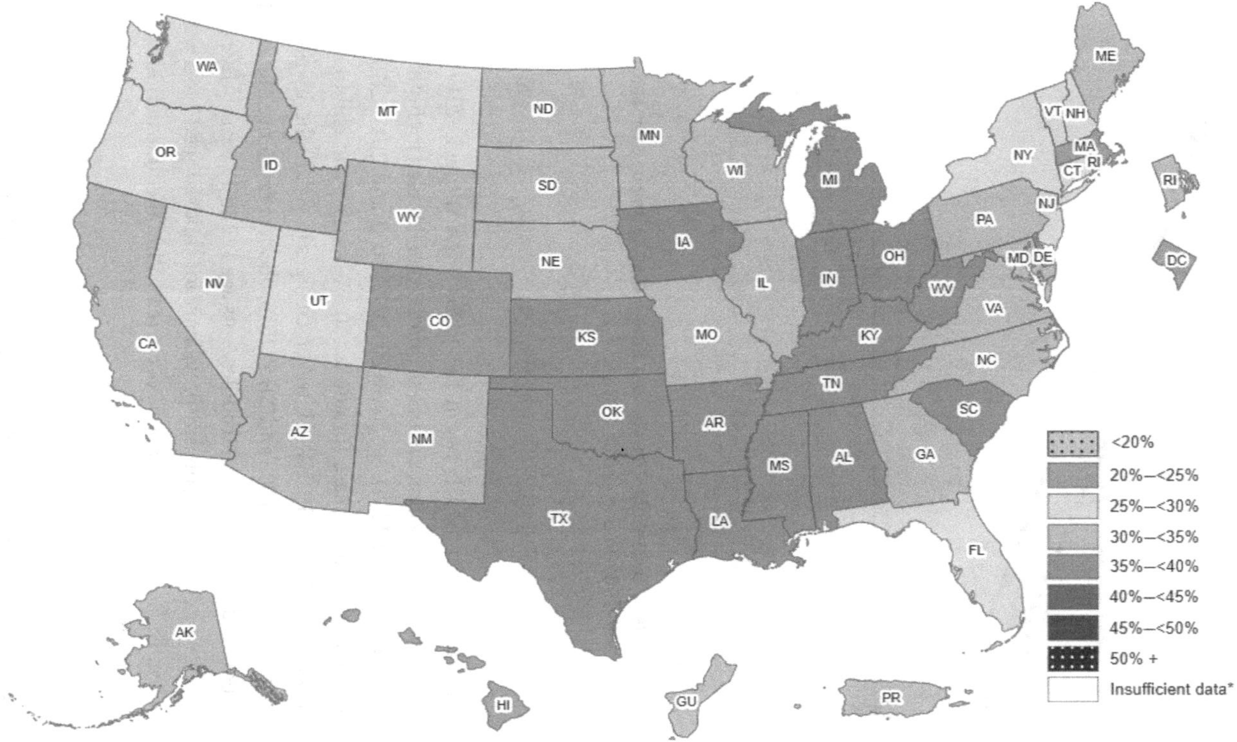

Source: Reprinted from CDC.[52]

**Prevalence* estimates reflect BRFSS methodological changes started in 2011. These estimates should not be compared to prevalence estimates before 2011. + Sample size was less than 50, the relative standard error (dividing the standard error by the prevalence) was 30% or greater, or there was no data in a specific year. Obesity is defined as body mass index of 30 kg/m^2 or higher.

Figure 11-2. Prevalence of Self-Reported Obesity Among US Adults by State and Territory, BRFSS, 2020

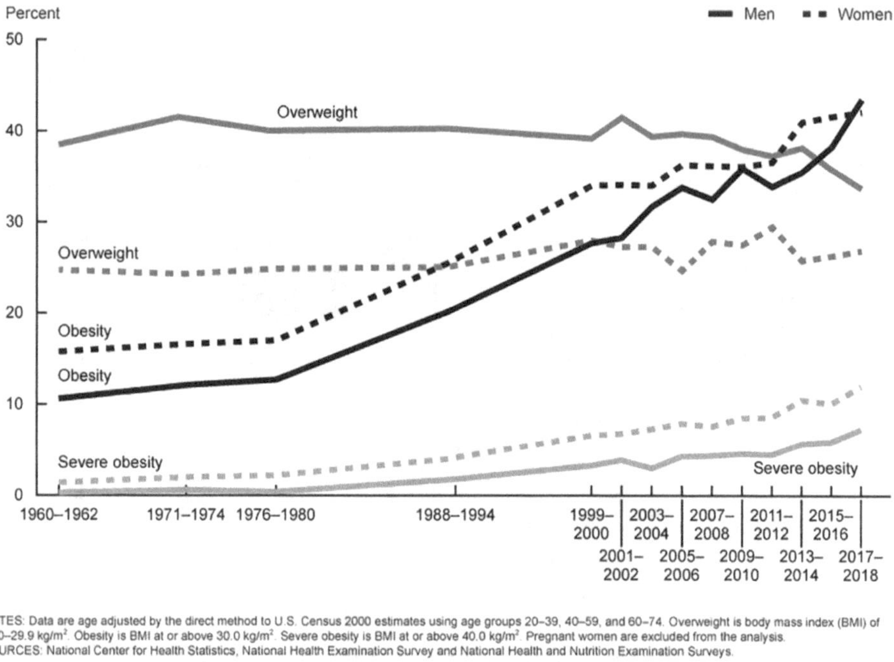

Source: Reprinted from Fryar et al.[55]

Figure 11-3. Age-Adjusted Trends in Overweight, Obesity, and Severe Obesity Among Men and Women Aged 20–74: United States, 1960–1962 Through 2017–2018

Time Trends

Trends in obesity have been examined between the early 1960s through 2017–2018. Between the 1960s and 1990s, the prevalence of obesity more than doubled for both adults (Figure 11-3) and children (Figure 11-4).[55,56] Between 1999–2000 and 2017–2018, the prevalence of obesity continued to increase for adults (30.5%–42.4%) and children and adolescents aged 2 to 19 years (13.9%–19.3%). However, changes in youth obesity prevalence have varied by age. Between 1999–2002 and 2015–2018, obesity prevalence increased significantly for children aged 6 to 11 years and adolescents aged 12 to 19 years.[57] By contrast, between 1999–2002 and 2015–2018, obesity prevalence for children aged 2 to 5 years did not change significantly. However, fluctuations occurred within the time period.

CAUSES

Conceptually, excessive weight gain is ultimately caused by an imbalance between energy intake and energy expenditure. However, a complex interplay of multiple factors at the individual level (e.g., genetics, knowledge, attitudes, health status, physiology) and the population level (e.g., environments and policies that support a healthful diet and

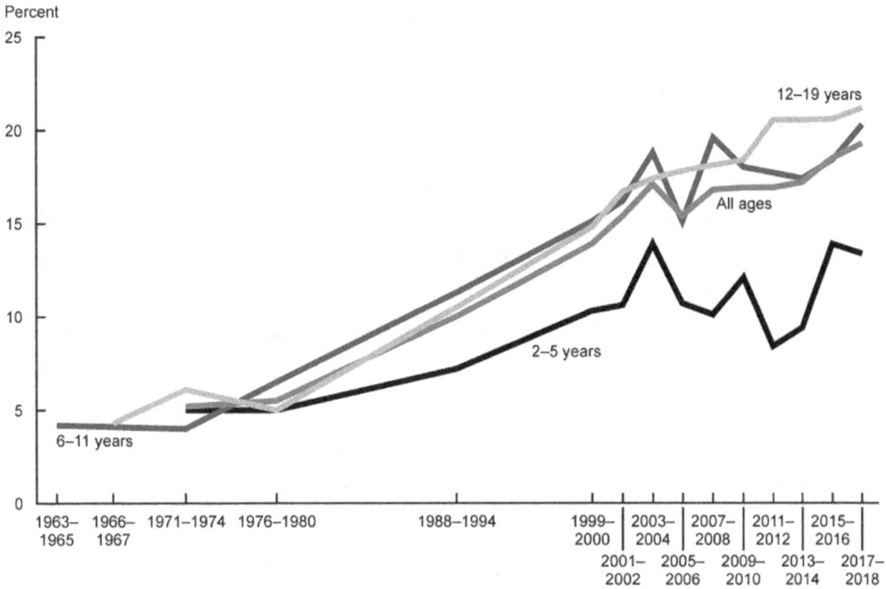

NOTE: Obesity is body mass index (BMI) at or above the 95th percentile from the sex-specific BMI-for-age 2000 CDC Growth Charts.
SOURCES: National Center for Health Statistics, National Health Examination Surveys II (ages 6–11), III (ages 12–17); and National Health and Nutrition Examination Surveys (NHANES) I–III, and NHANES 1999–2000, 2001–2002, 2003–2004, 2005–2006, 2007–2008, 2009–2010, 2011–2012, 2013–2014, 2015–2016, and 2017–2018.

Source: Reprinted from Fryar et al.[56]

Figure 11-4. Trends in Obesity Among Children and Adolescents Aged 2–19 Years by Age: United States, 1963–1965 Through 2017–2018

physical activity) can affect energy intake, metabolism, and expenditure.[58,59] This section briefly describes key modifiable risk factors at the individual level as well as how social determinants of health may affect obesity.

Modifiable Risk Factors

Diet, particularly as it relates to the overconsumption of calories, is one modifiable risk factor for obesity. Calories are obtained from four dietary sources: carbohydrates, proteins, fats, and alcohol. In general, the energy density of fats (9 kcal/g) and alcohol (7 kcal/g) are approximately twice that of carbohydrates (4 kcal/g) and proteins (4 kcal/g).[60] As such, one strategy promoted to prevent weight gain is reducing the consumption of high-calorie, low-nutrient foods or increasing the consumption of lower-calorie, nutrient-dense foods. An evidence review conducted for the 2020–2025 Dietary Guidelines for Americans concluded that there was moderate evidence that dietary patterns that are

- higher in vegetables, fruits, and whole grains,
- inclusive of seafood and legumes,
- moderate in dairy products (particularly low and non-fat dairy),

- moderate in alcohol intake,
- lower in meats (including red and processed meats),
- low in sugar-sweetened foods and beverages, and
- low in refined grains

are associated with favorable outcomes related to healthy body weight (including lower BMI, waist circumference, or percent body fat) or risk of obesity for adults.[61] A similar dietary pattern is associated with better adiposity outcomes in children. However, the evidence is more limited.[61]

Whether the consumption of specific foods or types of foods leads to weight gain is not clear, however, in part because foods are not consumed in isolation. One recent meta-analysis of cohort studies that examined individual foods and food groups reported that higher consumption of refined grains, red meat, or sugar-sweetened beverages was associated with higher levels of at least one measure of adiposity. By contrast, higher consumption of fruits, vegetables, whole grains, and potentially fish was associated with lower levels of at least one measure of adiposity.[62] However, these findings are not always consistent with findings from studies that change the consumption of these foods.[62] In addition to their relative contribution to calorie intake, these individual foods potentially affect weight gain by increasing satiety (e.g., fruits, vegetables, and whole grains) or by being very palatable and easily overconsumed (e.g., sugar-sweetened beverages and refined grains).

Another modifiable risk factor for obesity is low physical activity. Total daily energy expenditure consists of three components: basal and resting metabolic expenditure, the thermic effect of eating, and physical activity.[63] As the most modifiable component of energy expenditure, physical activity is the target of interventions to alter energy expenditure. Evidence reviewed for the 2018 Physical Activity Guidelines for Americans focused on longitudinal and experimental studies and found benefits of increased physical activity for both youth and adults. Among youth, greater amounts of physical activity are associated with better measures of weight status/adiposity or reduced risk of excessive weight gain in children 6 to 17 years of age as well as children 3 to 5 years of age.[64] Among adults, greater amounts of physical activity are associated with less weight gain, particularly when the activity is of moderate-to-vigorous intensity.[64] (For more on physical activity, see Chapter 9).

In addition to the direct effects of energy intake via diet and energy expenditure through physical activity, other modifiable risk factors for weight gain have been proposed. Sedentary time—that is, time spent in sitting or supine positions while awake that burns few calories—may be a risk factor independent of lower physical activity. The relationship between sedentary time or sedentary behaviors (e.g., television viewing) and measures of adiposity have been studied for both adults and children. Evidence for the association is mixed. Among adults, one meta-analysis found a significant association between sedentary behaviors and incident overweight and obesity but not changes in weight.[65] Among children, a systematic review of reviews found small associations between screen time and adiposity in cross-sectional studies, inconsistent evidence in longitudinal studies, and evidence of small changes in measures of adiposity with changes in sedentary behaviors in intervention studies.[66]

Another modifiable risk factor for obesity is sleep duration; less sleep is associated with an increased risk of obesity or larger increase in weight status for adults,[67] infants, children, and adolescents.[68] Potential mechanisms for this association include changes in hormones that control appetite and may increase calorie intake, increased opportunities for eating because of longer waking hours, or increased fatigue, which might reduce physical activity.[67,68]

Prenatal or early childhood exposures are also modifiable risk factors for childhood obesity. Maternal risk factors for childhood obesity or higher weight include excessive weight gain during pregnancy,[69] gestational diabetes,[70] tobacco use during pregnancy,[70,71] and pre-pregnancy weight status.[70,72] During infancy breastfeeding, particularly if done for six months or more, is associated with lower risk of obesity during childhood.[61] By contrast, early introduction (before 4mo of age) of complementary foods or maternal feeding practices (e.g., restrictive feeding) may be associated with greater risk for childhood obesity.[61,73]

An emerging area of modifiable risk factors is the role of the gut microbiome, the bacterial composition of the gut. The gut microbiome appears to be different for those with obesity and those without.[74,75] The microbiome is thought to affect obesity either by producing different metabolites when the bacteria act on dietary components or by modifying metabolites produced by the body; these metabolites may affect the energy and nutrients available, the regulation of energy in the body, and the inflammatory response.[74,75]

Another evolving area is the role certain environmental chemicals may have on obesity. These chemicals, called obeseogens, are postulated to affect adiposity through at least three mechanisms: directly altering adipocytes or their regulation, altering hormones that affect appetite or satiety, or altering energy metabolism.[76,77] Effects are hypothesized to occur both during fetal development and after birth.[76] Examples of environmental chemicals associated with obesity include bisphenol A and polychlorinated biphenyls, the latter commonly referred to as PCBs.[78]

Social Determinants of Health

Like the individual-level determinants of obesity, the conditions in the environments where people are born and spend their time can affect their health; these conditions are called social determinants of health.[79] These determinants include economic stability, health care access and quality, education access and quality, social and community context, and the built environment.[79] (For more detailed discussion of the social determinants of health, see Chapter 6). Although the social determinants do not necessarily directly cause obesity, they can affect whether people can engage in behaviors related to healthy weight, as described earlier, obtain needed care for obesity treatment and its related comorbidities, or experience weight-related discrimination. How social determinants could affect obesity can be illustrated with three examples. First, food insecurity, a marker of economic insecurity, is associated with obesity in adults, particularly among women.[80] Second, community design, a measure of the built environment, can affect physical activity levels by making it easier or more difficult to walk for transportation.[81] Third, weight discrimination in health care may affect the quality of health care patients receive as well as their care-seeking behaviors.[82]

EVIDENCE-BASED INTERVENTIONS

Prevention

Obesity prevention focuses on limiting unhealthy weight gain. For children, this is the prevention of weight gain beyond that needed for growth and development. For adults, this is the prevention of weight gain among those of normal weight as well as the prevention of further weight gain among those with overweight or obesity. Prevention can be accomplished with the specific goal of addressing weight or can be an indirect effect of interventions that change obesity-related behaviors without a goal of changing weight status. Although individuals can take actions to prevent obesity, this section focuses on two population-level strategies for addressing obesity and obesity-related behaviors: (1) community-level interventions implemented in community settings where people spend their time and (2) broad-scale policies or programs that affect large numbers of places or people.

Community-Level Interventions

One way obesity can be addressed in communities is through interventions implemented in specific community settings. Setting-specific interventions to address obesity have been recommended by expert bodies for child-care settings, schools, and worksites.[58,83,84] Systematic reviews that have examined these settings-based interventions have found limited-to-moderate evidence of improvements in weight status in the child-care setting,[85–87] moderate-to-strong evidence in the school setting or when the school setting was combined with other settings,[87,88] and limited-to-moderate evidence in worksite settings.[89–91] In general, the most effective interventions address multiple obesity-related behaviors (e.g., diet and physical activity) and are multicomponent. Multicomponent interventions provide individuals the knowledge and skills they need to make behavior changes and also alter the environment to make the behavior changes easier—for example, by limiting the amount of unhealthy foods served in the cafeteria.

Multicomponent interventions shown to improve weight status include the Nutrition and Physical Activity Self-Assessment for Child Care (NAP SACC)[92] and, for schools, the El Paso Coordinated Approach to Child Health (CATCH).[93]

Communities can also implement interventions outside of these specific settings to address obesity-related behaviors such as physical activity or diet. For example, community-level interventions that improve physical activity include those that simultaneously improve transportation systems and land use polices to create activity-friendly routes to everyday destinations, those that provide and promote places to be active (such as parks and trails), and those that provide community members opportunities for social support such as walking clubs.[81]

Large-Scale Policies and Programs

In addition to interventions implemented in a specific community or setting, states and federal governments or large private institutions can implement policies or programs to address obesity or obesity-related behaviors across multiple facilities within their jurisdiction. These policies and programs create environments or conditions that support behavioral change or obesity treatment. They can create minimal standards all facilities must meet. As part of the licensing requirements for childcare, for example, states can include the high-impact components identified by the National Resource Center for Health and Safety in Child Care and Early Education to set minimal standards related to breastfeeding support, food served, and opportunities for physical activity in childcare.[94] States can also set standards about the minimum time and frequency for physical education, an evidence-based strategy to improve physical activity.[81] Worksites can influence the types of foods sold or served across all their facilities by setting standards in their procurement processes using guidelines such as the *Food Service Guidelines for Federal Facilities.*[95]

These policies and programs can also address systematic barriers to access. For example, federal programs such as the Child and Adult Care Food Program[96] and the National School Lunch Program[97] address barriers to access to healthier foods for children in childcare and schools by requiring that healthier foods be served as a stipulation of funding.

Screening

Clinical screening for obesity is recommended for both adults and children. For adults, the US Preventive Services Task Force recommends that all patients be screened for obesity using BMI and that those with a BMI of 30 kg/m^2 or higher be offered intensive, multicomponent behavioral interventions.[98] High-intensity interventions occur over 12 to 24 months and include at least 12 contacts in the first year. Multicomponent interventions tend to address both diet and physical activity; they also address techniques for behavioral modification (e.g., goal setting) and can include support tools such as pedometers.

For children and adolescents aged 6 to 18 years, the US Preventive Services Task Force also recommends screening for obesity and offering or referring children with obesity to intensive and comprehensive interventions.[99] The recommended measure of assessment for youth is an age- and sex-adjusted BMI. Intensive interventions involve at least 26 contact hours over 2 to 12 months. Comprehensive interventions include components such as addressing multiple weight-related topics, working with both parents and children, and incorporating behavioral modification techniques.

Treatment

Weight loss attempts are common in the United States, with approximately half of adults with overweight and two-thirds of adults with obesity attempting weight loss.[100] Weight loss, when intentional, is associated with short- and long-term health effects.

Weight loss improves metabolic health. Evidence from systematic reviews suggests that among adults, weight loss in the range of 5% to 10% of baseline weight is associated with improvements in blood pressure, lipid profiles, and blood glucose.[15] Among children, it is associated with improvements in blood pressure and lipid profiles.[101] Weight loss also appears to improve function in persons suffering from osteoarthritis.[27]

Whether weight loss affects chronic disease outcomes long term is less clear.[102–104] Interventions such as bariatric surgery, which result in substantive weight loss, are associated with reductions in mortality, cardiovascular disease, morbidity,[105] and potentially some cancers.[103] The strongest evidence for health effects for more modest reductions in weight loss exists for type 2 diabetes, where lifestyle interventions result in reductions in diabetes risk for high-risk individuals.[15]

For both adults and children, a variety of approaches can be used to facilitate weight loss. These include lifestyle change, pharmacotherapy, and surgery. The effectiveness and appropriateness of each modality have been extensively reviewed and are summarized here.

Lifestyle Change

Lifestyle change aims to reduce weight by modifying weight-related behaviors, primarily diet and physical activity. The individual can address these behaviors with or without the support of formal weight loss programs. The recommended strategy for both adults and children combines diet and physical activity with supporting behavioral therapies. Although for children and adults alike some reviews suggest diet-only interventions and diet-plus-physical-activity interventions may be equally effective in the short term,[106,107] the addition of physical activity appears to benefit long-term weight loss. For example, for adults, one meta-analysis found that at 12 to 18 months, interventions that combined diet and physical activity resulted in an average of 1.7 kg more weight loss when compared with diet-only interventions and 6.3 kg when compared with physical activity-only interventions.[107] The addition of physical activity may also benefit metabolic health for both adults[108] and children.[106]

Dietary Modification

A primary goal of dietary modification for weight loss is to reduce energy intake. For adults, on the basis of evidence from randomized controlled weight-loss trials, calorie reductions in the range of 500 to 750 calories per day or total caloric intake of 1,200 to 1,500 calories per day for women and 1,500 to 1,800 calories per day for men facilitate weight losses in the range of one to two pounds per week.[15] The required calorie change in children needs to take into account the increased calorie needs of children as they age. For example, to maintain their weight, two-year-old males who are not active need approximately 1,000 calories per day, whereas those same males at age 17 would need 2,400 calories.[109]

A variety of dietary approaches (e.g., diets with different macronutrient profiles, meal replacement programs, and restriction of food intake during certain times of day) can be used. In general, when calories are held constant, none appears more effective than others for both adults and children.[15,110]

Physical Activity

Because it increases energy expenditure, physical activity has a role in weight loss. The amount or type of physical activity needed for weight loss is unclear and, in part, depends on whether and to what extent calories are also being reduced. The use of physical activity as the sole weight-loss strategy in volumes realistic for most people can result in only very modest weight loss for both adults[111] and children.[112] For example, reviews have found that physical activity levels in the range of current recommendations for adults (~150 min/week) resulted in weight loss of 2 kg or less, an amount not sufficient to result in the clinically meaningful 5% to 10% weight loss for a person with obesity.[111,113] Another review concluded that 225 to 420 minutes of physical activity per week may be needed to achieve more clinically meaningful weight loss.[114]

Behavioral Change Strategies

Weight loss appears to be enhanced when persons develop strategies to address the day-to-day challenges of changing their diet or physical activity habits, and thus inclusion of these strategies is a recommended component of weight loss therapies for both adults[98,115] and children.[99] Examples of these strategies include tracking weight, the amount of food consumed, and the frequency of physical activity; limiting one's exposure to calorie-dense foods or situations in which they are served; setting realistic and specific goals; and problem-solving.

Pharmacological and Surgical Therapies

For high-risk individuals who have not successfully lost weight through behavioral change alone, pharmacological and surgical interventions can be considered. As of 2022 five drugs are approved by the US Food and Drug Administration for the long-term treatment of obesity, including orlistat and liraglutide for persons 12 and older and phentermine-topiramate, naltrexone-bupropion, and semaglutide for adults.[116] Orlistat works by reducing fat absorption, and the others reduce appetite. A meta-analysis that included four of the drugs found that pharmacotherapy, when combined with behavioral therapy, resulted in 2.5 to 9.0 times greater odds of 5% weight loss than the placebo alone.[117] In general, for adults, drugs are recommended as an adjunct to lifestyle interventions and for potential use in those with a BMI of 27 or higher with comorbidities or a BMI of 30 or higher when behavioral therapies alone have been ineffective.[118]

The purpose of surgical interventions is to reduce caloric intake by changing the structure of the gastrointestinal tract. These changes limit the intake of food or limit the absorption of nutrients.[119] Examples of procedures include sleeve gastrectomy and proximal Roux-en-Y gastric bypass. These surgeries result in substantial weight loss for adults and adolescents and are associated with reductions in risk factors for chronic disease, including for blood pressure, lipids, and diabetes-related parameters.[15,105,120] Long term, surgery is associated with reductions in all-cause mortality, CVD mortality, and CVD morbidity.[105] Because procedures are associated with medical complications and require a major lifestyle change related to food consumption, surgical interventions are recommended as an option only for select persons—adult or adolescent—with severe obesity who have been unsuccessful in using less-invasive methods of weight loss.[115,121] For adults, these are individuals with a BMI of 40 or higher or those with a BMI of 35 or higher with other comorbidities.[115] For adolescents, these are individuals with a BMI in the 140% or higher of CDC growth charts or BMI in the 120% or higher with comorbidities.[121]

Weight Loss Maintenance

Once weight is lost, an important next step is long-term maintenance. Continued attention to diet, physical activity, and behavioral support strategies appears to be important for weight maintenance.[122] Among persons who lost weight in structured comprehensive weight loss programs, continued use of the program also appears to reduce weight regain for adults.[15,104]

MOVING FORWARD

Given the magnitude and impact of obesity, continued and enhanced efforts will be needed to make progress on changing the upward trajectory of recent trends. At least four opportunities exist and are described next.

Obtaining and Providing More Data for Decision Makers

Decision makers in multiple settings and sectors need data to address public health problems, a need particularly highlighted during the COVID-19 pandemic. However, gaps in these data exist related to solving the problem of obesity. For example, although high-quality measured data on obesity exist at the national level, much less data exist at the state and local levels. When it does exist, it may be limited to self-report or not regularly collected. In addition, at these local levels, practitioners often do not have access to data to understand whether the solutions they implement work. Opportunities exist to take advantage of large sources of data (i.e., big data) and national efforts on data modernization to address these gaps. For example, when primary data collection is not feasible, data from electronic health records have the potential to be used to document the burden of obesity and obesity-related conditions in local settings. When linked to program data, these data can also potentially be used to evaluate the effectiveness of programs. However, issues related to data quality and privacy will need to be addressed. Refinement of statistical techniques such as small-area estimates may also allow scientists to estimate prevalence at the local level. New data sources for human movement such as those available from global positioning systems have the potential to enhance physical activity surveillance. Analysis of social media interactions could inform attitudes related to obesity-related policies.

Better data on the environmental conditions that facilitate or deter obesity-related behaviors is also needed. Opportunities exist to use new technologies to determine, for example, the presence and quality of sidewalks in communities or to use citizen science to conduct rapid assessments of community conditions.

Addressing Health Disparities and Improving Health Equity

Disparities in the prevalence of obesity and obesity-related behaviors exist and deserve attention. This will require working with individuals in affected communities and groups such as Black or Hispanic women to better understand how culture, environment, and day-to-day experiences affect them and how this information can be used to design more effective interventions. It will also require a better understanding of how more distal determinants of health, such as federal and state policies, racism, and food and housing insecurity, affect the context in which people make decisions about obesity-related behaviors. Researchers and practitioners can also work to ensure that population-level interventions do not exacerbate disparities because of unequal access, uptake, or effectiveness. Having data specific enough to understand the magnitude of the problem in different subgroups of the population is also a gap. For example, while national data identify the prevalence of obesity in Asian American and Hispanic persons overall, the data may be masking heterogeneity in subgroups of these populations. Understanding ways to address obesity-related discrimination could also affect disparities.

Scaling Up Evidence-Based Interventions

Numerous research-tested interventions exist to address obesity, but all are not widely implemented. A better understanding of the facilitators and barriers to moving these interventions to real-world settings could accelerate their use. For example, learning how reimbursement, access to quality programs, and patient characteristics might prevent health care providers from following the recommendation to refer adults and children with obesity to intensive lifestyle programs could enhance their adoption. When interventions move to the field, adaptations may be necessary to address the needs of the specific population or settings such as language barriers or limited budgets, respectively. Understanding which components of research-tested multicomponent interventions are necessary for success and ensuring these components are included with fidelity will help ensure that adaptations in the field do not diminish their impact. Scaling and spreading interventions may also need to consider multiple perspectives in complex systems. For example, practitioners implementing obesity-related interventions in schools may need to get buy-in from students, teachers, and school administrators while also considering local and state policies for curriculum. Ensuring equitable access to interventions will also be important.

Finding New Ways to Affect Obesity

Opportunities exist to identify and implement new interventions to address obesity and obesity-related behaviors. This starts with identifying and designing interventions that address new or emerging risk factors for weight gain. Another opportunity is designing interventions for new subgroups or settings. For example, increased attention is being paid to how lifelong diet, physical activity, and obesity are affected by experiences in the 1,000 days following conception; a better understanding of these influences and how to change them could be an area of focus. Another area to explore is the effectiveness of new ways to deliver interventions. Examples include determining how to implement obesity-related worksite interventions in the hybrid and remote environments occurring post-pandemic or how to use opportunities such as telehealth or new digital platforms to change obesity-related behaviors. Finally, evaluating the impact of innovative strategies being tried in the field through natural experiments could uncover new ways to address obesity.

In conclusion, in the United States obesity is a common, serious, and costly problem that will continue to require the attention of individuals, settings, and sectors across the country.

DISCUSSION QUESTIONS

1. What factors might explain the disparities in obesity by education? By race/ethnicity?
2. As a public health practitioner, you would like to work with your local school to implement an obesity prevention intervention that was shown to be effective in a research setting. What things would you need to consider to ensure its success in your community?
3. As a policy maker, if you had a limited amount of money to budget toward obesity, would you focus on children or adults? Why?

DISCLAIMER

The findings and conclusions in this chapter are those of the authors and do not necessarily represent the official position of the Centers for Disease Control and Prevention.

REFERENCES

1. Schwartz MW, Seeley RJ, Zeltser LM, et al. Obesity pathogenesis: an Endocrine Society scientific statement. *Endocr Rev.* 2017;38(4):267–296. doi:10.1210/er.2017-00111
2. Heymsfield SB, Wadden TA. Mechanisms, pathophysiology, and management of obesity. *N Engl J Med.* 2017;376(3):254–266. doi:10.1056/NEJMra1514009
3. Hopkins BD, Goncalves MD, Cantley LC. Obesity and cancer mechanisms: cancer metabolism. *J Clin Oncol.* 2016;34(35):4277–4283. doi:10.1200/jco.2016.67.9712
4. Centers for Disease Control and Prevention. Overweight and obesity: defining adult overweight and obesity. Available at: https://www.cdc.gov/obesity/adult/defining.html. Accessed January 16, 2023.
5. Centers for Disease Control and Prevention. Overweight and obesity: defining childhood weight status. December 14, 2022. Available at: https://www.cdc.gov/obesity/childhood/defining.html. Accessed January 16, 2023.
6. Stierman B, Afful J, Carroll MD, et al. National Health and Nutrition Examination Survey 2017–March 2020 prepandemic data files—development of files and prevalence estimates for selected health outcomes. National Health Statistics Report no 158. Hyattsville, MD: National Center for Health Statistics; 2021.
7. Moradi M, Mozaffari H, Askari M, Azadbakht L. Association between overweight/obesity with depression, anxiety, low self-esteem, and body dissatisfaction in children and adolescents:

a systematic review and meta-analysis of observational studies. *Crit Rev Food Sci Nutr.* 2022;62(2):555–570. doi:10.1080/10408398.2020.1823813

8. Sikorski C, Luppa M, Luck T, Riedel-Heller SG. Weight stigma "gets under the skin"—evidence for an adapted psychological mediation framework: a systematic review. *Obesity (Silver Spring).* 2015;23(2):266–276. doi:10.1002/oby.20952
9. Spahlholz J, Baer N, König HH, Riedel-Heller SG, Luck-Sikorski C. Obesity and discrimination—a systematic review and meta-analysis of observational studies. *Obes Rev.* 2016;17(1):43–55. doi:10.1111/obr.12343
10. Reiband HK, Heitmann BL, Sørensen TIA. Adverse labour market impacts of childhood and adolescence overweight and obesity in Western societies—a literature review. *Obes Rev.* 2020;21(8):e13026. doi:10.1111/obr.13026
11. Amiri M, Ramezani Tehrani F. Potential adverse effects of female and male obesity on fertility: a narrative review. *Int J Endocrinol Metab.* 2020;18(3):e101776. doi:10.5812/ijem.101776
12. Marchi J, Berg M, Dencker A, Olander EK, Begley C. Risks associated with obesity in pregnancy, for the mother and baby: a systematic review of reviews. *Obes Rev.* 2015;16(8): 621–638. doi:10.1111/obr.12288
13. D'Souza R, Horyn I, Pavalagantharajah S, Zaffar N, Jacob CE. Maternal body mass index and pregnancy outcomes: a systematic review and metaanalysis. *Am J Obstet Gynecol MFM.* 2019;1(4):100041. doi:10.1016/j.ajogmf.2019.100041
14. Vats H, Saxena R, Sachdeva MP, Walia GK, Gupta V. Impact of maternal pre-pregnancy body mass index on maternal, fetal and neonatal adverse outcomes in the worldwide populations: a systematic review and meta-analysis. *Obes Res Clin Pract.* 2021;15(6):536–545. doi:10.1016/j.orcp.2021.10.005
15. National Institutes of Health (NIH). Managing overweight and obesity in adults: systematic evidence review from the Obesity Expert Panel, 2013. Available at: https://www.nhlbi.nih.gov/sites/default/files/media/docs/obesity-evidence-review.pdf. Accessed January 16, 2023.
16. Güngör NK. Overweight and obesity in children and adolescents. *J Clin Res Pediatr Endocrinol.* 2014;6(3):129–143. doi:10.4274/Jcrpe.1471
17. Amin MN, Hussain MS, Sarwar MS, et al. How the association between obesity and inflammation may lead to insulin resistance and cancer. *Diabetes Metab Syndr.* 2019;13(2): 1213–1224. doi:10.1016/j.dsx.2019.01.041
18. Ellulu MS, Patimah I, Khaza'ai H, Rahmat A, Abed Y. Obesity and inflammation: the linking mechanism and the complications. *Arch Med Sci.* 2017;13(4):851–863. doi:10.5114/aoms.2016.58928
19. Riaz H, Khan MS, Siddiqi TJ, et al. Association between obesity and cardiovascular outcomes: a systematic review and meta-analysis of Mendelian randomization studies. *JAMA Netw Open.* 2018;1(7):e183788. doi:10.1001/jamanetworkopen.2018.3788
20. Strazzullo P, D'Elia L, Cairella G, Garbagnati F, Cappuccio FP, Scalfi L. Excess body weight and incidence of stroke: meta-analysis of prospective studies with 2 million participants. *Stroke.* 2010;41(5):e418–e426. doi:10.1161/strokeaha.109.576967
21. Lauby-Secretan B, Scoccianti C, Loomis D, Grosse Y, Bianchini F, Straif K. Body fatness and cancer—viewpoint of the IARC Working Group. *N Engl J Med.* 2016;375(8):794–798. doi:10.1056/NEJMsr1606602

22. Bendor CD, Bardugo A, Pinhas-Hamiel O, Afek A, Twig G. Cardiovascular morbidity, diabetes and cancer risk among children and adolescents with severe obesity. *Cardiovasc Diabetol.* 2020;19(1):79. doi:10.1186/s12933-020-01052-1
23. Qu Y, Hu HY, Ou YN, et al. Association of body mass index with risk of cognitive impairment and dementia: a systematic review and meta-analysis of prospective studies. *Neurosci Biobehav Rev.* 2020;115:189–198. doi:10.1016/j.neubiorev.2020.05.012
24. Danat IM, Clifford A, Partridge M, et al. Impacts of overweight and obesity in older age on the risk of dementia: a systematic literature review and a meta-analysis. *J Alzheimers Dis.* 2019;70(suppl 1):S87–S99. doi:10.3233/jad-180763
25. Luppino FS, de Wit LM, Bouvy PF, et al. Overweight, obesity, and depression: a systematic review and meta-analysis of longitudinal studies. *Arch Gen Psychiatry.* 2010;67(3):220–229.
26. Sutaria S, Devakumar D, Yasuda SS, Das S, Saxena S. Is obesity associated with depression in children? Systematic review and meta-analysis. *Arch Dis Child.* 2019;104(1):64–74. doi:10.1136/archdischild-2017-314608
27. Bliddal H, Leeds AR, Christensen R. Osteoarthritis, obesity and weight loss: evidence, hypotheses and horizons—a scoping review. *Obes Rev.* 2014;15(7):578–586. doi:10.1111/obr.12173
28. Zhao X, Gang X, He G, et al. Obesity increases the severity and mortality of influenza and COVID-19: a systematic review and meta-analysis. *Front Endocrinol (Lausanne).* 2020;11(595):109. doi:10.3389/fendo.2020.595109
29. Mitra AK, Bhuiyan AR, Jones EA. Association and risk factors for obstructive sleep apnea and cardiovascular diseases: a systematic review. *Diseases.* 2021;9(4):88. doi:10.3390/diseases9040088
30. Beuther DA, Sutherland ER. Overweight, obesity, and incident asthma: a meta-analysis of prospective epidemiologic studies. *Am J Respir Crit Care Med.* 2007;175(7):661–666. doi:10.1164/rccm.200611-1717OC
31. Shan LS, Zhou QL, Shang YX. Bidirectional association between asthma and obesity during childhood and adolescence: a systematic review and meta-analysis. *Front Pediatr.* 2020;8:576858. doi:10.3389/fped.2020.576858
32. National Guideline Center (UK). Non-alcoholic fatty liver disease: assessment and management. National Institute for Health and Care Excellence. Available at: https://www.ncbi.nlm.nih.gov/books/NBK384735. Accessed January 16, 2023.
33. Aune D, Norat T, Vatten LJ. Body mass index, abdominal fatness and the risk of gallbladder disease. *Eur J Epidemiol.* 2015;30(9):1009–1019. doi:10.1007/s10654-015-0081-y
34. Simmonds M, Llewellyn A, Owen CG, Woolacott N. Predicting adult obesity from childhood obesity: a systematic review and meta-analysis. *Obes Rev.* 2016;17(2):95–107. doi:10.1111/obr.12334
35. Umer A, Kelley GA, Cottrell LE, Giacobbi P Jr., Innes KE, Lilly CL. Childhood obesity and adult cardiovascular disease risk factors: a systematic review with meta-analysis. *BMC Public Health.* 2017;17(1):683. doi:10.1186/s12889-017-4691-z
36. Reilly JJ, Kelly J. Long-term impact of overweight and obesity in childhood and adolescence on morbidity and premature mortality in adulthood: systematic review. *Int J Obes (Lond).* 2011;35(7):891–898. doi:10.1038/ijo.2010.222

37. Dobbins M, Decorby K, Choi BC. The association between obesity and cancer risk: a meta-analysis of observational studies from 1985 to 2011. *ISRN Prev Med.* 2013:680536. doi:10.5402/2013/680536
38. Mongraw-Chaffin ML, Peters SAE, Huxley RR, Woodward M. The sex-specific association between BMI and coronary heart disease: A systematic review and meta-analysis of 95 cohorts with 1.2 million participants. *Lancet Diabetes Endocrinol.* 2015;3(6):437–449. doi:10.1016/s2213-8587(15)00086-8
39. Yu HJ, Ho M, Liu X, Yang J, Chau PH, Fong DYT. Association of weight status and the risks of diabetes in adults: a systematic review and meta-analysis of prospective cohort studies. *Int J Obes (Lond).* 2022;46(6):1101–1113. doi:10.1038/s41366-022-01096-1
40. Berrington de Gonzalez A, Hartge P, Cerhan JR, et al. Body-mass index and mortality among 1.46 million white adults. *N Engl J Med.* 2010;363(23):2211–2219. doi:10.1056/NEJMoa1000367
41. McGee DL. Body mass index and mortality: a meta-analysis based on person-level data from twenty-six observational studies. *Ann Epidemiol.* 2005;15(2):87–97. doi:10.1016/j.annepidem.2004.05.012
42. Whitlock G, Lewington S, Sherliker P, et al. Body-mass index and cause-specific mortality in 900 000 adults: collaborative analyses of 57 prospective studies. *Lancet.* 2009;373(9669):1083–1096. doi:10.1016/s0140-6736(09)60318-4
43. Global BMI Mortality Collaboration; Di Angelantonio E, Bhupathiraju S, et al. Body-mass index and all-cause mortality: individual-participant-data meta-analysis of 239 prospective studies in four continents. *Lancet.* 2016;388(10046):776–786. doi:10.1016/s0140-6736(16)30175-1
44. Flegal KM, Graubard BI, Williamson DF, Gail MH. Excess deaths associated with underweight, overweight, and obesity. *JAMA.* 2005;293(15):1861–1867. doi:10.1001/jama.293.15.1861
45. Mahamat-Saleh Y, Fiolet T, Rebeaud ME, et al. Diabetes, hypertension, body mass index, smoking and COVID-19-related mortality: a systematic review and meta-analysis of observational studies. *BMJ Open.* 2021;11(10):e052777. doi:10.1136/bmjopen-2021-052777
46. Bolnick HJ, Bui AL, Bulchis A, et al. Health-care spending attributable to modifiable risk factors in the USA: an economic attribution analysis. *Lancet Public Health.* 2020;5(10):e525–e535. doi:10.1016/s2468-2667(20)30203-6
47. Ward ZJ, Bleich SN, Long MW, Gortmaker SL. Association of body mass index with health care expenditures in the United States by age and sex. *PLoS One.* 2021;16(3):e0247307. doi:10.1371/journal.pone.0247307
48. Finkelstein EA, Graham WC, Malhotra R. Lifetime direct medical costs of childhood obesity. *Pediatrics.* 2014;133(5):854–862. doi:10.1542/peds.2014-0063
49. Finkelstein EA, DiBonaventura M, Burgess SM, Hale BC. The costs of obesity in the workplace. *J Occup Environ Med.* 2010;52(10):971–976. doi:10.1097/JOM.0b013e3181f274d2
50. Villarroel MA, Blackwell DL, Jen A. Tables of summary health statistics for US adults: 2018 National Health Interview Survey. National Center for Health Statistics. November 5, 2019. Available at: http://www.cdc.gov/nchs/nhis/SHS/tables.htm. Accessed January 16, 2023.
51. Centers for Disease Control and Prevention. 1991–2019 High School Youth Risk Behavior Survey data: United States, 2019 results. US Dept of Health and Human Services. Available at: https://nccd.cdc.gov/Youthonline. Accessed Janaury 16, 2023.

52. Centers for Disease Control and Prevention. Overweight and obesity: adult obesity maps. Updated September 27, 2022. Available at: https://www.cdc.gov/obesity/data/prevalence-maps.html. Accessed January 16, 2023.
53. Hales CM, Fryar CD, Carroll MD, Freedman DS, Aoki Y, Ogden CL. Differences in obesity prevalence by demographic characteristics and urbanization level among adults in the United States, 2013–2016. *JAMA*. 2018;319(23):2419–2429. doi:10.1001/jama.2018.7270
54. Ogden CL, Fryar CD, Hales CM, Carroll MD, Aoki Y, Freedman DS. Differences in obesity prevalence by demographics and urbanization in US children and adolescents, 2013–2016. *JAMA*. 2018;319(23):2410–2418. doi:10.1001/jama.2018.5158
55. Fryar C, Carroll M, Afful J. Prevalence of overweight, obesity, and severe obesity among adults aged 20 and over: United States, 1960–1962 through 2017–2018. NCHS Health E-Stats. 2020. Available at: https://www.cdc.gov/nchs/data/hestat/obesity-adult-17-18/overweight-obesity-adults-H.pdf. Accessed January 16, 2023.
56. Fryar C, Carroll M, Afful J. Prevalence of overweight, obesity, and severe obesity among children and adolescents aged 2–19 years: United States, 1963–1965 through 2017–2018. NCHS Health E-Stats. 2020. Available at: https://www.cdc.gov/nchs/data/hestat/obesity-child-17-18/overweight-obesity-child-H.pdf. Accessed January 16, 2023.
57. Ogden CL, Fryar CD, Martin CB, et al. Trends in obesity prevalence by race and Hispanic origin—1999–2000 to 2017–2018. *JAMA*. 2020;324(12):1208–1210. doi:10.1001/jama.2020.14590
58. Institute of Medicine. *Accelerating Progress in Obesity Prevention: Solving the Weight of the Nation*. Washington DC: National Academies Press; 2012.
59. US Department of Health and Human Services. *The Surgeon General's Vision for a Healthy and Fit Nation*. Rockville, MD: Office of the Surgeon General; 2010. Available at: https://www.ncbi.nlm.nih.gov/books/NBK44660. Accessed January 16, 2023.
60. National Research Council Committee on Diet Health. *Diet and Health: Implications for Reducing Chronic Disease Risk*. Washington, DC: National Academies Press; 1989.
61. Dietary Guidelines Advisory Committee. *Scientific Report of the 2020 Dietary Guidelines Advisory Committee. Advisory Report to the Secretary of Agriculture and the Secretary of Health and Human Services*. Washington DC: US Dept of Agriculture, Agricultural Research Service; 2020.
62. Schlesinger S, Neuenschwander M, Schwedhelm C, et al. Food groups and risk of overweight, obesity, and weight gain: a systematic review and dose–response meta-analysis of prospective studies. *Adv Nutr*. 2019;10(2):205–218. doi:10.1093/advances/nmy092
63. Bouchard CE, Shephard RJ, Stephens TE. *Physical Activity, Fitness, and Health: International Proceedings and Consensus Statement*. Champaign, IL: Human Kinetics Publishers; 1994.
64. 2018 Physical Activity Guidelines Advisory Committee. *2018 Physical Activity Guidelines Advisory Committee Scientific Report*. Washington, DC: US Dept of Health and Human Services; 2018. Available at: https://health.gov/paguidelines/second-edition/report. Accessed January 16, 2023.
65. Campbell SDI, Brosnan BJ, Chu AKY, et al. Sedentary behavior and body weight and composition in adults: a systematic review and meta-analysis of prospective studies. *Sports Med*. 2018;48(3):585–595. doi:10.1007/s40279-017-0828-6
66. Biddle SJ, García Bengoechea E, Wiesner G. Sedentary behaviour and adiposity in youth: a systematic review of reviews and analysis of causality. *Int J Behav Nutr Phys Act*. 2017;14(1):43. doi:10.1186/s12966-017-0497-8

67. Guimarães KC, Silva CM, Latorraca COC, Oliveira R, Crispim CA. Is self-reported short sleep duration associated with obesity? a systematic review and meta-analysis of cohort studies. *Nutr Rev*. 2021;80(5):983–1000. doi:10.1093/nutrit/nuab064
68. Miller MA, Kruisbrink M, Wallace J, Ji C, Cappuccio FP. Sleep duration and incidence of obesity in infants, children, and adolescents: a systematic review and meta-analysis of prospective studies. *Sleep*. 2018;41(4). doi:10.1093/sleep/zsy018
69. Mamun AA, Mannan M, Doi SA. Gestational weight gain in relation to offspring obesity over the life course: a systematic review and bias-adjusted meta-analysis. *Obes Rev*. 2014;15(4): 338–347. doi:10.1111/obr.12132
70. Woo Baidal JA, Locks LM, Cheng ER, Blake-Lamb TL, Perkins ME, Taveras EM. Risk factors for childhood obesity in the first 1,000 days: a systematic review. *Am J Prev Med*. 2016;50(6):761–779. doi:10.1016/j.amepre.2015.11.012
71. Ino T. Maternal smoking during pregnancy and offspring obesity: meta-analysis. *Pediatr Int*. 2010;52(1):94–99. doi:10.1111/j.1442-200X.2009.02883.x
72. Heslehurst N, Vieira R, Akhter Z, et al. The association between maternal body mass index and child obesity: a systematic review and meta-analysis. *PLoS Med*. 2019;16(6):e1002817. doi:10.1371/journal.pmed.1002817
73. Spill MK, Callahan EH, Shapiro MJ, et al. Caregiver feeding practices and child weight outcomes: a systematic review. *Am J Clin Nutr*. 2019;109(suppl 7):s990–s1002. doi:10.1093/ajcn/nqy276
74. Sanmiguel C, Gupta A, Mayer EA. Gut microbiome and obesity: a plausible explanation for obesity. *Curr Obes Rep*. 2015;4(2):250–261. doi:10.1007/s13679-015-0152-0
75. Geng J, Ni Q, Sun W, Li L, Feng X. The links between gut microbiota and obesity and obesity related diseases. *Biomed Pharmacother*. 2022;147:112678. doi:10.1016/j.biopha.2022.112678
76. Darbre PD. Endocrine disruptors and obesity. *Curr Obes Rep*. 2017;6(1):18–27. doi:10.1007/s13679-017-0240-4
77. Heindel JJ, Blumberg B. Environmental obesogens: mechanisms and controversies. *Annu Rev Pharmacol Toxicol*. 2019;59:89–106. doi:10.1146/annurev-pharmtox-010818-021304
78. Aaseth J, Javorac D, Djordjevic AB, et al. The role of persistent organic pollutants in obesity: a review of laboratory and epidemiological studies. *Toxics*. 2022;10(2). doi:10.3390/toxics10020065
79. Healthy People 2030. Social determinants of health. US Dept of Health and Human Services. Available at: https://health.gov/healthypeople/priority-areas/social-determinants-health. Accessed January 16, 2023.
80. Moradi S, Mirzababaei A, Dadfarma A, et al. Food insecurity and adult weight abnormality risk: a systematic review and meta-analysis. *Eur J Nutr*. 2019;58(1):45–61. doi:10.1007/s00394-018-1819-6
81. Community Preventive Services Task Force. The Community Guide: physical activity. Available at: https://www.thecommunityguide.org/topic/physical-activity. Accessed January 16, 2023.
82. Phelan SM, Burgess DJ, Yeazel MW, Hellerstedt WL, Griffin JM, van Ryn M. Impact of weight bias and stigma on quality of care and outcomes for patients with obesity. *Obes Rev*. 2015;16(4):319–326. doi:10.1111/obr.12266
83. Khan LK, Sobush K, Keener D, et al. Recommended community strategies and measurements to prevent obesity in the United States. *MMWR Recomm Rep*. 2009;58(7):1–29.

84. Division of Adolescent and School Health, National Center for Chronic Disease Prevention and Health Promotion. School health guidelines to promote healthy eating and physical activity. *MMWR Recomm Rep*. 2011;60(Rr-5):1–76.
85. Sisson SB, Krampe M, Anundson K, Castle S. Obesity prevention and obesogenic behavior interventions in child care: a systematic review. *Prev Med*. 2016;87:57–69.
86. Zhou YE, Emerson JS, Levine RS, Kihlberg CJ, Hull PC. Childhood obesity prevention interventions in childcare settings: systematic review of randomized and nonrandomized controlled trials. *Am J Health Promot*. 2014;28(4):e92–e103. doi:10.4278/ajhp.121129-LIT-579
87. Wang Y, Cai L, Wu Y, et al. What childhood obesity prevention programmes work? A systematic review and meta-analysis. *Obes Rev*. 2015;16(7):547–565.
88. Langford R, Bonell CP, Jones HE, et al. The WHO Health Promoting School framework for improving the health and well-being of students and their academic achievement. *Cochrane Database Syst Rev*. 2014;(4):CD008958. doi:10.1002/14651858.CD008958.pub2
89. Anderson LM, Quinn TA, Glanz K, et al. The effectiveness of worksite nutrition and physical activity interventions for controlling employee overweight and obesity: a systematic review. *Am J Prev Med*. 2009;37(4):340–357. doi:10.1016/j.amepre.2009.07.003
90. Verweij LM, Coffeng J, van Mechelen W, Proper KI. Meta-analyses of workplace physical activity and dietary behaviour interventions on weight outcomes. *Obes Rev*. 2011;12(6): 406–429. doi:10.1111/j.1467-789X.2010.00765.x
91. Gudzune K, Hutfless S, Maruthur N, Wilson R, Segal J. Strategies to prevent weight gain in workplace and college settings: a systematic review. *Prev Med*. 2013;57(4):268–277. doi:10.1016/j.ypmed.2013.03.004
92. Alkon A, Crowley AA, Neelon SE, et al. Nutrition and physical activity randomized control trial in child care centers improves knowledge, policies, and children's body mass index. *BMC Public Health*. 2014;14:215. doi:10.1186/1471-2458-14-215
93. Coleman KJ, Tiller CL, Sanchez J, et al. Prevention of the epidemic increase in child risk of overweight in low-income schools: the El Paso coordinated approach to child health. *Arch Pediatr Adolesc Med*. 2005;159(3):217–224. doi:10.1001/archpedi.159.3.217
94. National Resource Center for Health and Safety in Child Care and Early Education. Healthy weight. Available at: https://nrckids.org/HealthyWeight. Accessed January 16, 2023.
95. Food Service Guidelines Federal Workgroup. *Food Service Guidelines for Federal Facilities*. Washington, DC: US Dept of Health and Human Services; 2017. Available at: https://www.cdc.gov/obesity/downloads/guidelines_for_federal_concessions_and_vending_operations.pdf. Accessed January 16, 2023.
96. US Department of Agriculture. Child and Adult Care Food Program: child day care centers. US Department of Agriculture, Food and Nutrition Service. Updated March 31, 2019. Available at: https://www.fns.usda.gov/cacfp/child-day-care-centers. Accessed January 16, 2023.
97. US Department of Agriculture. National School Lunch Program. US Dept of Agriculture, Food and Nutrition Service. Available at: https://www.fns.usda.gov. Accessed January 17, 2023.
98. Curry SJ, Krist AH, Owens DK, et al. Behavioral weight loss interventions to prevent obesity-related morbidity and mortality in adults: US Preventive Services Task Force recommendation statement. *JAMA*. 2018;320(11):1163–1171. doi:10.1001/jama.2018.13022

99. Grossman DC, Bibbins-Domingo K, Curry SJ, et al. Screening for obesity in children and adolescents: US Preventive Services Task Force recommendation statement. *JAMA*. 2017;317(23):2417–2426. doi:10.1001/jama.2017.6803

100. Martin CB, Herrick KA, Sarafrazi N, Ogden CL. Attempts to lose weight among adults in the United States, 2013–2016. NCHS data brief 313. Updated July 12, 2018. Available at: https://www.cdc.gov/nchs/products/databriefs/db313.htm. Accessed January 17, 2023.

101. Rajjo T, Almasri J, Al Nofal A, et al. The association of weight loss and cardiometabolic outcomes in obese children: systematic review and meta-regression. *J Clin Endocrinol Metab*. 2017;102(3):758–762. doi:10.1210/jc.2016-2575

102. Ma C, Avenell A, Bolland M, et al. Effects of weight loss interventions for adults who are obese on mortality, cardiovascular disease, and cancer: systematic review and meta-analysis. *BMJ*. 2017;359:j4849. doi:10.1136/bmj.j4849

103. Birks S, Peeters A, Backholer K, O'Brien P, Brown W. A systematic review of the impact of weight loss on cancer incidence and mortality. *Obes Rev*. 2012;13(10):868–891. doi:10.1111/j.1467-789X.2012.01010.x

104. LeBlanc EL, Patnode CD, Webber EM, Redmond N, Rushkin M, O'Connor EA. *Behavioral and Pharmacotherapy Weight Loss Interventions to Prevent Obesity-Related Morbidity and Mortality in Adults: An Updated Systematic Review for the US Preventive Services Task Force*. Evidence Synthesis 168. AHRQ publication 18-05239-EF-1. Rockville, MD: Agency for Healthcare Research and Quality; 2018.

105. Cosentino C, Marchetti C, Monami M, Mannucci E, Cresci B. Efficacy and effects of bariatric surgery in the treatment of obesity: network meta-analysis of randomized controlled trials. *Nutr Metab Cardiovasc Dis*. 2021;31(10):2815–2824. doi:10.1016/j.numecd.2021.06.018

106. Ho M, Garnett SP, Baur LA, et al. Impact of dietary and exercise interventions on weight change and metabolic outcomes in obese children and adolescents: a systematic review and meta-analysis of randomized trials. *JAMA Pediatr*. 2013;167(8):759–768. doi:10.1001/jamapediatrics.2013.1453

107. Johns DJ, Hartmann-Boyce J, Jebb SA, Aveyard P. Diet or exercise interventions vs combined behavioral weight management programs: a systematic review and meta-analysis of direct comparisons. *J Acad Nutr Diet*. 2014;114(10):1557–1568. doi:10.1016/j.jand.2014.07.005

108. Swift DL, McGee JE, Earnest CP, Carlisle E, Nygard M, Johannsen NM. The effects of exercise and physical activity on weight loss and maintenance. *Prog Cardiovasc Dis*. 2018;61(2):206–213. doi:10.1016/j.pcad.2018.07.014

109. US Department of Agriculture; US Department of Health and Human Services. *Dietary Guidelines for Americans, 2020–2025*. 9th ed. 2020. Available at: https://www.dietaryguidelines.gov. Accessed January 17, 2023.

110. Gow ML, Ho M, Burrows TL, et al. Impact of dietary macronutrient distribution on BMI and cardiometabolic outcomes in overweight and obese children and adolescents: a systematic review. *Nutr Rev*. 2014;72(7):453–470. doi:10.1111/nure.12111

111. Swift DL, Johannsen NM, Lavie CJ, Earnest CP, Church TS. The role of exercise and physical activity in weight loss and maintenance. *Prog Cardiovasc Dis*. 2014;56(4):441–447. doi:10.1016/j.pcad.2013.09.012

112. Kelley GA, Kelley KS, Pate RR. Effects of exercise on BMI z-score in overweight and obese children and adolescents: a systematic review with meta-analysis. *BMC Pediatr.* 2014;14:225. doi:10.1186/1471-2431-14-225

113. Twells LK, Harris Walsh K, Blackmore A, et al. Nonsurgical weight loss interventions: a systematic review of systematic reviews and meta-analyses. *Obes Rev.* 2021;22(11):e13320. doi:10.1111/obr.13320

114. Donnelly JE, Blair SN, Jakicic JM, Manore MM, Rankin JW, Smith BK. American College of Sports Medicine position stand: appropriate physical activity intervention strategies for weight loss and prevention of weight regain for adults. *Med Sci Sports Exerc.* 2009;41(2): 459–471. doi:10.1249/MSS.0b013e3181949333

115. Jensen MD, Ryan DH, Apovian CM, et al. 2013 AHA/ACC/TOS guideline for the management of overweight and obesity in adults: a report of the American College of Cardiology/ American Heart Association Task Force on Practice Guidelines and the Obesity Society. *Circulation.* 2 014;129(25 suppl 2):S102–S138. doi:10.1161/01.cir.0000437739.71477.ee

116. National Institutes of Health (NIH). Prescription medications to treat overweight and obesity. National Institute of Diabetes and Digestive and Kidney Diseases. Available at: https://www.niddk.nih.gov/health-information/weight-management/prescription-medications-treat-overweight-obesity. Accessed January 17, 2023.

117. Khera R, Murad MH, Chandar AK, et al. Association of pharmacological treatments for obesity with weight loss and adverse events: a systematic review and meta-analysis. *JAMA.* 2016;315(22):2424–2434. doi:10.1001/jama.2016.7602

118. Garvey WT, Mechanick JI, Brett EM, et al. American Association of Clinical Endocrinologists and American College of Endocrinology comprehensive clinical practice guidelines for medical care of patients with obesity. *Endocr Pract.* 2016;22(3):1–203. doi:10.4158/ep161365.Gl

119. Public Education Committee of the American Society for Metabolic and Bariatric Surgery. Bariatric surgery procedures. Updated May 2021. Available at: https://asmbs.org/patients/bariatric-surgery-procedures. Accessed January 17, 2023.

120. Shoar S, Mahmoudzadeh H, Naderan M, et al. Long-term outcome of bariatric surgery in morbidly obese adolescents: A systematic review and meta-analysis of 950 patients with a minimum of 3 years follow-up. *Obes Surg.* 2017;27(12):3110–3117. doi:10.1007/s11695-017-2738-y

121. Pratt JSA, Browne A, Browne NT, et al. ASMBS pediatric metabolic and bariatric surgery guidelines, 2018. *Surg Obes Relat Dis.* 2018;14(7):882–901. doi:10.1016/j.soard.2018.03.019

122. Ramage S, Farmer A, Eccles KA, McCargar L. Healthy strategies for successful weight loss and weight maintenance: a systematic review. *Appl Physiol Nutr Metab.* 2014;39(1):1–20. doi:10.1139/apnm-2013-0026

12

Diabetes

Michael Fang, PhD, MHS, Rozalina G. McCoy, MD, MS,
Patrick J. O'Connor MD, MA, MPH, and Elizabeth Selvin, PhD, MPH

LEARNING OBJECTIVES

After completing this chapter, readers should be able to

1. Identify public health and clinical factors that have contributed to the epidemic of type 2 diabetes.
2. Comprehend integrated public health and clinical strategies for primary prevention of type 2 diabetes.
3. Understand how changes in the definition of diabetes and in diabetes screening guidelines may have affected estimates of diabetes incidence and prevalence.
4. Grasp the magnitude of disparities in type 2 diabetes incidence, prevalence, management, and complications related to race, ethnicity, and socioeconomic status and appreciate the need to design diabetes prevention and care interventions for maximal effectiveness in high-risk groups.

INTRODUCTION

Diabetes mellitus (subsequently referred to as diabetes) is a group of chronic conditions characterized by high blood glucose, or hyperglycemia. Type 2 diabetes makes up 90% to 95% of all cases of diabetes and is most common among older adults, persons with obesity, and racial or ethnic minority populations (Figure 12-1).[1] Genetic, social, and environmental factors are the major determinants of type 2 diabetes. Over time, hyperglycemia leads to complications across multiple body systems, impaired quality of life, high direct and indirect costs, and premature mortality. The prevalence of type 2 diabetes in the United States has grown significantly over the past three decades, making prevention and effective management critical public health priorities.

Characterizing the burden of diabetes and its complications is challenging. In the United States, population-based studies such as the National Health and Nutrition Examination Survey (NHANES) and the National Health Interview Survey (NHIS) are important data sources. Yet, definitions of diabetes used in national prevalence studies do not always align with how diabetes is diagnosed in clinical practice. Cohort studies,

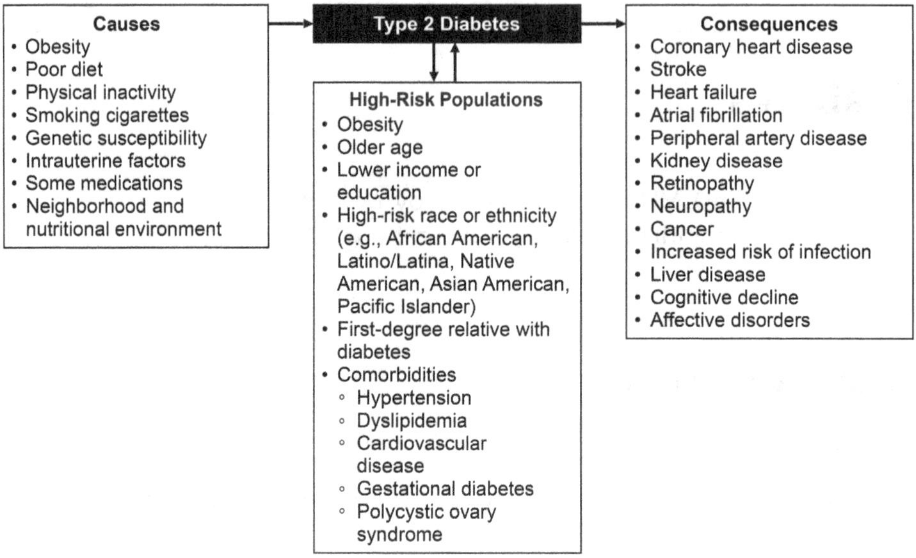

Figure 12-1. Type 2 Diabetes: Causes, Consequences, and High-Risk Populations

while useful to monitor the risk of diabetes complications, are often unable to assess the full array of clinical outcomes associated with diabetes because of the lack of long-term and complete surveillance, nor can they capture the nonclinical risk factors for diabetes and its complications, especially on a national scale. Moreover, awareness and screening of diabetes, along with the criteria of the diagnosis of diabetes, have changed substantially over time. This context has implications for estimating the burden of diabetes, establishing the drivers of its increased incidence and prevalence, and understanding disparities in diabetes management and outcomes, and it is critical for correctly interpreting epidemiologic data and effectively using this information to inform public health efforts.

DIABETES DIAGNOSIS AND EPIDEMIOLOGY

Standardized definitions of diabetes were first introduced in 1979. The National Diabetes Data Group recommended diagnosing diabetes using fasting glucose of higher than 140 mg/dL or two-hour glucose of higher than 200 mg/dL on a 75-gram oral glucose tolerance test.[2] These cut points were based on data showing that the prevalence of diabetic retinopathy, an eye disease that is highly specific to diabetes, appeared to increase significantly above these critical glucose values. However, the diagnostic overlap between the two-hour glucose and fasting glucose criteria was imperfect, with the two tests identifying different populations of people with hyperglycemia. In 1997 an expert panel lowered the fasting glucose diagnostic cut point to 126 mg/dL, bringing the two-hour glucose and fasting glucose criteria into better alignment.[3] In 2009 glycated hemoglobin (HbA1c) of 6.5% or greater was added to the diagnostic criteria for diabetes, representing a new, more specific, and less burdensome way to measure criterion for diabetes diagnosis.[4] These three criteria are currently the recommended approaches for screening and diagnosing diabetes (Table 12-1).

These shifting definitions reflect the somewhat arbitrary nature of diabetes cut points. The risk of major complications increases continuously with increasing glucose

Table 12-1. Advantages, Disadvantages, and Diagnostic Cut Points for Diabetes Diagnostic Tests

Diagnostic Test	Brief Description of Test	Current Recommended Cut Point[a]	Major Advantages	Major Disadvantages
2 hr oral glucose tolerance test	Patients are asked to fast ≥8 hr prior to testing. On the day of the test, providers first collect a blood sample to measure baseline fasting glucose levels. After the first sample is taken, patients consume a beverage containing a specific amount of glucose (usually 75 g). Patients then wait a specific amount of time (usually 2 hr) before having their glucose levels retested.	≥200 mg/dL	Most sensitive test; identifies the most cases of diabetes.	• Requires fasting. • Involves a large time commitment. • Patients sometimes experience nausea from the glucose drink. • Has low reproducibility.
Fasting glucose	Patients are asked to fast ≥8 hr prior to testing. On the day of the test, providers collect a blood sample to measure fasting glucose levels.	≥126 mg/dL	Inexpensive and widely available.	• Requires fasting. • Test not standardized across instruments or labs.
HbA1c	Providers collect a blood sample from patients, regardless of fasting status.	≥6.5%	• Convenient, no fasting required. • Most specific, generally identifies patients at highest risk for complications. • High reproducibility. • Test standardized across labs. • Reflects "average."	• Is the least sensitive test: can miss patients with milder forms of diabetes. • May be inaccurate for patient health conditions that influence red blood cells (e.g., anemia).

[a] Unless a patient has clear clinical symptoms of diabetes (e.g., hyperglycemic crisis), the American Diabetes Association requires 2 elevated test results, either from the same sample or in 2 separate test samples, for diagnosis.

concentrations, and no single value perfectly distinguishes where diabetes truly "begins." Instead, diagnostic cut points represent a balance between identifying persons at high risk for diabetes complications and minimizing false detection. Cut points are necessary in clinical practice to define who should receive treatment and closer monitoring.

All three glycemic tests for diabetes have variability. To reduce the likelihood of false positive diagnoses, clinical guidelines recommend confirming any elevated reading with a second test,[5] which can be done at the same time (different diagnostic tests) or on different days (same or different diagnostic tests). In large epidemiologic studies, short-term repeat testing is often not feasible, making it difficult to estimate the burden of diabetes in a manner entirely consistent with clinical practice.[6,7]

All three diagnostic tests also have strengths and limitations (Table 12-1). For example, the two-hour glucose test identifies the most cases of diabetes but has the lowest reproducibility and requires patients to consume an unpleasant, highly concentrated glucose drink. The different tests also measure different aspects of diabetes: impaired fasting glucose represents hepatic insulin resistance with increased liver glucose production; impaired glucose tolerance as measured by the oral glucose tolerance test assesses for skeletal muscle insulin resistance; and elevated HbA1c is an indirect measure of average blood glucose levels over the course of approximately two to three months irrespective of the mechanism for glucose elevation. Because individuals may differ in their specific phenotype of diabetes, results of these three tests are sometimes discordant. Importantly, results of all three tests have been linked to increased risk of complications, making them all "correct." Researchers and practitioners should keep these issues in mind when screening and diagnosing diabetes and when designing and interpreting epidemiologic studies.

Incidence

From 1980 to the late 1990s the rate of new cases (incidence) of diagnosed diabetes remained stable at around 4 per 1,000 person-years (Figure 12-2).[8] In the late 1990s cases began rising sharply, reaching 8 per 1,000 person-years in 2008. Part of these trends were likely related to rising levels of diabetes risk factors, obesity in particular. The lower fasting glucose criteria (140–126 mg/dL) introduced in 1997, coupled with rising awareness and screening, likely also contributed to earlier diagnosis of diabetes in the population.

In the late 2000s the incidence of diabetes began declining, reaching ~6 per 1,000 persons in 2016. It is possible that preventive efforts contributed to this decline; however, during this same period there was no evidence of increases in physical activity and prevalence of obesity continued to grow, raising questions about this explanation. The introduction of the HbA1c criteria in 2009 may have influenced trends, though the net impact of this change is uncertain. The HbA1c test generally identifies fewer people with diabetes because the 6.5% cut point is highly specific but is less sensitive than the

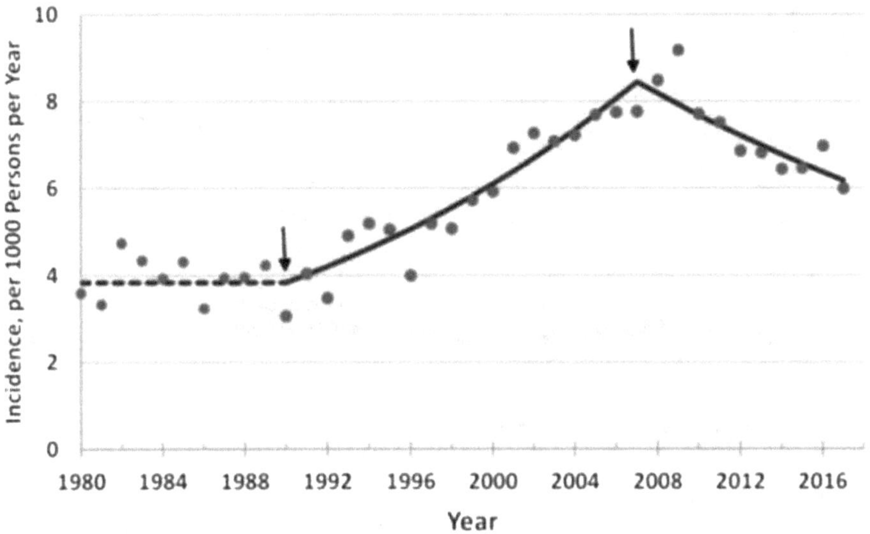

Source: Benoit et al.[8] Reprinted with permission of BMJ Publishing Group Ltd.

Note: Data are from the Centers for Disease Control and Prevention's National Health Interview Survey. Dots are observed annual values; the lines are modeled using Joinpoint Trend Analysis Software. The dotted lines indicate no significant trend; solid lines indicate a significant annual percentage change. Arrows indicate joinpoints (changes in trend). The 2000 US Census was used for age adjustment using age groups 18–44, 45–64, and 65–79 years.

Figure 12-2. Trends in the Age-Adjusted Incidence of Diabetes Among US Adults Aged 18–79 Years, 1980–2017

other criteria. It is nonetheless a convenient test that does not require fasting, potentially allowing more patients to be screened. The lowering of the fasting glucose cut point, along with increased diabetes awareness and screening, may have resulted in better detection of diabetes in the general US adult population. After a decade of more intensive testing, incidence may have declined because fewer high-risk patients remained undiagnosed.[9] The underlying reasons for the declining incidence of diabetes in the United States therefore remain unclear.

Prevalence

From 1999 to 2016 the Centers for Disease Control and Prevention (CDC) reported that the age-adjusted prevalence of total diabetes (undiagnosed and diagnosed diabetes) rose from 9.5% to 12.0% (Figure 12-3).[1] This growth has been driven by increased prevalence of diagnosed diabetes, while the prevalence of undiagnosed diabetes has remained relatively stable. Although the *proportion* of diabetes that remains undiagnosed has declined significantly, the CDC estimates that as many as 22% of US diabetes cases remain undiagnosed.

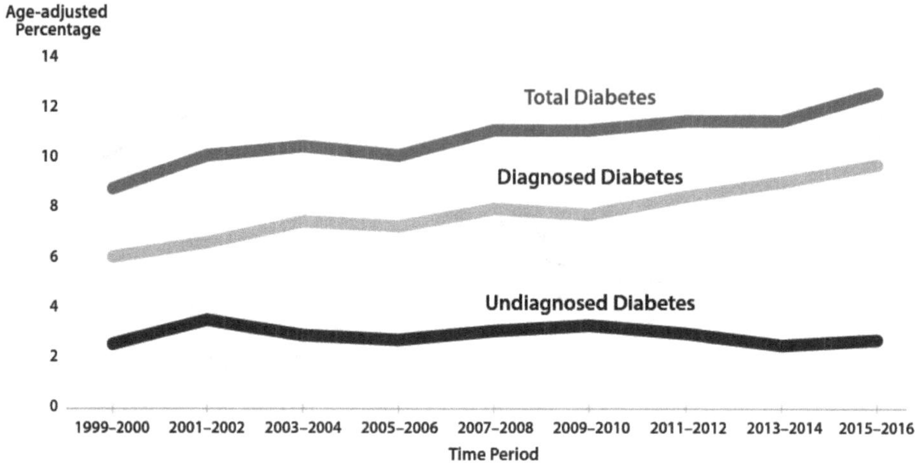

Source: Reprinted from CDC.[1]
Note: Data are from the National Health and Nutrition Examination Surveys. Diagnosed diabetes was based on self-report. Undiagnosed diabetes was based on fasting plasma glucose and A1C levels among people self-reporting no diabetes.

Figure 12-3. Trends in Age-Adjusted Prevalence of Diagnosed Diabetes, Undiagnosed Diabetes, and Total Diabetes Among Adults Aged 18 Years and Older: United States, 1999–2016

To accurately estimate the prevalence of undiagnosed diabetes using epidemiological data, it is critical to use definitions of diabetes that are consistent with approaches to screening and diagnosis of diabetes in clinical practice (i.e., with confirmatory testing). Many previous studies have used broad definitions of undiagnosed diabetes (i.e., without confirmatory testing) inconsistent with diagnostic practices, leading to overestimates of the prevalence of undiagnosed diabetes. A recent study suggests that the fraction of the total diabetes population that remains undiagnosed may be as low as 9.5% as a result of increased screening and diagnosis of diabetes in the general US adult population.[7] Nonetheless, major disparities in diabetes screening and diagnosis remain, with a high burden of undiagnosed diabetes in younger adults, racial and ethnic minority populations, and persons who lack health insurance or are underinsured.[7]

DIABETES RISK FACTORS AND PATHOPHYSIOLOGY

Normal Physiology

Blood glucose levels are driven by hepatic glucose production, dietary intake of carbohydrates and other macronutrients, and glucose utilization in the peripheral tissues. Insulin is the primary driver of this balance, with additional inputs by glucagon, neural signaling, and other metabolic signals. In the fasting state and when blood glucose levels are low, low levels of insulin and high levels of glucagon promote hepatic glucose production through gluconeogenesis and glycogenolysis, raising available glucose levels. After eating, blood glucose levels rise sharply and stimulate pancreatic insulin secretion while dampening glucagon levels. Insulin then facilitates glucose utilization by skeletal muscle and other tissues. Thus, in the absence of insulin or in the presence of insulin resistance, glucose cannot be metabolized properly, resulting in measurable hyperglycemia (i.e., glucose is left in the bloodstream, where it is not supposed to be) and absent glucose in the cells. High glucose levels in the blood and low glucose levels in the tissues all contribute to the development of diabetes complications.

Insulin is produced by beta cells of the pancreatic Islets of Langerhans as a precursor molecule, preproinsulin, which is metabolized to proinsulin and then into co-secreted insulin and c-peptide molecules. The c-peptide level is therefore an effective indicator of endogenous insulin secretion and may be used clinically to differentiate type 1 from type 2 diabetes (i.e., c-peptide levels are low or undetectable in type 1 diabetes). However, it is often difficult or not feasible to differentiate type 1 and type 2 diabetes in epidemiologic studies, where such laboratory data are not available. Glucose is the primary regulator of insulin secretion (i.e., higher glucose levels stimulate greater insulin secretion, typically starting when glucose is >70 mg/dL), but amino acids, ketones, different nutrients, gastrointestinal peptides, and neurotransmitters can stimulate insulin secretion as well. Glucagon is produced by alpha cells of the pancreatic islets in inverse relation to insulin.

Type 1 Diabetes

Type 1 diabetes is characterized by absolute insulin deficiency resulting from the destruction of insulin-producing pancreatic beta cells caused by a constellation of autoimmune, genetic, and environmental causes. Most often, this is mediated by autoimmune beta cell dysfunction by one or more autoantibodies against islet cells. Polymorphisms of multiple genes influence the risk of type 1 diabetes; known genetic loci contribute to 48% of familial aggregation, and genes in the major histocompatibility complex contribute another 41% to familial aggregation.[10] As a result, the lifelong risk of type 1 diabetes is approximately 6% in children, 5% in siblings, and 50% in identical twins, compared with 0.4% in individuals with no family history of diabetes.[11] People with type 1 diabetes are also at increased risk for other autoimmune disorders such as autoimmune thyroid disease (i.e., Hashimoto thyroiditis, Graves disease), celiac disease, autoimmune adrenalitis (Addison disease), vitiligo, autoimmune hepatitis, myasthenia gravis, and pernicious anemia.

Several environmental factors have been proposed to influence the risk of developing type 1 diabetes in susceptible individuals, but they remain poorly understood. Pregnancy-related and perinatal factors include older maternal age, preeclampsia, neonatal respiratory disease, jaundice, and high birth weight. Exposure to enteroviruses, both in utero and in childhood, can induce beta cell damage. SARS-Co-V2 is similarly linked to increased risk of type 1 diabetes. Data on dietary risk factors are weak; there is inconsistent evidence regarding exposure to cow's milk and increased risk of type 1 diabetes,[12] while exposure to vitamin D and omega-3 fatty acids may be protective.[13,14] There is no evidence of any association between childhood immunization and type 1 diabetes.[15]

Important to note is the increasing recognition that while previously referred to as juvenile-onset diabetes, type 1 diabetes can develop at any age and there is heterogeneity in the rate of beta cell destruction leading to complete insulin deficiency. Children with type 1 diabetes often present with the classic symptoms of hyperglycemia (frequent urination, thirst, weight loss) and nearly half present with diabetic ketoacidosis, a life-threatening acute complication of diabetes.[16] Adults with type 1 diabetes are less likely to present with these classic symptoms and may even experience temporary remission from the need for insulin.[17,18] The most important feature of type 1 diabetes, and what distinguishes it from type 2 diabetes, is therefore the absolute lack of endogenous insulin production and consequent requirement of insulin treatment for survival. Features most useful in discrimination of type 1 from type 2 diabetes are younger age at diagnosis (<35 y), lower body mass index (BMI <25 kg/m^2), presentation with weight loss, glucose higher than 360 mg/dL, or diabetic ketoacidosis.[19] However, some individuals cannot be clearly classified as having type 1 or type 2 diabetes at the time of diagnosis, may be misdiagnosed (usually as type 2 diabetes), or may have clinical features of both conditions.

Type 2 Diabetes

The pathogenesis of type 2 diabetes is complex, multifactorial, and incompletely understood (Figure 12-1). It is characterized by a combination of (1) progressive insulin resistance, considered to be the primary driver of type 2 diabetes and typically attributed to environmental factors (e.g., excess adiposity, sedentary lifestyle, and poor nutrition); (2) defective insulin secretion (beta cell dysfunction that is largely the result of genetic factors and the aging process); and (3) excessive hepatic glucose production. More than 500 distinct genetic signals have been associated with type 2 diabetes, though each gene individually confers a small increase in risk.[20]

Unlike in type 1 diabetes, environmental factors are known to be major contributors to type 2 diabetes, explaining 50% to 60% of patients' health outcomes vis-à-vis their impacts on obesity, insulin resistance, and systemic inflammation.[21] Socioeconomic status, a multidimensional construct that includes educational (educational quality and quantity, health literacy and numeracy), economic (income, wealth), and occupational (employment status, job stability, job type, working conditions, shift work) status, is a strong predictor of diabetes onset, progression, and severity both at the individual and the neighborhood level. Neighborhood and physical environment factors that influence diabetes risk include housing (stability, safety, quality), built environment (walkability, greenspace), and environmental exposures (environmental toxins, air pollution, ambient noise). Both individual and community food environments, defined by the availability, accessibility, and affordability of nutritious food, are associated with diabetes incidence, prevalence, control, and complications risk. There is emerging evidence that social cohesion, social capital, and social support further influence diabetes risk through their impacts on stress and health behaviors. Social context influences racism and discrimination and contributes to persistent disparities in diabetes incidence and care.[22,23] This includes historical and pervasive discrimination within the medical field (chattel slavery, eugenics movement, experimentation on Black and other vulnerable individuals without consent, closure of medical schools training Black physicians in the early 20th century), causing mistrust of the health care system. Health care provider bias toward patients of minority backgrounds contributes to decreased access to and quality of care. Policies such as redlining and predatory lending have resulted in racial residential segregation and housing insecurity, while continued disinvestments in education, employment, public spaces, and infrastructure in Black and other minority neighborhoods have resulted in environments that lack safe spaces for physical activity, healthy food, affordable housing, high-quality education, stable employment, and high-quality health care. As such, structural and institutional racism have amplified diabetes risk factors (obesity, poor nutrition, inadequate physical activity, high stress) and reduced access to care for diabetes and other conditions (lack of health care, mistrust in the health care system, uninsurance and underinsurance, poor health literacy).[23]

Type 2 diabetes generally develops gradually, progressing from normal glucose levels to prediabetes to diabetes. Prediabetes progresses to overt diabetes at rates depending on the definition of prediabetes and also demographic and clinical factors. Meta-analyses suggest that about 5% to 10% of people with prediabetes develop type 2 diabetes each year; however, risk is not equal across all people with prediabetes and range from about 4% to 19% per year.[24] Type 2 diabetes is a progressive disease, and response to treatment varies over time. People with type 2 diabetes may have insulin levels that are normal or elevated, though as the disease progresses some people may develop insulin deficiency. Lifetime risk of type 2 diabetes from age 20 ranges from 40% to 50% in various demographic groups.[25]

Gestational Diabetes

Gestational diabetes refers to hyperglycemia that develops during pregnancy and reflects underlying beta cell dysfunction that confers increased risk for developing diabetes (usually type 2 diabetes, but potentially also type 1 diabetes) later in life.[26] Gestational diabetes occurs in 14% of pregnancies,[27] and between 20% and 60% of women who had gestational diabetes will progress to diabetes within 5 to 10 years.[24] Risk factors for gestational diabetes include older maternal age, family history of type 2 diabetes, gestational diabetes in a previous pregnancy, and excess adiposity.[28] High-risk individuals (Figure 12-1) should be screened for type 2 diabetes prior to or at onset of pregnancy. All women should also be screened for gestational diabetes between 24 and 28 weeks of gestational age. Those with gestational diabetes should have glucose levels rechecked six weeks after delivery to ensure restoration of normal glucose levels, be monitored closely for recurrent gestational diabetes during subsequent pregnancies, and be screened for type 2 diabetes annually thereafter.

High-Risk Populations and Diabetes Health Disparities

Racial and ethnic disparities in type 2 diabetes and gestational diabetes stem from multiple factors. Black, Hispanic, and Indigenous populations have higher rates of obesity than White individuals.[1] Black and Latino/Latina individuals also have greater hyperinsulinemia and insulin resistance independent of adiposity. While there are limited data on genetic susceptibility to type 2 diabetes in non-European ancestry populations, available studies do not suggest that genetic risk factors for type 2 diabetes differ substantially across racial/ethnic groups. Factors such as acculturation, health behaviors, racism, neighborhood factors, occupation, socioeconomic disparities, exposure to environmental toxins as the result of residential segregation and sequelae of redlining, and stress contribute to historical inequities and diabetes risk.[29] Substantial data also indicate that rural residents experience higher rates of diabetes, obesity, and diabetes complications than do urban populations.[30]

PUBLIC HEALTH IMPACT

Mortality

Diabetes is one of the leading causes of death in the United States. In 2020 diabetes was listed as the seventh leading cause of death, with over 100,000 deaths directly attributed to the condition.[31] These estimates are based on data from the National Vital Statistics System, which collects and processes death certificate information from registries in each US state. However, death certificate data may be subject to substantial misclassification. With the exception of its acute complications (e.g., diabetic ketoacidosis, hyperglycemic hyperosmolar state, and hypoglycemia), diabetes does not directly cause death. Instead, diabetes contributes to other diseases (e.g., cardiovascular disease, cancer, kidney disease, heightened risk of infection) that may be an immediate cause of death and listed as such on the death certificate. Clinicians may also not be aware of an individual's diabetes status when completing the death certificate. Vital statistics are an important resource to tell us about the burden of disease, but their reliability depends on accurate coding.

An alternative approach to estimating the national mortality burden of diabetes involves linking data from cohorts of individuals with (and without) diabetes to mortality data. For example, the NHIS and NHANES systems have been linked to the National Vital Statistics System. An important advantage of this approach for understanding the

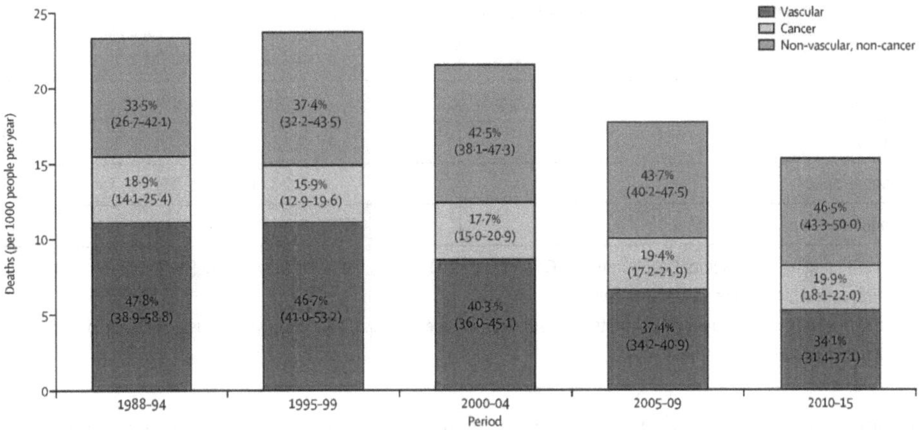

Source: Gregg et al.[32] Reprinted with permission of Elsevier Science & Technology Journals.
Note: Numbers in bars represent the percentage of total deaths (95% confidence intervals).

Figure 12-4. Deaths From Vascular, Cancer, and Nonvascular, Non-Cancer Causes Among US Adults Diagnosed With Diabetes

mortality burden of diabetes is that diabetes status is known for nearly all participants. Nationally representative cohort studies show higher mortality rate in persons with diabetes versus without diabetes, with declining mortality in both groups over time (Figure 12-4).[32] These gains appear to be driven largely by cardiovascular mortality, which declined significantly over time in the general population as well as in people with diabetes. As a result, the underlying causes of death for people with diabetes may be changing, with noncardiovascular causes becoming relatively more common.

Other mortality data come from prospective cohort studies that do not rely solely on death certificates. Instead, causes of death are adjudicated by experts using additional sources of information, such as medical records. Because of the intensity of this process, these studies tend to be smaller than national studies such as NHANES and NHIS and cannot be said to be nationally representative. Nonetheless, they offer robust evidence of the relationship between diabetes and different causes of mortality. A meta-analysis of cohort studies suggests that the risk of mortality was 70% higher for those with (vs. without) diabetes after adjusting for confounders such as age and smoking status (Table 12-2).[33] Diabetes was associated with an increased risk for different causes of death and was especially pronounced for cardiovascular mortality (hazard ratio 2.13).

Complications

Diabetes complications can be classified as acute complications stemming from severely abnormal glucose levels at a single point in time (i.e., severe hypoglycemia and severe hyperglycemia, which includes both diabetic ketoacidosis and hyperglycemic

Table 12-2. Association Between Diabetes (Versus No Diabetes) and Mortality

	Hazard Ratio (95% CI)
All-cause mortality	1.70 (1.62 to 1.79)
Vascular death	2.13 (1.96 to 2.32)
Cancer death	1.24 (1.17 to 1.31)
Noncancer, nonvascular death	1.64 (1.54 to 1.75)

Source: Emerging Risk Factors Collaboration.[33] Copyright © 2011 Massachusetts Medical Society. Reprinted with permission of Massachusetts Medical Society.

Note: CI = confidence interval. All estimates are adjusted for age, sex, smoking, body mass index, systolic blood pressure, and total cholesterol.

hyperosmolar state) and chronic complications related to prolonged exposure to hyperglycemia, recurrent hypoglycemia, and high glycemic variability. Chronic complications can be further categorized as macrovascular, microvascular, and nonvascular complications and can affect nearly every organ system (Figure 12-1).

For most nonpregnant adults with diabetes, glucose levels should be maintained between 70 and 180 mg/dL to prevent hypoglycemia (glucose levels < 70 mg/dL) and hyperglycemia (glucose levels > 180 mg/dL). Hypoglycemia is most often caused by excessive doses of insulin or insulin secretagogue (e.g., sulfonylurea) medications relative to what is required in the context of the individual's dietary carbohydrate intake (which raises glucose levels) and physical activity (which lowers glucose levels). Patients who are not treated with insulin or sulfonylurea are at low risk for hypoglycemia. Risk factors for severe hypoglycemia include type 1 (rather than type 2) diabetes, older age, having multiple or advanced comorbidities (including chronic kidney disease, heart disease, liver disease, and dementia), and prior history of hypoglycemia.[34] Black individuals, patients with low income, and people who live in disadvantaged neighborhoods also face heightened hypoglycemia risk.[34,35] Severe hypoglycemic events most often occur in patients who have poorly controlled diabetes (elevated HbA1c) and high glycemic variability.[34,36]

Risk factors for severe hyperglycemic events include type 1 diabetes, need for insulin therapy, younger age, multiple comorbidities (including mental health conditions), and poor medication adherence.[34,35] As in severe hypoglycemia, Black patients, individuals with low income, and those who live in socioeconomically deprived areas are at increased risk for severe hyperglycemia.[34,35] Severe hyperglycemia generally occurs in the setting of insufficient doses of glucose-lowering medications (particularly insulin) and/or increased physiologic stress (acute illness, infection, or ischemic events). Patients with type 1 diabetes generally experience diabetic ketoacidosis, while patients with type 2 diabetes can experience either diabetic ketoacidosis or hyperglycemic hyperosmolar state, potentially with overlapping presentations. Both events are medical emergencies that require immediate medical attention and can be fatal, with hyperglycemic hyperosmolar state having a nearly tenfold higher risk of death than diabetic ketoacidosis.[37]

Typical macrovascular (large vessel) complications of diabetes include accelerated atherosclerotic cardiovascular disease (ASCVD) resulting in coronary heart disease, cerebrovascular disease, and peripheral vascular disease. ASCVD is the leading cause of morbidity and mortality among people with diabetes. Drivers of excess macrovascular complications in diabetes include hypertension, dyslipidemia (high low-density lipoprotein cholesterol, low high-density lipoprotein cholesterol), tobacco use, and increased thrombotic risk. Heart failure, with either diastolic or systolic dysfunction, is also an important and common complication of diabetes, with emerging evidence suggesting a bidirectional relationship between heart failure and diabetes, as people with heart failure are more likely to develop type 2 diabetes, and people with both type 1 and type 2 diabetes are more likely to develop heart failure.[38] Heart failure in diabetes can develop in the absence of traditional heart failure risk factors (e.g., hypertension, coronary artery disease, valve disease), underscoring the independent impact of diabetes on this disease.[38] Microvascular (small-vessel) complications include diabetic eye disease (diabetic retinopathy, macular edema), neuropathy (sensory and motor peripheral neuropathies, autonomic neuropathy), and nephropathy (diabetic kidney disease). Diabetes is the leading causes of blindness, nontraumatic lower extremity amputation, and end-stage kidney disease in the United States.

Nonvascular complications of diabetes include gastrointestinal dysfunction (gastroparesis, diarrhea, constipation), genitourinary dysfunction (uropathy, sexual dysfunction in both men and women), dermatologic complications, heightened infection risk, nonvascular eye complications (cataracts, glaucoma), cancer, cognitive decline, and dementia.[39] Glycemic control (HbA1c levels < 7%–8%) lowers the risks of nearly all chronic diabetes complications, though reducing the risks of macrovascular events also requires control of other ASCVD risk factors, including blood pressure, lipids, smoking, and obesity.

Diabetes in pregnancy (including gestational diabetes and preexisting type 1 or type 2 diabetes) confers risk to the mother, fetus, and neonate related to the degree of hyperglycemia and coexistence of chronic complications and comorbidities of diabetes. Hyperglycemia-associated maternal complications include spontaneous pregnancy loss, preeclampsia, and preterm delivery. Fetal and neonatal complications include congenital anomalies, fetal demise, macrosomia, neonatal hypoglycemia, hyperbilirubinemia, and neonatal respiratory distress syndrome, among others. In addition, diabetes in pregnancy may increase the risk of obesity, hypertension, and type 2 diabetes in the offspring later in life.

PREVENTION, SCREENING, AND TREATMENT

Prevention

Although there is no durable cure for type 1 diabetes, several clinical trials have explored preventing or reversing type 1 diabetes. Recent and current investigations can be divided into (1) primary prevention: before the development of autoimmunity or hyperglycemia; (2) secondary prevention: after autoantibodies are present, but before the onset of beta cell dysfunction and hyperglycemia; and (3) tertiary prevention: after disease onset, but early enough in the process that there are still beta cells to be preserved. Interventions have ranged from dietary modifications, primarily targeting primary prevention in infants and children at genetic risk for type 1 diabetes, to immunotherapies targeting secondary and tertiary prevention. Despite a growing number of large studies, to date there are no trials that have successfully delayed or prevented type 1 diabetes.[40]

Successful prevention or delay in onset of type 2 diabetes has been clearly demonstrated in large clinical trials including the US Diabetes Prevention Program (DPP).[41–44] These studies, with follow-up times ranging between three and seven years, demonstrated that both lifestyle and pharmacological interventions prevent or delay the onset of type 2 diabetes in high-risk patients with prediabetes. In these trials the development of diabetes was reduced 25% to 60% at follow-up, with the largest reductions typically seen with intensive lifestyle interventions that resulted in substantial weight loss and increased physical activity.[45]

The DPP Research Group randomized 3,234 adults with prediabetes (impaired fasting glucose) and a BMI greater than 24 kg/m^2 to placebo, metformin (850 mg twice daily), or a lifestyle modification program. Goals of the DPP lifestyle intervention are a minimum of 7% weight loss or weight maintenance and a minimum of 150 minutes per week of physical activity.[46] The DPP included (1) individual case managers or "lifestyle coaches"; (2) frequent contact; (3) a structured, 16-session core curriculum, including behavioral self-management strategies; (4) supervised physical activity; (5) a maintenance intervention; (6) a "toolbox" of adherence strategies; (7) tailoring of materials and strategies to address ethnic diversity; and (8) an extensive network of training, feedback, and clinical support to reach these goals.[47,48] At an average follow-up of 2.8 years, diabetes incidence in the placebo, metformin, and lifestyle groups was 11.0, 7.8, and 4.8 per 100 person-years, respectively. This represents a 58% and 31% risk reduction in the lifestyle and metformin groups compared with the placebo. The lifestyle intervention reduced risk in all age, sex, and racial/ethnic groups, but it was especially effective in those aged 60 to 85 years, whereas metformin was more effective in younger adults.

In the DPP Outcomes Study (2002–2014) of the DPP (1996–2001), participants in the lifestyle and metformin groups were encouraged to continue their interventions, and all participants were offered a group-lifestyle intervention.[45] At 15-year follow-up, aggregate microvascular outcomes between the treatment groups and the placebo were not significantly different.[49] However, compared with no intervention, diabetes incidence was 27% lower for the lifestyle group and 18% lower for the metformin group. The DPP has been recognized as effective by the CDC and is reimbursed for those with prediabetes by many health insurance plans, including Medicare.

Several pharmacological agents, including metformin, α-glucosidase inhibitors, orlistat, thiazolidinedione, and the GLP-1 receptor agonists liraglutide and semaglutide have shown various levels of success in preventing or delaying onset of type 2 diabetes. Of these, metformin has the strongest evidence base for effectiveness and long-term safety for diabetes prevention.[50,51] Other drugs used in pharmacological interventions are more costly, have potentially dangerous side effects, or may be no more effective than lifestyle interventions. Moreover, weight loss, healthy diet, and physical activity have proven benefits for prevention and/or management of many diseases other than diabetes.

The DPP has been adapted for adolescents.[52] Preventing type 2 diabetes in children and adolescents is important because they experience diabetes complications and comorbidities at an accelerated rate. Studies of lifestyle change conducted with children in school settings have attempted to reduce or prevent the onset of obesity in high-risk youth through physical activity or dietary interventions. In school-based and clinic-based interventions, longer duration of intervention and inclusion of a strong parental component were associated with successful lifestyle change and weight loss.[53]

Screening

Although clinical trials have not found direct benefits of diabetes or prediabetes screening,[54] screening asymptomatic adults is important for timely detection and treatment of prediabetes and diabetes.[55] Availability of effective approaches to delay progression from prediabetes to diabetes also supports screening as an important first step for type 2 diabetes prevention.

Current diabetes screening guidelines vary widely. The US Preventive Services Task Force recommends screening asymptomatic adults aged 35 to 70 years with BMI of 25 kg/m^2 or higher, while the American Diabetes Association recommends screening adults aged 35 or older or with a BMI of 25 kg/m^2 or higher and one or more risk factors (Table 12-3).[5,54] The more sensitive approach, used by the American Diabetes Association, captures more cases of prediabetes and diabetes but requires testing a larger number of people, resulting in higher costs. The more specific US Preventive Services Task Force approach reduces costs and the number screened but identifies a lower proportion of those with prediabetes and diabetes.[56] Discordance between these two major guidelines is a source of confusion to clinicians and the public. Thus, bringing recommendations into closer alignment is an important public health priority. The "optimal" screening strategy depends on public health priorities and resources available.

Treatment

The goal of diabetes treatment is to implement lifestyle changes and, as appropriate, pharmacologic treatments to control hyperglycemia, prevent or delay diabetes-related

Table 12-3. Eligibility for Prediabetes and Diabetes Screening According to the US Preventive Services Task Force 2021 and American Diabetes Association 2022 Guidelines

Guidelines	Criteria
US Preventive Services Task Force 2021	Aged 35–70 y with BMI ≥25 kg/m^2
American Diabetes Association 2022	1. Aged ≥35 y; or 2. BMI ≥25 kg/m^2 and 1 additional risk factor, including • High-risk racial/ethnic background (non-White) • Physically inactive • Family history of diabetes in first-degree relative • Hypertension (>140/90 mm Hg or use of blood pressure–lowering medication) • Dyslipidemia (HDL cholesterol <35 mg/dL or triglycerides >250 mg/dL) • History of cardiovascular disease • History of gestational diabetes • Women with polycystic ovary syndrome • Other clinical conditions associated with insulin resistance (e.g., severe obesity, acanthosis nigricans)

Source: Based on ADA PCPC[5] and Davidson et al.[54]
Note: BMI = body mass index; HDL = high-density lipoprotein.

macrovascular and microvascular complications, and minimize the risks and burden of treatment. Regardless of the need for insulin or other pharmacotherapy, medical nutrition therapy is foundational to the management of diabetes. Pharmacologic treatment options for type 1 and type 2 diabetes are heterogeneous and should be tailored to the clinical goals and needs of each patient. In addition to adequate glucose control, there is abundant evidence from well-designed randomized clinical trials that adequate blood pressure, cholesterol, and tobacco control are critically important to prevent or delay major macrovascular and microvascular complications for all patients with diabetes.

Updated clinical guidelines on lifestyle and pharmacologic management of patients with diabetes (type 1, type 2, and gestational diabetes) are published annually by the American Diabetes Association and periodically by other organizations such as the US Preventive Services Task Force. In considering guideline recommendations, one should consider potential conflicts of interest of the sponsoring organization, board of director members, and guideline authors, as advised by the National Academy of Medicine.[57]

People with type 1 diabetes and some people with long-standing type 2 diabetes and relative insulin deficiency need insulin. Basal (i.e., intermediate-acting or long-acting) insulin provides a steady supply of insulin over the course of the day to moderate glucose release by the liver and facilitate glucose use at the cellular level. Bolus or prandial (i.e., short-acting or rapid-acting) insulin is administered before meals to cover the glucose content of that meal. Patients treated with insulin pumps receive continuous subcutaneous delivery of rapid-acting insulin plus intermittent boluses of rapid-acting insulin for meals. There are many available formulations of basal and bolus insulins, each with a different pharmacologic profile, and doses must be carefully and closely adjusted to each individual patient's needs, routines, and circumstances. Interruption in insulin availability or incorrect dosing of insulin can be fatal.

Metformin has been and continues to be recommended as first-line treatment for nonpregnant adults with type 2 diabetes because of its efficacy, safety, tolerability, and low cost. However, guidelines increasingly recommend preferential use of GLP-1 receptor agonists or SGLT2 inhibitors by patients with diabetes who also have cardiovascular disease, kidney disease, or heart failure because these medication classes have low risk of hypoglycemia, may induce weight loss, and improve cardiovascular, kidney, and heart failure outcomes independent of their ability to lower HbA1c. Thus, GLP-1 receptor agonists and SGLT2 inhibitors reduce the risks of diabetes complications through multiple pathways, making them highly attractive treatment options. The choice of medications for an individual patient with type 2 diabetes is guided by the patient's clinical goals and comorbidity profiles but is often constrained by affordability considerations. For example, some GLP-1 receptor agonists and, to a lesser extent, SGLT2 inhibitors remain very costly, with list prices approaching $400 to $1,500 for a month's supply. The high cost of these medications—and most insulins—is increasingly recognized as a common barrier to optimal diabetes management that leads to cost-related nonadherence and suboptimal clinical outcomes.[58]

Weight management is a core issue in diabetes care. In adults with type 2 diabetes and a BMI of 35 kg/m^2 or higher, metabolic/bariatric surgery has substantial clinical benefits, including 30% average weight loss at 2 years, diabetes remission in about 60% of those with type 2 diabetes at 2 years, substantially reduced 10-year mortality, and substantially lower rates of heart attack, stroke, and microvascular complications of diabetes.[59] However, the magnitude of these benefits varies greatly from patient to patient. With recent progress in surgical technique, risks of metabolic/bariatric surgery are now comparable to gallbladder surgery or appendectomy, but geographic and financial barriers to metabolic/bariatric surgery are common.

Recent advances in diabetes technology such as continuous glucose monitoring and insulin pumps have been revolutionary for people with type 1 diabetes. Some insulin-treated patients with type 2 diabetes may also benefit from continuous glucose monitoring.[60] Technology that connects home-based glucose, blood pressure, weight, and lifestyle monitoring with clinicians and care managers has considerable potential to reduce clinical inertia and may help reduce the burden of treatment for those with diabetes and related conditions. However, such intensive monitoring can also increase treatment burden, which can manifest as burnout or diabetes distress among people with diabetes and their caregivers. Burden of treatment can have substantial impact on quality of life and health outcomes and should therefore be discussed with individuals when establishing care goals and treatment plans.

The cost of care for patients with diabetes is 200% to 300% higher than for age- and sex-matched patients without diabetes, and in human terms high costs of care often correlate with distress and suffering.[61] The economic and human burdens of diabetes care underscore the extreme importance of developing and implementing more effective public health efforts to prevent or delay onset of type 2 diabetes and to treat it effectively and efficiently when it occurs.

MOVING FORWARD

Primary Prevention

More effective strategies are needed to prevent or delay onset of type 2 diabetes using lifestyle or pharmacologic strategies. Prevention of type 2 diabetes is inextricably linked to control of the obesity epidemic, and strategies to prevent or manage obesity are of extreme importance. Broad dissemination of successful prevention strategies such as the DPP to individuals and populations at high risk of diabetes, particularly minority, rural, and underserved populations, is needed.

Secondary Prevention

Although healthy lifestyle choices combined with pharmacologic management has the potential to prevent or delay most diabetes complications, fewer than 25% of adults with diabetes simultaneously reach recommended levels of glucose, blood pressure, cholesterol, and tobacco control.[62] Innovations that improve the quality and delivery of chronic disease care, especially in primary care settings, are urgently needed. Although electronic health records have potential to support novel approaches to patient-centered care and shared decision-making, these hopes have not yet been fully realized. Experimentation with new approaches to shared decision-making, combatting therapeutic inertia, and diabetes self-management are needed. Mapping the clinical decision space of diabetes care, identifying clinician-specific care improvement opportunities, and providing simulated case-based training or personalized clinical decision support can also improve diabetes care quality. Metabolic bariatric surgery and medications (e.g., GLP-1 receptor agonists, SGLT2 inhibitors, tirzepatide) offer new options for effective glucose and weight management.

The Need for Improved Policy Approaches

There is robust evidence that fee-for-service payment models dampen innovation in chronic disease care, and organizations that are not dependent on fee-for-service financing, such as Kaiser Permanente and the Veterans Administration, have often been leaders in diabetes care improvement.[63] The impact of innovative financing mechanisms and of financial incentives for patients, clinicians, and care systems to improve the quality of chronic disease care deserves further attention. While public reporting of diabetes quality measures is a commonly used strategy to motivate improvement, there is little evidence that publicly reported diabetes quality-of-care measures improve quality of diabetes care on a sustained basis.[64]

DISCUSSION QUESTIONS

1. Describe recent trends in incidence and prevalence of diabetes and discuss factors that may be driving these trends.
2. How effective are the strategies tested in the DPP at preventing progression from prediabetes to diabetes? Discuss why DPP results in community practice have not been as robust as results in published DPP randomized clinical trials.
3. Identify strategies to modify the physical and social environment in ways that may reduce the burden of diabetes in urban and rural areas. Describe how you would evaluate the effectiveness of the strategies you propose.
4. In the last decade new and effective medication classes and more sophisticated ways to monitor glucose have been developed, but there is little evidence of sustained national improvement in glucose control. Suggest an integrated public health and clinical strategy to improve community-wide glucose, blood pressure, cholesterol, tobacco, and weight management in adults and adolescents with diabetes.
5. Some experts recommend universal screening for diabetes in adults, while others favor a more targeted approach based on age, body mass index, and other factors. Discuss how these two approaches might differ in terms of sensitivity, positive predictive value, cost, and cost-effectiveness.

REFERENCES

1. Centers for Disease Control and Prevention. National diabetes statistics report, 2020. Available at: https://www.cdc.gov/diabetes/pdfs/data/statistics/national-diabetes-statistics-report.pdf. Accessed January 18, 2023.
2. National Diabetes Data Group. Classification and diagnosis of diabetes mellitus and other categories of glucose intolerance. *Diabetes*. 1979;28(12):1039–1057.
3. Gavin JR III, Alberti K, Davidson MB, DeFronzo RA. Report of the expert committee on the diagnosis and classification of diabetes mellitus. *Diabetes Care*. 1997;20(7):1183.
4. International Expert Committee. International Expert Committee report on the role of the A1C assay in the diagnosis of diabetes. *Diabetes Care*. 2009;32(7):1327–1334.
5. American Diabetes Association Professional Practice Committee. 2. Classification and diagnosis of diabetes: *Standards of Medical Care in Diabetes—2022. Diabetes Care*. 2022; 45(suppl 1):S17–S38.

6. Geiss LS, Bullard KM, Brinks R, Gregg EW. Considerations in epidemiologic definitions of undiagnosed diabetes. *Diabetes Care.* 2018;41(9):1835–1838.
7. Fang M, Wang D, Coresh J, Selvin E. Undiagnosed diabetes in US adults: prevalence and trends. *Diabetes Care.* 2022;45(9):1994–2002. doi:10.2337/dc22-0242
8. Benoit SR, Hora I, Albright AL, Gregg EW. New directions in incidence and prevalence of diagnosed diabetes in the USA. *BMJ Open Diabetes Res Care.* 2019;7(1):e000657. doi:10.1136/bmjdrc-2019-000657
9. Selvin E, Ali MK. Declines in the incidence of diabetes in the US—real progress or artifact? *Diabetes Care.* 2017;40(9):1139–1143.
10. Todd JA, Walker NM, Cooper JD, et al. Robust associations of four new chromosome regions from genome-wide analyses of type 1 diabetes. *Nat Genet.* 2007;39(7):857–64.
11. Atkinson MA, Maclaren NK. The pathogenesis of insulin-dependent diabetes mellitus. *N Engl J Med.* 1994;331(21):1428–36. doi:10.1056/nejm199411243312107
12. Hummel M, Füchtenbusch M, Schenker M, Ziegler AG. No major association of breast-feeding, vaccinations, and childhood viral diseases with early islet autoimmunity in the German BABYDIAB Study. *Diabetes Care.* 2000;23(7):969–74. doi:10.2337/diacare.23.7.969
13. Vitamin D supplement in early childhood and risk for Type I (insulin-dependent) diabetes mellitus. The EURODIAB Substudy 2 Study Group. *Diabetologia.* 1999;42(1):51–54. doi:10.1007/s001250051112
14. Norris JM, Yin X, Lamb MM, et al. Omega-3 polyunsaturated fatty acid intake and islet autoimmunity in children at increased risk for type 1 diabetes. *JAMA.* 2007;298(12):1420–1428. doi:10.1001/jama.298.12.1420
15. Morgan E, Halliday SR, Campbell GR, Cardwell CR, Patterson CC. Vaccinations and childhood type 1 diabetes mellitus: a meta-analysis of observational studies. *Diabetologia.* 2016;59(2):237–243. doi:10.1007/s00125-015-3800-8
16. Jensen ET, Stafford JM, Saydah S, et al. Increase in prevalence of diabetic ketoacidosis at diagnosis among youth with type 1 diabetes: the SEARCH for Diabetes in Youth Study. *Diabetes Care.* 2021;44(7):1573–1578. doi:10.2337/dc20-0389
17. Thomas NJ, Lynam AL, Hill AV, et al. Type 1 diabetes defined by severe insulin deficiency occurs after 30 years of age and is commonly treated as type 2 diabetes. *Diabetologia.* 2019;62(7):1167–1172. doi:10.1007/s00125-019-4863-8
18. Hope SV, Wienand-Barnett S, Shepherd M, et al. Practical classification guidelines for diabetes in patients treated with insulin: a cross-sectional study of the accuracy of diabetes diagnosis. *Br J Gen Pract.* 2016;66(646):e315–322. doi:10.3399/bjgp16X684961
19. Holt RIG, DeVries JH, Hess-Fischl A, et al. The management of type 1 diabetes in adults: a consensus report by the American Diabetes Association (ADA) and the European Association for the Study of Diabetes (EASD). *Diabetes Care* 2021;44(11):2589–2625. doi:10.2337/dci21-0043
20. Vujkovic M, Keaton JM, Lynch JA, et al. Discovery of 318 new risk loci for type 2 diabetes and related vascular outcomes among 1.4 million participants in a multi-ancestry meta-analysis. *Nat Genet.* 2020;52(7):680–691. doi:10.1038/s41588-020-0637-y
21. Hill-Briggs F, Adler NE, Berkowitz SA, et al. Social determinants of health and diabetes: a scientific review. *Diabetes Care.* 2020;44(1):258–279. doi:10.2337/dci20-0053

22. Williams DR, Lawrence JA, Davis BA. Racism and health: evidence and needed research. *Annu Rev Public Health*. 2019;40:105–125. doi:10.1146/annurev-publhealth-040218-043750
23. Golden SH, Joseph JJ, Hill-Briggs F. Casting a health equity lens on endocrinology and diabetes. *J Clin Endocrinol Metab*. 2021;106(4):e1909–e1916.
24. Tabák AG, Herder C, Rathmann W, Brunner EJ, Kivimäki M. Prediabetes: a high-risk state for diabetes development. *Lancet*. 2012;379(9833):2279–2290.
25. Gregg EW, Zhuo X, Cheng YJ, Albright AL, Narayan KV, Thompson TJ. Trends in lifetime risk and years of life lost due to diabetes in the USA, 1985–2011: a modelling study. *Lancet Diabetes Endocrinol*. 2014;2(11):867–874.
26. Jarvela IY, Juutinen J, Koskela P, et al. Gestational diabetes identifies women at risk for permanent type 1 and type 2 diabetes in fertile age: predictive role of autoantibodies. *Diabetes Care*. 2006;29(3):607–612.
27. Wang H, Li N, Chivese T, et al. IDF diabetes atlas: estimation of global and regional gestational diabetes mellitus prevalence for 2021 by International Association of Diabetes in Pregnancy Study Group's criteria. *Diabetes Res Clin Pract*. 2022;183:109050. doi:10.1016/j.diabres.2021.109050
28. Zhang C, Ning Y. Effect of dietary and lifestyle factors on the risk of gestational diabetes: review of epidemiologic evidence. *Amer J Clin Nutr*. 2011;94(6 suppl):1975S–1979S.
29. Golden SH, Brown A, Cauley JA, et al. Health disparities in endocrine disorders: biological, clinical, and nonclinical factors—an Endocrine Society scientific statement. *J Clin Endocrinol Metab*. 2012;97(9):E1579– E1639. doi:10.1210/jc.2012-2043
30. Dugani SB, Mielke MM, Vella A. Burden and management of type 2 diabetes in rural United States. *Diabetes/Metabolism Res* Rev. 2021;37(5):e3410.
31. Ahmad FB, Anderson RN. The leading causes of death in the US for 2020. *JAMA*. 2021;325(18):1829–1830.
32. Gregg EW, Cheng YJ, Srinivasan M, et al. Trends in cause-specific mortality among adults with and without diagnosed diabetes in the USA: an epidemiological analysis of linked national survey and vital statistics data. *Lancet*. 2018;391(10138):2430–2440.
33. Emerging Risk Factors Collaboration. Diabetes mellitus, fasting glucose, and risk of cause-specific death. *N Engl J Med*. 2011;364(9):829–841.
34. McCoy RG, Lipska KJ, Van Houten HK, Shah ND. Association of cumulative multimorbidity, glycemic control, and medication use with hypoglycemia-related emergency department visits and hospitalizations among adults with diabetes. *JAMA Netw Open*. 2020;3(1):e1919099. doi:10.1001/jamanetworkopen.2019.19099
35. Kurani SS, Heien HC, Sangaralingham LR, et al. Association of area-level socioeconomic deprivation with hypoglycemic and hyperglycemic crises in US adults with diabetes. *JAMA Netw Open*. 2022;5(1):e2143597. doi:10.1001/jamanetworkopen.2021.43597
36. Umpierrez GE, Kovatchev BP. Glycemic variability: how to measure and its clinical implication for type 2 diabetes. *Amer J Med Sci*. 2018;356(6):518–527.
37. McCoy RG, Galindo RJ, Swarna KS, et al. Sociodemographic, clinical, and treatment-related factors associated with hyperglycemic crises among adults with type 1 or type 2 diabetes in the US from 2014 to 2020. *JAMA Netw Open*. 2021;4(9):e2123471–e2123471.

38. Pop-Busui R, Januzzi JL, Bruemmer D, et al. Heart failure: an underappreciated complication of diabetes: a consensus report of the American Diabetes Association. *Diabetes Care.* 2022;45(7):1670–1690. doi:10.2337/dci22-0014
39. Tomic D, Shaw JE, Magliano DJ. The burden and risks of emerging complications of diabetes mellitus. *Nat Rev Endocrinol.* 18(9):525-539. doi:10.1038/s41574-022-00690-7
40. Michels A, Zhang L, Khadra A, Kushner JA, Redondo MJ, Pietropaolo M. Prediction and prevention of type 1 diabetes: update on success of prediction and struggles at prevention. *Pediatr Diabetes.* 2015;16(7):465–484. doi:10.1111/pedi.12299
41. Knowler WC, Barrett-Connor E, Fowler SE, et al. Reduction in the incidence of type 2 diabetes with lifestyle intervention or metformin. *N Engl J Med.* 2002;346(6):393–403.
42. Tuomilehto J, Lindström J, Eriksson JG, et al. Prevention of type 2 diabetes mellitus by changes in lifestyle among subjects with impaired glucose tolerance. *N Engl J Med.* 2001;344(18): 1343–1350.
43. Lindström J, Ilanne-Parikka P, Peltonen M, et al. Sustained reduction in the incidence of type 2 diabetes by lifestyle intervention: follow-up of the Finnish Diabetes Prevention Study. *Lancet.* 2006;368(9548):1673–1679.
44. Pan XR, Li GW, Hu YH, et al. Effects of diet and exercise in preventing NIDDM in people with impaired glucose tolerance: the Da Qing IGT and Diabetes Study. *Diabetes Care.* 1997;20(4): 537–544.
45. Diabetes Prevention Program Research Group. 10-year follow-up of diabetes incidence and weight loss in the Diabetes Prevention Program Outcomes Study. *Lancet.* 2009;374(9702): 1677–1686.
46. Knowler WC, Barrett-Connor E, Fowler SE, et al. Reduction in the incidence of type 2 diabetes with lifestyle intervention or metformin. *N Engl J Med.* 2002;346(6):393-403. doi:10.1056/NEJMoa012512
47. Thompson VLS, Johnson-Jennings M, Baumann AA, Proctor E. Peer reviewed: use of culturally focused theoretical frameworks for adapting diabetes prevention programs: a qualitative review. *Prev Chronic Dis.* 2015;12:e60. doi:10.5888/pcd12.140421
48. Tabak RG, Sinclair KA, Baumann AA, et al. A review of diabetes prevention program translations: use of cultural adaptation and implementation research. *Transl Behav Med.* 2015;5(4): 401–414. doi:10.1007/s13142-015-0341-0
49. Diabetes Prevention Program Research Group. Long-term effects of lifestyle intervention or metformin on diabetes development and microvascular complications over 15-year follow-up: the Diabetes Prevention Program Outcomes Study. *Lancet Diabetes Endocrinol.* 2015;3(11): 866–875.
50. Diabetes Prevention Program Research Group. The 10-year cost-effectiveness of lifestyle intervention or metformin for diabetes prevention: an intent-to-treat analysis of the DPP/DPPOS. *Diabetes Care.* 2012;35(4):723–730.
51. Hostalek U, Gwilt M, Hildemann S. Therapeutic use of metformin in prediabetes and diabetes prevention. *Drugs.* 2015;75(10):1071–1094.
52. Hingle MD, Turner T, Kutob R, et al. The EPIC Kids Study: a randomized family-focused YMCA-based intervention to prevent type 2 diabetes in at-risk youth. *BMC Public Health.* 2015;15(1):1–12.

53. Gonzalez-Suarez C, Worley A, Grimmer-Somers K, Dones V. School-based interventions on childhood obesity: a meta-analysis. *Am J Prev Med.* 2009;37(5):418–427.
54. Davidson KW, Barry MJ, Mangione CM, et al. Screening for prediabetes and type 2 diabetes: US Preventive Services Task Force recommendation statement. *JAMA.* 2021;326(8):736–743.
55. Fang M, Selvin E. Thirty-year trends in complications in US adults with newly diagnosed type 2 diabetes. *Diabetes Care.* 2021;44(3):699–706.
56. Fang M, Wang D, Echouffo-Tcheugui JB, Selvin E. Prediabetes and diabetes screening eligibility and detection in US adults after changes to US Preventive Services Task Force and American Diabetes Association recommendations. *JAMA.* 2022;327(19):1924–1925. doi:10.1001/jama.2022.5185
57. Institute of Medicine Committee on Standards for Developing Trustworthy Clinical Practice; Graham R, Mancher M, Miller Wolman D, Greenfield S, Steinberg E, eds. *Clinical Practice Guidelines We Can Trust.* Washington, DC: National Academies Press; 2011.
58. Taha MB, Valero-Elizondo J, Yahya T, et al. Cost-related medication nonadherence in adults with diabetes in the United States: the National Health Interview Survey 2013–2018. *Diabetes Care.* 2022;45(3):594-603. doi:10.2337/dc21-1757
59. Fisher DP, Johnson E, Haneuse S, et al. Association between bariatric surgery and macrovascular disease outcomes in patients with type 2 diabetes and severe obesity. *JAMA.* 2018; 320(15):1570–1582.
60. Martens T, Beck RW, Bailey R, et al. Effect of continuous glucose monitoring on glycemic control in patients with type 2 diabetes treated with basal insulin: a randomized clinical trial. *JAMA.* 2021;325(22):2262–2272.
61. American Diabetes Association. Economic costs of diabetes in the US in 2017. *Diabetes Care.* 2018;41(5):917–928.
62. Fang M, Wang D, Coresh J, Selvin E. Trends in diabetes treatment and control in US adults, 1999–2018. *N Engl J Med.* 2021;384(23):2219–2228.
63. Kanter MH, Lindsay G, Bellows J, Chase A. Complete care at Kaiser Permanente: transforming chronic and preventive care. *Jt Comm J Qual Patient Saf.* 2013;39(11):484–494. doi:10.1016/s1553-7250(13)39064-3
64. Jiang DH, O'Connor PJ, Huguet N, Golden SH, McCoy RG. Modernizing diabetes care quality measures. *Health Aff (Millwood).* 2022;41(7):955–962. doi:10.1377/hlthaff.2022.00233

13

Hypertension

Leonelo E. Bautista, MD, DrPH, MPH, and Oscar L. Rueda, MD, PhD

LEARNING OBJECTIVES

After completing this chapter, readers should be able to

1. Identify the main mechanisms of blood pressure regulation and explain how hypertension is defined and diagnosed.
2. Describe the frequency of hypertension in different populations and its health impact in the United States and the world.
3. Recognize the most important risk factors for the development of hypertension and understand the role of preventive and therapeutic interventions in reducing the health burden of hypertension.

INTRODUCTION

Arterial blood pressure is the force that circulating blood exerts on the walls of the larger, low-resistance arteries of the vascular system. High blood pressure, also called hypertension, is asymptomatic because blood pressure cannot be perceived. However, hypertension has a large impact on morbidity and mortality in almost all populations as a result of its high prevalence and strong association with the incidence of cardiovascular and renal disease (Figure 13-1). Fortunately, hypertension is fairly easy to diagnose, and blood pressure control results in significant health benefits.

The precise blood pressure levels defining hypertension are those above which blood pressure–lowering interventions result in significant reduction of the risk of stroke and coronary heart disease.[2,3] Accordingly, the definition of hypertension has changed over time as new knowledge on the consequences of hypertension and on the benefits of lowering blood pressure has accumulated. Although somewhat arbitrary, the definition of hypertension is very useful for clinicians making treatment decisions, for research, for epidemiologic surveillance, and for public health policy formulation.

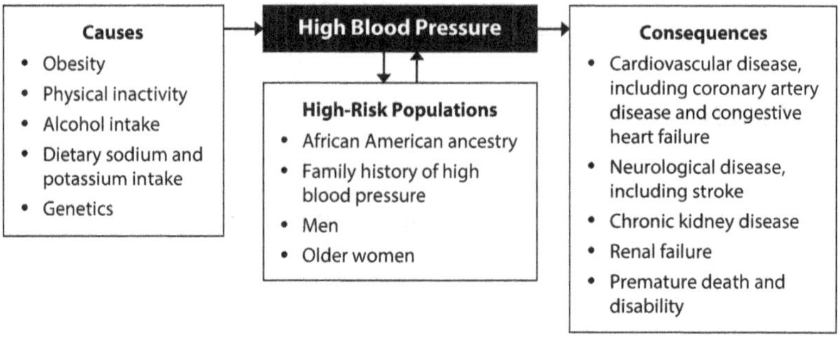

Source: Based on CDC.[1]

Figure 13-1. High Blood Pressure: Causes, Consequences, and High-Risk Populations: National Health and Nutrition Examination Survey, United States, 2009–2020

PATHOPHYSIOLOGY

Mean arterial pressure is the product of cardiac output, the volume of blood pumped by the heart per unit of time, and systemic vascular resistance, the force that small peripheral arteries oppose to the circulation of the blood. Essential hypertension, which accounts for about 95% of the cases of hypertension, is defined as elevated blood pressure that is not a consequence of an underlying medical condition. The mechanisms causing essential hypertension are not completely understood. However, it is well recognized that the kidney, the sympathetic nervous system, and the renin-angiotensin system play central roles in blood pressure regulation. Under normal conditions, the human body maintains a precise balance between the intake and output of fluids and electrolytes. If this balance were compromised, the volume of body fluids could expand or contract to a point at which the circulatory system would fail. The long-term regulation of body fluid volume depends greatly on the ability of the kidneys to excrete and reabsorb sodium chloride. When the extracellular concentration of sodium increases, blood volume increases, leading to an elevation in cardiac output and blood pressure. In response to the rise in blood pressure, the kidney increases sodium excretion, leading to lower blood volume, reduced cardiac output, and normal blood pressure. Conversely, when blood pressure falls below normal, the kidney retains water and sodium as a way to increase blood volume and cardiac output and reestablish normal blood pressure.

All forms of essential hypertension are characterized by impaired pressure natriuresis, a condition in which a blood pressure higher than normal is required to stimulate the kidney to excrete sodium as a way to maintain normal body fluid volumes. Impaired pressure natriuresis could be caused by factors within or outside the kidney. A reduced glomerular filtration rate or an increased tubular reabsorption of sodium are kidney mechanisms that may lead to hypertension. When the intrinsic balance between glomerular filtration rate and tubular reabsorption is altered, blood pressure increases as a way to increase natriuresis and preserve normal body fluid volume.

Increased activity of the sympathetic nervous system is a mechanism outside the kidney often associated with the pathogenesis of hypertension. In fact, increased sympathetic activity has been proposed as a mechanism for obesity- and stress-related hypertension. Activation of the sympathetic nervous system can cause short-term increases in blood pressure by increasing heart rate, heart contractility, and cardiac output and by increasing vasoconstriction and systemic vascular resistance. More important, activation of renal sympathetic activity could lead to hypertension by increasing sodium retention and impairing pressure natriuresis.

Disorders that induce arterial vasoconstriction or sodium retention can also play a role in the pathogenesis of hypertension. For example, an increased activity of the renin-angiotensin system results in high levels of angiotensin II, a powerful vasoconstrictor that helps to maintain blood pressure in situations in which blood volume or cardiac contractility are low. High levels of angiotensin II increase vasoconstriction and systemic vascular resistance and impair pressure natriuresis. This may lead to chronic hypertension because higher levels of blood pressure would be needed to preserve normal sodium excretion and body fluid volume. Finally, vasodilating (e.g., nitric oxide) and vasoconstricting (e.g., endothelin-1) factors, produced by the vascular endothelium in response to mechanical and biochemical agonists, participate in blood pressure control, but their role on the pathogenesis of hypertension has yet to be fully elucidated.

Blood Pressure Measurement and Diagnosis of High Blood Pressure

Owing to blood pressure's intrinsic variability, the diagnosis of hypertension has traditionally been based on the average of at least two blood pressure measurements made on at least two sequential clinic visits, using a mercury sphygmomanometer. In the last decade or so automated oscillometric devices have become widely used in the clinical setting and have provided more precise estimates of blood pressure levels and their relationship with cardiovascular risk. However, the accuracy of oscillometric devices in clinical practice is uncertain in some groups of patients, such as pregnant women, elderly patients with arrhythmias, and patients with a low heart rate. Therefore, oscillometric devices should be validated in specific groups of patients, following standard protocols. Online lists of validated oscillatory devices are provided by different professional associations.[4]

Oscillometric automated devices to measure blood pressure in the absence of medical personnel have become key in the diagnosis and management of hypertension, and the use of ambulatory blood pressure measurement (ABPM) and home blood pressure measurement (HBPM) has been recently endorsed in hypertension management guidelines.[4,5] ABPM and HBPM are used mainly to identify individuals whose blood pressure is high in a medical setting but normal in an ambulatory setting (white coat hypertension), individuals whose blood pressure is high in an ambulatory but not medical setting (masked hypertension), and individuals with a poor response to antihypertensive treatment.[4,5]

ABPM is usually conducted over a 24-hour period and measurements are taken regularly every 20 to 30 minutes while patients go about their usual daily activities. Average blood pressure is obtained during awake and sleep periods. ABPM predicts long-term cardiovascular outcomes, beyond the effect of office blood pressure, and in some settings is considered the best method for out-of-office blood pressure measurement.[4,5] A main hurdle for the replacement of office blood pressure by ambulatory blood pressure is that most of our knowledge on the impact of blood pressure on cardiovascular risk, risk stratification, and blood pressure management has been guided by office blood pressure. For this reason, the diagnosis of hypertension and threshold targets for treatment still rely on office measurements.[4,5] Although there is limited trial evidence on the cost-effectiveness of ABPM, modeling studies indicate that ABPM is cost-effective in adult patients compared with office measurements and HBPM.[6] This has helped to dispel previous concerns about its role in the management of hypertension.

HBPM devices were originally developed as a product for consumers. However, HBPM has been recommended as a tool to confirm the diagnosis of hypertension after initial in-office diagnosis and for blood pressure monitoring.[4,5] Although guidance for HBPM varies in clinical practice, patients should take at least two readings one minute apart in the morning and in the evening, for a period of one to two weeks before a clinic visit; they should also receive adequate training and follow specific instructions when measuring their blood pressure.

HBPM does not seem a reliable approach for the diagnosis of hypertension. In a systematic review of studies using ABPM as the reference standard, the sensitivity of HBPM was higher than that of office measurements (86%–95% CI, 78–91 vs. 75%–95% CI, 61–85). However, this improvement in sensitivity resulted in lower specificity of HBPM: 62% (95% CI, 48–75) versus 75% (95% CI, 48–90).[7] Although HBPM seems to be a better predictor of cardiovascular outcomes than office blood pressure, the evidence remains inconclusive.[8]

Current hypertension guidelines recommend initial screening with office blood pressures and following with ABPM or HBPM for confirmation. Although the diagnosis, staging, and treatment of hypertension still rely on conventional office measurements, evidence in support of the use of automatic devices, ABPM, and HBPM has accumulated in the last decade. Current guidelines concur on screening for hypertension in the clinical setting and recommend using ABPM and office blood pressure for the diagnosis of white coat and masked hypertension.[4,5] However, recommended protocols are inconsistent, and there is evidence that obtaining multiple automated office measurements could expedite the diagnosis of these conditions and reduce human error and the need for out-of-office blood pressure measurements.[9]

The Use of Standard Guidelines for Measuring Blood Pressure

Regardless of the measuring approach and diagnostic procedures, standard guidelines must be followed to obtain accurate and reliable clinic and ambulatory blood pressure measurements. Multiple studies now suggest that automated office blood pressures, when taken following standard guidelines, with the patient alone in a quiet place, are more accurate than regular office blood pressures and are similar to awake ABPM values.[5,9] This and the phasing out of mercury sphygmomanometers have made automatic devices the preferred method of blood pressure measurement in the clinical setting.

For more than three decades individuals aged 18 years and older who are not acutely ill and have systolic blood pressure (SBP) of 140 millimeters of mercury (mm Hg) or higher or diastolic blood pressure (DBP) of 90 mm Hg or higher have been diagnosed as hypertensive, because they have an important increase in cardiovascular risk and they benefit from additional examinations or blood pressure–lowering interventions. This definition of hypertension is used throughout this chapter. However, current guidelines vary significantly in terms of the approach and cut points used for diagnosing and staging hypertension. Current US guidelines[5] categorize blood pressure levels (systolic/diastolic, mm Hg) as normal (<120/80), elevated (120–129/<80), Stage 1 hypertension (130–139/80–89) and Stage 2 hypertension (≥140/≥90), as shown in Table 13-1. ABPM and HBPM are recommended to confirm the diagnosis of hypertension and for titration of blood pressure–lowering medication. Supportive interventions to improve adherence to treatment and blood pressure control, such as team-based care and telehealth strategies, are also recommended. ABPM or HBPM is recommended in adults with an untreated systolic blood pressure (SBP) higher than 130 but lower than 160 mm Hg or diastolic blood pressure (DBP) higher than 80 but lower than 100 mm Hg, to screen for white coat hypertension before the start of treatment. In adults with elevated office blood pressure (120–129/75–79) but not meeting the criteria for hypertension, screening for masked hypertension with daytime ABPM or HBPM is also reasonable.[5]

PUBLIC HEALTH SIGNIFICANCE

The Worldwide Impact of High Blood Pressure

Hypertension imposes an extraordinary health burden in almost all populations because of its high prevalence and the large increase in the risk of cardiovascular and renal disease in individuals with this condition.

Estimates of the prevalence of hypertension come mostly from epidemiologic studies in which cases are defined by using the average of multiple blood pressure readings taken in a single evaluation, instead of multiple sequential clinic visits. Prospective studies linking blood pressure and cardiovascular risk have relied on this epidemiologic definition of hypertension. The Noncommunicable Disease Risk Factor Collaboration (NCD-RisC)

Table 13-1. Office Blood Pressure (Systolic/Diastolic, mm Hg) Staging According to International Guidelines for the Evaluation and Treatment of High Blood Pressure Among Adults

Stage	2017 ACC/AHA[5]	2018 Canada[10]	2018 ESC[11]	2019 UK-NICE[12]	2019 JSH[13]	2020 ISH[14]
Optimal	NA	NA	<120/<80	NA	NA	NA
Normal	<120/80	NA	120–129/80–84	<135/<85	<120/<80	<13/85
High normal	NA	NA	130–139/85–89	NA	120–129/<80	130–139/85–89
Elevated	120–129/<80	NA	NA	NA	130–139/80–89	NA
Hypertension		≥140/90[b]				
Stage 1	130–139/80–89[a]	NA	140–159/90–99[c]	≥140/90[d]	140–159/90–99	140–159/90–99
Stage 2	≥140/≥90	NA	160–179/100–109	≥160/100	160–179/100–109	≥160/≥100
Stage 3	NA	NA	≥180/≥110	≥180/120	≥180/≥110	NA

Note: ABPM = ambulatory blood pressure measurement; ACC = American College of Cardiology; AHA = American Heart Association; ESC = European Society of Cardiology; JSH = Japanese Society of Hypertension; ISH = International Society of Hypertension; NA= not applicable.

[a]ACC/AHA also considers as hypertensive patients with a mean daytime ABPM of ≥135/85, a mean nighttime ABPM of ≥120/70, or 24-hr ABPM of ≥130/80.

[b]Canadian guidelines also consider as hypertensive patients with an automated office blood pressure or daytime ABPM of ≥135/85, a 24-hr ABPM of ≥130/80, or a home blood pressure of ≥135/85.

[c]ESC guidelines also consider as hypertensive patients with a mean 24-hr ABPM of ≥130/80, a mean daytime ABPM of ≥135/85, or a mean nighttime ABPM of ≥120/70.

[d]NICE-UK defines Stage 1 as an ABPM of ≥135/85 and Stage 2 as an ABPM ≥150/95 in a 24-hr period. Stage 3 does not require an ABPM.

conducted a recent analysis of data from more than 100 million participants aged 30 to 79 years, from studies conducted in 1990 to 2019. The worldwide prevalence of hypertension was 32% (95% credible interval [CrI]: 30, 34) in women and 34% in men (95% CrI: 32, 37). Those values were similar to prevalence levels in 1990.[15] However, during that period the number of hypertensive individuals doubled, independently of age, from 331 to 626 million in women, and from 317 to 652 million in men. The stable global prevalence of hypertension in those aged 30 to 79 years seems to be attributable to a decrease in high-income countries and an increase in low-income and middle-income countries.[15,16] However, NCD-RisC has also reported a decrease in age-standardized prevalence of hypertension: by 29.5% in 1975 to 24.1% in 2015 in men aged 18 years or older and by 26.1 to 20.1% in women aged 18 years or older.[17] This decline of about six percentage points was also observed in those aged 30 to 79 years.

Among men and women aged 18 years and older, global age-standardized SBP remained stable from 1975 to 2015 (126.6–127.0 and 123.9–121.3 mm Hg, respectively).[17] DBP has also remained stable during this period, with a mean of 78.7 mm Hg in men and 76.7 mm Hg in women. In general, blood pressure has declined in high-income and some middle-income countries, but it has increased or remained stable in other middle-income and low-income countries.[17] These findings are consistent with previous studies.

White coat hypertension has been detected in 20% to 40% of all hypertensive patients. In a meta-analysis of 12 cohort studies in random samples of the population, the prevalence of white coat hypertension was 36.0% (95% CI, 34.1–37.9).[18] However, when multiple blood pressure measures are taken in at least two clinic visits, following standard protocols, the prevalence of white coat hypertension is closer to 9% in individuals without a previous diagnosis of hypertension.[19]

Health Effects

Ample evidence suggests hypertension is a strong risk factor for the development of ischemic heart disease, stroke, sudden death, heart failure, atrial fibrillation, peripheral arterial disease, abdominal aortic aneurysm, and chronic kidney disease.

Hypertension is also strongly associated with cardiovascular mortality in all ages. The effect of blood pressure on cardiovascular mortality has been estimated in a meta-analysis of cohort studies in more than one million adults.[20] In that study, an increase of 20 mm Hg in SBP increased the coronary heart disease death rate from 50% to 100%, and stroke death rate by 50% to 180%, depending on age. Similarly, an increase of 10 mm Hg in DBP increased coronary heart disease mortality from 40% to 110% and stroke mortality by 60% to 190%, depending on age (Table 13-2). These results show that the relative effect of hypertension on cardiovascular mortality is higher in younger individuals. However, absolute differences in mortality are larger in older individuals because cardiovascular

Table 13-2. Percent Increase in Coronary Heart Disease and Stroke Mortality Rate by Age Group Due to an Increase of 20 mm Hg in Systolic Blood Pressure or 10 mm Hg in Diastolic Blood Pressure.

Age, y	Systolic Blood Pressure		Diastolic Blood Pressure	
	CHD	Stroke	CHD	Stroke
80–89	50	50	40	60
70–79	70	100	60	110
60–69	90	130	80	150
50–59	100	160	90	190
40–49	100	180	110	190

Source: Based on Lewington.[20]
Note: CHD = chronic heart disease. The increase is due to an increase of 20 mm Hg in systolic blood pressure or 10 mm Hg in diastolic blood pressure.

disease mortality increases with age. The relative increase in mortality associated with an absolute difference in blood pressure was the same at all levels of blood pressure down to at least 115 mm Hg of SBP and 75 mm Hg of DBP.[20]

In addition, it is estimated that 3.5 billion people aged 25 years or older (77%–86% of all individuals in this group) have SBP of at least 110 to 115 mm Hg,[21] which is considered the minimum level of SBP associated with an increase in the risk of cardiovascular disease.[20] According to worldwide studies conducted a decade ago, SBP above 110 to 115 mm Hg was the leading single contributor to the global burden of disease.[22] At that time about 9.4 million deaths per year (13% of all deaths in the world) were caused by hypertension, which was responsible for at least 45% of deaths attributed to ischemic heart disease and 51% of deaths attributed to stroke. The number of disability-adjusted life years (DALYs) attributed to hypertension was 173.6 million (7.0% of the total), considerably larger than that for smoking (136.9 million), alcohol intake (120.6 million), obesity (93.6 million), high fasting plasma glucose (89.0 million), and high total cholesterol (40.9 million).[22] According to more recent estimates, in 2015 the number of deaths reached 10.7 million per year (19% of all deaths in the world), and the number of DALYs reached 211 million per year—8.6% of the total.[21]

DESCRIPTIVE EPIDEMIOLOGY

Blood Pressure Patterns by Gender, Age, and Race

Average blood pressure and prevalence of hypertension depend strongly on age, gender, and race/ethnicity. Average blood pressure increases with age in most populations, except isolated populations with low sodium intake. Age-related changes in blood pressure are mostly explained by the loss of elasticity of the aorta and other large arteries

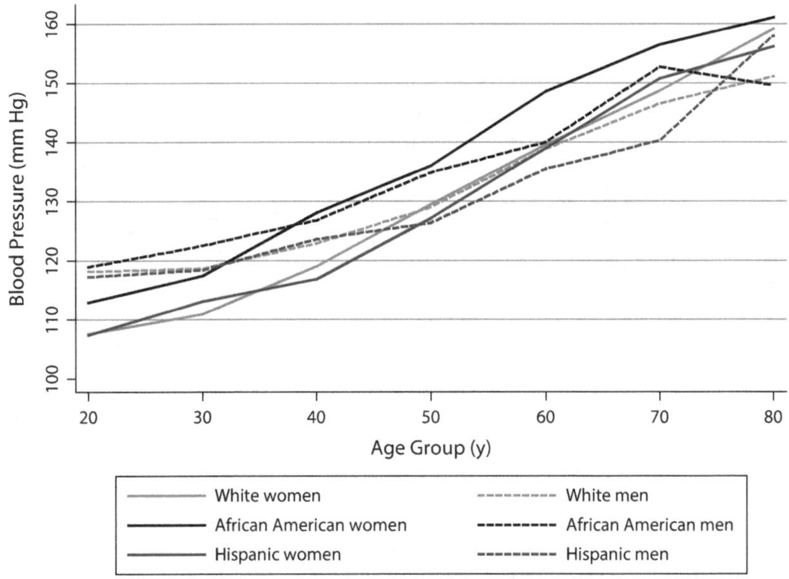

Source: Based on CDC.[1]

Figure 13-2. Average Systolic Blood Pressure by Age, Gender, and Race: National Health and Nutrition Examination Survey, United States, 2009–2020

(arterial stiffness) that occurs normally with aging. Age- and gender-related changes in blood pressure are illustrated here with data from the National Health and Nutrition Examination Survey (NHANES, 2009–2020) in the United States.[1]

Systolic and diastolic blood pressure levels strongly depend on age, gender, and race. SBP increases with age in both men and women, from 109 mm Hg in women aged 20 years to about 141 mm Hg at 80 years, and from about 118 mm Hg in men aged 20 years to about 134 mm Hg at 80 years. Therefore, SBP is higher in young men than in young women, but it becomes higher in women than in men around 65 years in all races (Figure 13-2).[1] Among adults younger than 65 years, age-adjusted SBP is 5.7 mm Hg higher in men than in women, but in those aged 65 or older it is 3.9 mm Hg lower. Age-adjusted SBP is higher in men than in women across all races and ethnicities, from 3.6 mm Hg higher in Whites to 6.4 mm Hg higher in Mexican Americans. Age- and gender-adjusted SBP is similar in Asians, about 1 mm Hg higher in Hispanics and Mexican Americans, but about 5 mm Hg higher in Blacks than in Whites.

In contrast to the steady age-related increase in SBP, in men and women from all ethnic/racial groups average DBP increases with age until about 50 years of age and starts decreasing shortly after, around 55 years of age (Figure 13-3).[1] Among Whites and Hispanics, DBP peaks and then levels off at around 40 years of age in men and 50 years of age in women. Corresponding changes occur around 50 and 60 years of age

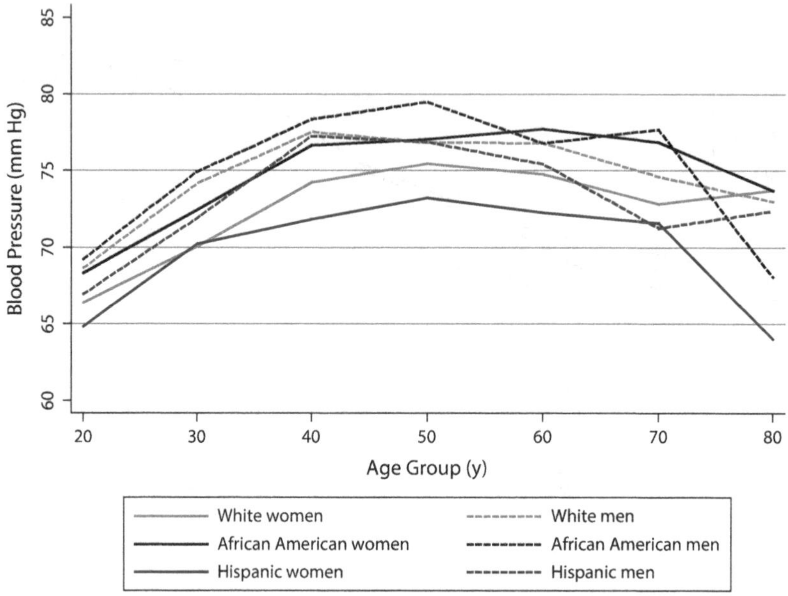

Source: Based on CDC.[1]

Figure 13-3. Average Diastolic Blood Pressure by Age, Gender, and Race: National Health and Nutrition Examination Survey, United States, 2009–2020

among Blacks. Average age-adjusted DBP is similar in Black men and women, but is 1.5 to 2.5 mm Hg higher in men than in women in other ethnic/racial groups. While age- and gender-adjusted DBP is similar in other ethnic/racial groups; it is about 1 mm Hg lower in Mexican Americans and Hispanics than in Whites.

Estimates of the prevalence of hypertension in the United States come from NHANES data collected between 2015 and March 2020 (Table 13-3).[1] The overall prevalence of HBP in adults 20 years or older was 29.2% but ranged from about 4% in those aged 20 to 29 years to 75% in those aged 80 to 89 years. Similar to average SBP, the prevalence of hypertension increases with age and is higher in young men than in young women, but it is higher in older women than in older men (Table 13-3; Figure 13-4). This gender pattern is consistent in all racial/ethnic groups, with the exception of Blacks, among whom young women have similar or higher prevalence than young men.

Data on the incidence of hypertension are limited because ascertaining incident cases requires active follow-up of populations with frequent blood pressure measurements for a long time. Among participants aged 20 to 69 years participants in the Framingham Cohort Study, followed for 3.8 years, the incidence of hypertension was 3.84 and 3.41 per 100 person-years in men and women, respectively.[23] In the Atherosclerosis Risk in Communities Study (ARIC), the incidence of hypertension in White men and

Table 13-3. Prevalence of Hypertension by Gender and Age: National Health and Nutrition Examination Survey, United States, 2015-March 2020

Age, y	Women (95% CI)	Men (95% CI)	All (95% CI)
20-29	3.1 (1.4-3.7)	5.6 (4.3-6.8)	4.4 (3.2-5.5)
30-39	12.6 (9.6-15.6)	18.3 (14.1-22.4)	15.5 (12.9-18.1)
40-49	22.1 (18.3-25.8)	30.5 (25.4-35.6)	26.2 (22.6-29.8)
50-59	41.7 (37.2-46.1)	45.3 (40.0-50.6)	43.4 (39.9-46.9)
60-69	59.4 (54.6-64.2)	57.9 (53.7-62.2)	58.7 (55.2-62.3)
70-79	74.3 (69.9-78.7)	62.0 (56.4-67.6)	68.7 (65.1-72.4)
80-89	78.2 (73.4-83.1)	69.4 (62.8-75.9)	74.7 (71.7-77.8)
All	29.6 (27.9-31.3)	28.8 (27.0-30.6)	29.2 (27.7-30.7)

Source: Based on CDC.[1]

Note: CI = confidence interval. Hypertension was defined as systolic blood pressure ≥140 mm Hg or diastolic blood pressure ≥90 mm Hg or self-reported history of a diagnosis of hypertension plus current use of antihypertensive medication. Blood pressure measures for 2017–March 2020 were taken with an oscillometric device. Pregnant women were excluded.

women aged 45 to 64 years, followed for 6 years, was 2.82 and 2.60 per 100 person-years in men and women, respectively.[24] When combined, data from these studies show an incidence of 3.15 (95% CI, 2.64–3.66) cases per 100 person-years, which is about 30% lower than the 4.45 cases per 100 person-years observed among Whites aged 45 to 64 years enrolled in the Multi-Ethnic Study of Atherosclerosis (MESA) and followed for 4.8 years.[25]

Race/ethnicity has a large impact in hypertension incidence. In the ARIC study, the incidence per 100 person-years was 2.70 and 4.32 per 100 person-years in Whites and Blacks, respectively,[24] while in the MESA study the incidence was 5.68 for Whites, 8.49 for Blacks, 6.57 for Hispanics, and 5.22 for Chinese aged 45 to 84 years.

The age-cumulative risk of hypertension in participants in the Framingham Study free of the condition at 55 or 65 years was about 90% in their median residual lifetime expectancy: 20 years for 65-year-old adults and 25 years for 55-year-old adults.[26] Similarly, in 45-year-old adults participating in MESA, the 40-year risk of developing hypertension was 92.7% for Blacks, 92.4% for Hispanics, 86.0% for Whites, and 84.1% for Chinese adults.

In addition to age, the incidence of hypertension depends greatly on starting blood pressure values. Among Framingham Study participants with optimum (SBP <120 mm Hg and DBP <80 mm Hg), normal (SBP <130 and DBP <85 mm Hg), or high-normal blood pressure (SBP 130–139 mm Hg and DBP 85–89 mm Hg),[27] the four-year risk of hypertension was 5.1%, 18.1%, and 39.4% in adults aged 35 to 64 years and 18.5%, 29.0%, and 52.5% in those aged 65 to 94 years, respectively.[28]

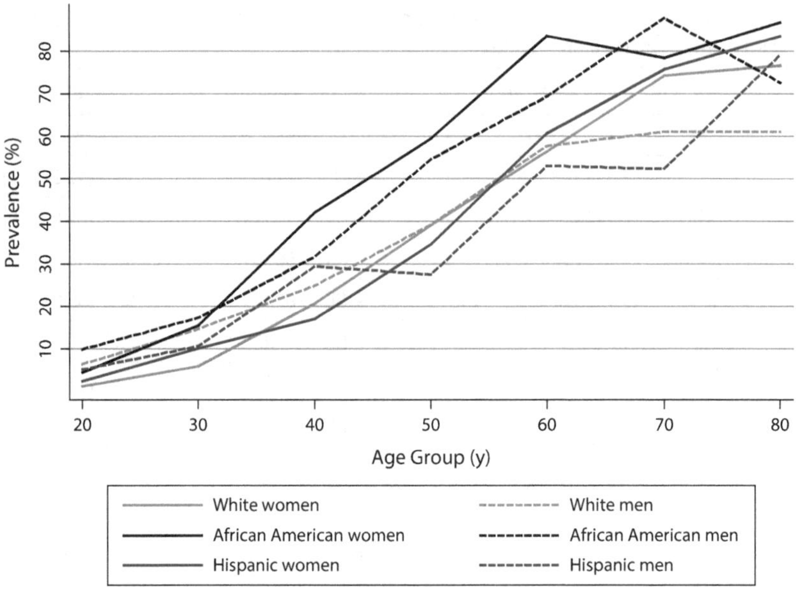

Source: Based on CDC.[1]

Figure 13-4. Prevalence of Hypertension by Age, Gender, and Race: National Health and Nutrition Examination Survey, United States, 2009–2020

In 2019 in the United States 102,072 deaths were attributed to hypertension, for a crude death rate of 31.1 per 100,000: 40.6 in Blacks, 31.0 in Whites, 14.9 in Asian Americans, and 12.6 in Hispanics.[29] From 2009 to 2019, the age-adjusted death rate for hypertension increased 34.2%, increasing 44.1% in Whites, 22.6% in Hispanics, and 5.2% in Blacks.[29] In the last decade age-adjusted hypertensive heart disease mortality has increased in Black and White men and women. Although the absolute mortality rate continues to be higher in Blacks, the increase in mortality has been highest in White women and men.[30]

The annual average total cost of hypertension in 2017 to 2018 was $51.1 billion.[29]

Geographic Trends

The prevalence of hypertension is higher in states and communities with a higher proportion of Blacks, such as the South and southeastern United States. Hypertension prevalence seems to be higher in Whites in the central Southeast and in Blacks in the western Southeast, and there is evidence members of these racial groups living or born in southern states are at higher risk of developing hypertension than those born in other areas of the United States.[31]

Time Trends

A downward trend in the prevalence of hypertension was observed from 1971 to 1991 in the US population across all age, gender, and racial/ethnic groups, with the exception of Black men aged 50 and older, who experienced a small increase.[32] This trend reversed during 1998 to 2000, when the age-adjusted prevalence increased from 25.0% to 28.7% across all groups.[33] More recent data indicate the prevalence of hypertension has stabilized or decreased.[34] Prevalence estimates were 24.1% in 1988 to 1994, 30.2% in 1999 to 2002, 32.1% in 2003 to 2006, and 32.2% in 2009 to 2012, with 2015 to 2020 seeing a 2% absolute decrease in age-adjusted prevalence.[34] In NHANES data from 2015 to 2020, hypertension prevalence was 28.9 % (95% CI, 27.5–30.5), an increase of 8% compared with 2009 to 2014, when it was 26.8% (95% CI, 25.6–28.1). However, the change in prevalence depended on age. In adults younger than 70 years, there was an increase of 10% (95% CI, 2.4–18.1), while in those 70 years and older, there was a decrease of 5% (95% CI, 0.4–9.6).

Impact on Morbidity and Mortality

A considerable fraction of all new cases of cardiovascular and renal disease in the United States is attributable to hypertension. Table 13-4 shows the relative risk and the attributable risk for the main diseases associated with hypertension.

Among middle-class White participants in the Framingham Study, those with hypertension were about two times more likely than those without to develop coronary heart disease.[36] However, in a recent large cohort study hypertension increased the risk of coronary heart disease by 4.8, 2.0, 2.1, and 1.6 times in Black women, Black men, White women, and White men, respectively.[37] Pooled estimates from cohort studies result in a relative risk of 1.81 (95% CI, 1.62–2.00).[37–40]

Hypertension is the strongest independent risk factor for stroke. The relative risk of stroke associated with hypertension has been remarkably consistent in several cohort studies.[41–45] The pooled relative risk in those studies indicate that stroke incidence is 2.38 (95% CI, 2.07–2.70) times higher in hypertensive than in normotensive individuals. The relative effect of hypertension on stroke incidence does not seem to depend on race or gender.

Hypertension increases the risk of congestive heart failure by 2.02 times (95% CI, 1.39–2.65).[46–48] Although the increase in risk is similar in men and women, it is currently uncertain whether it varies significantly by race.

Hypertension can also lead to the development of chronic kidney disease (see Chapter 23), a progressive loss of renal function, and to end-stage renal disease, an advanced stage of chronic kidney disease requiring dialysis or renal transplant as a form of renal replacement therapy. Individuals with hypertension are 3.56 times (95% CI, 2.72–4.39) more likely to develop chronic kidney disease (glomerular filtration rate

Table 13-4. Relative Risk and Population Attributable Risk for Diseases Associated With Hypertension in Men (M) and Women (W) by Race/Ethnicity: National Health and Nutrition Examination Survey, United States, 2015–March 2020

		Population Attributable Risk, %[a]							
		White		Black		Hispanic		All	
Disease	Relative Risk[b,c]	M	W	M	W	M	W	M	W
Coronary heart disease	1.81 (1.62–2.00)	19.1 (15.0–23.1)	19.3 (15.1–23.3)	28.1 (10.6–39.8)	31.4 (12.2–43.7)	19.2 (8.3–28.8)	20.0 (8.7–28.8)	17.1 (12.7–21.2)	22.7 (10.1–32.2)
Stroke	2.38 (2.07–2.70)	29.5 (24.5–34.0)	29.7 (24.7–34.3)	31.3 (26.1–36.0)	34.8 (29.3–39.7)	24.4 (20.0–28.4)	25.3 (20.8–29.5)	29.0 (24.9–33.5)	28.4 (23.5–32.9)
Congestive heart failure	2.02 (1.39–2.65)	23.6 (10.6–33.4)	23.8 (10.7–33.6)	25.2 (11.4–35.3)	28.3 (13.1–39.0)	19.2 (8.3–27.8)	20.0 (8.7–28.8)	23.2 (10.3–32.2)	22.7 (10.1–32.2)
Chronic kidney disease	3.56 (2.72–4.39)	43.7 (34.3–50.7)	44.0 (34.5–51.0)	45.8 (36.2–52.8)	49.8 (40.0–56.8)	37.4 (28.6–44.2)	38.6 (29.7–45.4)	43.1 (33.7–50.1)	42.2 (33.1–49.4)

Source: Based on CDC.[1]

[a]Population-attributable risks were calculated using Levin's formula.[35] Estimates of the prevalence of hypertension were taken from Table 13-2, and 95% confidence intervals were calculated using the 95% confidence bounds from the pooled risk ratios.

[b]Relative risks were calculated by the author by pooling the estimates from references cited in text (for coronary heart disease the relative risks were 1.78 in Whites, 2.18 in Blacks, 2.02 in Hispanics, 1.70 in men, and 2.02 in women).

[c]Overall prevalence of hypertension was as follows: White men/women: 30.4%/30.7%; Black men/women: 33.0%/38.8%; Hispanic men/women: 23.3%/24.6%.

<60 mL/min per 1.73 m^2) than those with normal blood pressure,[49–53] and the risk increases progressively with higher levels of blood pressure. The strength of the association between blood pressure and chronic kidney disease is similar in men and women[52] and in Blacks and Whites.[54]

About 20% of all cases of coronary heart disease are attributable to hypertension (Table 13-4). However, the proportion of attributable cases seems to be higher in Black women (31%) and men (28%) than in other race/gender groups. The larger absolute impact in Black men and women is attributable to both a higher relative risk and a higher prevalence of hypertension. Approximately 28% of all strokes, 23% of all cases of congestive heart failure, and 42% of all cases of chronic kidney disease are attributable to hypertension, and the impact is higher in Blacks than in all other racial/ethnic groups. Overall, about one out of every four cases of cardiovascular disease in the United States could theoretically be prevented by eliminating hypertension.

The population attributable risks presented in Table 13-4 likely underestimate the impact of elevated blood pressure because they do not take into account that the risk of developing cardiovascular and renal disease increases even with blood pressure levels within the "normal range" (SBP <140 mm Hg and DBP <90 mm Hg). Indeed, according to Vasan et al.[55] individuals with SBP between 130 and 139 mm Hg and DBP between 85 and 89 mm Hg are 2.5 and 1.6 times more likely to develop cardiovascular disease, respectively, than are those with SBP less than 120 mm Hg and DBP less than 80 mm Hg. In the ARIC study, the risk of ischemic stroke increased about 50% for each increase of 19 mm Hg in SBP.[42] In addition, in the Framingham cohort an increase of 20 mm Hg in SBP or 10 mm Hg in DBP was associated with corresponding increases of 56% and 24%, respectively, in the incidence of congestive heart failure.[56] Finally, an increase of 16 mm Hg in SBP or 10 mm Hg in DBP resulted in a similar increase of 76% in the risk of end-stage renal disease.[49]

Given the differences in baseline risk of cardiovascular and renal disease, the relative effect of blood pressure is larger in younger persons, but the absolute effect is larger in older individuals. The impact of blood pressure on disease incidence also depends on the type of blood pressure. In adults younger than 50, DBP is the strongest predictor of coronary heart disease. From 50 to 59 years of age, SBP, DBP, and their difference (pulse pressure) are equally predictive of coronary heart disease. For those 60 years and older, pulse pressure becomes a better predictor than SBP, and for them higher levels of DBP are associated with lower risk of coronary heart disease.[57] Moreover, SBP seems to be a better predictor of stroke incidence than DBP and pulse pressure.[58] SBP and pulse pressure also confer a greater risk of congestive heart disease than DBP.[56] Although all blood pressure measurements are directly associated with increased risk of chronic kidney disease, results from a large observational study and from several clinical trials suggest that SBP is a stronger predictor of chronic kidney disease than DBP and pulse pressure.[59]

RISK FACTORS

Various genetic and environmental factors promote the development and persistence of hypertension (Figure 13-1). Nonmodifiable risk factors include age, gender, and genetic susceptibility. Known modifiable risk factors include high dietary intake of sodium and low dietary intake of potassium, alcohol intake, obesity, and low levels of physical activity. Other potential risk factors have been identified, but it remains uncertain whether they have an independent effect on blood pressure levels. These potential risk factors include low birthweight; socioeconomic status; insulin resistance; dietary intake of fat, protein, calcium, and fiber; mild chronic inflammation; and psychological and emotional stress.

Genetic Factors

Blood pressure level aggregates in families, partly because of shared genetic predisposition. About 40% of the variability in blood pressure is explained by genetic factors, and the risk of developing hypertension in persons younger than 50 years doubles for each first-degree relative with a history of hypertension.[60] However, identifying genetic causes has been particularly difficult because blood pressure is regulated by multiple mechanisms involving multiple nonallelic genes with small additive effects. The altered mechanism cannot be identified in 90% of the cases because hypertension looks the same in all individuals. This compromises our ability to identify gene variants (alleles) or combinations of variants (haplotypes) associated with the development of hypertension.

Obesity

Excessive accumulation of body fat commonly leads to higher blood pressure. This effect could be mediated by overactivation of the sympathetic nervous system and the renin-angiotensin system and by alterations in endothelial and renal function. The prevalence of hypertension in US adults (NHANES 2009–2020) increases progressively with body mass index (BMI: weight in kilograms/[height in meters]^2), from 13.5% in those with normal BMI (<25 kg/m^2) to 32.4% in those with overweight (BMI ≥25 and <30 kg/m^2) and 44.1% in those with obesity (BMI ≥30 kg/m^2). Combining data from two large cohort studies, Field et al.[61] showed that the risk of hypertension increased 2.1, 2.7, 2.4, and 3.9 times in overweight women, obese women, overweight men, and obese men, respectively, compared to those with normal BMI. About 46% of all new cases of hypertension in men and women in the United States could be attributed to overweight (Table 13-5). The population-attributable risk is slightly higher in men than in women among Whites and Hispanics. However, among Blacks the population-attributable risk is

Table 13-5. Relative Risk and Population Attributable Risk for Risk Factors for Hypertension: National Health and Nutrition Examination Survey (NHANES), United States, 2009–March 2020

Risk Factor	Relative Risk[a]	Population-Attributable Risk, %
Overweight and obesity	2.5	46.5
Salt intake (>4.6 g/d)	1.5[b]	30.4
Alcohol intake in men[c]	1.2	15.5
Alcohol intake in women[c]	1.5	5.0
Low physical activity[d]	1.7	16.6

Source: Based on CDC[1] and Khaw et al.[62]

[a]Relative risks were calculated by pooling the estimates mentioned in the text, and prevalence of risk factors came from NHANES 2015-2020.

[b]This is a conservative estimate based on the report of Khaw et al.[62]

[c]Exposure corresponds to ≥1 drink/d in men and ≥4 drinks/d in women.

[d]Exposure corresponds to < 3 hr/wk of moderate or vigorous physical activity.

about 50% in men and 45% in women. Corresponding figures are 38% and 33% in Asian Americans. Multiple randomized controlled trials of nonpharmacological weight reduction interventions have corroborated the effect of obesity on blood pressure (see Lifestyle Modifications).[63]

Salt Intake

A high dietary intake of salt (sodium chloride) is associated with the development of hypertension. A high intake of salt over prolonged periods compromises the kidneys' capacity to excrete sodium, leading to a persistent increase in blood volume and blood pressure. The International Study of Salt and Blood Pressure (INTERSALT), a standardized epidemiologic study of more than 10,000 persons from 32 countries, showed that an increase of 100 millimoles (mmol) per day of urinary sodium (an additional intake of ~5 g of salt) increased SBP by 3 to 6 mm Hg and DBP by 0 to 3 mm Hg.[64] In a prospective study of more than 23,000 individuals, SBP and DBP were 7.2 and 3.0 mm Hg higher, respectively, in those with a daily salt intake 12.6 grams or more per day compared to 4.6 grams or less.[62] Accordingly, the risk of having a SBP equal to or greater than 160 mm Hg was about 2.5 times higher in those in the highest compared to those in the lowest salt intake. These findings were consistent with those from a multinational cohort study based on urinary sodium excretion.[65] For each increase of 1g in estimated daily sodium intake, SBP increased by 1.30 and 2.49 mm Hg and DBP by 0.58 and 0.91 mm Hg in normotensive and hypertensive individuals, respectively. In fact, the population-attributable risk of hypertension for a salt intake of more than 4.6 grams per day is about 30% in the United States (Table 13-5). The effect of salt intake on blood pressure increases with age[64,65] and has been confirmed in multiple randomized controlled trials of sodium intake reduction.[66] The reduction in blood pressure seems to be stronger when the reduction in salt intake is combined with other dietary changes.[67]

Potassium Intake

Increased dietary intake of potassium has been associated with lower blood pressure. Administration of dietary potassium increases renal sodium and chloride excretion, reduces blood volume, and decreases blood pressure. A concurrent decrease of 1.24 mm Hg in SBP (95% CI, 0.31–2.70) per 1,000 mg per day increase in potassium intake was observed in a large representative sample of the US population, with an average intake of 2,745 mg per day.[68] Individuals in the upper quartile of potassium intake were 28% less likely to be hypertensive (95% CI, 0.03–0.47). These associations were consistent across age, gender, race/ethnicity, obesity, and education. However, in a large international cohort study, systolic and diastolic blood pressure increased by 1.08 (95% CI, 0.97–1.19) and 0.09 mm Hg for each increment of 1 g per day in estimated potassium excretion.[65] The lack of a significant effect of potassium intake in this study could be explained by sodium intake and by a low sensitivity of the method used, since urinary excretion of dietary potassium is lower than that of dietary sodium. An inverse relationship between potassium intake and blood pressure has been corroborated in multiple studies.[69]

Alcohol Intake

There is ample evidence linking alcohol intake and hypertension. Although the biological mechanisms of its long-term effect on blood pressure are unclear, the hypertensive effect of alcohol intake has been documented in cross-sectional and cohort studies.[24] In the ARIC study, participants who drank three or more drinks per day were 1.2 to 2.3 times more likely to develop hypertension after six years of follow-up.[24] In addition, a low-to-moderate alcohol intake (≤3 drinks/d) was associated with higher incidence of hypertension or increased blood pressure in Blacks but not in Whites, suggesting higher alcohol sensitivity among Blacks.

In a recent meta-analysis of cohort studies, including more than 90,000 incident cases, the relative risks of hypertension were 1.19 (95% CI, 1.07–1.31), 1.51 (1.30–1.76), and 1.74 (1.35–2.24) for men consuming one to two, three to four, and five or more drinks/day (12 g of pure ethanol/drink).[70] However, the relative risks were 0.94 (95% CI, 0.88–1.01) and 1.42 (1.22–1.66) in women consuming one to two and more than two drinks per day, respectively. Thus, alcohol intake seems to have a stronger effect in men than in women, and light-to-moderate alcohol intake seems to be protective in women but not in men.

The effect of alcohol intake on blood pressure has also been demonstrated in randomized clinical trials of alcohol reduction[71] and increase[72] in alcohol intake.

Physical Activity

Leisure time physical activity is inversely associated with blood pressure level. Long-term physical activity lowers blood pressure by reducing stroke volume, systemic arterial resistance, sympathetic activity, urinary sodium retention, and insulin resistance. In a meta-analysis of cohort studies including 330,222 participants and 67,698 new cases, people with high versus low leisure-time physical activity were 16% (95% CI, 10–22) less likely to develop hypertension.[73] The risk of hypertension was 6% lower (95% CI, 3–8) per each 10 additional metabolic equivalents of activity per hour per week. Findings were similar for leisure-time and total physical activity and for men and women.

No beneficial effects of physical activity on blood pressure were observed in Blacks from the ARIC[74] and the Coronary Artery Risk Development in (Young) Adults (CARDIA) cohorts.[75] However, in a study using a physical activity questionnaire validated for use with Blacks, the hazard ratio was 0.76 (95% CI, 0.58–0.99) when comparing participants with ideal versus poor levels of moderate-to-vigorous physical activity.[76]

Multiple randomized clinical trials have shown that aerobic physical training results in significant reductions in systolic and diastolic blood pressure.[77] Low physical activity carries a population-attributable risk for hypertension of about 17% (Table 13-5).

EVIDENCE-BASED INTERVENTIONS

Prevention

Interventions to diminish the health burden of hypertension could and should be implemented at the individual and population levels. At the individual level, preventive interventions are aimed at high-risk persons, with the goal of limiting their risk of becoming hypertensive (primary prevention). Preventive interventions are also aimed at hypertensive and prehypertensive individuals, with the goal of avoiding the cardiovascular, neurological, renal, and ocular consequences of hypertension (secondary prevention). At the population level, prevention is aimed at a collection of individuals, with the goal of shifting the whole blood pressure distribution to lower values.

Significance of Primary Prevention Strategies

Primary and secondary prevention are complementary strategies. Even modest decreases in average blood pressure can delay the onset of hypertension and substantially reduce hypertension-related morbidity and mortality. A considerably larger reduction on disease burden could be achieved through primary prevention interventions in the whole population than by secondary prevention because the number of persons with normal blood pressure is considerably larger than the number of those with pre-hypertension and hypertension. A population-wide hypothetical reduction of 2 mm Hg in SBP in

Whites participating in the ARIC study would result in a decrease of 27, 24, and 41 cases of coronary heart disease, stroke, and heart failure per 100,000 person-years, respectively.[78] Corresponding reductions in Blacks would be 18, 19, and 27 cases per 100,000 person-years. In contrast, a 10% proportional reduction in unaware, untreated, or uncontrolled blood pressure would achieve significantly smaller reductions.

Lifestyle Modifications (Nonpharmacological Interventions)

Primary prevention of hypertension involves detection and management of modifiable risk factors through lifestyle changes. Lifestyle modifications recommended for primary prevention in individuals are also recommended as interventions to reduce blood pressure in the general population.[5,29] The efficacy of lifestyle changes in decreasing blood pressure and reducing the incidence of hypertension has been shown in randomized clinical trials.[79]

Weight Reduction

In a meta-analysis of 25 randomized clinical trials of weight control, bodyweight reduction of 1 kg was associated with a decrease of approximately 1 mm Hg in both SBP and DBP (Table 13-6).[63] Similar to other lifestyle modification interventions, the beneficial effect of weight loss tends to be larger in hypertensive patients than in non-hypertensives and to weaken with time. In a meta-analysis of trials with longer follow-up (≥2 years) the

Table 13-6. Effects of Lifestyle Interventions to Reduce Blood Pressure, Quantified in Randomized Controlled Trials

Intervention	Change in Risk Factor	Reduction in Blood Pressure (mm Hg)		Recommended Level
		Systolic	Diastolic	
Weight loss[58]	−1 kg	1.0	1.0	BMI 18.5–24.9 kg/m^2
Reduce sodium intake[80]	75 mmol/d urinary sodium	4.2	2.1	100 mmol/d (5.7 g salt/day)
Increase potassium Intake[81,82]	75 mmol/d (supplement)	3.1	2.0	120 mmol/d (4.7 g/day, diet)
Moderation in alcohol intake[83]	−50%	5.5	4.0	≤2 drinks/d in men ≤1 drink/d in women
Aerobic physical activity[84]	≥3 sessions/wk 30–60 min	5.1	2.2	30 min/d, most d of the wk
DASH diet[85]	Diet rich in fruits, vegetables, and low-fat dairy products, and low in saturated and total fat	5.5	3.0	Regularly

Note: BMI = body mass index; DASH = Dietary Approach to Stop Hypertension.

decrease in blood pressure was about half that observed in shorter trials.[84] However, in a trial in individuals with high-normal blood pressure, body weight was similar in both groups, but the incidence of hypertension was still 77% lower in the weight loss intervention group than in the control group. Randomized clinical trials also suggest that patients require less intensive antihypertensive drug therapy if they follow a weight-reducing diet.[85] The American Heart Association (AHA) recommends maintaining a BMI of less than 25 kg/m^2 in those 20 years or older.[29]

Reduction in Salt Intake

Numerous studies support a blood pressure-lowering effect of reduced salt intake. In a meta-analysis of 34 studies, an average urinary sodium decrease of 75 mmol per day (~4.4 g/d of salt) reduced diastolic and systolic blood pressure 4.2 and 2.1 mm Hg, respectively (Table 13-6).[86] Blood pressure reduction was at least two times larger in hypertensive than in normotensive subjects (SBP: –5.39 vs. –2.42 mm Hg; DBP: –2.82 vs. –1.00 mm Hg). The effect of reduced sodium intake seems to be stronger in older and non-White individuals. These findings are consistent with those from a more recent meta-analysis.[87] In addition, hypertensive patients following a low-salt diet have a lower need for antihypertensive medication.[88]

AHA currently recommends a maximum sodium intake of 1.5 g per day (3.8 g/d of salt) in all persons with hypertension, all middle-aged and older adults, and all Blacks, and a maximum of 2.3 g per day (5.8 g/d of salt) in the rest of the population.[29]

Increase in Potassium Intake

A consistently inverse relationship between increased potassium intake and blood pressure has been shown in cohort studies[65] and randomized trials (Table 13-6). In a meta-analysis, potassium supplementation (median: 75 mmol/d) reduced systolic and diastolic blood pressure by 3.1 mm Hg and 2.0 mm Hg, respectively.[89] The average effect size was larger in hypertensive subjects and in Blacks. Moreover, the effect of potassium supplementation on blood pressure is larger in the context of a concurrent high intake of sodium and vice versa. However, in a meta-analysis of trials with a duration of four weeks or longer, a low (30 mmol/d) and high (>80 mmol/d) urinary potassium excretion increased blood pressure, particularly in participants with hypertension,[90] and cohort studies of the effect of potassium intake on cardiovascular diseases have given mixed results.[91]

On the basis of findings from randomized clinical trials, AHA sets the recommended potassium intake level of about 4.7 gr per day in healthy individuals.[92] It is important to note that this level of potassium intake can and should be achieved through consumption of fruits, vegetables, and nuts in the diet, instead of diet pill supplements.

Reduction in Alcohol Intake

A dose-dependent association between high alcohol intake (≥1 drink/d) and risk of hypertension has been documented in observational and experimental studies. Light-to-moderate alcohol consumption seems to decrease hypertension risk in women and increase it in men, with cut points for harmful effects of four or more drinks per day in women and only one or more drinks per day in men. Results from a meta-analysis including 36 trials with 2,865 participants indicated that SBP decreases by 5.50 mm Hg and DBP by 3.97 mm Hg in participants who drank six or more drinks per day and reduced their intake by half (Table 13-6).[81] The effect of alcohol reduction in hypertensive individuals with low intake and in women remains uncertain. Alcohol intake should be limited to no more than two drinks per day in most men and no more than one drink per day in women and lighter-weight persons (1 drink = 12 oz of regular beer, 5 oz of wine, or 1.5 oz of 80-proof distilled spirits).[92]

Increase in Physical Activity

Regular physical activity lowers blood pressure and prevents the development of hypertension. In a recent meta-analysis of 24 trials, aerobic physical training decreased SBP and DBP by 5.09 and 2.20 mm Hg, respectively (Table 13-6).[82] These effects were stronger in individuals aged 65 years or older. The effect of physical activity on blood pressure seems to be slightly greater in hypertensive subjects, independent of baseline body weight and weight loss. AHA recommends 150 or more minutes per week of moderate-intensity, 75 minutes per week of vigorous-intensity, or 150 minutes or more per week of moderate-plus vigorous-intensity physical activity.[93]

The DASH Diet

A considerable proportion of the between-population variability in blood pressure could be explained not by differences in single nutrients but by large variations in dietary patterns. The effect of three dietary patterns on blood pressure was evaluated in the Dietary Approach to Stop Hypertension (DASH) trial, a controlled dietary intervention study.[67,83] The DASH trial included 133 hypertensive and 326 normotensive adults who received carefully controlled diets for 11 weeks. One group received a control diet low in fruits, vegetables, and dairy products, with a fat content typical of the average diet in the United States; the second group received a diet rich in fruits and vegetables; and the third group received the DASH diet (i.e., a combination diet rich in fruits, vegetables, and low-fat dairy products and with reduced saturated and total fat). The DASH diet significantly reduced SBP and DBP by 5.5 and 3.0 mm Hg more, respectively, than the control diet (Table 13-6). The effect of the DASH diet was significantly larger among participants with hypertension (reductions of 11.4 and 5.5 mm Hg in SBP and DBP, respectively) and among Blacks compared with Whites (6.9 vs. 3.3 mm Hg in SBP and 3.7 vs. 2.4 mm Hg in DBP, respectively).[83] Importantly, the effect of the DASH diet was evident within the first two weeks of the trial. The benefits of the DASH diet have been confirmed in meta-analyses of randomized trials,[94] and it is currently recommended by AHA as a way to prevent and treat hypertension.[29]

Screening

Screening for hypertension has a substantial net benefit because blood pressure can be reliably and safely measured, and treating hypertensive patients significantly reduces their risk of cardiovascular morbidity and mortality. The US Preventive Services Task Force recommends screening for hypertension in adults 18 years or older with office blood pressure measurement and obtaining blood pressure measurements outside of the clinical setting for diagnostic confirmation before starting treatment. Screening should be conducted yearly in adults 40 years or older and in all adults at increased risk for hypertension, and every three to five years, as appropriate, for adults aged 18 to 39 years without a high risk of hypertension.[95] Although high salt and low potassium intake are also risk factors for hypertension, they are difficult to identify in the context of a regular clinic visit.

As a consequence of regular screening, hypertension awareness improved progressively in the United States, from 68% in 1990 to 2000 to 83% in 2011 to 2012, to 85.3% in 2013 to 2014. However, it decreased to 79.7% in 2017 to 2020. The United States also experienced a decrease in the proportion of treated patients, from 96.8% in 2009 to 2010 to 92.6% in 2017 to 2020, and in the proportion of treated patients with controlled blood pressure, from 51.2% in 2009 to 2014 to 45.9% in 2017 to 2020.

Treatment

Strategies for treating patients with hypertension include nonpharmacological and pharmacological therapy. Their goal is to prevent the development of hypertension-related cardiovascular and renal disease (secondary prevention). Nonpharmacologic interventions are based on the lifestyle prevention strategies already described. Lifestyle interventions decrease SBP and DBP by 4 to 5 mm Hg and 2 to 4 mm Hg, respectively.[79] However, the DASH diet could decrease SBP by approximately 11 mm Hg.[83]

Nonpharmacologic interventions are recommended in adult patients with Stage 1 hypertension (130–139/80–89 mm Hg, systolic/diastolic) and otherwise at low risk of atherosclerotic cardiovascular disease (ASCVD). These patients should be reevaluated after three to six months of nonpharmacologic therapy.[5]

Pharmacological therapy, which involves blood pressure–lowering drugs, is recommended for all adults with an average SBP of 140 mm Hg or higher or DBP of 90 mm Hg

Table 13-7. Management of High Blood Pressure According to American College of Cardiology and the American Heart Association 2017 Guidelines

BP Stage	Systolic BP (mm Hg)		Diastolic BP (mm Hg)	Starting Treatment
Normal	<120	and	<80	NPT (encourage lifestyle modifications)
Elevated	120–129	or	<80	NPT
Stage 1 hypertension	130–139	or	80–89	• 10-y risk of CVD <10% and no or ASCVD→ NPT • 10-y risk of CVD ≥10% or ASCVD→ NPT + BPLD
Stage 2 hypertension	≥140	or	≥90	NPT + BPLD

Source: Based on Whelton et al.[5]

Note: ASCVD = atherosclerotic cardiovascular disease; BP = blood pressure; BPLD = blood pressure-lowering drugs; CVD = cardiovascular disease; NPT = nonpharmacological therapy. All patients with BP≥120/80 mm Hg and a compelling indication (heart failure, post-myocardial infarction, high risk of coronary heart disease, diabetes, chronic kidney disease, or recurrent stroke) should receive drugs for the compelling indication independently of their BP level.

or higher (Table 13-7), regardless of their baseline risk of ASCVD, and in adults 65 years or older with a SBP of 130 mm Hg or higher, those with Stage 1 hypertension at high risk of ASCVD, and those with diabetes or chronic kidney disease.[5] A high risk of ASCVD corresponds to a probability of 10% or greater of developing a cardiovascular event in the next 10 years.[96] A reevaluation of blood pressure levels should be conducted in one month in all patients receiving pharmacological therapy, and treatment should be adjusted, if needed, in order to achieve therapeutic targets.

Initial first-line therapy for Stage 1 hypertension includes thiazide diuretics, calcium channel blockers, angiotensin-converting enzyme inhibitors, or angiotensin receptor blockers. Two first-line drugs of different classes are recommended for patients with Stage 2 hypertension and an average blood pressure 20/10 mm Hg above their blood pressure target.[5] Most hypertensive patients requiring pharmacological therapy should be initially treated with two drugs of different classes. Improved adherence can be achieved with once-daily drug dosing, rather than multiple dosing, and with combination therapy rather than separate administration of each individual drug. The therapeutic target for drug-treated hypertensive patients with previous cardiovascular disease or a ten-year risk of 10% or greater is an SBP/DBP less than 130/80 mm Hg. This is also a desirable target in patients without other conditions and a risk of ASCVD less than 10% in 10 years.[5]

Adults with Stage 2 hypertension should be evaluated by a primary care provider within one month of initial diagnosis. They should be treated with a combination of nonpharmacologic therapy and two antihypertensive drugs of different classes. In individuals with SBP of 160 mm Hg or higher or DBP of 100 mm Hg or higher, expeditious evaluation and drug treatment, followed by careful monitoring and upward dose adjustment, is recommended.[5]

Every adult with hypertension should have a clear, detailed, and current evidence-based plan of care that ensures the achievement of treatment and self-management goals, effective management of comorbid conditions, and timely health care follow-up. Effective behavioral and motivational strategies are recommended to promote lifestyle modification.[97] A structured team-based approach, including a physician, nurse, and pharmacist, is also recommended, along with integrating home-based monitoring and telehealth interventions.[5]

There is irrefutable evidence that treatment of hypertensive patients with commonly used drugs greatly reduces the risk of cardiovascular events and that the reduction in risk is proportional to the reduction in blood pressure, and this occurs in patients with both low and high cardiovascular risk and in those with and without diabetes.[98] In spite of the proven benefit of blood pressure lowering, current rates of hypertension treatment and control in the United States remain unsatisfactory, particularly in young people, men, minority groups, and those with low socioeconomic status.[34] In addition, there has been a decrease in recent years in the proportion of people with hypertension who are aware, treated, and have controlled blood pressure (see Screening section earlier in this chapter). Failure by patients to use medications as prescribed is a major contributor to poor blood pressure control and is largely the result of treatment nonadherence.

MOVING FORWARD

In spite of significant progress in the diagnosis and management of hypertension in the past few decades, hypertension prevalence remains high in middle- and high-income countries and is increasing in low-income countries. Knowledge of factors driving the increase and persistence of hypertension in most world populations is needed to develop and implement ethnic/racial and culturally appropriate interventions. Little is known about heterogeneity in the prevalence and in the effect of established risk factors, such as obesity and increased salt intake across diverse populations. Research efforts should also be focused on the identification of genetic, environmental, and behavioral factors that lead to a persistent impaired pressure natriuresis early in life, even before the diagnosis of hypertension. Promising avenues include the role of vascular oxidative stress, adhesion molecules, inflammatory cytokines, and psychosocial stress on blood pressure regulation.

Poor medication adherence, which occurs in about 50% of newly treated hypertensive patients within the first year of treatment, is a main cause of uncontrolled hypertension, which in turn increases overall mortality, hospitalization, and cost of care. Further research on factors useful to predict short- and long-term adherence could have a significant impact on designing adherence-enhancing interventions, targeting patients who may benefit from those interventions, and reducing hypertension-related morbidity and mortality.

Self-monitoring of blood pressure seems to have a limited effect on blood pressure control in treated individuals. However, most available studies did not take into account the discrepancies between office and out-of-office measurements, and repeated self-measurements following a standard protocol are more likely to detect smaller but clinically important changes in blood pressure than office measurements. Therefore, more studies are needed to clarify the role of self-monitoring on blood pressure control.

In addition, there is clear evidence that treating hypertensive patients to lower blood pressure targets results in a large (~25%) reduction in the risk of cardiovascular and all-cause mortality. This begs the question of whether current cut points to define hypertension and blood pressure therapeutic targets should be lowered, and among whom, as a way to improve cardiovascular disease prevention.

Further research is also needed to clarify the relative benefits of treating patients to a target blood pressure or to a target level of cardiovascular risk.

DISCUSSION QUESTIONS

1. Which factors may be major contributors to the high prevalence of hypertension in middle- and high-income countries?
2. Out of the available interventions for primary prevention of hypertension, which ones do you think could be more cost-effective in the United States? What about middle- and low-income countries?
3. Out of the available interventions for secondary prevention, in patients with hypertension, which ones do you think could be more cost-effective in the United States?
4. Discuss why high blood pressure is one of the top three strongest determinants of the global burden of health.

REFERENCES

1. Centers for Disease Control and Prevention, National Center for Health Statistics. The National Health and Nutrition Examination Survey: NHANES survey methods and analytic guidelines. 2006. Available at: https://wwwn.cdc.gov/nchs/nhanes/analyticguidelines.aspx. Accessed May 10, 2023.
2. Evans JG, Rose G. Hypertension. *BrMed Bull.* 1971;27(1):37–42.
3. Zanchetti A, Mancia G. Longing for clinical excellence: a critical outlook into the NICE recommendations on hypertension management—is nice always good? *J Hypertens.* 2012; 30(4):660–668. doi:10.1097/HJH.0b013e328351b4e4
4. Stergiou GS, Palatini P, Parati G, et al. 2021 European Society of Hypertension practice guidelines for office and out-of-office blood pressure measurement. *J Hypertens.* 2021;39(7): 1293–1302.
5. Whelton PK, Carey RM, Aronow WS, et al. 2017 ACC/AHA/AAPA/ABC/ACPM/AGS/ APhA/ASH/ASPC/NMA/PCNA Guideline for the prevention, detection, evaluation, and

management of high blood pressure in adults. *J Am Coll Cardiol.* 2018; 71(19):e127–e248. doi:10.1016/j.jacc.2017.11.006

6. Krakoff LR. Blood pressure out of the office: its time has finally come. *Am J Hypertens.* 2016;29(3):289–295. doi:10.1093/ajh/hpv179
7. Hodgkinson J, Mant J, Martin U, et al. Relative effectiveness of clinic and home blood pressure monitoring compared with ambulatory blood pressure monitoring in diagnosis of hypertension: systematic review. *BMJ.* 2011;342:d3621. doi:10.1136/bmj.d3621
8. Piper MA, Evans CV, Burda BU, Margolis KL, O'Connor E, Whitlock EP. Diagnostic and predictive accuracy of blood pressure screening methods with consideration of rescreening intervals: a systematic review for the US Preventive Services Task Force. *Ann Intern Med.* 2015;162(3):192–204. doi:10.7326/M14-1539
9. Roerecke M, Kaczorowski J, Myers MG. Comparing automated office blood pressure readings with other methods of blood pressure measurement for identifying patients with possible hypertension: a systematic review and meta-analysis. *JAMA IntMed.* 2019;179(3):351–362. doi:10.1001/jamainternmed.2018.6551
10. Rabi DM, McBrien KA, Sapir-Pichhadze R, et al. Hypertension Canada's 2020 comprehensive guidelines for the prevention, diagnosis, risk assessment, and treatment of hypertension in adults and ahildren. *Can J Cardiol.* 2020;36(5):596–624. doi:10.1016/j.cjca.2020.02.086
11. Williams B, Mancia G, Spiering W, et al. 2018 ESC/ESH guidelines for the management of arterial hypertension. *Eur Heart J.* 2018;39(33):3021–3104. doi:10.1093/eurheartj/ehy339
12. Jones NR, McCormack T, Constanti M, McManus RJ. Diagnosis and management of hypertension in adults: NICE guideline update 2019. *Br J Gen Pract.* 2020;70(691):90. doi:10.3399/bjgp20X708053
13. Umemura S, Arima H, Arima S, et al. The Japanese Society of Hypertension Guidelines for the Management of Hypertension (JSH 2019). *Hypertens Res.* 2019;42(9):1235–1481. doi:10.1038/s41440-019-0284-9
14. Unger T, Borghi C, Charchar F, et al. 2020 International Society of Hypertension Global Hypertension Practice Guidelines. *Hypertension.* 2020;75(6):1334–1357. doi:10.1161/HYPERTENSIONAHA.120.15026
15. Zhou B, Carrillo-Larco RM, Danaei G, et al. Worldwide trends in hypertension prevalence and progress in treatment and control from 1990 to 2019: a pooled analysis of 1201 population-representative studies with 104 million participants. *Lancet.* 2021;398(10304):957–980. doi:10.1016/S0140-6736(21)01330-1
16. NCD Risk Factor Collaboration. Contributions of mean and shape of blood pressure distribution to worldwide trends and variations in raised blood pressure: a pooled analysis of 1018 population-based measurement studies with 88.6 million participants. *Int J Epidemiol.* 2018; 47(3):872–883i. doi:10.1093/ije/dyy016
17. Zhou B, Bentham J, Di Cesare M, et al. Worldwide trends in blood pressure from 1975 to 2015: a pooled analysis of 1479 population-based measurement studies with 19.1 million participants. *Lancet.* 2017;389(10064):37–55. doi:10.1016/S0140-6736(16)31919-5
18. Asayama K, Thijs L, Li Y, et al. Setting thresholds to varying blood pressure monitoring intervals differentially affects risk estimates associated with white-coat and masked hypertension

in the population. *Hypertension.* 2014;64(5):935–942. doi:10.1161/HYPERTENSIONAHA.114.03614

19. Shimbo D, Kuruvilla S, Haas D, Pickering TG, Schwartz JE, Gerin W. Preventing misdiagnosis of ambulatory hypertension: algorithm using office and home blood pressures. *J Hypertens.* 2009;27(9):1775–1783. doi:10.1097/HJH.0b013e32832db8b9
20. Lewington S, Clarke R, Qizilbash N, Peto R, Collins R. Age-specific relevance of usual blood pressure to vascular mortality: a meta-analysis of individual data for one million adults in 61 prospective studies. *Lancet.* 2002;360(9349):1903–1913. https://doi.org/10.1016/S0140-6736(02)11911-8
21. Forouzanfar MH, Liu P, Roth GA, et al. Global burden of hypertension and systolic blood pressure of at least 110 to 115 mm Hg, 1990–2015. *JAMA.* 2017;317(2):165–182. doi:10.1001/jama.2016.19043
22. Lim SS, Vos T, Flaxman AD, et al. A comparative risk assessment of burden of disease and injury attributable to 67 risk factors and risk factor clusters in 21 regions, 1990–2010: a systematic analysis for the Global Burden of Disease Study 2010. *Lancet.* 2012;380(9859):2224–2260. doi:10.1016/S0140-6736(12)61766-8
23. Parikh NI, Pencina MJ, Wang TJ, et al. A risk score for predicting near-term incidence of hypertension: the Framingham Heart Study. *Ann Intern Med.* 2008;148(2):102–110. doi:10.7326/0003-4819-148-2-200801150-00005
24. Fuchs FD, Chambless LE, Whelton PK, Nieto FJ, Heiss G. Alcohol consumption and the incidence of hypertension: the Atherosclerosis Risk in Communities Study. *Hypertension.* 2001;37(5):1242–1250. doi:10.1161/01.HYP.37.5.1242
25. Carson AP, Howard G, Burke GL, Shea S, Levitan EB, Muntner P. Ethnic differences in hypertension incidence among middle-aged and older adults: the multi-ethnic study of atherosclerosis. *Hypertension.* 2011;57(6):1101–1107. doi:10.1161/HYPERTENSIONAHA.110.168005
26. Vasan RS, Levy D. Rates of progression to hypertension among non-hypertensive subjects: implications for blood pressure screening. *Eur Heart J.* 2002;23(14):1067–1070. doi:10.1053/euhj.2002.3223
27. Sheps SG, Black HR, Cohen JD, et al. The sixth report of the Joint National Committee on prevention, detection, evaluation, and treatment of high blood pressure. *Arch Intern Med.* 1997;157(21):2413–2446.
28. Vasan RS, Larson MG, Leip EP, Kannel WB, Levy D. Assessment of frequency of progression to hypertension in non-hypertensive participants in the Framingham Heart Study: a cohort study. *Lancet.* 2001;358(9294):1682–1686. doi:10.1016/S0140-6736(01)06710-1
29. Tsao CW, Aday AW, Almarzooq ZI, et al. Heart disease and stroke statistics—2022 update: a report from the American Heart Association. *Circulation.* 2022;145(8):e153–e639. doi:10.1161/CIR.0000000000001052
30. Shah NS, Molsberry R, Rana JS, et al. Heterogeneous trends in burden of heart disease mortality by subtypes in the United States, 1999–2018: observational analysis of vital statistics. *BMJ.* 2020;370:m2688. doi:10.1136/bmj.m2688
31. Kershaw KN, Diez Roux AV, Carnethon M, et al. Geographic variation in hypertension prevalence among Blacks and Whites: the multi-ethnic study of atherosclerosis. *Am J Hypertens.* 2010;23(1):46–53. https://doi.org/10.1038/ajh.2009.211

32. Burt VL, Cutler JA, Higgins M, et al. Trends in the prevalence, awareness, treatment, and control of hypertension in the adult US population. data from the health examination surveys, 1960 to 1991. *Hypertension*. 1995;26(1):60–69. doi:10.1161/01.HYP.26.1.60
33. Hajjar I, Kotchen TA. Trends in prevalence, awareness, treatment, and control of hypertension in the United States, 1988–2000. *JAMA*. 2003;290(2):199–206. doi:10.1001/jama.290.2.199
34. Whelton PK. The elusiveness of population-wide high blood pressure control. *Annu Rev Public Health*. 2015;36:109–130. doi:10.1146/annurev-publhealth-031914-122949
35. Levin ML. The occurrence of lung cancer in man. *Acta-Unio Internationalis Contra Cancrum*. 1953;9(3):531–541.
36. Kannel WB. Blood pressure as a cardiovascular risk factor: prevention and treatment. *JAMA*. 1996;275(20):1571–1576. doi:10.1001/jama.1996.03530440051036
37. Jones DW, Chambless LE, Folsom AR, et al. Risk factors for coronary heart disease in African Americans: the atherosclerosis risk in communities study, 1987–1997. *Arch Intern Med*. 2002;162(22):2565–2571. doi:10.1001/archinte.162.22.2565
38. Nilsson PM, Nilsson JÅ, Berglund G. Population-attributable risk of coronary heart disease risk factors during long-term follow-up: the Malmö Preventive Project. *J Intern Med*. 2006;260(2):134–141. doi:10.1111/j.1365-2796.2006.01671.x
39. Hu G, Jousilahti P, Tuomilehto J. Joint effects of history of hypertension at baseline and type 2 diabetes at baseline and during follow-up on the risk of coronary heart disease. *Eur Heart J*. 2007;28(24):3059–3066. doi:10.1093/eurheartj/ehm501
40. D'Agostino RB, Sr., Grundy S, Sullivan LM, Wilson P. Validation of the Framingham coronary heart disease prediction scores: results of a multiple ethnic groups investigation. *JAMA*. 2001;286(2):180–187. doi:10.1001/jama.286.2.180
41. Li C, Engstrom G, Hedblad B, Berglund G, Janzon L. Blood pressure control and risk of stroke: a population-based prospective cohort study. *Stroke*. 2005;36(4):725–730. doi:10.1161/01.STR.0000158925.12740.87
42. Ohira T, Shahar E, Chambless LE, Rosamond WD, Mosley TH Jr., Folsom AR. Risk factors for ischemic stroke subtypes: the Atherosclerosis Risk in Communities study. *Stroke*. 2006;37(10):2493–2498. doi:10.1161/01.STR.0000239694.19359.88
43. Qureshi AI, Suri MF, Mohammad Y, Guterman LR, Hopkins LN. Isolated and borderline isolated systolic hypertension relative to long-term risk and type of stroke: a 20-year follow-up of the National Health and Nutrition Survey. *Stroke*. 2002;33(12):2781–2788. doi:10.1161/01.str.0000039402.05613.0f
44. Liu K, Colangelo LA, Daviglus ML, et al. Can antihypertensive treatment restore the risk of cardiovascular disease to ideal levels? *J Am Heart Assoc*. 2015;4(9):e002275. doi:10.1161/JAHA.115.002275
45. Madsen TE, Howard G, Kleindorfer DO, et al. Sex differences in hypertension and stroke risk in the REGARDS Study: a longitudinal cohort study. *Hypertension*. 2019;74(4):749–755. doi:10.1161/HYPERTENSIONAHA.119.12729
46. Levy D, Larson MG, Vasan RS, Kannel WB, Ho KK. The progression from hypertension to congestive heart failure. *JAMA*. 1996;275(20):1557–1562. doi:10.1001/jama.1996.03530440037034

47. McNeill AM, Katz R, Girman CJ, et al. Metabolic syndrome and cardiovascular disease in older people: the cardiovascular health study. *J Am Geriatr Soc.* 2006;54(9):1317–1324. doi:10.1111/j.1532-5415.2006.00862.x
48. Williams SA, Kasl SV, Heiat A, Abramson JL, Krumholz HM, Vaccarino V. Depression and risk of heart failure among the elderly: a prospective community-based study. *Psychosom Med.* 2002;64(1):6–12. doi:10.1097/00006842-200201000-00002
49. Klag MJ, Whelton PK, Randall BL, et al. Blood pressure and end-stage renal disease in men. *N Engl J Med.* 1996;334(1):13–18. doi:10.1056/NEJM199601043340103
50. Fox CS, Larson MG, Leip EP, Culleton B, Wilson PW, Levy D. Predictors of new-onset kidney disease in a community-based population. *JAMA.* 2004;291(7):844–850. doi:10.1001/jama.291.7.844
51. Kurella M, Lo JC, Chertow GM. Metabolic syndrome and the risk for chronic kidney disease among nondiabetic adults. *J Am Soc Nephrol.* 2005;16(7):2134–2140. doi:10.1681/ASN.2005010106
52. Haroun MK, Jaar BG, Hoffman SC, Comstock GW, Klag MJ, Coresh J. Risk factors for chronic kidney disease: a prospective study of 23,534 men and women in Washington County, Maryland. *J Am Soc Nephrol.* 2003;14(11):2934–2941. doi:10.1097/01.ASN.0000095249.99803.85
53. Hsu CY, McCulloch CE, Darbinian J, Go AS, Iribarren C. Elevated blood pressure and risk of end-stage renal disease in subjects without baseline kidney disease. *Arch Intern Med.* 2005;165(8):923–928. doi:10.1001/archinte.165.8.923
54. Klag MJ, Whelton PK, Randall BL, Neaton JD, Brancati FL, Stamler J. End-stage renal disease in African-American and White men. 16-year MRFIT findings. *JAMA.* 1997;277(16):1293–1298. doi:10.1001/jama.1997.03540400043029
55. Vasan RS, Larson MG, Leip EP, et al. Impact of high-normal blood pressure on the risk of cardiovascular disease. *N Engl J Med.* 2001;345(18):1291–1297. doi:10.1056/NEJMoa003417
56. Haider AW, Larson MG, Franklin SS, Levy D. Systolic blood pressure, diastolic blood pressure, and pulse pressure as predictors of risk for congestive heart failure in the Framingham Heart Study. *Ann InternMed.* 2003;138(1):10–16. doi:10.7326/0003-4819-138-1-200301070-00006
57. Franklin SS, Larson MG, Khan SA, et al. Does the relation of blood pressure to coronary heart disease risk change with aging? the Framingham Heart Study. *Circulation.* 2001;103(9):1245–1249. doi:10.1161/01.CIR.103.9.1245
58. Bowman TS, Gaziano JM, Kase CS, Sesso HD, Kurth T. Blood pressure measures and risk of total, ischemic, and hemorrhagic stroke in men. *Neurology.* 2006;67(5):820–823. doi:10.1212/01.wnl.0000233981.26176.e
59. Mentari E, Rahman M. Blood pressure and progression of chronic kidney disease: importance of systolic, diastolic, or diurnal variation. *Curr Hypertens Rep.* 2004;6(5):400–404.
60. Hopkins PN, Hunt SC. Genetics of hypertension. *Genet Med.* 2003;5(6):413–429. doi:10.1097/01.gim.0000096375.88710.a6
61. Field AE, Coakley EH, Must A, et al. Impact of overweight on the risk of developing common chronic diseases during a 10-year period. *Arch Intern Med.* 2001;161(13):1581–1586. doi:10.1001/archinte.161.13.1581

62. Khaw KT, Bingham S, Welch A, et al. Blood pressure and urinary sodium in men and women: the Norfolk Cohort of the European Prospective Investigation into Cancer (EPIC-Norfolk). *Am J Clin Nutr.* 2004;80(5):1397–1403. doi:10.1093/ajcn/80.5.1397
63. Neter JE, Stam BE, Kok FJ, Grobbee DE, Geleijnse JM. Influence of weight reduction on blood pressure: a meta-analysis of randomized controlled trials. *Hypertension.* 2003;42(5):878–884. doi:10.1161/01.HYP.0000094221.86888.AE
64. Stamler J. The INTERSALT Study: background, methods, findings, and implications. *Am J Clin Nutr.* 1997;65(2 suppl):626S–642S. doi:10.1093/ajcn/65.2.626S
65. Mente A, O'Donnell MJ, Rangarajan S, et al. Association of urinary sodium and potassium excretion with blood pressure. *N Engl J Med.* 2014;371(7):601–611. doi:10.1056/NEJMoa1311989
66. He FJ, MacGregor GA. Effect of longer-term modest salt reduction on blood pressure. *Cochrane Database Syst Rev.* 2004;(3):CD004937. doi:10.1002/14651858.CD004937.pub2
67. Sacks FM, Svetkey LP, Vollmer WM, et al. Effects on blood pressure of reduced dietary sodium and the Dietary Approaches to Stop Hypertension (DASH) diet. *N Engl J Med.* 2001;344(1):3–10. doi:10.1056/NEJM200101043440101
68. Zhang Z, Cogswell ME, Gillespie C, et al. Association between usual sodium and potassium intake and blood pressure and hypertension among US adults: NHANES 2005–2010. *PLoS One.* 2013;8(10):e75289. doi:10.1371/journal.pone.0075289
69. Aburto NJ, Hanson S, Gutierrez H, Hooper L, Elliott P, Cappuccio FP. Effect of increased potassium intake on cardiovascular risk factors and disease: systematic review and meta-analyses. *BMJ.* 2013;346:f1378. doi:10.1136/bmj.f1378
70. Roerecke M, Tobe SW, Kaczorowski J, et al. Sex-specific associations between alcohol consumption and incidence of hypertension: a systematic review and meta-analysis of cohort studies. *J Am Heart Assoc.* 2018/07/03 2018;7(13):e008202. doi:10.1161/JAHA.117.008202
71. Xin X, He J, Frontini MG, Ogden LG, Motsamai OI, Whelton PK. Effects of alcohol reduction on blood pressure: a meta-analysis of randomized controlled trials. *Hypertension.* 2001;38(5):1112–1117. doi:10.1161/hy1101.093424
72. McFadden CB, Brensinger CM, Berlin JA, Townsend RR. Systematic review of the effect of daily alcohol intake on blood pressure. *Am J Hypertens.* 2005;18(2 pt 1):276–286. doi:10.1016/j.amjhyper.2004.07.020
73. Liu X, Zhang D, Liu Y, et al. Dose–response association between physical activity and incident hypertension. *Hypertension.* 2017;69(5):813–820. doi:10.1161/HYPERTENSIONAHA.116.08994
74. Pereira MA, Folsom AR, McGovern PG, et al. Physical activity and incident hypertension in Black and White adults: the Atherosclerosis Risk in Communities Study. *Prev Med.* 1999;28(3):304–312. doi:10.1006/pmed.1998.0431
75. Dyer AR, Liu K, Walsh M, Kiefe C, Jacobs DR Jr., Bild DE. Ten-year incidence of elevated blood pressure and its predictors: the CARDIA study: Coronary Artery Risk Development in (Young) Adults. *J Hum Hypertens.* 1999;13(1):13–21. doi:10.1038/sj.jhh.1000740
76. Diaz KM, Booth JN, Seals SR, et al. Physical activity and incident hypertension in African Americans. *Hypertension.* 2017;69(3):421–427. doi:10.1161/HYPERTENSIONAHA.116.08398
77. Bersaoui M, Baldew S-SM, Cornelis N, Toelsie J, Cornelissen VA. The effect of exercise training on blood pressure in African and Asian populations: a systematic review and meta-analysis

of randomized controlled trials. *Eur J of Preve Cardiol.* 2020;27(5):457–472. doi:10.1177/2047487319871233

78. Hardy ST, Loehr LR, Butler KR, et al. Reducing the blood pressure–related burden of cardiovascular disease: impact of achievable improvements in blood pressure prevention and control. *J Am Heart Assoc.* 2015;4(10):e002276. doi:10.1161/JAHA.115.002276
79. Dickinson HO, Mason JM, Nicolson DJ, et al. Lifestyle interventions to reduce raised blood pressure: a systematic review of randomized controlled trials. *J Hypertens.* 2006;24(2):215–233. doi:10.1097/01.hjh.0000199800.72563.26
80. Geleijnse JM, Kok FJ, Grobbee DE. Blood pressure response to changes in sodium and potassium intake: a metaregression analysis of randomised trials. *J Hum Hypertens.* 2003;17(7):471–480. doi:10.1038/sj.jhh.1001575
81. Roerecke M, Kaczorowski J, Tobe SW, Gmel G, Hasan OSM, Rehm J. The effect of a reduction in alcohol consumption on blood pressure: a systematic review and meta-analysis. *Lancet Public Health.* 2017;2(2):e108–e120. doi:10.1016/S2468-2667(17)30003-8
82. Herrod PJJ, Doleman B, Blackwell JEM, et al. Exercise and other nonpharmacological strategies to reduce blood pressure in older adults: a systematic review and meta-analysis. *J Am Soc Hypertens.* 2018;12(4):248–267. doi:10.1016/j.jash.2018.01.008
83. Appel LJ, Moore TJ, Obarzanek E, et al. A clinical trial of the effects of dietary patterns on blood pressure. DASH Collaborative Research Group. *N Engl J Med.* 1997;336(16):1117–1124. doi:10.1056/NEJM199704173361601
84. Aucott L, Rothnie H, McIntyre L, Thapa M, Waweru C, Gray D. Long-term weight loss from lifestyle intervention benefits blood pressure? *Hypertension.* 2009;54(4):756–762. doi:10.1161/HYPERTENSIONAHA.109.135178
85. Mulrow CD, Chiquette E, Angel L, et al. Dieting to reduce body weight for controlling hypertension in adults. *Cochrane Database Syst Rev.* 2000;(2):CD000484. doi:10.1002/14651858.CD000484
86. He FJ, Li J, MacGregor GA. Effect of longer term modest salt reduction on blood pressure: Cochrane systematic review and meta-analysis of randomised trials. *BMJ.* 2013;346:f1325. doi:10.1136/bmj.f1325
87. Huang L, Trieu K, Yoshimura S, et al. Effect of dose and duration of reduction in dietary sodium on blood pressure levels: systematic review and meta-analysis of randomised trials. *BMJ.* 2020;368:m315. doi:10.1136/bmj.m315
88 Whelton PK, Appel LJ, Espeland MA, et al. Sodium reduction and weight loss in the treatment of hypertension in older persons: a randomized controlled trial of nonpharmacologic interventions in the elderly (TONE). TONE Collaborative Research Group. *JAMA.* 1998;279(11):839–846. doi:10.1001/jama.279.11.839
89. Whelton PK, He J, Cutler JA, et al. Effects of oral potassium on blood pressure: meta-analysis of randomized controlled clinical trials. *JAMA.* 1997;277(20):1624–1632. doi:10.1001/jama.1997.03540440058033
90. Filippini T, Naska A, Kasdagli MI, et al. Potassium intake and blood pressure: a dose–response meta-analysis of randomized controlled trials. *J Am Heart Assoc.* 2020;9(12):e015719. doi:10.1161/JAHA.119.015719

91. Whelton PK. Sodium and potassium intake in US adults. *Circulation*. 2018;137(3):247–249. doi:10.1161/CIRCULATIONAHA.117.031371
92. Appel LJ, Brands MW, Daniels SR, Karanja N, Elmer PJ, Sacks FM. Dietary approaches to prevent and treat hypertension: a scientific statement from the American Heart Association. *Hypertension*. 2006;47(2):296–308. doi:10.1161/01.HYP.0000202568.01167.B6
93. Franklin BA, Thompson PD, Al-Zaiti SS, et al. Exercise-related acute cardiovascular events and potential deleterious adaptations following long-term exercise training: placing the risks into perspective—an update: a scientific statement from the American Heart Association. *Circulation*. 2020;141(13):e705–e736. doi:10.1161/CIR.0000000000000749
94. Filippou CD, Tsioufis CP, Thomopoulos CG, et al. Dietary Approaches to Stop Hypertension (DASH) diet and blood pressure reduction in adults with and without hypertension: a systematic review and meta-analysis of randomized controlled trials. *Adv Nutr*. 2020;11(5): 1150–1160. doi:10.1093/advances/nmaa041
95. US Preventive Services Task Force. Screening for hypertension in adults: US Preventive Services Task Force reaffirmation recommendation statement. *JAMA*. 2021;325(16):1650–1656. doi:10.1001/jama.2021.4987
96. Goff, Jr., Lloyd-Jones DM, Bennett G, et al. 2013 ACC/AHA Guideline on the assessment of cardiovascular risk. a report of the American College of Cardiology/American Heart Association Task Force on Practice Guidelines. *J Am Coll Cardiol*. 2014;63(25 pt B):2935–2959 doi:10.1016/j.jacc.2013.11.005
97. Artinian NT, Fletcher GF, Mozaffarian D, et al. Interventions to promote physical activity and dietary lifestyle changes for cardiovascular risk factor reduction in adults: a scientific statement from the American Heart Association. *Circulation*. 2010;122(4):406–441. doi:10.1161/CIR.0b013e3181e8edf1
98. Thomopoulos C, Parati G, Zanchetti A. Effects of blood-pressure-lowering treatment on outcome incidence in hypertension. 11. Effects of total cardiovascular risk and achieved blood pressure: overview and meta-analyses of randomized trials. *J Hypertens*. 2017;35(11): 2138–2149. doi:10.1097/HJH.0000000000001548

14

Dyslipidemia

Angela M. Thompson-Paul, PhD, MSPH, Ahlia Sekkarie, PhD, MPH, and Fleetwood Loustalot, PhD, FNP

LEARNING OBJECTIVES

After completing this chapter, readers should be able to

1. Describe the role of dyslipidemia in atherosclerotic cardiovascular disease.
2. Identify primary contributing factors to dyslipidemia.
3. Describe the population impact of dyslipidemia.
4. Describe nonpharmacologic and pharmacological treatment options for dyslipidemia.

INTRODUCTION

Nearly half of all US adults (49.2%) have cardiovascular disease (CVD).[1] Atherosclerotic cardiovascular disease (ASCVD) includes myocardial infarction (MI), coronary heart disease (CHD), stroke, angina, and peripheral arterial disease (PAD). Coronary heart disease and stroke are the first and fifth leading causes of death in the United States, responsible for 41.3% and 17.3% of deaths, respectively, in 2019.[1] Atherosclerosis is a condition in which areas on the surface of arteries become encrusted or hardened by the deposition of calcium, altering the endothelial cells and intruding into the inner lining of the artery as the fatty streak expands, which may restrict or obstruct blood flow to the heart, brain, or lower extremities or lead to acute thrombosis or plaque rupture.[2,3] Dyslipidemia, a condition in which one or more lipid profile measures fall outside the recommended ranges, contributes to atherosclerosis and is a leading risk factor for ASCVD. Abnormal lipid profile measures can result from an unhealthy lifestyle, other metabolic factors, certain medications, or genetics (Figure 14-1). Factors such as inter-individual variability in lipid measurements taken at different visits, age when exposure to abnormal lipid levels began, and number of years an individual was exposed to abnormal lipid levels can moderate the risk of adverse outcomes, such as ASCVD morbidity and mortality and higher health care and societal costs.[1,4–6] Certain populations may also be at higher risk for adverse outcomes as a result of abnormal lipid levels. The risk of these adverse outcomes may be reduced through lipid management, including lifestyle modifications and, if required, an appropriate medication regimen.

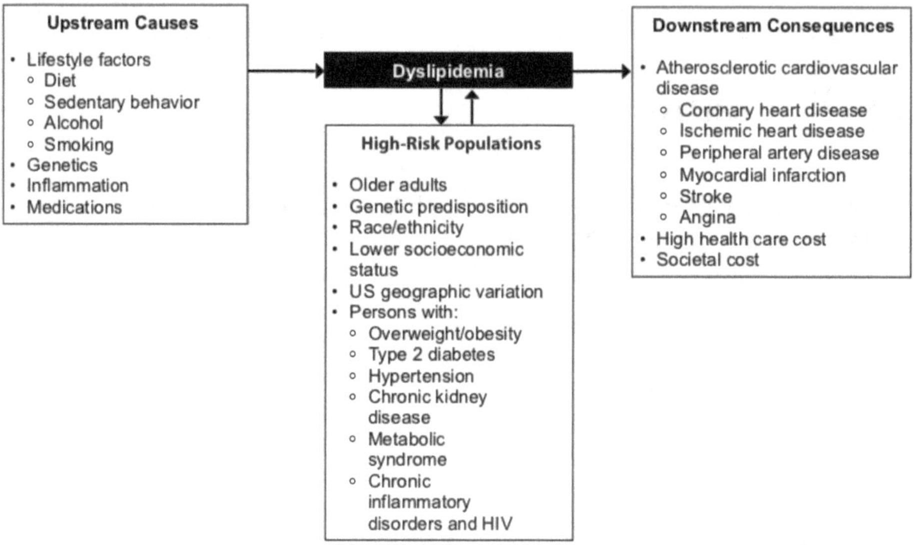

Figure 14-1. Dyslipidemia: Causes, Consequences, and High-Risk Populations

PATHOPHYSIOLOGY

Cholesterol is a waxy, fatlike substance present in the cell membrane. Cholesterol, which is carried in the blood, comes from two sources: the body (endogenous) and diet (exogenous). The body's production of cholesterol maintains cell membranes, cell growth, and steroid hormone synthesis.[7] If there is too much cholesterol in the blood, it can begin to build up on the walls of the blood vessels and produce deposits called plaque. Plaque buildup can produce inflammation and scar tissue limiting or blocking the flow of blood, a condition referred to as atherosclerosis.[8]

Cholesterol travels in the blood on proteins called lipoproteins, classified as low-density lipoprotein cholesterol (LDL-C), very low-density lipoprotein cholesterol (VLDL-C), and high-density lipoprotein cholesterol (HDL-C). Both LDL-C and VLDL-C are atherogenic, meaning that they tend to promote formation of fatty plaques in arteries. LDL-C is the dominant cholesterol form, while VLDL-C is the primary carrier of triglycerides (TGs).[9] LDL-C is responsible for the plaque buildup in the blood vessels that develops into atherosclerosis. HDL-C helps to manage LDL-C storage and clear the cholesterol out of the bloodstream through reverse cholesterol transport to the liver. LDL-C and HDL-C have been labeled as "bad" and "good" cholesterol, respectively. Total cholesterol may be directly measured or calculated using the commonly used Friedewald equation (where TC = LDL-C + HDL-C + 20% of TGs), or newer equations that may more accurately estimate LDL-C when TGs are 150 mg/dL or greater.[10,11]

Risk of CVD increases when any lipid profile measure is abnormal, but the risk is greatest when HDL-C, LDL-C, and TG are outside of the normal range (Table 14-1).[12]

Table 14-1. Adjusted Hazard Ratios for 10-Year Cardiovascular Disease Outcomes Among Participants: Framingham Heart Study, United States, 1987–2011

Sex	Lipid Profile Measures			Hazard Ratio (95% CI)
	HDL-C	LDL-C	Triglycerides	
Overall	Normal	Normal	Normal	Reference
	Normal	High	Normal	1.28 (1.03-1.59)
	Normal	Normal	High	1.35 (0.91-1.98)
	Normal	High	High	1.52 (1.12-2.07)
	Low	Normal	High	1.74 (1.28-2.38)
	Low	High	Normal	1.82 (1.33-2.49)
	Low	Normal	Normal	1.93 (1.37-2.71)
	Low	High	High	2.28 (1.73-3.02)
Men	Normal	Normal	Normal	Reference
	Normal	High	Normal	1.42 (1.03-1.97)
	Normal	Normal	High	1.21 (0.67-2.17)
	Normal	High	High	1.64 (1.07-2.52)
	Low	Normal	High	1.58 (1.06-2.35)
	Low	High	Normal	1.81 (1.23-2.66)
	Low	Normal	Normal	1.96 (1.30-2.93)
	Low	High	High	2.41 (1.67-3.46)
Women	Normal	Normal	Normal	Reference
	Normal	High	Normal	1.16 (0.86-1.57)
	Normal	Normal	High	1.54 (0.91-2.59)
	Normal	High	High	1.44 (0.91-2.27)
	Low	Normal	High	2.55 (1.48-4.37)
	Low	High	Normal	2.33 (1.23-4.40)
	Low	Normal	Normal	2.04 (0.94-4.44)
	Low	High	High	2.09 (1.27-3.44)

Source: Based on Andersson et al.[12]

Note: CI = confidence interval; HDL-C = high-density lipoprotein cholesterol; LDL-C = low-density lipoprotein cholesterol; TG = triglycerides. Abnormal cholesterol levels were defined using the National Cholesterol Education (NCEP) III standards: high LDL-C = ≥130 mg/dL, high TG = ≥150 mg/dL, and low HDL-C = <40 mg/dL.

Therefore, each lipid profile measure may add information to an individual's risk profile, and their combined role in development of ASCVD has become the focus of treatment, research, and public health efforts. Total cholesterol associated with CVD had been the main focus of lipid research in the past. However, TC assumes an additive effect of LDL-C, HDL-C, and TGs and may not adequately distinguish the protective effect of HDL-C or the inverse association of TGs with HDL-C.[13] Non-HDL-C is a measure of all athero-genic particles in the blood and is calculated as TC minus HDL cholesterol. Non-HDL-C concentrations in the blood are associated with long-term risk of ASCVD. As the effects of HDL-C and non-HDL-C on ischemic heart disease mortality are independent of each other, the ratio of HDL-C to non-HDL-C tends to be more informative than either one alone.[14] Although increasing HDL-C is associated with lower CHD risk, there may be a potential threshold of benefit at very high HDL-C levels; however, the HDL-C-to-non-HDL-C ratio shows no evidence of threshold effect.[8,15] The TC-to-HDL-C ratio has also been found to highly correlate with severity of coronary artery calcification (CAC), a proxy measure for the amount of atherosclerosis in the arteries that supply the heart muscle.[16] Calcium is deposited in areas of inflammation, such as an active or inflamed plaque, and therefore CAC is an estimate of plaque burden.[8] CAC has been associated with incident cardiovascular events and is considered an ASCVD risk factor.[9]

Familial Hypercholesterolemia

Familial hypercholesterolemia (FH) is a genetic disorder in which the capacity to clear LDL-C from the blood is decreased. It is an autosomal-dominant condition characterized by elevated serum LDL-C present from birth. It may present as heterozygous or homozygous with a dose effect; people who are homozygous have much higher LDL-C and earlier onset of CVD than those who are heterozygous.[17] The LDL-C can range from 155 to 500 mg/dL among heterozygotes and can be greater than 400 mg/dL in homozygotes.[17] Clinical manifestations of FH may not begin until adulthood, but high concentrations of LDL-C beginning in childhood result in the deleterious effects of prolonged exposure, premature development of atherosclerotic plaques, and premature CVD events. FH is estimated to be responsible for 20% of heart attacks that occur in those younger than 45 years.[18]

PUBLIC HEALTH IMPACT

Dyslipidemia constitutes a tremendous public health burden. It is a well-established risk factor for ASCVD morbidity and mortality, having both direct and indirect associations with cardiovascular outcomes (Table 14-2). Following high systolic blood pressure and dietary risk, dyslipidemia is estimated to be the third leading attributable risk for CVD globally.[19] Dyslipidemia was found to be the most important risk factor for first MI in the INTERHEART Study, a large, multicenter study that included approximately 15,000 cases and controls from 52 countries.[20] Total cholesterol has a strong graded relationship with CHD,[21] ischemic heart disease,[14] and MI, with higher TC levels incurring greater risk. Low HDL-C concentrations and high visit-to-visit variability of HDL-C concentrations are associated with increased risk of MI, stroke, and cardiovascular mortality.[22]

Being exposed to abnormal LDL-C levels during childhood or adolescence is an important predictor of onset and severity of ASCVD outcomes in middle-age and

Table 14-2. Potential Outcomes of Dyslipidemia

	Outcome						
Lipid Measure	Coronary Heart Disease	Ischemic Heart Disease	Myocardial Infarction	Stroke	Health Care Cost	ASCVD Morbidity	ASCVD Mortality
Any dyslipidemia	↑	↑	↑	↑	↑	↑	↑
Elevated total cholesterol	↑[a]	↑[a]	↑	NA	NA	↑	↑
Low HDL-C	NA	NA	↑	↑	NA	↑	↑
Elevated LDL-C	NA	NA	↑	↑	↑	↑[a]	↑
Elevated triglycerides	NA	NA	NA	NA	NA	↑	NA

Note: ASCVD = atherosclerotic cardiovascular disease; HDL-C = high-density lipoprotein cholesterol; LDL-C = low-density lipoprotein cholesterol; NA = not available.

[a] Risk increases in dose-dependent manner.

older adulthood.[4,5] Multiple studies have demonstrated an association between intra-individual variability in cholesterol measures and adverse cardiovascular outcomes (including all-cause mortality, MI, and stroke).[6] Greater cumulative exposure to high LDL-C levels appears to confer greater risk for ASCVD later in life. Therefore, emphasis on achieving and maintaining optimal cholesterol levels beginning earlier is important for better cardiovascular health later in life.

There is a great deal of work to be done to improve awareness, prevention, and control of blood cholesterol levels. Awareness of high cholesterol and use of cholesterol-lowering treatment among those eligible is low. In one report, 68% of US adults eligible for cholesterol-lowering therapies but not taking any medication were not aware of their condition.[23] Use of cholesterol-lowering medication is also suboptimal. Nationally representative data from 2011 to 2018 showed that 41.5% of US adults aged 20 years and older were recommended or should be considered for cholesterol-lowering treatment, yet less than half of those recommended in this age group were taking cholesterol-lowering medication.[24]

Data from the Medical Expenditures Panel Survey (MEPS, 2017–2018) estimated $226.2 billion in direct costs and $151.8 billion in indirect costs attributed to premature CVD mortality.[1] Hyperlipidemia accounts for approximately $30.2 billion in direct costs annually.[1] The highest costs were associated with inpatient care following a cardiovascular event, followed by ambulatory care and pharmaceutical costs in the first three years following the event.[25] Globally, elevated LDL-C concentrations are estimated to account for 98.6 million disability-adjusted life years (DALYs) and 4.4 million deaths.[19]

Dyslipidemia prevention and management deserves increased attention from clinicians and public health practitioners, given dyslipidemia's high burden, significant association with CVD, underutilized treatment, and high costs, as well as the effective management strategies that are not being optimally implemented.

DESCRIPTIVE EPIDEMIOLOGY

Approximately one-third of adults (29.0%) have elevated LDL-C (defined as LDL-C ≥130 mg/dL), with the highest prevalence among persons aged 40 to 64 years (36.4%) and lowest prevalence among those 20 to 39 years (21.9%; Table 14-3).[24] Low HDL-C (<40 mg/dL in men, <50 mg/dL in women) was identified among one in four adults (26.2%), with higher prevalence among those of Hispanic ethnicity (31.9%) and those without health insurance coverage (31.5%) or less than a high school education (32.8%). One in five adults (21.6%) has elevated TG (≥150 mg/dL), with highest prevalence among men (25.2%) and persons aged 40 to 64 years, and lowest prevalence among non-Hispanic Black adults (9.8%). Severe hyperlipidemia (LDL-C ≥190 mg/dL) was identified among 2.3% of adults, and the highest prevalence was among middle-aged adults (3.2%).

More than half of US adults have at least one blood cholesterol measure that is not in the normal range (Table 14-4).[24] Elevated LDL-C was the most common single abnormal lipid measure. The most common combinations of more than one abnormal lipid level included low HDL-C plus elevated TG or low HDL-C plus elevated LDL-C and elevated TG. Men were more likely than women to have elevated TG alone or in combination with severely elevated LDL-C. Women were more likely than men to have low HDL-C in combination with elevated LDL-C or elevated TG.

High-Risk Populations

Familial Hypercholesterolemia

The prevalence of FH is estimated to be 0.32% worldwide in the general population (1 in 313 persons), 3.2% among people with ischemic heart disease (IHD, 1 in 31 persons), 6.7% among those with premature IHD (1 in 15 persons), and 7.2% among persons with severe hypercholesterolemia (1 in 14 persons).[26] Prevalence may be higher in certain countries or specific ethnic subpopulations[26,27] In the United States, FH has been estimated to range from 620,000 to 1,500,000 people based on a prevalence of 1 in 250 to 500.[27]

Comorbidities

Dyslipidemia directly affects cardiovascular outcomes and also indirectly affects these outcomes by increasing other cardiovascular risk factors, such as hypertension, diabetes,

Table 14-3. Prevalence of Abnormal Serum Blood Cholesterol Levels Among Adults Aged 20 Years and Older: National Health and Nutrition Examination Survey, United States, 2011–2018

Characteristic		Prevalence of Abnormal Serum Lipid Levels, % (SE)							
		Low HDL-C[a]		Elevated LDL-C[b]		Severe Hyperlipidemia[c]		Elevated TG[d]	
	N = 8,958	%	(SE)	%	(SE)	%	(SE)	%	(SE)
Overall	8,958	26.2	(0.8)	29.0	0.6	2.3	0.2	21.6	0.7
Sex									
Men	4,340	23.2	(0.9)	28.4	0.9	2.2	0.3	25.2	1.1
Women	4,618	29.0	(1.1)	29.6	(0.8)	2.3	(0.3)	18.3	(0.8)
Age, y									
20–39	2,865	27.5	(1.3)	21.9	(0.8)	1.3	(0.2)	14.7	(0.9)
40–64	3,946	26.9	(1.1)	36.4	(0.9)	3.2	(0.4)	26.4	(1.0)
≥65	2,147	22.3	(1.4)	25.0	(1.2)	1.8	(0.3)	23.1	(1.6)
Race/ethnicity									
Non-Hispanic White	3,387	25.6	(1.0)	29.3	(0.8)	2.3	(0.3)	23.0	(0.9)
Non-Hispanic Black	1,881	22.8	(1.3)	28.0	(1.2)	2.5	(0.4)	9.8	(0.7)
Asian	1,178	22.0	(1.4)	28.3	(1.7)	1.9	(0.5)	22.2	(1.5)
Hispanic	2,199	31.9	(1.2)	29.2	(1.3)	2.1	(0.3)	24.0	(1.0)
Other	313	29.7	(3.8)	26.4	(3.8)	2.3	(1.1)	21.9	(3.9)
Educational attainment									
<HS education	1,988	32.8	(1.6)	29.1	(1.4)	2.4	(0.4)	24.2	(1.2)
HS graduation/GED	1,980	27.0	(1.8)	30.8	(1.6)	2.4	(0.5)	23.8	(1.4)
>HS education	4,985	24.3	(1.0)	28.3	(0.7)	2.2	(0.3)	20.2	(0.9)
Health insurance coverage									
Public	4,518	23.3	(1.0)	29.8	(0.8)	2.0	(0.3)	20.7	(0.8)
Private	2,615	29.8	(1.1)	25.2	(1.1)	2.6	(0.3)	23.0	(1.2)
None	1,773	31.5	(1.6)	31.3	(1.6)	2.8	(0.6)	22.8	(1.5)

Source: Based on Thompson-Paul et al.[24]

Note: HDL-C = high-density lipoprotein cholesterol; HS = high school; LDL-C = low-density lipoprotein cholesterol; SE = standard error; TG = triglycerides. Pregnant women were excluded. Fasting adults (≥20 y) were included with complete data for LDL-C, HDL-C, and TG. Participants missing education attainment or type of health insurance are included in the analysis but not reported as subgroups.

[a]Low HDL-C: <40 mg/dL in men, <50 mg/dL in women.

[b]Elevated LDL-C: ≥130 mg/dL.

[c]Severe hyperlipidemia: LDL-C ≥190 mg/dL.

[d]Elevated TG: ≥150 mg/dL.

Table 14-4. Prevalence of Abnormal Lipid Measures Among Adults: National Health and Nutritional Examination Survey, United States, 2011–2018

Lipid Profile Measures			Men		Women			
HDL-C[a]	LDL-C[b,c]	Triglycerides[d]	%	(SE)	%	(SE)	aPR	(95% CI)
Normal	Normal	Normal	47.5	(1.0)	46.5	(1.1)	1.0	(1.0–1.1)
Normal	Elevated	Normal	15.3	(0.8)	16.0	(0.7)	1.0	(0.8–1.1)
Normal	Severe	Normal	0.8	(0.2)	1.2	(0.2)	0.9	(0.6–1.3)
Normal	Normal	Elevated	6.9	(0.5)	3.8	(0.4)	1.8	(1.4–2.4)
Normal	Elevated	Elevated	5.2	(0.5)	3.4	(0.4)	1.6	(1.1–2.2)
Normal	Severe	Elevated	1.0	(0.2)	0.3	(0.1)	3.3	(1.5–7.2)
Low	Normal	Elevated	8.4	(0.6)	13.9	(0.7)	0.6	(0.5–0.7)
Low	Elevated	Normal	2.5	(0.3)	4.2	(0.4)	0.6	(0.4–0.8)
Low	Normal	Normal	0.2	(0.1)	0.1	(0.0)	1.0	(0.5–2.0)
Low	Elevated	Elevated	8.7	(0.6)	6.2	(0.5)	1.4	(1.1–1.8)
Low	Severe	Elevated	3.1	(0.3)	3.8	(0.4)	0.8	(0.6–1.1)

Note: aPR = adjusted prevalence ratio; CI = confidence interval; HDL-C = high-density lipoprotein cholesterol; LDL-C = low-density lipoprotein cholesterol; SE = standard error. The prevalence ratio comparing men with women has been adjusted (aPR) for age group (20–39, 40–64, ≥65 y) and race/Hispanic origin (non-Hispanic White, non-Hispanic Black, non-Hispanic Asian, Hispanic, other).

[a]HDL-C is <40 mg/dL in men and <50 mg/dL in women.

[b]Elevated LDL-C is ≥130 mg/dL.

[c]Severe LDL-C is ≥190 mg/dL.

[d]Elevated TG is ≥150 mg/dL.

metabolic syndrome, and nonalcoholic fatty liver disease. The 2018 American College of Cardiology/American Heart Association Clinical Practice Guidelines for cholesterol management identified ASCVD risk enhancers, which are assessed to help clinicians and patients determine primary prevention for people who may be at borderline or intermediate ASCVD risk.[9] Risk enhancers are factors that have strong associations with ASCVD and include certain conditions such as chronic kidney disease (CKD), metabolic syndrome, inflammatory diseases, preeclampsia, and premature menopause, as well as family history of premature ASCVD and certain biomarker measures.[9] For secondary prevention of ASCVD, the presence of certain comorbid conditions may categorize an individual who previously had a cardiovascular event as very high risk. Being categorized as very high risk is defined as a history of multiple major ASCVD events or one major event plus multiple high-risk conditions (heterozygous familial hypercholesterolemia, diabetes mellitus, hypertension, CKD, history of congestive heart failure, LDL-C that is persistently ≥100 mg/dL despite maximally tolerated statin therapy and ezetimibe, current smoking, or history of prior coronary artery bypass surgery).[9] Individuals categorized as very high risk are recommended to begin high-intensity or maximally tolerated HMG-CoA reductase inhibitors (statin) therapy.

Many chronic conditions coexist with dyslipidemia because of similar cardiometabolic risk factors, and combined they may have an additive effect on ASCVD risk.[28] Among older adults with peripheral arterial disease, having comorbid dyslipidemia, diabetes mellitus, and hypertension was associated with a threefold increased risk of a major adverse cardiovascular event.[28] The prevalence of dyslipidemia among those with type 2 diabetes was twice that of adults with normal glucose tolerance.[29] In particular, the combination of high TG and low HDL-C is prevalent among people with type 2 diabetes and is associated with higher risks of adverse CVD outcomes.[30,31] An increase of one standard deviation of LDL-C (26–29 mg/dL) has been associated with a 50% increased risk of CVD hospitalization among adults with type 2 diabetes.[32] However, the ratio of non-HDL-C to HDL-C may be a better predictor of CHD than LDL-C alone because this ratio had a consistent increasing linear association with CHD rate among adults with diabetes.[31]

People with dyslipidemia have a three times higher risk of hypertension than those with normal lipids.[33] Hypertension is associated with both increased ASCVD risk and dyslipidemia. Systolic blood pressure is about 2.4 millimeters of mercury (mm Hg) higher for every 1 mmol/L increase of TC after taking into account age, sex, and study population.[14] In children and adolescents, having blood pressure levels in the 95th percentile or higher was associated with an increased likelihood of having abnormal levels of TC and non-HDL-C compared with those with an average blood pressure reading, independent of body mass index (BMI).[34] Furthermore, the association between TC and ischemic heart disease mortality varies with systolic blood pressure; at higher levels of systolic blood pressure, the association between increased TC and ischemic heart disease mortality is stronger than at lower systolic blood pressure readings, and having greater systolic blood pressure is more detrimental for CVD-related outcomes at greater levels of TC versus lower TC levels.[14]

CKD is associated with increased risk for CVD. Persons with an estimated glomerular filtration rate (eGFR, measured in units of mL/min/1.73m^2) between 15 and 29 have more than threefold increased risk of cardiovascular mortality compared with people with an eGFR of 60 or greater.[35] Among people with CKD, cardiovascular event rates differed across tertiles of VLDL-C, TG, HDL-C, and apolipoprotein A-I; further, this effect was modified by eGFR level.[36] People with suboptimal eGFR and low HDL-C were at increased risk for ASCVD events. In a cohort of more than 1.9 million US veterans, those with a more advanced stage of CKD and serum LDL-C 160 mg/dL or greater were found to be at increased risk for all-cause and cardiovascular mortality compared with people without CKD.[37]

People living with HIV have a higher risk of CVD[38] and excess heart age[39] compared with people living without HIV. After adjusting for traditional cardiovascular risk factors, comorbidities, and substance use, people living with HIV had a 48% increased risk of MI. Factors that may contribute to this excess risk may include inflammation, endothelial dysfunction, metabolic changes resulting from antiretroviral therapy, and abnormal fat distribution.[40] These metabolic changes then lead to high prevalence of dyslipidemia among persons living with HIV. Because of drug interactions, not all statins are appropriate for use in people living with HIV; therefore clinicians should be aware of recommendations and contraindications related to statin use for CVD prevention among these individuals.[9,41]

Sex and Age Differences

Dyslipidemia presents differently in men and women and changes during different life stages. Data collected from 2015 to 2018 for the National Health and Nutrition Examination Survey (NHANES) showed that the prevalence of elevated total cholesterol was greater for women (12.1% ≥240 mg/dL and 40.4% ≥200 mg/dL) than men (10.5% ≥240 mg/dL and 35.3% ≥200 mg/dL), but prevalence of low HDL-C (<40 mg/dL) was higher among men (26.6%) than women (8.5%).[1] The prevalence of LDL-C of 130 mg/dL or higher was similar between men (27.4%) and women (28.1%) in the United States over this same time period.

Hormonal changes from pregnancy or menopause or conditions such as polycystic ovarian syndrome (PCOS) may affect blood lipid levels over a woman's lifetime. TC and LDL-C levels vary by 5% to 8% throughout the menstrual cycle. PCOS is associated with increased prevalence of dyslipidemia. Cholesterol levels increase during pregnancy. LDL-C levels increase an average of 2 mg/dL per year during the pre- and peri-menopausal periods and 1.2 mg/dL after menopause, and TC increases 1.5 mg/dL each year after menopause.[42] Although blood lipid measures change with age, in women the changes associated with menopause are independent of age.

Mean TC, LDL-C, and TG increase with each decade of age, with the greatest values occurring between 40 and 70 years and declining thereafter.[43] Prevalence of low HDL-C is higher among adults younger than 50 years compared with those older than 50 years.[44] Even with age-related changes in serum lipid levels, adults older than 70 still have greater mean TC, LDL-C, TGs, and HDL-C levels than those in the youngest age group (<20).[44] Cumulative exposure to elevated LDL-C levels during young adulthood (18–39 y) increases risk for CHD in later life in a dose-dependent manner independent of later life exposures.[45] Studies have reported conflicting evidence on the association of LDL-C and CVD risk for adults in the oldest age groups, and further research is therefore needed in this area.[43–46]

Hormones and hormonal changes during childhood and adolescence also affect serum lipid levels. Fatty streaks in arteries can be clinically found during childhood, and the presence of abnormal lipid levels increases the risk of developing atherosclerosis in the presence of fatty streaks. During 2009 to 2016, 19.2% of US children and adolescents had at least one abnormal cholesterol measure, including 7.1% with TC of 200 mg/dL or greater, 12.1% with HDL-C less than 40 mg/dL, and 6.4% with non-HDL-C of 145 mg/dL or greater.[1]

In 2015 to 2018, among US children (6–11 y) mean TC was 157.4 mg/dL for males and 157.1 mg/dL for females; among adolescents (12–19 y), mean TC was 155.1 mg/dL for males and 152.7 mg/dL for females.[1] Prevalence of abnormal TC and lipid subfractions is low among children and adolescents. Prevalence of TC of 200 mg/dL or greater was 7.1% among children aged 6 to 19. Among adolescents, elevated LDL-C occurs in 6.1% of males and 3.0% of females, and low HDL-C is found in 18.4% of males and 7.4% of females.[1] Mean HDL-C decreases with increasing age in boys and remains similar from age 3 to 19 in girls.[34] Non-HDL cholesterol levels fluctuate in children and are greatest among children aged 9 to 11 and 17 to 19 years compared with other age groups.[46] TG levels tend to be higher among girls than boys before the age of 12, then decrease to similar levels from ages 12 to 19 years. Abnormal lipid levels are negatively associated with carotid intima-media thickness (CIMT) and early development of atherosclerosis in children and adolescents. Measures associated with CVD morbidity and mortality in adulthood, including CIMT, concentric left ventricular remodeling and left ventricular hypertrophy, CAC, and cardiometabolic risk factors, are associated with pediatric hyperlipidemia.[47]

Race/Ethnicity

Disparities in dyslipidemia are seen among racial/ethnic groups in presentation and severity of abnormal cholesterol levels that should be kept in mind when considering treatments or interventions for specific populations. Mean serum cholesterol levels have decreased for all adults between 1999 and 2018; however, data from NHANES shows that TC was higher for non-Hispanic White adults and Mexican Americans compared with non-Hispanic Black adults.[1] In 2017 to 2018 the age-adjusted prevalence of serum TC of 200 mg/dL or greater in US adults 20 years of age or older was highest among non-Hispanic White women (40.0%) and non-Hispanic Asian men (40.8%) and lowest among non-Hispanic Black women (32.3%) and non-Hispanic Black men (31.8%).[1] NHANES data from 2015 to 2018 show that the prevalence of low HDL-C (<40 mg/dL) was higher among Hispanic males (32.0%) and Hispanic females (12.3%) compared with other races and ethnicities.

Factors such as socioeconomic status and acculturation have been associated with a difference in dyslipidemia prevalence among racial/ethnic subgroups.[48] There is great variation within subgroups of Hispanic adults with the prevalence of LDL-C of 130 mg/dL or greater ranging from 31.6% among Dominican adults to 44.5% among Cuban adults. TG level of 200 mg/dL or greater ranged from 7.6% among Dominicans to 18.3% among those from Central America.[48] Similarly, there are differences in lipid profile measures among various Asian American subgroups. For example, the prevalence of ever having LDL-C of 130 mg/dL or greater was highest among Filipino men (73.1%) and women (63.0%) but lowest in Chinese men (55.3%) and women (45.8%).[49]

The racial/ethnic differences in dyslipidemia prevalence seen in adults also occur among children and adolescents. Among US children aged 6 to 11 years, mean TC was highest among non-Hispanic Asian males (167.5 mg/dL) and females (159.0 mg/dL) and lowest among non-Hispanic White males (156.1 mg/dL) and Hispanic females (154.8 mg/dL).[1] Among adolescents aged 12 to 19, TC was highest among non-Hispanic Black males (155.8 mg/dL) and non-Hispanic Asian females (165.0 mg/dL) and lowest among non-Hispanic White males (151.2 mg/dL) and Hispanic females (153.8 mg/dL).

Social Determinants of Health

Factors such as socioeconomic status, insurance status, health care access, and social and community context have been associated with health disparities for many conditions, including dyslipidemia. Awareness, treatment, and control of elevated LDL-C were found to be similar among publicly and privately insured adults but were significantly greater among insured adults compared with uninsured adults.[50] Other factors associated with LDL-C control included greater frequency of health care visits, having hypertension, and having higher income. Data from the Reasons for Geographic and Racial Differences in Stroke (REGARDS) study found that statin use and LDL-C control was greatest for White men compared with Black men, Black women, and White women even after adjusting for CVD risk factors and factors that influence health care utilization, concluding that differences in prescribing patterns, such as more aggressive prescription of statins to White men potentially because they may have been perceived to be at higher risk for adverse CHD outcomes, may explain some of this difference.[51] Access to resources and factors influencing educational attainment also influence the lipid profiles of young adults. Data collected from more than 4,000 students who attended a private southeastern US college between 2003 and 2015 demonstrated that college students have healthier lipid profiles than age-matched controls from the general US population.[52]

Geographic Distribution

Globally in 2019, high LDL-C was the third leading modifiable risk factor attributable to CVD.[19] Although blood lipid levels and LDL-C vary across countries, notably according to higher socioeconomic status,[53] the association between ischemic heart disease mortality and cholesterol does not differ across countries after differences in age distribution are taken into account.[14]

In the United States, cholesterol screening, awareness, and treatment prevalence varies geographically.[54] US states that have older populations and populations with higher

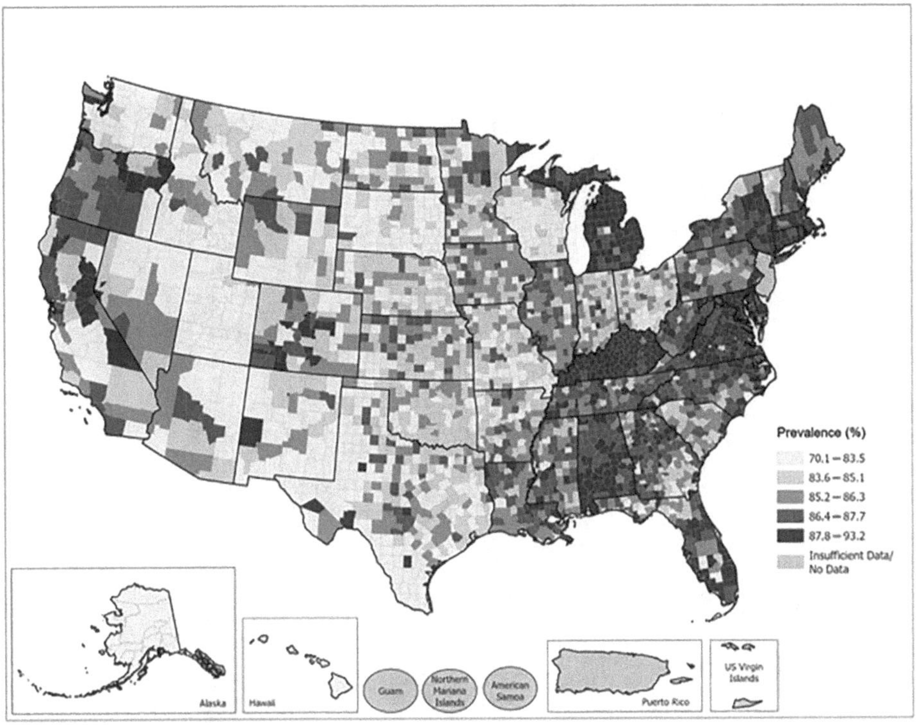

Source: Based on CDC.[55]

Note: The numerator pertains to respondents aged ≥18 years who report having their cholesterol checked within the previous 5 years. The denominator pertains to respondents aged ≥18 years (excluding those who refused to answer, had a missing answer, or answered "don't know/not sure").

Figure 14-2. Cholesterol Screening Among Adults Aged 18 Years and Older: Behavioral Risk Factor Surveillance System Survey, United States, 2019

rates of Medicare-insured people are more likely to perform cholesterol screenings and prescribe cholesterol-lowering medication.[55] The prevalence of cholesterol screenings among adults 18 years or older is greatest in the Northeast, upper Midwest, and Southeast (Figure 14-2),[55] whereas the highest prevalence of high cholesterol is concentrated in the "Stroke Belt"[56] (Figure 14-3). Urban and rural disparities also exist that are compounded by sex and race. Rural women, for example, have 3.3 greater odds of elevated LDL-C compared with urban men.[57]

Time Trends

The prevalence of high TC, high LDL-C, and low HDL-C levels has been declining among US adults for decades.[58] The proportion of adults with TC of 240 mg/dL or greater declined from 18.3% in 1999 to 2000 to 10.5% in 2017 to 2018.[59] Although the prevalence

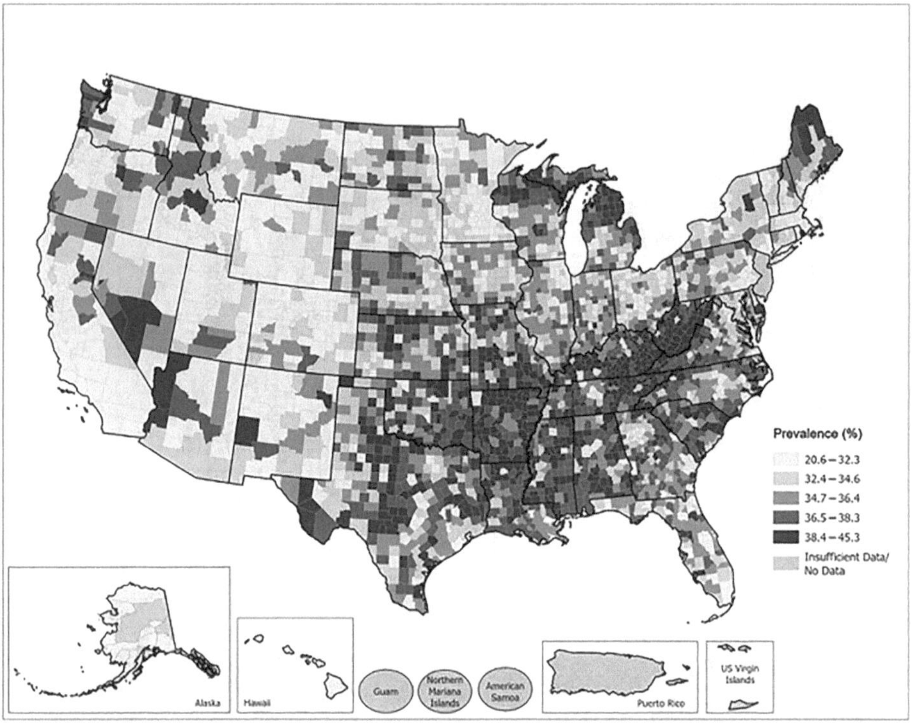

Source: Based on CDC.[55]

Note: The numerator pertains to respondents aged ≥18 years who report having been told by a doctor, nurse, or other health professional that they had high cholesterol. The denominator pertains to respondents aged ≥18 years who report having their cholesterol checked within the past 5 years (excluding those who refused to answer, had a missing answer, or answered "don't know/not sure").

Figure 14-3. High Cholesterol Among Adults Aged 18 Years and Older Who Have Been Screened in the Past Five Years: Behavioral Risk Factor Surveillance System Survey, United States, 2019

of high LDL-C decreased from 59% to 27% from the late 1970s through 2010 among the general US adult population,[60] there has been little or no change in the proportion who have their LDL-C at or below recommended levels among adults with CHD or who have had a stroke.[58] Prevalence of low HDL-C has decreased from 22.2% in 2007 to 2008 to 16.0% in 2017 to 2018.[59]

CAUSES

Modifiable Risk Factors

Increased risk factors for cholesterol-associated conditions such as stroke and hypertension include overweight/obesity, poor dietary intake, and a sedentary lifestyle or lack of physical activity. Alcohol consumption and smoking also pose risks for cholesterol-associated conditions. However, these particular risk factors can be modified, as explained in the following sections.

Overweight or Obesity

Being overweight or having obesity is associated with increased risk of CVD and CVD risk factors such as hypertension, type 2 diabetes, and dyslipidemia.[1] That risk is further increased through the interaction between dyslipidemia and overweight.[33] Hypertriglyceridemia in obesity is in part attributable to impaired metabolic processes, with increased free fatty acids released from adipose tissue and free fatty acid clearance reduced. TGs accumulate in the liver, HDL-C concentrations are reduced, and TG concentrations are reduced in LDL-C, leaving small, dense LDL-C particles.[61] Categories of overweight or obesity have been associated with lower levels of HDL-C and higher levels of LDL-C and TGs in a dose-response relationship in which the various lipid levels worsen with higher levels of obesity compared with normal or healthy weight. Abdominal and visceral adiposity are positively associated with higher TGs and lower HDL-C.[62] When different measures of adult body composition were compared, waist-to-hip ratio was a better estimator of HDL-C and LDL-C than BMI, waist-to-height ratio, and body adiposity index.[63] Waist-to-hip ratio, waist-to-height ratio, and BMI were all significant estimators of TG levels.

In children and adolescents, higher BMI percentiles are significantly associated with HDL-C and LDL-C, and the prevalence of high non-HDL-C is consistently greater among children with overweight or obesity and for those with waist circumference in the 90th percentile or higher.[46] The prevalence of HDL-C lower than 40 mg/dL increases with the degree of overweight or obesity (6.8% for normal weight, 14.8% for overweight, and 33.2% for obesity) among children, as does non-HDL-C greater than or equal to 145 mg/dL (5.7% for normal weight, 9.7% for overweight, and 16.7% for obesity).[64]

Dietary Intake

An unhealthy diet has been associated with a variety of chronic diseases and their risk factors, including dyslipidemia. Conversely, healthy dietary patterns focus on key foods and nutrients that promote cardiovascular health. The 2020 to 2025 Dietary Guidelines for Americans recommend aiming to increase intake of nutrient-dense foods such as fruits and vegetables while limiting consumption of foods high in saturated fatty acids (SFA), added sugar, and sodium.[65] Current Dietary Guidelines recommend that less than 10% of daily calories come from SFA; healthy oils, such as monounsaturated fatty acids and polyunsaturated fatty acids, should be used instead.

The American Heart Association identified five primary and three secondary metrics in their healthy diet pattern.[1] Primary metrics include fruits and vegetables (≥4.5 cups/d), fish and shellfish (≥2 3.5 oz servings/wk), sodium (≤1,500 mg/d), sugar-sweetened beverages (≤36 fl oz/wk), and whole grains (≥3 1 oz equivalent servings/d). Secondary metrics include nuts, seeds, and legumes (≥4 servings/wk), processed meats (≤2 1.75 oz servings/week), and saturated fat (≤7% energy). Meeting more of these target metrics equates to a higher healthy diet score and is correlated with better cardiovascular health.

Many studies investigating associations of diet with lipid profile measures have focused on dietary fat intake. A meta-analysis showed that a long-term low-fat diet is associated with a decline in serum TC and LDL-C, but a high-fat diet was associated with an increase in HDL-C and reduction in TGs.[66] However, the type of fat consumed matters. Lower TC was associated with lower intake of saturated fats and higher intake of polyunsaturated fats.[66] Although reducing SFA consumption results in decreases in TC and LDL-C, if reduction in SFA consumption alone is associated with any changes in HDL-C or TGs remains unclear.[67,68] It is also unclear if improvement in lipid profiles from dietary changes affects long-term outcomes. These associations may depend on the population of interest. For example, among a population of elderly women, there was a strong positive association between high SFA intake and ASCVD mortality, as well as a strong association between SFA intake and LDL-C; however, LDL-C was not associated with ASCVD mortality.[67] Reduced dietary saturated fat has been shown to significantly reduce risk of cardiovascular events but not significantly affect all-cause mortality, fatal or nonfatal MI, or stroke.[68]

Physical Activity/Sedentary Behavior

The many health benefits of physical activity are well established, including lowering ASCVD risk, improving glycemic control, and improving lipid profile measures.[69,70] Frequency, intensity, time spent being physically active, and type of activity (aerobic or muscle-strengthening exercise) are associated with beneficial changes in lipid levels.[69] Increased physical fitness levels in young adulthood are associated with lower incidence of low HDL-C, high LDL-C, and high TGs in middle age.[70] Conversely, sedentary behavior has been associated with a decrease in HDL-C and replacing short bouts of sedentary behavior with light or moderate activity may improve HDL-C levels.[71] Although most of the physical activity evidence associated with dyslipidemia is related to HDL-C and TGs, the effects it has on LDL-C and TC are less consistent.[69]

The Physical Activity Guidelines for Americans recommend that each week adults should engage in at least 150 to 300 minutes of moderate-intensity or 75 to 150 minutes of vigorous-intensity aerobic physical activity or an equivalent combination to achieve or maintain good health.[72] Muscle-strengthening activities are also recommended at least two days per week. Children and adolescents aged 6 to 17 years should get at least 60 minutes of physical activity daily.[72] People who do not meet the guidelines for physical activity tend to have lower HDL-C than those meeting the guidelines.[73]

For children and adolescents, evidence exists of physical activity's impact on all lipid profile measures. Total physical activity (min/d) is significantly associated with lower TGs and LDL-C and greater HDL-C.[74] By contrast, sedentary behavior (min/d) was associated with higher levels of TG and lower HDL-C in children and adolescents.[74,75] Even light-intensity physical activity is associated with higher HDL-C than no activity.[75]

Alcohol Consumption and Smoking

The association between alcohol intake and blood cholesterol levels is mixed. Alcohol consumption (drinks/d) has been positively associated with HDL-C and inversely associated with LDL-C, and it may have a J-shaped association with TC-to-HDL-C ratio.[76,77] The type of alcohol consumed (beer, wine, or spirits/mixed drinks) does not affect the positive association with HDL-C.[78] However, beer consumption has been associated with higher levels of TGs, most likely because of its carbohydrate content. To help Americans move toward a healthy dietary pattern and minimize risks associated with drinking, the 2020 to 2025 Dietary Guidelines for Americans recommends that adults of legal drinking age choose not to drink or to drink in moderation by limiting intakes to two drinks or less in a day for men and one drink or less in a day for women, on days when alcohol is consumed.[65]

Along with being a risk factor for CVD and stroke, smoking is also associated with markers of inflammation, development and progression of subclinical atherosclerosis, and lower HDL-C levels.[79] Serum cotinine (through smoking or secondhand exposure) is associated with increased risk of dyslipidemia.[80] People who smoke tend to have lower HDL-C and higher TGs than nonsmokers, with an apparent dose-dependent association between these measures and daily tobacco consumption.[81] Although former smokers have similar HDL-C levels as nonsmokers, former smokers tend to have higher levels of LDL-C and TC compared with nonsmokers and even current smokers.[81] The favorable association between alcohol consumption and HDL-C has been shown to be attenuated by active smoking in that an individual who currently smokes and has moderate alcohol consumption has similar HDL-C levels as an individual who is a nonsmoker and nondrinker.[78]

Population-Attributable Risk

Globally, there were an estimated 523 million prevalent cases of CVD and 18.6 million deaths from CVD in 2019.[19] Among the top 10 modifiable risk factors to which CVD burden was attributed, elevated LDL-C ranked third.[19] The population-attributable fraction refers to the fraction of all cases of a particular disease or other adverse condition, such as CVD morbidity or mortality, in a population that is attributable to a specific exposure, for example, dyslipidemia.[82] In 2020 the population-attributable fraction was 7.96 for mortality resulting from elevated LDL-C, ranging from 7.55 for men to 8.45 for women.[1]

Population-attributable risk refers to the proportion of all CVD events that could have been prevented if abnormal lipid levels were not present in the population. Analysis of data from the Framingham Heart Study demonstrated that population-attributable risk ranged from 3.0% to 7.5% depending on the combination of abnormal lipid measurements present, but the risk was highest for persons with elevated LDL-C, particularly in the presence of other abnormal lipid levels.[12] Approximately 6.4% of CVD events are attributable to elevated LDL-C alone, and 7.5% of CVD events are attributable to having the combination of elevated LDL-C, low HDL-C, and elevated TG. Among adults with diabetes but without CVD, 12.6% of all CVD morbidity, 19.6% of MI, and 13.7% of stroke were attributed to LDL-C of 100 mg/dL or greater.[83] Among those individuals with a history of CVD, 2.1% of all CVD, 5.1% of MI, and 5.5% of stroke were attributed to this level of LDL-C.

PREVENTION

For the prevention and management of dyslipidemia and its downstream complications, following a lifestyle that promotes cardiovascular health is essential. Lifestyle modifications form the cornerstone for improving lipid profile measures and reducing ASCVD risk and are recommended both before initiation of, and concurrently with, pharmacological interventions.[9,84] Multicomponent interventions that focus on comprehensive lifestyle changes, including increased physical activity, weight reduction, reduced sodium intake, and a reduced fat/calorie diet, as well as some components that focus on psychosocial factors, have a beneficial effect on cholesterol levels and coronary atherosclerosis.[85] Lifestyle interventions among children and adolescents with obesity, for example, have also resulted in beneficial changes in lipid profiles.[86]

In addition to primary prevention, primordial prevention is another important area of focus that works by preserving low risk in early life and preventing the development of CVD risk factors. Exposure to lower lipid levels earlier in life is associated with better cardiovascular health as an adult.[87] Sustaining a healthy lifestyle, from young adulthood through middle age, is associated with lower CVD risk in later years. The Coronary Artery Risk Development in Young Adults (CARDIA) prospective cohort study examined five healthy lifestyle factors (not smoking cigarettes; being physically active; and maintaining a healthy BMI, low alcohol intake, and a healthy diet) and found that having a greater number of healthy lifestyle factors as a young adult was positively associated with having a lower CVD risk and with changes in measures of subclinical atherosclerosis, such as CAC and CIMT, 20 years later.[88]

Dyslipidemia is of concern among children and adolescents in the United States. Long-term exposure to unhealthy cholesterol levels in childhood and young adulthood can increase risk for CHD in middle age.[4] Therefore, it is important to check lipid profile measures and provide lifestyle modification assistance when necessary during childhood and young adulthood to reduce the burden of ASCVD later in life.

Screening

Adults With Risk Factors

In the United States, the Multisociety Guideline on the Management of Blood Cholesterol recommended that adults aged 20 years or older who are free from ASCVD have a blood lipid profile measured every four to six years, and more frequently for people at increased CVD risk.[9] According to 2019 data from the Behavioral Risk Factor Surveillance System (BRFSS), the majority of US adults reported having had their blood cholesterol checked in the past five years (86.6%), and 33.1% were aware they had high cholesterol (i.e., report having been told that they had high cholesterol by a health care provider).[1]

Differences in screening and awareness exist across gender, age, race/ethnicity, language, comorbid conditions, risk factors, geography (Figure 14-2), and structural factors such as health insurance, income level, and access to health care. Although more than half of the people who had their cholesterol tested were screened because of a health care provider recommendation, those who did not have their cholesterol tested were characterized by an increased number of risk factors such as smoking, sedentary behavior, excessive alcohol consumption, or low fruit and vegetable intake.[89] People facing more structural barriers were also more likely to report never having been screened for cholesterol.[90] In addition, men and adults younger than 65 years were less likely to have ever had a cholesterol screening compared with women and older adults.[91] In women, the prevalence of cholesterol screening was higher for nonsmokers, non-Hispanic Black adults, those who had health insurance, and those who had seen a health care provider within the recommended screening period of five years.[92] Non-Hispanic Black adults were more likely, and Hispanic adults less likely, to report having their cholesterol checked in the past five years compared with Asian/Pacific Islander adults and American Indian adults.[91] Among pregnant women in the United States, those who were less likely to receive cholesterol screening included younger women (18–29 years), uninsured women, those with a family income less than 200% of the federal poverty level, and those without a usual source of care.[93]

Children and Adolescents

For children and adolescents, universal lipid screening is recommended for ages 9 to 11 years and again for ages 17 to 21 years.[9,94] Despite these recommendations, screening rates are low.[34,95,96] Among children aged 9 to 11 who had continuous insurance coverage between 2013 and 2016, screening prevalence was 19.8%.[95] Of children and adolescents, those more likely to be screened for cholesterol were at an older age, had greater BMI and blood pressure percentiles, and were girls.[34] Targeted screening relying on family history of premature CVD or cholesterol disorders as the primary factor for determining lipid screening may miss 30% to 60% of children with dyslipidemia.[96]

Treatment

Lifestyle modification serves as the cornerstone of dyslipidemia treatment and is recommended for all patients. The current Cholesterol Management Guidelines, published in 2018, focus on four patient management groups (Table 14-5).[9] Along with lifestyle modification, cholesterol-lowering medications (including statins, bile acid sequestrants, fibrates, niacin, ezetimibe, and proprotein convertase subtilisin/kexin type 9 [PCSK9] inhibitors) may be recommended for people with dyslipidemia or who are at increased risk for ASCVD.

Evidence from randomized clinical trials demonstrates that the most efficient way to reduce ASCVD risk is through LDL-C lowering.[9] Therapies with a strong evidence-base for reducing LDL-C and risk of ASCVD include statins and add-on therapies including ezetimibe and PCSK9 inhibitors. Statins are first-line cholesterol-lowering therapy and work by interfering with cholesterol synthesis. The majority of people on cholesterol-lowering medications (≥90%) use statins.[24] As of 2018, guidelines also recommend ezetimibe and PCSK9 inhibitors for additional LDL-C lowering in patients who are statin intolerant or do not achieve sufficient LDL-C lowering on a maximally tolerated statin.[9] Specifically, guidelines on medication for blood cholesterol recommend that for patients with clinical ASCVD or severe primary hypercholesterolemia, high-intensity statins or

Table 14-5. Patient Management Groups Identified in the 2018 Guideline on the Management of Blood Cholesterol

Patient Management Group	Definition
Secondary ASCVD prevention	Adults with clinically established ASCVD, defined as acute coronary syndrome, history of myocardial infarction, stable and unstable angina, coronary or other arterial revascularization, stroke, transient ischemic attack, or peripheral arterial disease
Severe hypercholesterolemia	LDL-C levels ≥190 mg/dL (≥4.9 mmol/L)
Diabetes mellitus	Adults aged 40–75 y with diabetes and LDL-C levels 70–189 mg/dL
Primary prevention	Adults aged 40–75 y without diabetes having a 10-y pooled-cohort ASCVD risk score ≥7.5% and LDL-C levels 70–189 mg/dL

Source: Based on Grundy et al.[9]

Note: ASCVD = atherosclerotic cardiovascular disease; LDL-C = low-density lipoprotein cholesterol.

maximally tolerated statins should be prescribed first. In the highest-risk patients, an LDL-C threshold of 70 mg/dL should be used to consider addition of ezetimibe or PCSK9 inhibitors.

Statin therapy is categorized into three intensities based on percentage LDL-C lowering achieved, high (≥50%), moderate (30%–49%) or low (<30%).[9] Since statins have a dose-response relationship with reduction in LDL-C,[97] adults at highest ASCVD risk are recommended to take high-intensity statins rather than moderate-intensity statins, resulting in greater reductions in LDL-C levels. Depending on statin type and dosage, statins can reduce LDL-C anywhere from 10% to 58%, and because high-intensity statins are recommended for high-risk adults who tend to be at the high end of the population LDL-C distribution, cholesterol-lowering medication has played a key role in the population-level decrease in LDL-C and TC. Absolute LDL-C reduction in response to statin treatment is greatest among those with higher pretreatment LDL-C levels. However, percentage reduction is independent of the pretreatment LDL-C concentration.

Ezetimibe, which works by blocking cholesterol absorption in the small intestine, is considered a second-line add-on therapy for patients who are unable to tolerate statins or do not achieve adequate lowering of LDL-C on maximally tolerated statin.[9] Ezetimibe in addition to statin therapy may lower serum LDL-C by an additional 20%. The Improved Reduction of Outcomes: Vytorin Efficacy International Trial (IMPROVE IT) randomized clinical trial demonstrated the addition of ezetimibe to a statin therapy compared with statin therapy alone led to improved CVD outcomes in patients with acute coronary syndrome, regardless of baseline LDL-C levels.[98]

PCSK9 inhibitors, approved by the US Food and Drug Administration (FDA) in 2015, are monoclonal antibodies that lead to lower levels of circulating LDL-C in the blood.[99] Two randomized clinical trials demonstrated that PCSK9 inhibitors reduced LDL-C by an additional 43% to 64% and improved CVD outcomes in patients with acute coronary syndrome.[100,101] A network meta-analysis of 14 randomized control trials of add-on ezetimibe and PCSK9 inhibitors found they may reduce nonfatal MI and stroke in adults at the highest risk of CVD but not in those with moderate or low CVD risk.[102]

Persisting with treatment results in greater reductions in LDL-C concentrations and ischemic heart disease risk. An LDL-C reduction of 1.0 mmol/L (38.7 mg/dL) is associated with a reduction in risk of ischemic heart disease of 11% in the first year of treatment, 24% in the second year of treatment, 33% in years three to five, and 36% in the sixth year and beyond.[97] However, as with other chronic disease medications, adherence and persistence of cholesterol-lowering medication regimens can be a challenge, given numerous barriers that contribute to nonadherence, including side effects, regimen complexity, and comorbidities, among other factors.[103]

Cholesterol-lowering medication use has greatly increased in the past 30 years and is largely responsible for reducing population levels of TC and LDL-C.[23,60] National-level electronic health record prescription data from 2017 to 2022 show that total statin prescriptions have increased 22%, with the greatest increase for prescription of high-intensity statins alone (86%).[24] The total number of prescription fills for PCSK9 inhibitors has been increasing each quarter since their introduction to the market in 2015.[104] Their uptake may have accelerated after prices for PCSK9 inhibitors were reduced and they were included in updated national Cholesterol Management Guidelines, as well as after the FDA broadened indications for their use. Ezetimibe and PCSK9 inhibitors as add-on therapies for further LDL-C lowering are prescribed most frequently with high-intensity statins; the use of these lipid-lowering combination therapies has increased more than 200% and 2,000%, respectively, since 2017.[105]

Applying the 2018 multisociety cholesterol management guideline,[9] approximately one in four US adults (27.8%) would be recommended statin treatment, with prevalence varying by gender, age, and race/Hispanic origin (Table 14-6).[24] The highest prevalence was among males (21.9%), persons aged 65 years and older (36.3%), and non-Hispanic Black adults (24.0%). Prescriptions of, and adherence to, cholesterol-lowering

Table 14-6. Prevalence of Statin Recommendations Among Adults by Demographic Characteristics, 2018 Cholesterol Guidelines: National Health and Nutrition Examination Survey, United States, 2011–2018

	Unweighted n	Population N	Prevalence		
Characteristic	(Sample Size)	(Millions)	%	(SE)	N (Millions)
Total overall	8,642	231.6	19.9	(0.6)	46.1
Men	4,207	112.6	21.9	(0.9)	24.7
Women	4,435	119.0	18.0	(0.8)	21.5
Age, y					
20–39	2,767	82.4	2.2	(0.3)	1.8
40–64	3,799	104.0	26.8	(1.0)	27.9
≥65	2,076	45.2	36.3	(1.5)	16.4
65–75	1,286	29.9	54.8	(2.2)	16.4
>75	790	15.3	0.0	(0.0)	0.0
Race/Hispanic origin					
Non-Hispanic White	3,276	150.3	19.2	(0.8)	28.9
Non-Hispanic Black	1,817	26.2	24.0	(0.9)	6.3
Non-Hispanic Asian	1,124	12.5	17.9	(1.3)	2.2
Hispanic	2,121	34.7	19.0	(0.9)	6.6
Other	304	7.9	26.4	(3.6)	2.1

Source: Thompson-Paul et al.[24] Adapted with permission of Elsevier.
Note: SE = standard error.

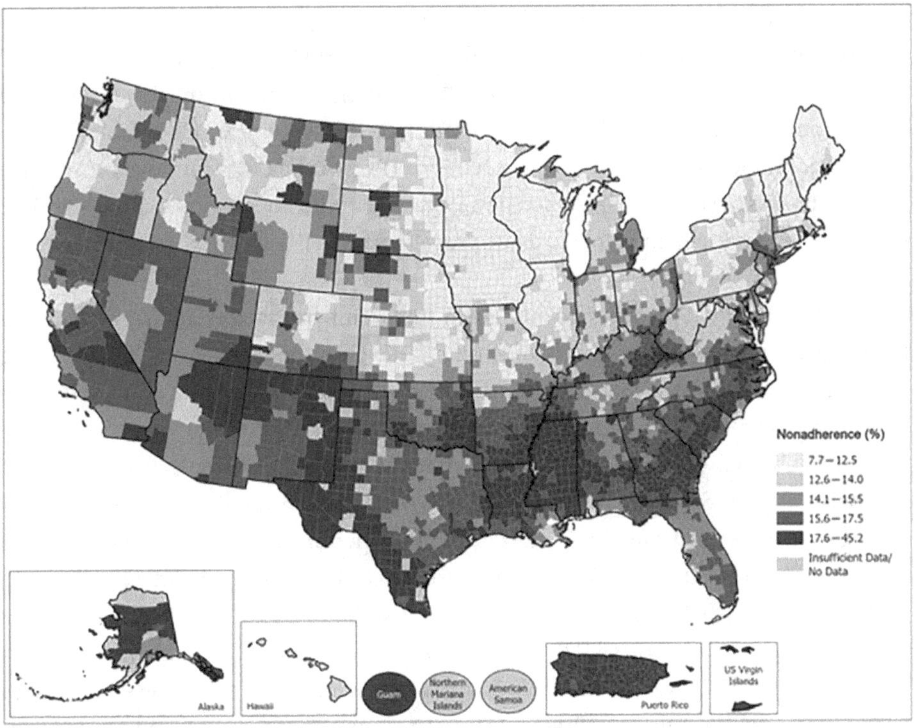

Source: Based on CDC.[107]

Note: Medication nonadherence is defined as the proportion of days a beneficiary was covered with medication of >80%, and was assessed using prescription drug claims data among Medicare Advantage or Medicare fee-for-service in beneficiaries aged ≥65 years with Medicare Part D coverage.

Figure 14-4. Cholesterol-Lowering Medication Nonadherence Among Medicare Part D Beneficiaries Aged 65 Years and Older: United States, 2019

medications vary by geographic region. In 2015 prescriptions of high-intensity statins were greatest among states in the New England region and lowest among those in the East South-Central and West South-Central regions.[106] Similarly, nonadherence was lowest in the New England region and highest in the East and West South-Central regions (Figure 14-4).[107]

Clinical Decision-Making and Risk Scores

Clinical decisions about treatment are based on both medical knowledge and a complete understanding of the patient, including the individual's risk factors, health concerns, treatment preferences, and health goals.

Dyslipidemia frequently co-occurs with other ASCVD risk factors and comorbidities. CVD researchers have long sought to develop easily understandable methods to quantify the risk of future ASCVD events in relation to an individual's risk factor profile. One of the first gender-specific 10-year CVD risk equations developed was based on the Framingham Heart Study and considered age, diabetes status, smoking status, blood pressure medication use, TC, and HDL-C.[108] However, this risk estimator did not take into account racial/ethnic differences when estimating 10-year CVD risk.[109] More recently developed, the pooled-cohort equations (PCE) used data from five prospective community-based studies, which include a larger and more diverse population. The PCE includes the Framingham risk calculator predictors as well as gender- and race-specific factors.[109]

Although the PCE incorporate additional important risk factors compared with the Framingham risk calculator, there remain limitations to these equations. For example, traditional risk equations may underestimate risk in certain high-risk populations such as individuals with HIV,[110] and these traditional equations may or may not be applicable to diverse subgroup populations across the United States, such as heterogeneous Hispanic and Asian groups. Studies have continued to investigate the validity of these equations among diverse populations. Validation of the PCE performed with a diverse US adult population found that as ASCVD risk increased, LDL-C levels slightly increased from a mean of 115.9 mg/dL for those with ASCVD risk less than 5% to 118.4 mg/dL for ASCVD risk 10% or greater, whereas HDL-C (59.5–49.7 mg/dL) and TC (197.2–194.6 mg/dL) levels decreased.[111] However, the PCE tends to overestimate risk, specifically for those adults with a PCE-estimated 10-year ASCVD risk of 10% or greater and among subgroups of Asian populations.[112] Researchers continue to examine additional factors that may improve individual risk prediction or those that could potentially be used in population health monitoring.[113]

Communicating risk to help guide recommendations for patients can be complicated. The concept of heart age was introduced to represent an alternative way of describing an individual's risk for having CVD events.[114] Heart age estimates the difference between the individual's chronological age and vascular age based on the risk factors traditionally used in CVD risk prediction equations. In the general US adult population, men and women were found to have heart ages 7.8 and 5.4 years in excess of their chronological age, respectively.[114] This difference of excess heart age was even greater in higher-risk populations such as those with cancer (8.5 y for men and 6.5 y for women) or people living with HIV (11.5 y for men and 13.5 y for women).[39]

MOVING FORWARD

Dyslipidemia is a well-known risk factor for CVD, yet prevalence of screening varies across populations and well-established, effective treatments are underutilized. Efforts to promote improved screening and management of blood cholesterol through all available avenues (e.g., community health workers, team-based care, patient-centered care, shared decision-making) may be important for addressing this gap. In addition, efforts to improve cholesterol-screening prevalence among children and adolescents may be a key opportunity. Cholesterol screening earlier in life may identify people who may be at increased risk for adverse ASCVD outcomes, providing opportunities to modify health behaviors or start pharmacologic treatment earlier and thereby reduce risk later in life. Efforts to address risk factors such as physical inactivity, poor diet, smoking, and obesity should be emphasized beginning early in life and continuing throughout adulthood.

In 2011 to 2018 less than half of people recommended or considered for statin treatment reported using statins, according to NHANES data.[24] Prescription of statins and other cholesterol lowering medications has increased, potentially indicating uptake and clinical implementation of the Cholesterol Management Guidelines.[115] However, improvements in the optimization of cholesterol management and ASCVD prevention through clinical practice and patient–provider discussion may still be beneficial.[116] It may be beneficial to explore factors associated with ASCVD risk such as lipoprotein (a) and CAC to better understand how they may be useful in helping to guide therapy decisions.[113]

During the course of the COVID-19 pandemic, the cardioprotective effects of the anti-inflammatory and antithrombotic properties of statins for persons infected with SARS-CoV-2 has been hypothesized, though findings have been mixed.[117] A meta-analysis including 12 studies and 72,881 participants found that statin therapy was associated with a 35% reduced risk of mortality among hospitalized COVID-19 patients.[118] However, a recent randomized clinical trial failed to find a reduction in certain cardiovascular events or mortality associated with statin use among patients with SARS-CoV-2.[119]

The awareness, prevention, screening, and management of dyslipidemia are influenced by a multitude of factors, from individual patient-level factors (e.g., health insurance coverage, adherence to medications/lifestyle) to provider and practice setting (e.g., communication skills, patient education/care coordination), up to local, state, and national policies (e.g., income inequality, hospital performance policies, Medicare reimbursement). Given the many intervention points for public health practitioners, selecting which areas to target depends on the setting, population, and program. Under these circumstances, public health practitioners are encouraged to use evidence-based recommendations to maximize their impact.

DISCUSSION QUESTIONS

1. How is dyslipidemia associated with atherosclerotic cardiovascular disease?
2. Which risk factors of dyslipidemia are preventable?
3. What proportion of ASCVD events in the US population are attributable to dyslipidemia?
4. What is the most common treatment used for dyslipidemia? What are some reasons that this treatment is commonly used?

ACKNOWLEDGMENTS

The authors would like to thank key team members from the Centers for Disease Control and Prevention, Division for Heart Disease and Stroke Prevention, for assistance in developing Tables 14-3, 14-4, and 14-6 and Figures 14-2, 14-3, and 14-4: Cathleen Gillespie and Wen Zhou (Statistical Unit), and Linda Schieb and Yui Fujii (Small Area Analysis Unit). The findings and conclusions in this chapter are those of the authors and do not necessarily represent the official position of the Centers for Disease Control and Prevention, the US Department of Health and Human Services, or the US Public Health Service. The authors have no disclosures nor any relationship with industry.

REFERENCES

1. Tsao CW, Aday AW, Almarzooq ZI, et al. Heart disease and stroke statistics—2022 update: a report from the American Heart Association. *Circulation.* 2022;145(8):e153–e639. doi:10.1161/cir.0000000000001052
2. Ross R. The pathogenesis of atherosclerosis: a perspective for the 1990s. *Nature.* 1993; 362(6423):801–809. doi:10.1038/362801a0
3. Bentzon JF, Otsuka F, Virmani R, Falk E. Mechanisms of plaque formation and rupture. *Circulation Res.* 2014;114(12):1852–1866. doi:10.1161/circresaha.114.302721
4. Zhang Y, Pletcher MJ, Vittinghoff E, et al. Association between cumulative low-density lipoprotein cholesterol exposure during young adulthood and middle age and risk of cardiovascular events. *JAMA Cardiol.* 2021;6(12):1406–1413. doi:10.1001/jamacardio.2021.3508
5. Navar-Boggan AM, Peterson ED, D'Agostino RB, Sr., Neely B, Sniderman AD, Pencina MJ. Hyperlipidemia in early adulthood increases long-term risk of coronary heart disease. *Circulation.* 2015;131(5):451–458. doi:10.1161/circulationaha.114.012477
6. Bangalore S, Fayyad R, Messerli FH, et al. Relation of variability of low-density lipoprotein cholesterol and blood pressure to events in patients with previous myocardial infarction from the IDEAL trial. *Am J Cardiol.* 2017;119(3):379–387. doi:10.1016/j.amjcard.2016.10.037
7. Helkin A, Stein JJ, Lin S, Siddiqui S, Maier KG, Gahtan V. Dyslipidemia part 1—review of lipid metabolism and vascular cell physiology. *Vasc Endovascular Surg.* 2016;50(2):107–118. doi:10.1177/1538574416628654
8. Otsuka F, Kramer MC, Woudstra P, et al. Natural progression of atherosclerosis from pathologic intimal thickening to late fibroatheroma in human coronary arteries: a pathology study. *Atherosclerosis.* 2015;241(2):772–782. doi:10.1016/j.atherosclerosis.2015.05.011
9. Grundy SM, Stone NJ, Bailey AL, et al. AHA/ACC/AACVPR/AAPA/ABC/ACPM/ADA/AGS/APhA/ASPC/NLA/PCNA guideline on the management of blood cholesterol: a report of the American College of Cardiology/American Heart Association Task Force on Clinical Practice Guidelines. *J Am Coll Cardiol.* 2018; 73(24):e285–e350. doi:10.1016/j.jacc.2018.11.003
10. Martin SS, Blaha MJ, Elshazly MB, et al. Friedewald-estimated versus directly measured low-density lipoprotein cholesterol and treatment implications. *J Am Coll Cardiol.* 2013; 62(8):732–739. doi:10.1016/j.jacc.2013.01.079

11. Whelton SP, Meeusen JW, Donato LJ, et al. Evaluating the atherogenic burden of individuals with a Friedewald-estimated low-density lipoprotein cholesterol <70 mg/dL compared with a novel low-density lipoprotein estimation method. *J Clin Lipidol.* 2017;11(4):1065–1072. doi:10.1016/j.jacl.2017.05.005
12. Andersson C, Lyass A, Vasan RS, Massaro JM, D'Agostino RB, Sr., Robins SJ. Long-term risk of cardiovascular events across a spectrum of adverse major plasma lipid combinations in the Framingham Heart Study. *Am Heart J.* 2014;168(6):878–883.e1. doi:10.1016/j.ahj.2014.08.007
13. Kolovou GD, Anagnostopoulou KK, Damaskos DS, et al. Gender differences in the lipid profile of dyslipidemic subjects. *Eur J Intern Med.* 2009;20(2):145–151. doi:10.1016/j.ejim.2008.06.011
14. Lewington S, Whitlock G, Clarke R, et al. Blood cholesterol and vascular mortality by age, sex, and blood pressure: a meta-analysis of individual data from 61 prospective studies with 55,000 vascular deaths. *Lancet.* 2007;370(9602):1829–1839. doi:10.1016/s0140-6736(07)61778-4
15. Wilkins JT, Ning H, Stone NJ, et al. Coronary heart disease risks associated with high levels of HDL cholesterol. *J Am Heart Assoc.* 2014;3(2):e000519. doi:10.1161/jaha.113.000519
16. Martin SS, Blaha MJ, Blankstein R, et al. Dyslipidemia, coronary artery calcium, and incident atherosclerotic cardiovascular disease: implications for statin therapy from the multi-ethnic study of atherosclerosis. *Circulation.* 2014;129(1):77–86. doi:10.1161/circulationaha.113.003625
17. Santos RD, Gidding SS, Hegele RA, et al. Defining severe familial hypercholesterolaemia and the implications for clinical management: a consensus statement from the International Atherosclerosis Society Severe Familial Hypercholesterolemia Panel. *Lancet Diabetes Endocrinol.* 2016;4(10):850–861. doi:10.1016/s2213-8587(16)30041-9
18. Hopkins PN, Toth PP, Ballantyne CM, Rader DJ. Familial hypercholesterolemias: prevalence, genetics, diagnosis and screening recommendations from the National Lipid Association Expert Panel on Familial Hypercholesterolemia. *J Clin Lipidol.* 2011;5(3 suppl):S9–S17. doi:10.1016/j.jacl.2011.03.452
19. Roth GA, Mensah GA, Johnson CO, et al. Global burden of cardiovascular diseases and risk factors, 1990–2019: update from the GBD 2019 study. *J Am Coll Cardiol.* 2020;76(25): 2982–3021. doi:10.1016/j.jacc.2020.11.010
20. Yusuf S, Hawken S, Ounpuu S, et al. Effect of potentially modifiable risk factors associated with myocardial infarction in 52 countries (the INTERHEART Study): case-control study. *Lancet.* 2004;364(9438):937–592. doi:10.1016/s0140-6736(04)17018-9
21. Stamler J, Wentworth D, Neaton JD. Is relationship between serum cholesterol and risk of premature death from coronary heart disease continuous and graded? findings in 356,222 primary screenees of the Multiple Risk Factor Intervention Trial (MRFIT). *JAMA.* 1986;256(20):2823–2828.
22. Han BH, Han K, Yoon KH, Kim MK, Lee SH. Impact of mean and variability of high-density lipoprotein-cholesterol on the risk of myocardial infarction, stroke, and mortality in the general population. *J Am Heart Assoc.* 2020;9(7):e015493. doi:10.1161/jaha.119.015493
23. Mercado C, DeSimone AK, Odom E, Gillespie C, Ayala C, Loustalot F. Prevalence of cholesterol treatment eligibility and medication use among adults—United States, 2005–2012. *MMWR Morb Mortal Wkly Rep.* 2015;64(47):1305–1311. doi:10.15585/mmwr.mm6447a1

24. Thompson-Paul AM, Gillespie C, Wall HK, Loustalot F, Sperling L, Hong Y. Recommended and observed statin use among US adults—National Health and Nutrition Examination Survey, 2011–2018. *J Clin Lipidol.* 2023;17(2):225–235.10. doi:1016/j.jacl.2022.12.005
25. Fox KM, Wang L, Gandra SR, Quek RGW, Li L, Baser O. Clinical and economic burden associated with cardiovascular events among patients with hyperlipidemia: a retrospective cohort study. *BMC Cardiovasc Dis.* 2016;16:13. doi:10.1186/s12872-016-0190-x
26. Beheshti SO, Madsen CM, Varbo A, Nordestgaard BG. Worldwide prevalence of familial hypercholesterolemia: meta-analyses of 11 million subjects. *J Am Coll Cardiol.* 2020;75(20): 2553–2566. doi:10.1016/j.jacc.2020.03.057
27. Goldberg AC, Hopkins PN, Toth PP, et al. Familial hypercholesterolemia: screening, diagnosis and management of pediatric and adult patients: clinical guidance from the National Lipid Association Expert Panel on Familial Hypercholesterolemia. *J Clin Lipidol.* 2011;5(3 suppl): S1–S8. doi:10.1016/j.jacl.2011.04.003
28. Park YS, Ryu GW, Choi M. Multiple metabolic comorbidities and their consequences among patients with peripheral arterial disease. *PLoS One.* 2022;17(5):e0268201. doi:10.1371/journal.pone.0268201
29. Isomaa B, Almgren P, Tuomi T, et al. Cardiovascular morbidity and mortality associated with the metabolic syndrome. *Diabetes Care.* 2001;24(4):683–689. doi:10.2337/diacare.24.4.683
30. Kaze AD, Santhanam P, Musani SK, Ahima R, Echouffo-Tcheugui JB. Metabolic dyslipidemia and cardiovascular outcomes in type 2 diabetes mellitus: findings from the Look AHEAD study. *J Am Heart Assoc.* 2021;10(7):e016947. doi:10.1161/jaha.120.016947
31. Eliasson B, Gudbjornsdottir S, Zethelius B, Eeg-Olofsson K, Cederholm J. LDL-cholesterol versus non-HDL-to-HDL-cholesterol ratio and risk for coronary heart disease in type 2 diabetes. *Eur J Prev Cardiol.* 2014;21(11):1420–1428. doi:10.1177/2047487313494292
32. Nichols GA, Joshua-Gotlib S, Parasuraman S. Independent contribution of A1C, systolic blood pressure, and LDL cholesterol control to risk of cardiovascular disease hospitalizations in type 2 diabetes: an observational cohort study. *J Gen Intern Med.* 2013;28(5):691–697. doi:10.1007/s11606-012-2320-1
33. Tang N, Ma J, Tao R, et al. The effects of the interaction between BMI and dyslipidemia on hypertension in adults. *Sci Rep.* 2022;12(1):927. doi:10.1038/s41598-022-04968-8
34. Margolis KL, Greenspan LC, Trower NK, et al. Lipid screening in children and adolescents in community practice: 2007 to 2010. *Circ Cardiovasc Qual Outcomes.* 2014;7(5):718–726. doi:10.1161/circoutcomes.114.000842
35. Matsushita K, van der Velde M, Astor BC, et al. Association of estimated glomerular filtration rate and albuminuria with all-cause and cardiovascular mortality in general population cohorts: a collaborative meta-analysis. *Lancet.* 2010;375(9731):2073–2081. doi:10.1016/s0140-6736(10)60674-5
36. Bajaj A, Xie D, Cedillo-Couvert E, et al. Lipids, apolipoproteins, and risk of atherosclerotic cardiovascular disease in persons with CKD. *Am J Kidney Dis.* 2019;73(6):827–836. doi:10.1053/j.ajkd.2018.11.010
37. Hashemi L, Hsiung JT, Arif Y, et al. Serum low-density lipoprotein cholesterol and cardiovascular disease risk across chronic kidney disease stages (data from 1.9 million United States veterans). *Am J Cardiol.* 2022;170:47–55. doi:10.1016/j.amjcard.2022.01.034

38. Freiberg MS, Chang CC, Kuller LH, et al. HIV infection and the risk of acute myocardial infarction. *JAMA Intern Med.* 2013;173(8):614–622. doi:10.1001/jamainternmed.2013.3728
39. Thompson-Paul AM, Palella FJ, Jr., Rayeed N, et al. Excess heart age in adult outpatients in routine HIV care. AIDS. 2019;33(12):1935–1942. doi:10.1097/qad.0000000000002304
40. Maggi P, Di Biagio A, Rusconi S, et al. Cardiovascular risk and dyslipidemia among persons living with HIV: a review. *BMC Infect Dis.* 2017;17(1):551. doi:10.1186/s12879-017-2626-z
41. Panel on Antiretroviral Guidelines for Adults and Adolescents. Guidelines for the use of antiretroviral agents in adults and adolescents with HIV. 2022. Department of Health and Human Services. Available at: https://clinicalinfo.hiv.gov/sites/default/files/guidelines/documents/adult-adolescent-arv/guidelines-adult-adolescent-arv.pdf. Accessed January 19, 2023.
42. Sharma J, McAlister J, Aggarwal NR, et al. Evaluation and management of blood lipids through a woman's life cycle. *Am J Prev Cardiol.* 2022;10:100333. doi:10.1016/j.ajpc.2022.100333
43. Mortensen MB, Nordestgaard BG. Elevated LDL cholesterol and increased risk of myocardial infarction and atherosclerotic cardiovascular disease in individuals aged 70–100 years: a contemporary primary prevention cohort. *Lancet.* 2020;396(10263):1644–1652. doi:10.1016/s0140-6736(20)32233-9
44. Sumner AD, Sardi GL, Reed JF, III. Components of the metabolic syndrome differ between young and old adults in the US population. *J Clin Hypertens (Greenwich, Conn).* 2012;14(8):502–506. doi:10.1111/j.1751-7176.2012.00647.x
45. Zhang Y, Vittinghoff E, Pletcher MJ, et al. Associations of blood pressure and cholesterol levels during young adulthood with later cardiovascular events. *J Am Coll Cardiol.* 2019;74(3):330–341. doi:10.1016/j.jacc.2019.03.529
46. Dai S, Yang Q, Yuan K, et al. Non-high-density lipoprotein cholesterol: distribution and prevalence of high serum levels in children and adolescents: United States National Health and Nutrition Examination Surveys, 2005–2010. *J Pediatr.* 2014;164(2):247–253. doi:10.1016/j.jpeds.2013.08.069
47. Pool LR, Aguayo L, Brzezinski M, et al. Childhood risk factors and adulthood cardiovascular disease: a systematic review. *J Pediatr.* 2021;232:118–126.e23. doi:10.1016/j.jpeds.2021.01.053
48. Rodriguez CJ, Daviglus ML, Swett K, et al. Dyslipidemia patterns among Hispanics/Latinos of diverse background in the United States. *Am J Med.* 2014;127(12):1186–1194.e1. doi:10.1016/j.amjmed.2014.07.026
49. Frank AT, Zhao B, Jose PO, Azar KM, Fortmann SP, Palaniappan LP. Racial/ethnic differences in dyslipidemia patterns. *Circulation.* 2014;129(5):570–579. doi:10.1161/circulationaha.113.005757
50. Egan BM, Li J, Sarasua SM, et al. Cholesterol control among uninsured adults did not improve from 2001–2004 to 2009–2012 as disparities with both publicly and privately insured adults doubled. *J Am Heart Assoc.* 2017;6(11):e006105. doi:10.1161/jaha.117.006105
51. Gamboa CM, Colantonio LD, Brown TM, Carson AP, Safford MM. Race-sex differences in statin use and low-density lipoprotein cholesterol control among people with diabetes mellitus in the Reasons for Geographic and Racial Differences in Stroke Study. *J Am Heart Assoc.* 2017;6(5):e004264. doi:10.1161/jaha.116.004264

52. Hudson SE, Feigenbaum MS, Patil N, Ding E, Ewing A, Trilk JL. Screening and socioeconomic associations of dyslipidemia in young adults. *BMC Public Health.* 2020;20(1):104. doi:10.1186/s12889-019-8099-9
53. Global Burden of Disease 2017 Risk Factor Collaborators. Global, regional, and national comparative risk assessment of 84 behavioural, environmental and occupational, and metabolic risks or clusters of risks for 195 countries and territories, 1990–2017: a systematic analysis for the Global Burden of Disease Study 2017. *Lancet.* 2018;392(10159):1923–1994. doi:10.1016/s0140-6736(18)32225-6
54. Hsia SH, Desnoyers ML, Lee ML. Differences in cholesterol management among states in relation to health insurance and race/ethnicity across the United States. *J Clin Lipidol.* 2013;7(6):675–682. doi:10.1016/j.jacl.2013.03.010
55. Centers for Disease Control and Prevention (CDC), Behavioral Risk Factor Surveillance System Survey and CDC National Center for Chronic Disease Prevention and Health Promotion, Division of Population Health. PLACES: Local Data for Better Health. Available at: https://www.cdc.gov/PLACES. Accessed January 19, 2023.
56. Howard G, Howard VJ. Twenty years of progress toward understanding the Stroke Belt. *Stroke.* 2020;51(3):742–750. doi:10.1161/strokeaha.119.024155
57. Weeda ER, Bishu KG, Ward R, Axon RN, Taber DJ, Gebregziabher M. Joint effect of race/ethnicity or location of residence and sex on low density lipoprotein-cholesterol among veterans with type 2 diabetes: a 10-year retrospective cohort study. *BMC Cardiovasc Dis.* 2020;20(1):449. doi:10.1186/s12872-020-01730-8
58. Pahigiannis K, Thompson-Paul AM, Barfield W, et al. Progress toward improved cardiovascular health in the United States. *Circulation.* 2019;139(16):1957–1973. doi:10.1161/circulationaha.118.035408
59. Carroll MD, Fryar CD. *Total and High-Density Lipoprotein Cholesterol in Adults: United States, 2015–2018.* National Center for Health Statistics; April 2020. NCHS Data Brief 363. Available at: https://www.cdc.gov/nchs/data/databriefs/db363-h.pdf. Accessed August 9, 2023.
60. Kuklina EV, Carroll MD, Shaw KM, Hirsch R. Trends in high LDL cholesterol, cholesterol-lowering medication use, and dietary saturated-fat intake: United States, 1976–2010. *NCHS Data Brief.* 2013;(117):1–8.
61. Klop B, Elte JW, Cabezas MC. Dyslipidemia in obesity: mechanisms and potential targets. *Nutrients.* 2013;5(4):1218–1240. doi:10.3390/nu5041218
62. Rosito GA, Massaro JM, Hoffmann U, et al. Pericardial fat, visceral abdominal fat, cardiovascular disease risk factors, and vascular calcification in a community-based sample: the Framingham Heart Study. *Circulation.* 2008;117(5):605–613. doi:10.1161/circulationaha.107.743062
63. Melmer A, Lamina C, Tschoner A, et al. Body adiposity index and other indexes of body composition in the SAPHIR study: association with cardiovascular risk factors. *Obesity (Silver Spring).* 2013;21(4):775–781. doi:10.1002/oby.20289
64. Nguyen D, Kit B, Carroll M. Abnormal cholesterol among children and adolescents in the United States, 2011–2014. *NCHS Data Brief.* 2015;(228):1–8.
65. US Department of Health and Human Services; US Department of Agriculture. *2020–2025 Dietary Guidelines for Americans.* December 2020. Available at: https://www.dietaryguidelines.gov/sites/default/files/2020-12/Dietary_Guidelines_for_Americans_2020-2025.pdf. Accessed January 19, 2023.

66. Schwingshackl L, Hoffmann G. Comparison of effects of long-term low-fat vs high-fat diets on blood lipid levels in overweight or obese patients: a systematic review and meta-analysis. *J Acad Nutr Diet*. 2013;113(12):1640–1661. doi:10.1016/j.jand.2013.07.010
67. Blekkenhorst LC, Prince RL, Hodgson JM, et al. Dietary saturated fat intake and atherosclerotic vascular disease mortality in elderly women: a prospective cohort study. *The Am J Clin Nutr*. 2015;101(6):1263–1268. doi:10.3945/ajcn.114.102392
68. Hooper L, Martin N, Abdelhamid A, Davey Smith G. Reduction in saturated fat intake for cardiovascular disease. *Cochrane Database Syst Rev*. 2015;(6):Cd011737. doi:10.1002/14651858.Cd011737
69. Barone Gibbs B, Hivert MF, Jerome GJ, et al. Physical activity as a critical component of first-line treatment for elevated blood pressure or cholesterol: who, what, and how?: a scientific statement from the American Heart Association. *Hypertension*. 2021;78(2):e26–e37. doi:10.1161/hyp.0000000000000196
70. Sarzynski MA, Schuna JM, Jr., Carnethon MR, et al. Association of fitness with incident dyslipidemias over 25 years in the Coronary Artery Risk Development in Young Adults study. *Am J Prev Med*. 2015;49(5):745–752. doi:10.1016/j.amepre.2015.04.022
71. Whitaker KM, Pettee Gabriel K, Buman MP, et al. Associations of accelerometer-measured sedentary time and physical activity with prospectively assessed cardiometabolic risk factors: the CARDIA study. *J Am Heart Assoc*. 2019;8(1):e010212. doi:10.1161/jaha.118.010212
72. US Department of Health and Human Services. *Physical Activity Guidelines for Americans, 2nd Edition*. 2018. Available at: https://health.gov/sites/default/files/2019-09/Physical_Activity_Guidelines_2nd_edition.pdf. Accessed January 19, 2023.
73. Everage NJ, Linkletter CD, Gjelsvik A, McGarvey ST, Loucks EB. Social and behavioral risk marker clustering associated with biological risk factors for coronary heart disease: NHANES 2001–2004. *Biomed Res Int*. 2014;2014:389853. doi:10.1155/2014/389853
74. Väistö J, Eloranta AM, Viitasalo A, et al. Physical activity and sedentary behaviour in relation to cardiometabolic risk in children: cross-sectional findings from the Physical Activity and Nutrition in Children (PANIC) Study. *Int J Behav Nutr Phys Act*. 2014;11:55. doi:10.1186/1479-5868-11-55
75. Cliff DP, Okely AD, Burrows TL, et al. Objectively measured sedentary behavior, physical activity, and plasma lipids in overweight and obese children. *Obesity (Silver Spring)*. 2013;21(2):382–385. doi:10.1002/oby.20005
76. Wakabayashi I. Alcohol intake and triglycerides/high-density lipoprotein cholesterol ratio in men with hypertension. *Am J Hypertens*. 2013;26(7):888–895. doi:10.1093/ajh/hpt033
77. Shimomura T, Wakabayashi I. Inverse associations between light-to-moderate alcohol intake and lipid-related indices in patients with diabetes. *Cardiovasc Diabetol*. 2013;12:104. doi:10.1186/1475-2840-12-104
78. Slagter SN, van Vliet-Ostaptchouk JV, Vonk JM, et al. Combined effects of smoking and alcohol on metabolic syndrome: the LifeLines cohort study. *PLoS One*. 2014;9(4):e96406. doi:10.1371/journal.pone.0096406
79. US Department of Health and Human Services. Smoking cessation: a report of the surgeon general—executive summary. Office of the Surgeon General. 2020. Available at: https://www.hhs.gov/sites/default/files/2020-cessation-sgr-executive-summary.pdf. Accessed January 19, 2023.

80. Theilen LH, McNeil RB, Hunter S, et al. Serum cotinine and adverse cardiovascular outcomes: a cross-sectional secondary analysis of the nuMoM2b Heart Health Study. *Am J Perinatol.* 2021. doi:10.1055/a-1580-3155
81. Slagter SN, van Vliet-Ostaptchouk JV, Vonk JM, et al. Associations between smoking, components of metabolic syndrome and lipoprotein particle size. *BMC Med.* 2013;11:195. doi:10.1186/1741-7015-11-195
82. Mansournia MA, Altman DG. Population attributable fraction. *BMJ.* 2018;360:k757. doi:10.1136/bmj.k757
83. Vazquez-Benitez G, Desai JR, Xu S, et al. Preventable major cardiovascular events associated with uncontrolled glucose, blood pressure, and lipids and active smoking in adults with diabetes with and without cardiovascular disease: a contemporary analysis. *Diabetes Care.* 2015;38(5):905–912. doi:10.2337/dc14-1877
84. Arnett DK, Blumenthal RS, Albert MA, et al. 2019 ACC/AHA Guideline on the primary prevention of cardiovascular disease: a report of the American College of Cardiology/American Heart Association Task Force on Clinical Practice Guidelines. *Circulation.* 2019;140(11):e596–e646. doi:10.1161/cir.0000000000000678
85. Dudum R, Juraschek SP, Appel LJ. Dose-dependent effects of lifestyle interventions on blood lipid levels: results from the PREMIER trial. *Patient Educ Couns.* 2019;102(10):1882–1891. doi:10.1016/j.pec.2019.05.005
86. Kelishadi R, Malekahmadi M, Hashemipour M, et al. Can a trial of motivational lifestyle counseling be effective for controlling childhood obesity and the associated cardiometabolic risk factors? *Pediatr Neonatol.* 2012;53(2):90–97. doi:10.1016/j.pedneo.2012.01.005
87. Ference BA, Yoo W, Alesh I, et al. Effect of long-term exposure to lower low-density lipoprotein cholesterol beginning early in life on the risk of coronary heart disease: a Mendelian randomization analysis. *J Am Coll Cardiol.* 2012;60(25):2631–2639. doi:10.1016/j.jacc.2012.09.017
88. Spring B, Moller AC, Colangelo LA, et al. Healthy lifestyle change and subclinical atherosclerosis in young adults: Coronary Artery Risk Development in Young Adults (CARDIA) study. *Circulation.* 2014;130(1):10–17. doi:10.1161/circulationaha.113.005445
89. Filippidis FT, Gerovasili V, Majeed A. Association between cardiovascular risk factors and measurements of blood pressure and cholesterol in 27 European countries in 2009. *Prev Med.* 2014;67:71–74. doi:10.1016/j.ypmed.2014.07.002
90. Heintzman JD, Bailey SR, Muench J, Killerby M, Cowburn S, Marino M. Lack of lipid screening disparities in obese Latino adults at health centers. *Am J Prev Med.* 2017;52(6):805–809. doi:10.1016/j.amepre.2016.12.020
91. Liao Y, Bang D, Cosgrove S, et al. Surveillance of health status in minority communities—Racial and Ethnic Approaches to Community Health Across the US (REACH US) Risk Factor Survey, United States, 2009. *MMWR Surveill Summ.* 2011;60(6):1–44.
92. Robbins CL, Dietz PM, Bombard JM, Gibbs F, Ko JY, Valderrama AL. Blood pressure and cholesterol screening prevalence among US women of reproductive age opportunities to improve screening. *Am J Prev Med.* 2011;41(6):588–595. doi:10.1016/j.amepre.2011.08.010
93. Mszar R, Gopal DJ, Chowdary R, et al. Racial/ethnic disparities in screening for and awareness of high cholesterol among pregnant women receiving prenatal care. *J Am Heart Assoc.* 2021;10(1):e017415. doi:10.1161/jaha.120.017415

94. Expert panel on integrated guidelines for cardiovascular health and risk reduction in children and adolescents: summary report. *Pediatrics.* 2011;128(suppl 5):S213–S256. doi:10.1542/peds.2009-2107C
95. Berger JH, Chen F, Faerber JA, O'Byrne ML, Brothers JA. Adherence with lipid screening guidelines in standard- and high-risk children and adolescents. *Am Heart J.* 2021;232:39–46. doi:10.1016/j.ahj.2020.10.058
96. Lozano P, Henrikson NB, Morrison CC, et al. Lipid screening in childhood and adolescence for detection of multifactorial dyslipidemia: evidence report and systematic review for the US Preventive Services Task Force. *JAMA.* 2016;316(6):634–644. doi:10.1001/jama.2016.6423
97. Law MR, Wald NJ, Rudnicka AR. Quantifying effect of statins on low density lipoprotein cholesterol, ischaemic heart disease, and stroke: systematic review and meta-analysis. *BMJ.* 2003;326(7404):1423. doi:10.1136/bmj.326.7404.1423
98. Oyama K, Giugliano RP, Blazing MA, et al. Baseline low-density lipoprotein cholesterol and clinical outcomes of combining ezetimibe with statin therapy in IMPROVE-IT. *J Am Coll Cardiol.* 2021;78(15):1499–1507. doi:10.1016/j.jacc.2021.08.011
99. PRALUENT [package insert]. Bridgewater, NJ: sanofi-aventis US; 2015. Available at: https://www.accessdata.fda.gov/drugsatfda_docs/label/2015/125559orig1s000lbledt.pdf. Accessed January 19, 2023.
100. Sabatine MS, Giugliano RP, Keech AC, et al. Evolocumab and clinical outcomes in patients with cardiovascular disease. *N Engl J Med.* 2017;376(18):1713–1722. doi:10.1056/NEJMoa1615664
101. Schwartz GG, Steg PG, Szarek M, et al. Alirocumab and cardiovascular outcomes after acute coronary syndrome. *N Engl J Med.* 2018;379(22):2097–2107. doi:10.1056/NEJMoa1801174
102. Khan SU, Yedlapati SH, Lone AN, et al. PCSK9 inhibitors and ezetimibe with or without statin therapy for cardiovascular risk reduction: a systematic review and network meta-analysis. *BMJ.* 2022;377:e069116. doi:10.1136/bmj-2021-069116
103. Ingersgaard MV, Helms Andersen T, Norgaard O, Grabowski D, Olesen K. Reasons for non-adherence to statins—a systematic review of reviews. *Patient Prefer Adherence.* 2020;14:675–691. doi:10.2147/ppa.S245365
104. Attipoe-Dorcoo S, Yang P, Sperling L, et al. Characteristics and trends of PCSK9 inhibitor prescription fills in the United States. *J Clin Lipidol.* 2021;15(2):332–338. doi:10.1016/j.jacl.2021.01.010
105. Sekkarie AP, Park S, Therrian NL, Jackson SL, Woodruff RC, Attipoe-Dorcoo S, Yang PK, Sperling L, Loustalot FV, Thompson-Paul AM. Trends in lipid-lowering prescriptions by statin intensity—United States, 2017–2022. *Am J Prev Med.* 2023;64(4):561–566. doi:10.1016/j.amepre.2022.10.010
106. Bittner V, Colantonio LD, Dai Y, et al. Association of region and hospital and patient characteristics with use of high-intensity statins after myocardial infarction among Medicare beneficiaries. *JAMA Cardiol.* 2019;4(9):865–872. doi:10.1001/jamacardio.2019.2481
107. Centers for Disease Control and Prevention. Interactive Atlas of Heart Disease and Stroke. Available at: http://nccd.cdc.gov/DHDSPAtlas. Accessed October 1, 2022.
108. D'Agostino RB, Sr., Vasan RS, Pencina MJ, et al. General cardiovascular risk profile for use in primary care: the Framingham Heart Study. *Circulation.* 2008;117(6):743–753. doi:10.1161/circulationaha.107.699579

109. Goff DC, Jr., Lloyd-Jones DM, Bennett G, et al. 2013 ACC/AHA Guideline on the assessment of cardiovascular risk: a report of the American College of Cardiology/American Heart Association Task Force on Practice Guidelines. *Circulation.* 2013;129:S49–S73. doi:10.1161/01.cir.0000437741.48606.98

110. Thompson-Paul AM, Lichtenstein KA, Armon C, et al. Cardiovascular disease risk prediction in the HIV Outpatient Study. *Clin Infect Dis.* 2016;63(11):1508–1516. doi:10.1093/cid/ciw615

111. Muntner P, Colantonio LD, Cushman M, et al. Validation of the atherosclerotic cardiovascular disease pooled cohort risk equations. *JAMA.* 2014;311(14):1406–1415. doi:10.1001/jama.2014.2630

112. Chia YC, Lim HM, Ching SM. Validation of the pooled cohort risk score in an Asian population—a retrospective cohort study. *BMC Cardiovasc Dis.* 2014;14:163. doi:10.1186/1471-2261-14-163

113. Mehta A, Vasquez N, Ayers CR, et al. Independent association of lipoprotein(a) and coronary artery calcification with atherosclerotic cardiovascular risk. *J Am Coll Cardiol.* 2022;79(8):757–768. doi:10.1016/j.jacc.2021.11.058

114. Yang Q, Zhong Y, Ritchey M, et al. Vital signs: predicted heart age and racial disparities in heart age among US adults at the state level. *MMWR Morb Mortal Wkly Rep.* 2015;64(34):950–958. doi:10.15585/mmwr.mm6434a6

115. Patel N, Bhargava A, Kalra R, et al. Trends in lipid, lipoproteins, and statin use among US adults: impact of 2013 cholesterol guidelines. *J Am Coll Cardiol.* 2019;74(20):2525–2528. doi:10.1016/j.jacc.2019.09.026

116. Martin SS, Sperling LS, Blaha MJ, et al. Clinician-patient risk discussion for atherosclerotic cardiovascular disease prevention: importance to implementation of the 2013 ACC/AHA Guidelines. *J Am Coll Cardiol.* 2015;65(13):1361–1368. doi:10.1016/j.jacc.2015.01.043

117. Rubin R. Could statins do more than lower cholesterol in patients with COVID-19? *JAMA.* 2021;325(24):2424–2425. doi:10.1001/jama.2021.8201

118. Kollias A, Kyriakoulis KG, Kyriakoulis IG, et al. Statin use and mortality in COVID-19 patients: updated systematic review and meta-analysis. *Atherosclerosis.* 2021;330:114–121. doi:10.1016/j.atherosclerosis.2021.06.911

119. INSPIRATION-S Investigators. Atorvastatin versus placebo in patients with COVID-19 in intensive care: randomized controlled trial. *BMJ.* 2022;376:e068407. doi:10.1136/bmj-2021-068407

IV. DOWNSTREAM CHRONIC DISEASES

15

Sleep Behaviors and Disorders

Paul E. Peppard, PhD, Erika W. Hagen, PhD, and Lauren Hale, PhD

LEARNING OBJECTIVES

After completing this chapter, readers should be able to

1. Understand the descriptive epidemiology of insufficient sleep.
2. Understand upstream factors and outcomes associated with insufficient sleep.
3. Understand the descriptive epidemiology of obstructive sleep apnea.
4. Understand upstream factors and outcomes associated with obstructive sleep apnea.

INTRODUCTION

Sleep in humans has many properties: it is a state of consciousness, a compulsory behavior, and a vital homeostatic process. Good sleep hygiene is required for learning and memory formation. Chronically insufficient sleep and disturbed sleep are associated with dysregulation of multiple physiologic systems and a host of pathologies. Yet, most adults steal time from sleep to engage in less vital behaviors such as television watching.[1]

Even though humans, on average, spend more time in sleep than engaged in any other specific behavior, systematic investigations of risk factors for and outcomes of sleep disorders began in earnest only in the later decades of the 20th century. Thus, adverse consequences of sleep problems remain a rapidly growing area of inquiry. Nevertheless, a sufficient body of work demonstrates both a high prevalence of and adverse consequences of several sleep disorders.

There are over 100 sleep disorders detailed in the most recent edition of the International Classification of Sleep Disorders.[2] The disorders are generally grouped as insomnia, sleep-related breathing disorders (e.g., obstructive sleep apnea), central disorders of hypersomnolence (e.g., narcolepsy, insufficient sleep syndrome), circadian rhythm sleep-wake disorders (e.g., shift work disorder), parasomnias (e.g., sleepwalking), and sleep-related movement disorders (e.g., restless legs syndrome).

This chapter focuses on two of the most prevalent sleep disorders: chronic insufficient sleep and sleep apnea. There are other common sleep disorders, including, for example, restless legs syndrome and insomnia; however, the depth and breadth of the evidence bases linking chronic insufficient sleep and sleep apnea to chronic disease outcomes is

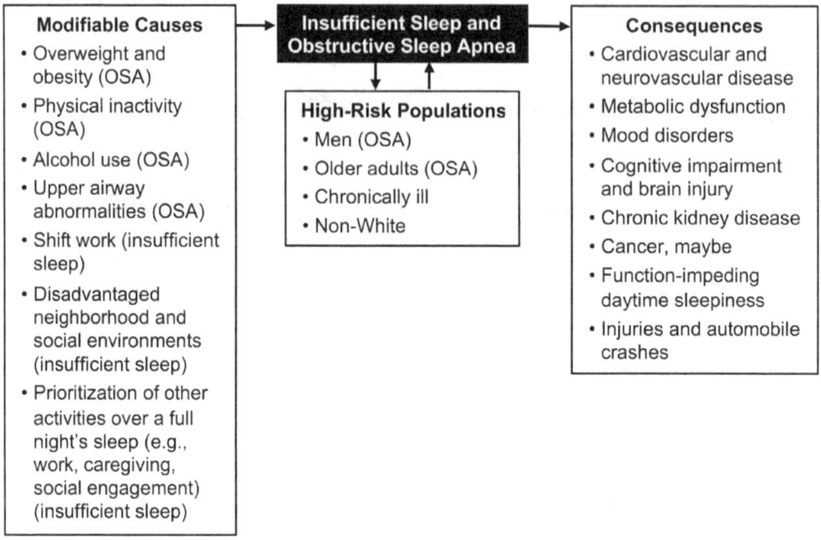

Note: OSA = obstructive sleep apnea.

Figure 15-1. Insufficient Sleep and Obstructive Sleep Apnea: Causes, Consequences, and High-Risk Populations

relatively robust compared with other common sleep disorders. Furthermore, this chapter examines these particular conditions in adults because the evidence bases for adverse chronic disease-related outcomes are distinct and more substantial in adults and the conditions are more prevalent in adulthood. Figure 15-1 illustrates the causes, high-risk populations, and outcomes of insufficient sleep and sleep apnea that we address in this chapter.

INSUFFICIENT SLEEP

Defined behaviorally, sleep is a reversible behavioral state characterized by disengagement from and unresponsiveness to the environment and is frequently characterized by postural recumbence, inactivity, and closed eyes.[3] Sleep can also be defined electrophysiologically: gold-standard clinical sleep assessment uses electrophysiologic information from electroencephalography (EEG, to measure brain activity), electrooculography (EOG, to assess eye movements) and electromyography (EMG, to measure muscle—chin or leg, for example—movements). Normal human sleep is characterized by two states, rapid eye movement (REM) sleep and non-rapid eye movement (NREM) sleep, that alternate cyclically across an episode of sleep. NREM sleep is divided into three stages, N1, N2, and N3, with N3 representing "deep" sleep—the stage of NREM sleep from which it is most difficult to arouse a sleeping person.[3]

Sleep is characterized as *insufficient* if it is inadequate to support alertness, performance, and health, the result of either inadequate total sleep time (i.e., insufficient sleep duration, the focus of this section) or sleep fragmentation that diminishes sleep quality.[4]

In the last decade, two separate expert consensus panels have recommended that for optimal health adults should sleep seven hours or more per night on a regular basis.[5,6] Insufficient sleep or short sleep duration is typically operationalized as less than seven hours, six hours or fewer, or less than six hours in a 24-hour period.

Pathophysiology

The characterization of mechanisms by which chronic insufficient sleep and poor sleep hygiene can lead to clinical morbidities is presently an area of active research. Insights into potential mechanisms are provided by short-term total sleep deprivation and longer-term partial sleep deprivation studies. These studies implicate multiple organ systems affected by sleep deprivation, including the central nervous, sympathetic nervous, endocrine, inflammatory, and cardiovascular systems, among others.[7,8] Chronic partial sleep deprivation negatively affects neurogenesis in the hippocampus—a brain structure crucial for learning and memory—and results in a variety of cognitive deficiencies (e.g., slowed reaction times, attentional lapses).[8] Sympathetic nervous system regulation of cardiovascular parameters is affected by sleep deprivation, a likely input into elevated blood pressures observed in sleep deprivation studies.[7] Endocrine effects are also consistently observed in sleep deprivation (complete or partial) studies, including activation of the hypothalamic-pituitary-adrenal axis and alterations to appetite-regulating hormones (e.g., elevation of ghrelin, suppression of leptin), leading to the increased appetite and eating observed in sleep-deprived conditions.[8] Inflammatory markers (e.g., CRP, IL-6, TNF-α) are also elevated in experimental sleep deprivation conditions. These and other (patho)physiologic responses to sleep deprivation likely underlie the development of the morbidities that are described next.

Public Health Burden

Mortality

While both short and long (frequently defined as >9 hr/night)[9] sleep are associated with higher risk of death,[10] this chapter will focus on short sleep duration—that is., insufficient sleep. Short sleep is consistently associated with higher risk of all-cause mortality. A recent meta-analysis suggested short sleep (<6 hr/night) is associated with a 12% (95% CI, 8–16) higher risk of all-cause mortality.[11]

Morbidity

Cardiovascular Disease and Stroke

Several large observational studies show an association between short sleep and risk of hypertension. The Sleep Heart Health Study and results from the 2007–2009 National

Health Interview Surveys showed cross-sectional associations between self-reported short sleep duration and higher risk for hypertension.[12] Sleeping less than six hours was associated with about 50% to 60% higher risk of hypertension compared with seven to eight hours of sleep. Short sleep is also associated with higher risk of incident hypertension. While there are some studies that do not find a significant association between sleep duration and hypertension risk, most studies, including two meta-analyses, do show a robust association.[12]

Studies of 24-hour blood pressure measurements suggest that sleep insufficiency interferes with the reductions in nighttime blood pressure that are normally observed during sleep as well as an amplification in morning blood pressure surges. These abnormalities in the diurnal blood pressure pattern are associated with higher risk of cardiovascular disease and cardiovascular disease–related death.[12]

Short sleep duration is associated with higher risk of cardiovascular disease and coronary heart disease, as well. A meta-analysis reported a 16% (95% CI, 10–23) higher risk of cardiovascular disease (including outcomes in both the heart and the brain) and a 26% (95% CI, 15–37) higher risk of coronary heart disease for short sleepers.[11] Studies show that prevalent coronary heart disease is higher among those with short sleep duration, and incidence of fatal and nonfatal coronary heart disease events is greater among short sleepers.[13] Studies with longer-term follow-up, such as the Nurses' Health Study, a community-based Chinese cohort, and the Framingham Offspring Cohort, report higher incidence of coronary heart disease events among those with short sleep durations.[13]

Evidence for whether short sleep duration is associated with higher risk of stroke is mixed. While one meta-analysis did not find a significantly higher risk of stroke,[11] another meta-analysis did find stroke risk to be higher among those with short sleep: prevalent stroke was 71% higher (95% CI, 39–102) and incident stroke risk was 13% higher (95% CI, 2–25) in this study.[14]

Metabolic Outcomes

Short sleep duration is consistently associated with greater risk of obesity. A review and meta-analysis showed that the large majority of studies examining the association of sleep duration and obesity found that short sleep (<5 or ≤5 hr/night over a 24-hr period in most studies) was associated with higher risk of obesity. The meta-analysis found the risk of obesity was 55% (95% CI, 43–68) higher among those with short sleep.[15]

There are many experimental studies that compare several days of restricted sleep with normal or extended periods of time in bed that demonstrate that insufficient sleep duration over several days is associated with dysregulation of appetite-regulating hormones and increased insulin resistance. Consistent with these laboratory-based findings, several cross-sectional studies find an association between short sleep duration and higher risk of obesity. In addition, a few prospective studies of this association have found increased risk of incident diabetes associated with short sleep duration at baseline.[16]

Experimental studies also show a relationship between sleep restriction—both total sleep deprivation and partial sleep restriction—and both hunger levels and caloric intake. Total sleep deprivation is associated with greater hunger levels than is partial sleep restriction, suggesting a possible dose–response relationship. Results from a meta-analysis of the association between partial sleep restriction and caloric intake suggest that participants under partial sleep restriction protocols consumed about 250 kcal more over a one-day period than controls with normal sleep conditions. In addition, several studies found that sleep restriction leads to higher calorie intake from snacks, with increased carbohydrate consumption.[17]

Notably, associations of insufficient sleep with metabolic dysregulation seen in adults are mirrored by those seen in studies of children.[18] This convergent evidence from different developmental phases strengthens the case for a causal connection between inadequate sleep and metabolic disruption.

Immune Response

Sleep insufficiency has also been demonstrated to influence immune function, including how the body responds to viral exposure and vaccination. In one well-controlled study,[19] participants were exposed to the rhinovirus and quarantined in a hotel for five days. Those with actigrapically assessed insufficient sleep (<6 hr) prior to the exposure were over four times more likely to develop cold symptoms than were those with seven or more hours of sleep (<5 hr vs. >7 hr, odds ratio [OR] 4.5; 95% CI, 1.1–18; 5–6 hr vs. >7 hr, OR 4.2; 95% CI, 1.1–17). Sleep sufficiency also boosts the immune response to vaccines; a study of the influenza vaccines showed that shorter sleep duration was associated with fewer antibodies one and four months later.[20]

Accidents and Falls

Insufficient sleep can lead to unintentional injuries and falls from myriad causes. Pooled results from a meta-analysis showed short sleep duration was associated with a 32% (95% CI, 21–46) increased risk of having one or more falls in the previous year.[21]

While few studies have specifically examined the risk of car accidents associated with insufficient sleep, epidemiologic research associates sleepiness, a reliable symptom of insufficient sleep, with a greater risk of motor vehicle crashes.[22] There are a few studies, however, that have directly assessed risk of traffic accidents with insufficient sleep. As noted, results from the Sleep Heart Health study show that sleeping fewer than six hours per night was associated with a 33% higher risk of having a crash compared with sleeping seven to eight hours per night.[23] Another study found drivers who slept five hours or less the previous night were almost three times as likely (OR 2.7;

95% CI, 1.4–5.4) to have a car crash in which someone was injured compared with those who slept more than five hours the previous night.[24] These observational results are corroborated by several lab-based sleep restriction studies that showed driving simulator performance was worse when sleep was restricted to between four and six hours of sleep per night.[25]

Psychological Outcomes

The relationship between insufficient sleep and psychological well-being is bidirectional. That is, insufficient sleep can be both a cause and consequence of mental distress. In support of the role of sleep duration in mental health, data from the China Health and Retirement Longitudinal Study demonstrated that short sleep duration (<5 and 5–6 hr/night, respectively) is predictive of both depression onset (OR 1.69 [95% CI, 1.36–2.11] and 1.48 [95% CI, 1.19–1.84], respectively) and recurrent depression (OR 1.44 [95% CI, 1.12–1.86] and 1.32 [95% CI, 1.00–1.74], respectively) compared with those who slept 7 to 8 hours per night.[26] In addition, a meta-analysis of randomized controlled trials shows a significant effect of interventions designed to improve sleep quality (not necessarily sleep duration) showed significant salutary effects on a range of mental health outcomes, including depression, anxiety, and rumination.[27] (For more information on mental disorders, see Chapter 19.)

Descriptive Epidemiology

Prevalence, Disparities, Geographic Distribution, and Time Trends

Insufficient sleep is common among US adults, with over a third of respondents from the 2014 Behavioral Risk Factor Surveillance System (BRFSS), which includes results from the 50 states and the District of Columbia, reporting fewer than seven hours of sleep over a 24-hour period.[28] Age-adjusted insufficient sleep duration was higher among non-Hispanic Blacks (46%), American Indians/Alaska Natives (40%), Native Hawaiians/Pacific Islanders (46%), and multiracial (46%) respondents but lower among non-Hispanic Whites (33%), Hispanics (35%), and Asians (38%).[28] Among all respondents, 12% reported sleep duration of five hours or fewer, 23% reported six hours, 30% reported seven hours, 28% reported eight hours, 4% reported nine hours, and 4% reported ten hours or more.[28] Married respondents had a lower prevalence of insufficient sleep duration (33%) compared with those who were divorced, widowed, or separated (44%) or never married (38%).[28]

The annual National Health Interview Survey is another source of data on self-reported sleep duration, analyzing data from over 400,000 individuals between 2004 and 2018. Consistent with the BRFSS data, self-reported short sleep duration (<7 hr/ night) was common among all individuals and higher among Asian and Black individuals compared with White and Hispanic individuals.[29]

Data from studies with objectively assessed actigraphy-measured sleep also provide evidence that insufficient sleep is common. A meta-analysis of sleep duration and age demonstrated that for adults aged 30 to 90 years, the average actigraphically assessed sleep duration is about 6.4 to 6.8 hours, depending on age, which is below the recommended sleep duration of 7 hours,[30] highlighting the high prevalence of insufficient sleep duration in adulthood. Another actigraphy study from the United Kingdom biobank of 82,000 participants shows that about 77% of midlife adults sleep seven or fewer hours, with 43% sleeping six or fewer hours.[31]

In the United States, prevalence of insufficient sleep does not vary substantially by sex. In the BRFSS study approximately 35% of both men and women reported sleeping fewer than seven hours per night.[28]

Data from the BRFSS suggest that the prevalence of insufficient sleep varies geographically across the United States. There is higher prevalence of insufficient sleep in southern states and along the Appalachian Mountains, while most of the Great Plains states show a lower prevalence of insufficient sleep.[28]

From 2004 to 2018, the prevalence of short sleep duration increased significantly, though this increase varied somewhat by race and ethnicity. Insufficient sleep prevalence increased more among Black and Hispanic individuals (~6%–7% increase over the time span) compared to the prevalence increase among White individuals (~3% increase over the time span).[29]

Causes

The 2009 BRFSS investigated social and behavioral predictors of insufficient sleep (<7 hr/night). The resulting self-reported data demonstrated that those who work more than 40 hours per week were about 65% more likely to have insufficient sleep; those who were caregivers to family/friends were about 50% more likely to have insufficient sleep; and those who lacked social and emotional support were about 25% more likely to have insufficient sleep.[28]

Shift work has also been associated with short sleep duration in many studies. Results from a meta-analysis show that permanent night shifts and rotating shifts result in shorter sleep duration than permanent day shift work. Rapidly rotating shift schedules result in shorter sleep than does a slower shift rotation.[32]

A growing body of research shows that like individual-level risk factors affecting sleep duration, neighborhood-level characteristics (measured by levels of disorder, safety, and social cohesion) and social environment (feelings of trust and safety) are associated with sleep duration and prevalence of insufficient sleep.[33,34]

Physical characteristics of the environment also matter for sleep health. For example, greater green space exposure is associated with lower risk for short sleep. Two of three cross-sectional studies that examined associations between short sleep duration and green space found a higher risk for short sleep with less green space exposure,[35,36] although a third study reported no significant association.[37] Another example of how physical environment affects sleep duration and quality is light at night. In one study using satellite assessment of artificial light at night, individuals who live in the highest quintile of light at night had 16% and 25% higher rates of short sleep duration (<7 hr/night) in women and men, respectively.[38] The association between light at night and short sleep duration is larger in neighborhoods with high poverty rates, underscoring the potential intersection of social and physical environments.

Over many decades, technological innovations—the invention and subsequent widespread availability of electric lighting being a particularly salient example—have had enormous impacts on sleep behaviors. Recent research in the technology–sleep arena has included a focus on "screen time" and social media use. Reviews of sleep and media use suggest that greater media use, especially at night, is associated with shorter sleep duration and worse sleep quality. Proposed mechanisms for these associations include bedtime delay because of screen usage; screen light exposure altering circadian rhythms, potentially altering sleep times; and increased cognitive arousal at bedtime.[39] There is a well-documented association of social media use with poorer sleep in adolescents; however, this association has also been observed in adults. In one study of 855 adults (mean age: 44 y), almost 70% of respondents engaged in in-bed electronic social media use, with almost 15% spending an hour or more per night. Participants with high in-bed social media use had 82% greater odds (95% CI, 20–156) of having shorter weeknight sleep duration (<6 hr/night) than those who did not use social media in bed.[40]

Evidence-Based Interventions

Treatment

Given the many forces that underlie sleep insufficiency, there is no one-size-fits-all approach to improving population-level sleep sufficiency. Instead, multilevel strategies must be embraced that encompass culturally sensitive and tailored approaches that address individual needs, social circumstances, and structural conditions.

At the individual level, there are cognitive and behavioral intervention approaches that can help improve sleep hygiene among individuals without sleep disorders. One meta-analysis of 11 studies (n = 1,082 participants) found that self-reported sleep quality and sleep duration improved significantly after cognitive and/or behavioral intervention.[41] These types of interventions involve activities such as providing handouts about sleep hygiene guidelines and using stimulus control.[42] Other approaches involve music therapy, relaxation training,[43] and mindfulness meditation.[44,45]

Given the growing evidence of the role neighborhood- and community-level influences play in sleep insufficiency, policy and neighborhood interventions may have an important role in creating social and contextual environments so that individuals can achieve the sleep they need.

Areas of Future Research

Whereas the many negative health consequences of insufficient sleep have been extensively investigated, strategies for improving (in most cases increasing) sleep duration in the population could be further investigated. In particular, future work could add to our understanding of which treatment interventions will work best for specific subpopulations, with a focus on being responsive to cultural, demographic, and social role–related characteristics and constraints. Future research could also investigate the extent to which various community-level changes in the physical environment and policy realm will lead to increasing sleep durations.

SLEEP APNEA

Sleep apnea—periodic cessations (apneas) and reductions (hypopneas) in breathing during sleep—has a variety of causes and ranges widely in severity. This section focuses on the most common form of sleep apnea: obstructive sleep apnea (OSA) in adults. Symptoms of OSA include loud and irregular snoring, choking, or gasping during sleep; excessive daytime sleepiness; unrefreshing sleep; morning headaches; and nocturia. Physical characteristics associated with OSA are obesity, large neck girth, and a "crowded" oropharynx.[46]

Gold-standard diagnosis of OSA is via polysomnography, either in a clinical laboratory or using ambulatory devices at home. Polysomnography measures multiple physiologic parameters, including brain activity (EEG) for identifying sleep state and stages; muscle and eye movements; body position; heart rhythm (electrocardiography); and blood oxygen saturation and additional breathing parameters (e.g., nasal air pressure, chest, and abdominal movements). OSA is typically characterized by the hourly rate of breathing events—apneas and hypopneas—during sleep. For example, the apnea-hypopnea index (AHI, the most commonly used OSA severity metric) is the average number of apnea plus hypopnea events per hour of sleep. There are a variety of approaches to defining and scoring apnea and hypopnea events; this abundance, effectively, results in different OSA severity thresholds for defining OSA cases and, consequently, contributes to variations in OSA prevalence estimates from different studies, populations, and time periods. Regardless of scoring method, OSA severity levels in adults are commonly defined by AHI cut points:

- No OSA: AHI <5 events per hour.
- Mild OSA: AHI from 5 to <15 events per hour.
- Moderate OSA: AHI from 15 to <30 events per hour.
- Severe OSA: AHI ≥30 events per hour.

Pathophysiology

As reviewed in Dempsey et al.,[47] OSA results from complete or partial collapse of the upper airway during sleep. These collapses are, in part, a consequence of the naturally reduced neuromuscular control of the upper airway during sleep, especially during REM sleep. This reduced defense of airway patency can combine with personal factors such as older age, excess body mass (obesity and/or excess adipose tissue in the neck region), anatomical predisposition (e.g., an unusually narrow upper airway), and acute factors such as back-sleeping, stuffy nose, and alcohol use near bedtime to episodically compromise the upper airway. In OSA-afflicted persons, these airway collapses result in intermittent hypoxia, sleep fragmentation, and exaggerated pressure swings in the chest. These proximal mechanisms—intermittent hypoxia, sleep fragmentation, and thoracic pressure swings—can then lead to a variety of downstream effects, including sympathetic nervous system and hypothalamic-pituitary-adrenal axis activation, systemic oxidative stress, and stresses on the heart and vasculature.[48] Over time these and other mechanisms lead to OSA-associated morbidities and mortality, discussed in the following sections.

Public Health Burden

OSA is a high public health burden disorder because of extensive OSA morbidities—themselves high-burden conditions—that are likely causal outcomes of sleep apnea (described later) and because of the high and growing prevalence of OSA (described later). In addition to having health-related consequences, OSA has negative impacts on workplace productivity, interpersonal relationships, and academic performance as well as difficult-to-measure total economic costs minimally estimated in the tens of billions of dollars in the United States.[49,50] In addition, OSA contributes to health disparities, as the prevalence of disparities tends to be higher and OSA treatment access and uptake lower in disadvantaged populations.

OSA has both acute next-day effects (e.g., sleepiness) and long-term consequences. These outcomes likely arise from the underlying mechanisms related to the acute episodes of intermittent hypoxia, sleep disruption, and excessive pressure changes in the chest that directly result from (and define) apnea and hypopnea events; these proximal effects then lead to a host of downstream physiologic responses (see earlier Pathophysiology section) and, thereafter, to a broad range of morbidity and mortality outcomes.

Morbidity

Sleepiness

Excessive daytime sleepiness is a cardinal feature of OSA and is reported by approximately 50% of OSA patients. Sleepiness has deleterious effects on safety, cognitive and physical functioning, mood, and perceived quality of life; many OSA treatment studies have demonstrated reduced sleepiness following effective treatment of OSA.[51,52] However, sleepiness is not always eliminated by treatment of OSA; this may, in part, be because sleepiness has causes other than OSA (e.g., insufficient sleep time), and these other causes are not necessarily addressed by OSA treatment.

Injury and Motor Vehicle Crashes

As noted, a salient feature of OSA is sleepiness. Meta-analyses of sleepiness as a predictor of motor vehicle crashes from 14 studies published from 1980 to 2016 show that drowsy driving increases the odds of crashes by approximately 30% compared with driving while not drowsy (pooled OR 1.34; 95% CI, 1.25–1.43).[22]

In their prospective observational cohort study, nested within the Sleep Heart Health Study and published in 2018, Gottlieb et al.[23] examined both sleepiness and OSA as predictors of motor vehicle crashes. More than 3,200 adults, objectively assessed for OSA and self-reported sleepiness, were followed over a two-year period. Adjusting for multiple covariates, both sleepiness and OSA were significantly associated with a higher risk of motor vehicle crashes. OSA was associated with crashes in a dose–response manner such that each increment of ten events per hour in the apnea-hypopnea index was associated with 15% greater odds of motor vehicle crash (OR 1.15; 95% CI, 1.04–1.26). OSA was associated with a significantly increased risk of motor vehicle crashes even among persons with OSA who did not report excessive sleepiness.

Several studies have also associated OSA with work-related injuries. As reported in their study published in 2022, Chou et al.[53] meta-analyzed 15 OSA injury investigations. These studies collectively demonstrated a pooled odds ratio for work-related injuries (not including professional drivers) of 1.60 (95% CI, 1.13–2.26) for workers with diagnosed OSA compared with workers not diagnosed with OSA. Not all those studies adjusted for potentially confounding variables, however, and more robust research is required in this area.

Mood Disorders

A meta-analysis of 73 studies[54] examining depression and anxiety symptoms in OSA patients found relatively high prevalence of these disorders. The pooled prevalence of depressive symptoms was 35% (95% CI, 28–41) and for anxiety symptoms was 32% (95% CI, 22–42) in OSA patients. Edwards et al.[55] meta-analyzed five longitudinal studies of OSA predicting incident depressive symptoms. Their results, published in 2020, showed that the pooled risk ratio for developing depressive symptoms was 2.18 (95% CI, 1.47–2.88), indicating a greater than twofold elevated risk for developing depressive symptoms among persons with OSA relative to persons without OSA.

Heart and Vascular Outcomes

An American Heart Association scientific statement[56] published in 2021 reviewed evidence linking OSA to cardiovascular disease (CVD). A vast literature links OSA to a range of cardiovascular outcomes, among them hypertension, arrhythmias, heart failure, coronary artery disease, stroke, and diabetes. Likely mechanisms include the intermittent hypoxia, sleep fragmentation, and exaggerated intrathoracic pressure changes of OSA giving rise to autonomic dysfunction, endothelial dysfunction, systemic inflammation, and other adverse pathophysiologic sequelae that then can result in the various heart and vascular outcomes.[56]

Hypertension was among the first OSA outcomes examined, with early epidemiology studies published in the 1980s. OSA and hypertension are often comorbid conditions, as are OSA and hypertension that are resistant to pharmacologic therapy.[56] Unfortunately, despite a robust literature linking OSA and hypertension, treatment of OSA in hypertensive people is usually insufficient to normalize blood pressure.[56] A recent meta-analysis of the association of OSA and hypertension[57] in studies that minimally adjusted for age, sex, and a measure of body habitus estimated that compared with persons without OSA, mild, moderate, and severe OSA were associated with 18% (95% CI, 9–27), 31% (95% CI, 20–43), and 56% (95% CI, 29–84) greater odds of hypertension, respectively.

In addition to being connected with hypertension, OSA is associated with an increased risk of incident heart failure as well as heart failure–associated symptom progression, hospitalization, and death.[56] OSA is also associated with coronary artery calcification, plaque instability, cardiovascular events (including cardiovascular death) and cerebrovascular events, with a relatively elevated risk of events during sleeping hours or shortly after awakening.[56] In a 2013 meta-analysis of 12 cohort studies, Wang et al.[58] calculated pooled estimates of elevated risks of cardiovascular outcomes associated with severe OSA: compared with persons without OSA, persons with severe OSA had a 79% (95% CI, 47–118) greater risk for CVD and 115% (95% CI, 42–224) greater risk for incident stroke (including stroke fatalities).

Cognition and Brain Injury

A wide variety of brain-related outcomes (e.g., cognitive functioning, structural brain injury, elevated dementia-related biomarkers) have been examined in relation to OSA.

Both acute and long-term mechanisms and effects of OSA may lead to micro- and macroscopic brain injury and cognitive dysfunction.

As many instruments are used to assess cognitive function in investigations of cognitive functioning in OSA, it is difficult to quantitatively pool findings across multiple studies (e.g., by meta-analysis). However, in a 2020 review, Bubu et al.[59] reported that among middle-age adults, OSA has generally been associated with a mild impairment in attention, memory, and executive function. These findings were less consistent in older adult populations. In their 2020 review, Vanek et al.[60] concurred that available evidence indicates that attention, working memory, episodic memory, and executive functioning are impaired in OSA. Unfortunately, OSA treatment studies generally do not show substantial improvements in cognitive function following OSA remediation.[60]

Evidence of numerous OSA-associated MRI-assessed brain structure, function, and injury outcomes have been recently reviewed and meta-analyzed. In their 2019 meta-analysis, Huang et al.[61] identified significant relatively decreased brain gray matter volumes among OSA patients compared with persons without OSA in multiple regions (e.g., bilateral anterior cingulate gyrus, hippocampus, orbital frontal cortex), as well as functional alterations in OSA patients such as hypoactivation of the dorsolateral prefrontal cortex and hyperactivation of the insula.

Investigations of neuroimaging-assessed cerebral small vessel disease in relation to OSA were reviewed by Huang et al.,[62] who in their 2020 study meta-analyzed 20 studies comprising more than 6,036 people. Pooled results indicated that moderate-to-severe OSA was significantly positively associated with white matter hyperintensities and silent brain infarctions. No significant associations were identified between OSA and cerebral microbleeds or perivascular spaces, and no substantial associations were found between mild OSA and any of the investigated cerebral small vessel disease parameters.

Chronic Kidney Disease

The connection between OSA and chronic kidney disease is a nascent area of investigation with almost all studies published in the 2010s or later. Potential mechanisms linking OSA to kidney disease include sympathetic nervous system activation, hypertension, and direct effects of hypoxia on the kidney.[63] In a meta-analysis of 12 studies comprising over three million patients, Hansrivijit et al.[64] found a pooled prevalence of kidney disease among OSA patients of just over 8% (95% CI, 5–14) and twofold greater odds of kidney disease associated with OSA relative to persons without OSA (adjusted pooled OR = 2.1; 95% CI, 1.8–2.5).

Cancer

Another nascent area of investigation is the association of OSA with carcinogenesis and accelerated tumor growth, with potential mechanisms including deleterious effects of

OSA on immune functioning, DNA damage from OSA-generated reactive oxygen species, and hypoxia-induced angiogenesis, among others.[65] In the early 2010s animal models suggested that implanted melanoma tumors grow[66] and metastasize[67] more rapidly in mice experimentally exposed to intermittent hypoxia, a defining feature of OSA. These findings spurred investigations of OSA–cancer associations in human epidemiology studies.

Because the investigation of OSA as a risk factor for cancer in humans is a very recent phenomenon, published studies have not been performed in epidemiology cohorts purpose-built to study OSA–cancer associations. Thus, these studies have been handicapped by several study limitations, including, for example, lack of measurement of potentially important confounders of OSA–cancer associations such as poor diet quality, physical inactivity, or excessive alcohol consumption. Thus, unsurprisingly, reviews of these recent studies have shown mixed results. In a 2022 study, Tan et al.[68] meta-analyzed 20 epidemiology studies representing more than five million participants. Patients with objectively assessed severe OSA had a slightly higher rate of any incident cancer diagnosis (pooled hazard ratio [HR] = 1.18; 95% CI, 1.03–1.35) compared with persons without OSA; less severe OSA was not associated with a higher rate of cancer. Stronger associations were observed when OSA severity was characterized by hypoxic burden rather than by the apnea-hypopnea index. Adjusted for multiple covariates, patients with severe nocturnal hypoxemia (≥12% of sleep time exposed to ≤90% oxyhemoglobin saturation) had a 43% greater all-cancer rate (HR = 1.43, 95% CI, 1.16–1.76) compared with normoxemic patients. While the potential for a causal OSA–cancer association in humans is an urgent area of research, links between OSA and cancer growth and metastasis will be difficult to examine in epidemiologic studies, since the identification of solid tumor cancers will often immediately trigger medical interventions that alter the trajectory of tumor growth and spread in cancer patients. Thus, future OSA–cancer studies may be able to most robustly investigate OSA–carcinogenesis associations; this may be an important limitation if it turns out that the putative salient impact of OSA on solid tumor cancers is not via carcinogenic effects but rather by impact on post-carcinogenesis disease trajectories.

Mortality

Several studies have examined objectively assessed OSA in relation to all-cause and specific causes of mortality. A meta-analysis[69] pooling multivariate-adjusted associations from 27 studies found a 19% greater rate (95% CI, −14 to 65) of mortality in persons with mild OSA compared with those without OSA; a 28% (95% CI, −4 to 69) greater rate in those with moderate OSA compared with those without OSA; and a 113% greater mortality rate in those with severe OSA (95% CI, 94–168) compared with those without OSA. While the positive associations with mortality were not statistically significant for mild and moderate OSA, there is a dose–response association over the spectrum from mild to severe OSA. A similar, though stronger, dose–response association was observed for mortality resulting from cardiovascular causes; those with severe OSA had a pooled estimate of 173% greater rate (95% CI, 94–285) of cardiovascular mortality compared with those with no OSA. In a systematic review of the association of OSA and cancer-specific mortality, Tan et al.[70] found no statistically significant association between OSA characterized by the most traditional measure of OSA severity, AHI, though associations were in the direction of greater cancer mortality with greater OSA severity. However, using a hypoxia-specific measure of OSA severity (percent of night spent below 90% oxyhemoglobin saturation), a significant association between more severe nocturnal hypoxia and a greater rate of cancer mortality was observed.

Descriptive Epidemiology

Obstructive Sleep Apnea Prevalence by Age, Sex, Geography, and Time Trends

While OSA affects persons of all ages, sexes, and body weights, the prevalence of OSA is highest among middle- to older-age persons, men, and persons with excess body fat. Largely because of the strong relation of OSA to excess body fat, the prevalence of OSA has been increasing in tandem with the increased prevalence of overweight and obesity—the obesity epidemic—that has occurred in the United States over the last several decades. Using data from a population-based epidemiology study that has measured OSA objectively over time in a cohort initiated in the late 1980s, as well as information from the US National Health and Nutrition Examination Survey (NHANES), Peppard et al.[71] estimated that US early to mid-2010s prevalence of moderate or more severe OSA (AHI ≥15 events/hr using a conservative definition of hypopneas; a less conservative definition yields higher prevalence estimates) were 3% (95% CI, 2–4) and 10% (95% CI, 7–12) for women and men aged 30 to 49 years, respectively, and 9% (95% CI, 7–11) and 17% (95% CI, 15–21) for women and men aged 50 to 70 years, respectively. These figures are 14% to 55% higher, depending on subgroup, than were prevalences estimated for the United States two decades prior, in the early 1990s.

Benjafield et al.,[72] using OSA prevalence studies conducted around the world estimated that 425 million (95% CI, 399–450 million) adults aged 30 to 69 years have moderate-to-severe OSA globally. There was considerable variation among countries, even within continents; much of the variation was attributable to differences in age structures and obesity prevalences among countries. In this study the US prevalence for moderate-to-severe OSA was estimated to be 14.5%, a middling value among estimates for all countries; for example, China's analogous prevalence estimate was 8.8% and Brazil's was 26.0%.

High-Risk Populations and Health Disparities

As indicated in the foregoing explication, persons with chronic health conditions associated with OSA, older persons, men, and overweight persons have higher prevalences of OSA. No specific strong genetic risk factors for OSA have yet to be reproducibly identified, though OSA does show familial clustering.[73] In the United States, lower socioeconomic status is associated with higher prevalences of OSA in both women and men.[74] Higher prevalences of OSA are also seen in African American, Native American, and Hispanic populations relative to White populations, with some of the differences paralleling differences in obesity prevalences among those populations.[75] Furthermore, there are disparities in OSA diagnosis and treatment, with African Americans, on average, diagnosed at a greater OSA severity level than White persons.[75]

Causes

As described, salient risk factors for OSA include excess body weight, male sex, and older age. In 2020 Gottlieb and Punjabi[48] summarized the literature estimating odds ratios for these and other important OSA risk factors: odds ratios for overweight versus normal weight predicting OSA in the literature range from approximately 2.3 to 3.4 (that is, overweight persons have ~3 times greater odds of having OSA than normal-weight persons); odds ratios for obese versus normal weight range from approximately 4 to 10; odds ratios for male sex versus female sex range from approximately 1.7 to 3.0; odds ratios for a 10-year increment in age during adulthood range from approximately 1.4 to 3.2; and odds ratios for postmenopausal versus premenopausal state in women range from approximately 2.8 to 4.3. Enlarged upper airway soft tissue (e.g., tongue) and craniofacial abnormalities (e.g., retrognathia) are also consistent risk factors for OSA.[48] A lesser body of literature exists examining the relationship between physical inactivity and OSA and alcohol use and OSA; however, those studies that do exist have implicated physical inactivity, independent of body weight, as a risk factor for OSA, as well as excess alcohol use, especially near bedtime.[73,76]

Of the OSA risk factors considered modifiable from a public health promotion perspective, sufficiently robust data exist to estimate the approximate age- and sex-group-specific percentage of OSA prevalence attributable to overweight or obesity. Table 15-1 presents data from an investigation[71] of adults aged 30 to 70 years that combined information from the Wisconsin Sleep Cohort Study and NHANES to estimate group-specific OSA prevalences for sex, age, and body mass index (BMI). The first four columns of data in the table present estimated OSA prevalences—for both mild or worse OSA and moderate or worse OSA severity levels— by age group (30–49 y and 50–70 y) and sex for normal-weight persons (BMI <25 kg/m^2). Here, the prevalences for mild or worse OSA range from 1.4% of women in the younger age group to 19% of men in the older age

Table 15-1. Prevalence of Mild or Worse and Moderate or Worse Obstructive Sleep Apnea and Population-Attributable Prevalence of Obstructive Sleep Apnea Associated With Overweight and Obesity for Men and Women by Age Group

	OSA Prevalence (%) by Age Group and Sex (Normal Weight, BMI <25 kg/m^2)				OSA Prevalence (%) by Age Group and Sex (Overall)				Population-Attributable a Prevalence[a] (%) by Age Group and Sex (Overweight and Obesity, BMI ≥ 25 kg/m^2)			
	30–49 y		50–70 y		30–49 y		50–70 y		30–49 y		50–70 y	
OSA severity	M	W	M	W	M	W	M	W	M	W	M	W
Mild or worse OSA[b]	7.0	1.4	19	9.3	27	8.7	43	28	74	84	56	67
Moderate or worse OSA[c]	0.9	0.2	3.6	1.4	9.5	2.7	17	9.1	90	93	79	84

Source: Based on Peppard et al.[71]

Note: AHI = apnea-hypopnea index; M = men; OSA = obstructive sleep apnea; W = women.

[a]Calculated as ([$\text{Prevalence}_{\text{overall}}$ − $\text{Prevalence}_{\text{normal weight}}$]/$\text{Prevalence}_{\text{overall}}$)*100%.

[b]Defined on the AHI as ≥5 events/h.

[c]Defined on the AHI as ≥15/h.

group. Both age and sex heavily affect OSA prevalence, with older age groups showing approximately three- to sevenfold higher OSA prevalences than younger age groups (depending on sex and OSA severity level) and men having three- to fivefold higher OSA prevalences than women (depending on age group and OSA severity level). The next four columns of data present estimated OSA prevalences for the overall population of adults aged 30 to 70 years. For all age and sex groups, these overall prevalence estimates are several multiples of the OSA prevalences estimated for normal-weight persons alone, exhibiting the strong causal role of overweight and obesity in OSA. The final four columns of data present estimated population-attributable prevalences of OSA (i.e., prevalences of mild or worse OSA and moderate or worse OSA attributable to overweight or obesity) by age group and sex. Together, these data indicate that while older age and male sex are important risk factors for OSA, within any specified age or sex group overweight/obesity is a dominating factor contributing to prevalent OSA, explaining an estimated 56% to 93% of prevalent OSA in the adult populations, depending on subgroup.

Evidence-Based Interventions

Prevention

Robust literature on OSA prevention is lacking. However, based on studies of risk factors for OSA, as presented in the preceding text, and behavioral interventions for OSA, it is reasonable to infer that strong candidates for OSA prevention are maintaining a healthy body weight, losing body weight if overweight, engaging in routine physical activity and exercise, and avoiding alcohol use before bedtime.

Screening

Following a review of then-available literature, in 2017 the US Preventive Services Task Force (USPSTF)[77] stated that "it found insufficient evidence on screening for . . . OSA in asymptomatic adults or adults with unrecognized symptoms." In the updated recommendation statement dated November 2022, USPSTF indicated that more recently available data have not changed the 2017 finding of insufficient evidence to judge the value of screening in general population adults.[78] Thus, currently available evidence does not support general population screening for OSA.

Specific populations may benefit from OSA screening. A 2021 American Heart Association scientific statement[56] recommends screening for OSA in patients with: poorly controlled hypertension, pulmonary hypertension, recurrent atrial fibrillation after either cardioversion or ablation, New York Heart Association Class II to IV heart failure, and several other specific conditions (see Yeghiazarians et al.[56] for the entire set of recommendations).

Available screening instruments range from questionnaires to devices that continuously measure multiple physiologic parameters, including blood oxygen saturation, heart rate variability, and electroencephalographic signals. Many of these tools have well-characterized validity parameters and can be used in primary care clinical settings for patients reporting excessive daytime sleepiness or other features of OSA as described at the beginning of this section. Examples of commonly used screening questionnaires include the Berlin Questionnaire and the STOP-BANG (Snoring, Tiredness, Observed Apnea, Blood Pressure, Body Mass Index, Age, Neck Circumference, and Gender); these questionnaires have estimated sensitivities for OSA above 75% but have also estimated specificities of approximately 33%.[79]

Treatment

Treatment of OSA is recommended for persons with an AHI of 15 or greater events per hour and for persons with 5 or more events per hour co-occurring with excessive daytime sleepiness, impaired cognition, mood disorders, insomnia, or specific cardiovascular or cerebrovascular conditions.[46] Gottlieb and Punjabi[48] discuss treatment options available for OSA, including behavioral treatments (e.g., weight loss, physical activity), surgical interventions (e.g., uvulopalatopharyngoplasty, hypoglossal nerve stimulation), oral appliances, and continuous positive air pressure therapy (CPAP) to splint the upper airway open during sleep. Presently there are no effective pharmacological treatments for OSA.

Therapy effectiveness depends on specific patient characteristics and underlying causes of OSA in each patient as well as the severity of OSA. The most widely used and studied therapy, CPAP, is very effective for mitigating OSA if tolerated by patients; unfortunately, CPAP, is often not well tolerated.[46] Also, while CPAP is highly effective in treating OSA per se, evidence of the effectiveness of CPAP at mitigating downstream outcomes of OSA is mixed. Thus far, CPAP has shown only moderate (hypertension) or little (cardiovascular events, cognitive dysfunction) success in mitigating important outcomes of OSA.[46,80]

Areas of Future Research

The American Heart Association[56] recommends several focus areas for future OSA research and development. These include the following:

- Investigating and developing wearable devices and remote monitoring technologies for OSA screening and for evaluating OSA treatment effectiveness.
- Using machine learning tools for synthesizing and interpreting OSA-relevant data from patients to aid in developing personalized therapies.
- Investigating and addressing structural racism and health inequities that result in higher prevalence of OSA in disadvantaged populations.
- Developing effective therapies that are well tolerated by a majority of OSA patients.

Many other important areas of future research exist, including

- Elucidating the role of long-term exposure to mild-moderate sleep apnea in cardiovascular, metabolic, physical functioning, and cognitive functioning outcomes in older age.
- Quantifying the effects of specific potential OSA prevention strategies (e.g., regular physical activity, healthy weight maintenance).
- Characterizing the roles and mechanisms, if any, of OSA in the carcinogenesis of specific cancers as well as the role of OSA in tumor growth and metastasis in solid tumor cancers.

DISCUSSION QUESTIONS

1. What are the implications of the information about population health risks (presented in Table 15-1) for public health practitioners?
2. Insufficient sleep and OSA are not commonly included as leading public health concerns in communities. Why do you think this is?
3. Given the widespread use of social media and devices that permit people to be connected 24/7, are you confident that interventions to reduce screen time will be effective?

4. A large number of studies implicate OSA as a likely cause of cardiovascular disease and cognitive dysfunction. However, to date, many OSA treatment studies do not show substantial improvements in cardiovascular risk or cognitive functioning following OSA treatment. Why might that be?
5. Say you have a family member who sleeps an average of only 5 hours per night. After reading this chapter, what convincing case would you make to your family member that they should sleep more?

REFERENCES

1. Basner M, Fomberstein KM, Razavi FM, et al. American time use survey: sleep time and its relationship to waking activities. *Sleep*. 2007;30(9):1085–1095.
2. American Academy of Sleep Medicine. *International Classification of Sleep Disorders*. 3rd ed. Darien, IL: American Academy of Sleep Medicine; 2014.
3. Carskadon MA, Dement WC. Normal human sleep: an overview. In: Kryger MH, Roth T, Dement WC, eds. *Principles and Practice of Sleep Medicine*. 6th ed. Philadelphia, PA: Elsevier Saunders; 2017:15–24.
4. Cirelli C, Benca R, Eichler AF. Insufficient sleep: definition, epidemiology, and adverse outcomes. UpToDate. Available at: https://www.uptodate.com/contents/insufficient-sleep-definition-epidemiology-and-adverse-outcomes. Accessed July 15, 2022.
5. Hirshkowitz M, Whiton K, Albert SM, et al. National Sleep Foundation's sleep time duration recommendations: methodology and results summary. *Sleep Health*. 2015;1(1):40–43.
6. Watson NF, Badr MS, Belensky G, et al. Recommended amount of daily sleep for a healthy adult: a joint consensus statement of the American Academy of Sleep Medicine and Sleep Research Society. *Sleep*. 2015;38(6):843–844.
7. Mullington JM, Haack M, Toth M, Serrador JM, Meier-Ewert HK. Cardiovascular, inflammatory, and metabolic consequences of sleep deprivation. *Prog Cardiovasc Dis*. 2009;51(4):294–302.
8. Reynolds AC, Banks S. Total sleep deprivation, chronic sleep restriction and sleep disruption. *Prog Brain Res*. 2010;185:91–103.
9. Grandner MA, Drummond SPA. Who are the long sleepers? Towards an understanding of the mortality relationship. *Sleep Med Rev*. 2007;11(5):341–360.
10. Kripke DF, Garfinkel L, Wingard DL, Klauber MR, Marler MR. Mortality associated with sleep duration and insomnia. *Arch Gen Psychiatry*. 2002;59(2):131–136.
11. Itani O, Jike M, Watanabe N, Kaneita Y. Short sleep duration and health outcomes: a systematic review, meta-analysis, and meta-regression. *Sleep Med*. 2017;32:246–256.
12. Makarem N, Shechter A, Carnethon MR, Mullington JM, Hall MH, Abdall M. Sleep duration and blood pressure: recent advances and future directions. *Curr Hypertens Rep*. 2019;21(5):33.
13. Covassin N, Singh P. Sleep duration and cardiovascular disease risk: epidemiologic and experimental evidence. *Sleep Med Clin*. 2016;11(1):81–89.
14. Ge BH, Guo XM. Short and long sleep durations are both associated with increased risk of stroke: a meta-analysis of observational studies. *Int J Stroke*. 2015;10(3):177–184.

15. Cappuccio FP, Taggart FM, Kandala NB, et al. Meta-analysis of short sleep duration and obesity in children and adults. *Sleep*. 2008;31(5):619–626.
16. Van Cauter E, Holmback U, Knutson K, et al.. Impact of sleep and sleep loss on neuroendocrine and metabolic function. *Horm Res*. 2007;67(suppl 1):2–9.
17. Zhu B, Shi C, Park CG, Zhao X, Reutrakul S. Effects of sleep restriction on metabolism-related parameters in healthy adults: a comprehensive review and meta-analysis of randomized controlled trials. *Sleep Med Rev*. 2019;45:18–30.
18. Hagen EW, Starke SJ, Peppard PE. The association between sleep duration and leptin, ghrelin, and adiponectin among children and adolescents. *Curr Sleep Med Rep*. 2015;1:185–194.
19. Prather AA, Janicki-Deverts D, Hall MH, Cohen S. Behaviorally assessed sleep and susceptibility to the common cold. *Sleep*. 2015;28(9):1353–1359.
20. Prather AA, Pressman SD, Miller GE, Cohen S. Temporal links between self-reported sleep and antibody responses to the influenza vaccine. *Int J Behav Med*. 2021;28(1):151–158.
21. Wu L, Sun D. Sleep duration and falls: a systemic review and meta-analysis of observational studies. *J Sleep Res*. 2017;26(3):293–301.
22. Moradi A, Nazari SS, Rahmani K. Sleepiness and the risk of road traffic accidents: a systematic review and meta-analysis of previous studies. *Transp Res Part F Traffic Psychol Behav*. 2019;65:620–629.
23. Gottlieb DJ, Ellenbogen JM, Bianchi MT, Czeisler CA. Sleep deficiency and motor vehicle crash risk in the general population. *BMC Med*. 2018;16(1):44.
24. Connor J, Norton R, Ameratunga S, et al. Driver sleepiness and risk of serious injury to car occupants: population based case control study. *BMJ*. 2002;324(7346):1125.
25. Banks S, Dinges DF. Behavioral and physiological consequences of sleep restriction. *J Clin Sleep Med*. 2007;3(5):519–528.
26. Sun Y, Shi L, Bao Y, Sun Y, Shi J, Lu L. The bidirectional relationship between sleep duration and depression in community-dwelling middle-aged and elderly individuals: evidence from a longitudinal study. *Sleep Med*. 2018;52:221–229.
27. Scott AJ, Webb TL, Martyn-St James M, Rowse G, Weich S. Improving sleep quality leads to better mental health: a meta-analysis of randomised controlled trials. *Sleep Med Rev*. 2021;60:101556.
28. Liu Y, Wheaton AG, Chapman DP, Cunningham TJ, Lu H, Croft JB. Prevalence of healthy sleep duration among adults—United States, 2014. *MMWR Morb Mortal Wkly Rep*. 2016;65:137–141.
29. Caraballo C, Mahajan S, Valero-Elizondo J, et al. Evaluation of temporal trends in racial and ethnic disparities in sleep duration among US adults, 2004–2018. *JAMA Netw Open*. 2022;5(4):e226385.
30. Evans MA, Buysse DJ, Marsland AL, et al. Meta-analysis of age and actigraphy-assessed sleep characteristics across the lifespan. *Sleep*. 2021;44(9):zsab088.
31. Zhu G, Catt M, Cassidy S, et al. Objective sleep assessment in >80,000 UK mid-life adults: associations with sociodemographic characteristics, physical activity and caffeine. *PLoS ONE* 2019;14(12):e0226220.
32. Pilcher JJ, Lamber BJ, Huffcutt AI. Differential effects of permanent and rotating shifts on self-report sleep length: a meta-analytic review. *Sleep*. 2000;23(2):1–9.

33. DeSantis AS, Diez Roux AV, Moore K, Baron KG, Mujahid MS, Nieto FJ. Associations of neighborhood characteristics with sleep timing and quality: the multi-ethnic study of atherosclerosis. *Sleep*. 2013;36(10):1543–1551.
34. Johnson DA, Simonelli G, Moore K, et al. The neighborhood social environment and objective measures of sleep in the multi-ethnic study of atherosclerosis. *Sleep*. 2017;40(1):zsw016.
35. Astell-Burt T, Feng X, Kolt GS. Does access to neighborhood green space promote a health duration of sleep? novel findings from a cross-sectional study of 259 319 Australians. *BMJ Open*. 2013;3(8):e003094.
36. Johnson BS, Malecki KM, Peppard PE, Beyer KMM. Exposure to neighborhood green space and sleep: evidence from the Survey of the Health of Wisconsin. *Sleep Health*. 2018;4(5):413–419.
37. Chum A, O'Campo P, Matheson F. The impact of urban land use on sleep duration and sleep problems. *Can Geogr*. 2015;59:404–418.
38. Xiao Q, Gee G, Jones RR, Jia P, James P, Hale L. Cross-sectional association between outdoor artificial light at night and sleep duration in middle-to-older aged adults: the NIH-AARP Diet and Health Study. *Environ Res*. 2020;180:108823.
39. Scott H, Woods HC. Understanding links between social media use, sleep and mental health: recent progress and current challenges. *Curr Sleep Med Rep*. 2019;5:141–149.
40. Bhat S, Pinto-Zipp G, Upadhyay H, Polos PG. "To sleep, perchance to tweet": in-bed electronic social media use and its associations with insomnia, daytime sleepiness, mood, and sleep duration in adults. *Sleep Health*. 2018;4(2):166–173.
41. Murawski B, Wade L, Plotnikoff RC, Lubans DR, Ducnan MJ. A systematic review and meta-analysis of cognitive and behavioral interventions to improve sleep health in adults without sleep disorders. *Sleep Med Rev*. 2018;40:160–169.
42. Brown FC, Buboltz WC Jr., Soper B. Development and evaluation of the Sleep Treatment and Education Program for Students (STEPS). *J Am Coll Health*. 2006;54(4):231–237.
43. Gao R, Li X, Zhou K, Jin X, Dang S, Li N. Effects of comprehensive sleep management on sleep quality in university students in mainland China. *Sleep Biol Rhythms*. 2014;12(3):194–202.
44. Greeson JM, Juberg MK, Maytan M, James K, Rogers H. A randomized controlled trial of Koru: a mindfulness program for college students and other emerging adults. *J Am Coll Health*. 2014;62(4):194–202.
45. Jensen CG, Lansner J, Petersen A, et al. Open and calm—a randomized controlled trial evaluating a public stress reduction program in Denmark. *BMC Public Health*. 2015;15:1245.
46. Veasey SC, Rosen IM. Obstructive sleep apnea in adults. *N Engl J Med*. 2019;380(15):1442–1449.
47. Dempsey JA, Veasey SC, Morgan BJ, O'Donnell CP. Pathophysiology of sleep apnea. *Physiol Rev*. 2010;90(1):47–112.
48. Gottlieb DJ, Punjabi NM. Diagnosis and management of obstructive sleep apnea: a review. *JAMA*. 2020;323(14):1389–1400.
49. Morsy NE, Farrag NS, Zaki NF, et al. Obstructive sleep apnea: personal, societal, public health, and legal implications. *Rev Environ Health*. 2019;34(2):153–169.
50. Streatfeild J, Smith J, Mansfield D, Pezzullo L, Hillman D. The social and economic cost of sleep disorders. *Sleep*. 2021;44(11):zsab132.
51. Young T, Peppard PE, Gottleib D. Epidemiology of obstructive sleep apnea: a population health perspective. *Am J Respir Crit Care Med*. 2002;165:1217–1239.

52. Lal C, Weaver TE, Bae CJ, Strohl KP. Excessive daytime sleepiness in obstructive sleep apnea. mechanisms and clinical management. *Ann Am Thorac Soc.* 2021;18(5):757–768.
53. Chou KT, Tsai YL, Yeh WY, Chen YM, Huang N, Cheng HM. Risk of work-related injury in workers with obstructive sleep apnea: a systematic review and meta-analysis. *J Sleep Res.* 2022;31(1):e13446.
54. Garbarino S, Bardwell WA, Guglielmi O, Chiorri C, Bonanni E, Magnavita N. Association of anxiety and depression in obstructive sleep apnea patients: a systematic review and meta-analysis. *Behav Sleep Med.* 2020;18(1):35–57.
55. Edwards C, Almeida OP, Ford AH. Obstructive sleep apnea and depression: a systematic review and meta-analysis. *Maturitas.* 2020;142:45–54.
56. Yeghiazarians Y, Jneid H, Tietjens JR, et al. Obstructive sleep apnea and cardiovascular disease: a scientific statement from the American Heart Association. *Circulation.* 2021;144(3):e56–e67.
57. Hou H, Zhao Y, Yu W, et al. Association of obstructive sleep apnea with hypertension: a systematic review and meta-analysis. *J Glob Health.* 2018;8(1):010405.
58. Wang X, Ouyang Y, Wang Z, Zhao G, Liu L, Bi Y. Obstructive sleep apnea and risk of cardiovascular disease and all-cause mortality: a meta-analysis of prospective cohort studies. *Int J Cardiol.* 2013;169(3):207–214.
59. Bubu OM, Andrade AG, Umasabor-Bubu OQ, et al. Obstructive sleep apnea, cognition and Alzheimer's disease: a systematic review integrating three decades of multidisciplinary research. *Sleep Med Rev.* 2020;50:101250.
60. Vanek J, Prasko J, Genzor S, et al. Obstructive sleep apnea, depression and cognitive impairment. *Sleep Med.* 2020;72:50–58.
61. Huang X, Tang S, Lyu X, Yang C, Chen X. Structural and functional brain alterations in obstructive sleep apnea: a multimodal meta-analysis. *Sleep Med.* 2019;54:195–204.
62. Huang Y, Yang C, Yuan R, Liu M, Hao Z. Association of obstructive sleep apnea and cerebral small vessel disease: a systematic review and meta-analysis. *Sleep.* 2020;43(4):zsz264.
63. Lin CH, Lurie RC, Lyons OD. Sleep apnea and chronic kidney disease: a state-of-the-art review. *Chest.* 2020;157(3):673–685.
64. Hansrivijit P, Puthenpura MM, Ghahramani N, Thongprayoon C, Cheungpasitporn W. Bidirectional association between chronic kidney disease and sleep apnea: a systematic review and meta-analysis. *Int Urol Nephrol.* 2021;53(6):1209–1222.
65. Owens RL, Gold KA, Gozal D, et al. Sleep and breathing… and cancer? *Cancer Prev Res.* 2016;9(11):821–827.
66. Almendros I, Montserrat JM, Ramirez J, et al. Intermittent hypoxia enhances cancer progression in a mouse model of sleep apnoea. *Eur Resp J.* 2012;39(1):215–217.
67. Almendros I, Montserrat JM, Torres M, et al. Intermittent hypoxia increases melanoma metastasis to the lung in a mouse model of sleep apnea. *Respir Physiol Neurobiol.* 2013;186(3):303–307.
68. Tan NK, Yap DW, Tan BK, et al. The association of obstructive sleep apnea with melanoma incidence and mortality: a meta-analysis of 5,276,451 patients. *Sleep Med.* 2021;88:213–220.
69. Fu Y, Xia Y, Yi H, Xu H, Guan J, Yin S. Meta-analysis of all-cause and cardiovascular mortality in obstructive sleep apnea with or without continuous positive airway pressure treatment. *Sleep Breath.* 2017;21(1):181–189.

70. Tan BK, Teo YH, Tan NK, et al. Association of obstructive sleep apnea and nocturnal hypoxemia with all-cancer incidence and mortality: a systematic review and meta-analysis. *J Clin Sleep Med.* 2022;18(5):1427–1440.
71. Peppard PE, Young T, Barnet JH, Palta M, Hagen EW, Hla KM. Increased prevalence of sleep-disordered breathing in adults. *Am J Epidemiol.* 2013;177(9):1006–1014.
72. Benjafield AV, Ayas NT, Eastwood PR, et al.. Estimation of the global prevalence and burden of obstructive sleep apnoea: A literature-based analysis. *Lancet Respir Med.* 2019;7(8): 687–698.
73. Punjabi NM. The epidemiology of adult obstructive sleep apnea. *Proc Am Thorac Soc.* 2008;5(2):136–143.
74. Etindele Sosso FA, Matos E. Socioeconomic disparities in obstructive sleep apnea: a systematic review of empirical research. *Sleep Breath.* 2021;25(4):1729–1739.
75. Dudley KA, Patel SR. Disparities and genetic risk factors in obstructive sleep apnea. *Sleep Med.* 2016;18:96–102.
76. Mendelson M, Bailly S, Marillier M, et al. Obstructive sleep apnea syndrome, objectively measured physical activity and exercise training interventions: a systematic review and meta-analysis. *Front Neurol.* 2018;9:73.
77. Bibbins-Domingo K, Grossman DC, Curry SJ, et al.. Screening for obstructive sleep apnea in adults: US Preventive Services Task Force recommendation statement. *JAMA.* 2017;317(4): 407–414.
78. US Preventive Services Task Force. Final recommendation statement: obstructive sleep apnea in adults: screening. November 15, 2022. Available at: uspreventiveservicestaskforce.org/uspstf/recommendation/obstructive-sleep-apnea-in-adults-screening. Accessed January 19, 2023.
79. Chiu HY, Chen PY, Chuang LP, et al. Diagnostic accuracy of the Berlin questionnaire, STOP-BANG, STOP, and Epworth sleepiness scale in detecting obstructive sleep apnea: a bivariate meta-analysis. *Sleep Med Rev.* 2017;36:57–70.
80. Patil SP, Ayappa IA, Caples SM, Kimoff RJ, Patel SR, Harrod CG. Treatment of adult obstructive sleep apnea with positive airway pressure: an American Academy of Sleep Medicine systematic review, meta-analysis, and GRADE assessment. *J of Clin Sleep Med.* 2019;15(2): 301–334.

16

Cardiovascular Disease

Longjian Liu, MD, PhD, MSc, Julianne Nelson, PhD, MPH, and Craig J. Newschaffer, PhD

LEARNING OBJECTIVES

After completing this chapter, readers should be able to

1. Learn the basic concepts of cardiovascular disease.
2. Describe the principals of cardiovascular disease epidemiology.
3. Understand the main risk factors and prevention strategies for cardiovascular disease.

INTRODUCTION

Cardiovascular disease (CVD) refers to a wide variety of heart and blood vessel diseases, principally coronary heart disease, cerebrovascular disease (stroke), heart failure, and peripheral arterial disease (Figure 16-1). In the United States today, CVD is of paramount public health importance because of its widespread nature and the potential for intervention. Risk factors such as obesity, hypertension, dyslipidemia, dysglycemia, and diabetes can lead to a range of CVDs. The prevalence and severity of CVDs also differ by age, sex, and race, resulting in an increase in targeted public health prevention and treatment programs. The consequences of these diseases are beyond the physical (disability and death), including a significant economic burden (health care costs and loss of income).

Cardiovascular disease death rates have declined precipitously over the past two decades; from 1999 to 2019, death rates attributable to CVD declined 38.9%. In the same 21-year period the actual number of CVD deaths per year declined by 8.5%. Yet, in 2019 CVD still accounted for 30.5% (869,883) of all deaths in the United States. This decline has been driven by continuing reductions in mortality from both coronary heart disease (CHD) and, to a lesser extent, stroke (Figure 16-2).[1] Cardiovascular disease remains a major public health challenge, with heart disease the first and stroke the fourth leading overall causes of death in the United States.[1-3]

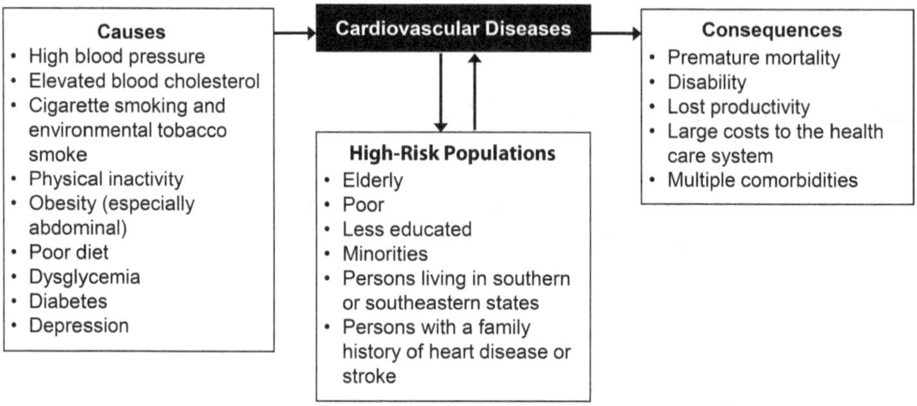

Figure 16-1. Cardiovascular Diseases: Causes, Consequences, and High-Risk Populations

Significance

Death rates for CVD vary markedly by age, race, sex, and social determinants.[4] In 2019 the age-adjusted death rates were 259.1 per 100,000 for men and 175.3 for women. The rates were 255.5 for non-Hispanic White men, 339.2 for non-Hispanic Black men, 189.2 for Hispanic men, 171.9 for non-Hispanic White women, 226.6 for non-Hispanic Black women, and 126.1 for Hispanic women.[1] The leading causes of death for both men

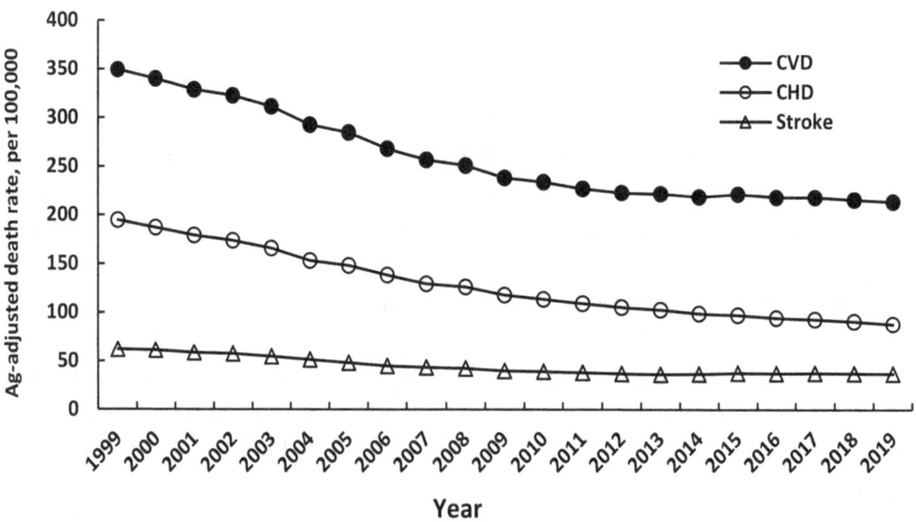

Source: Based on CDC.[1]

Note: CHD = coronary heart disease; CVD = cardiovascular disease. Data are from CDC WONDER multiple cause-of-death files, 1999–2019. Directly standardized to the age distribution of the 2000 US standard population. Coronary heart disease is defined as *ICD-10*: I20-I25. Stroke is defined as *ICD-10:* I60-I69.

Figure 16-2. Age-Adjusted Cardiovascular Disease Mortality by Year, 1999–2019

and women aged 65 years or older are (1) diseases of the heart, (2) cancer, (3) chronic lower respiratory disease, (4) stroke, and (5) Alzheimer's disease. Hispanics and Asian Americans appear to be at lower risk of heart disease and stroke mortality than Whites. However, CVD-related diseases remain the leading contributors to mortality for these racial and ethnic groups.[2]

Mortality captures only a portion of the health burden imposed by CVD. In 2018 cardiovascular disease was a primary diagnosis for more than 5 million inpatient hospital discharges and 7.1 million emergency department encounters. That year also saw 69.7 million physician office visits with a primary diagnosis of CVD. American adults self-reported heart trouble, stroke, or high blood pressure as the most common causes for their disability.[2] Cardiovascular disease accounted for 15% of total health expenditures in 2011 to 2012, more than any other major diagnostic group. The direct and indirect cost of CVD for 2017 to 2018 in the United States is an estimated $378 billion. This figure includes the cost of health care services, medicines, and lost productivity because of death.[4] Mortality rates from CVD remain higher in the United States than in many other industrialized nations; however, reflective of the worldwide spread of CVD, the United States (out of 204 countries) had only the 167th-highest 2019 age-adjusted CVD mortality per Our World in Data.[5] As estimated by the World Health Organization, 17.9 million people died from CVD in 2019, representing 32% of all global deaths. Of these deaths, 85% were the result of heart attack and stroke. More than 75% of CVD deaths take place in low- and middle-income countries. Out of the 17 million premature deaths (<70 years) from noncommunicable diseases in 2019, 38% were caused by CVD.[6]

Pathophysiology

Atherosclerosis, the underlying disease process of the major forms of CVD, is a slowly progressive condition in which the inner layers of the arterial walls become thick, irregular, and rigid. The process is complex, with contributing factors including deposition of fat and cholesterol, inflammation, migration and proliferation of smooth muscle cells, formation of raised fibrous lesions, and calcification. With the progression of atherosclerosis, the arteries narrow, the blood flow is decreased, and there is greater likelihood that the built-up material, or plaque, will disrupt, creating a traveling blood clot (or embolism; see also Chapter 14, Dyslipidemia).

Cardiovascular disease usually manifests clinically in middle age or later—the lifetime risk for incident CVD for men aged 40 years is about 66%, and it is just over 50% for like-aged women.[7] However, atherosclerosis typically initiates in childhood, and there is growing speculation that fetal factors may also be etiologically significant. Atherosclerosis is associated with several modifiable risk factors, including those well known as risk factors for CVD: high blood cholesterol, high blood pressure, cigarette smoking, physical inactivity, diabetes, obesity, and cardiometabolic syndrome.[8] The advent of noninvasive means of evaluating atherosclerosis has fostered the epidemiologic study of asymptomatic CVD. Control of modifiable risk factors, at both the population and individual levels, remains the key to primary and secondary prevention of CVD.

Coronary heart disease, heart failure, cerebrovascular disease (stroke), and peripheral arterial disease (PAD) share, but are not influenced equally by, many of the same CVD risk factors. Coronary heart disease is rarely found in populations without elevated cholesterol and body mass index. In contrast, stroke is a disease most strongly associated with high blood pressure with less contribution coming from cholesterol and other risk factors. Diabetes and smoking are most strongly associated with PAD. This chapter provides a detailed discussion of each of these four major types of CVD.

CORONARY HEART DISEASE

Introduction

Coronary heart disease (CHD), a disease of the blood vessels supplying the heart muscle, is the single-largest killer of American men and women today, accounting for 360,900 deaths in 2019. It represents almost half (>41%) of the CVD deaths and more than 13% of all-cause mortality.[2] Each year there are more than 805,000 new or recurrent heart attacks, and it is estimated that approximately 21% of these heart attacks are silent. Every 40 seconds someone in the United States has a heart attack. The American Heart Association (AHA) estimates that among American adults aged 20 years and older, 12.9% have a family history of CHD. About 1.3 million hospital admissions each year involve diagnoses of CHD, and the average annual costs associated with medical care, lost earnings, and lost productivity attributable to CHD were estimated at $219.6 billion for 2016 to 2017.[3,9] Even with the nationwide impact of the novel SARS-CoV-2 virus on mortality, heart disease remains the number one cause of death and is expected to remain so for many years to come, in part as a consequence of the long-term effects of SARS-CoV-2 and the global pandemic.[10,11]

Pathophysiology

Coronary heart disease, also called ischemic heart disease or coronary artery disease, is a term used to identify several disorders that reduce the blood supply to the heart muscle. This impairment of circulation to the heart is most frequently the result of narrowing of the coronary arteries by atherosclerosis. The onset, and much of the progression, of atherosclerosis is subclinical (i.e., without symptoms), with the most common emergent clinical manifestations of coronary atherosclerosis being angina pectoris (chest pain), myocardial infarction (heart attack), and sudden death.

Historically, CHD epidemiology has been dependent on studies of these clinical manifestations as endpoints. However, the incorporation of new technologies into epidemiologic investigations, such as the B-mode ultrasound of the carotid arteries used in the Atherosclerosis Risk in Communities (ARIC) studies, is allowing new insights about risk factors for early stage CHD. Those implicated through these studies thus far include conventional CHD risk factors, genetic changes at the cellular level, circulating markers of inflammation, infectious agents, micronutrients, and hemostatic factors.[12,13]

Descriptive Epidemiology

High-Risk Populations

Throughout life men have much higher CHD mortality rates than women. Overall, the age-adjusted death rate for CHD in the United States is almost twice as high for men as it is for women.[1] The incidence of CHD in women lags behind men by 7 to 10 years for total CHD and by 20 years for more serious clinical events such as myocardial infarction and sudden death.[9,14] However, in women CHD is still the single greatest mortality risk, with the age-adjusted mortality rate more than three times greater than that for breast cancer.[2,15]

Coronary heart disease risk increases with age independent of known CHD risk factors. Almost 21 per 1,000 Americans aged 65 years or older will experience heart failure, and 87% of the people who die of heart attacks are older than 65 years of age.[2,4] CHD is the leading cause of death for men and women older than 65 years of age and the third leading cause of disability in older men and women.[4] For men, major increases in CHD risk begin around 45 years of age, whereas for women, the marked increase is delayed until after menopause, around 55 years of age. Coronary heart disease incident rates in women after menopause are two to three times those of women the same age before menopause, and recent studies have shown that an earlier age at menopause is also associated with an increased risk of CHD. Subclinical CHD is more prevalent in older than in younger individuals and has been shown to be associated with the same risk factors linked to clinical disease at younger ages, thereby suggesting that risk factor modification in older individuals may still be a very cost-effective public health strategy.

For men and women combined, CHD death rates are higher among Blacks than Whites until 85 years of age and older, at which point they are higher among Whites. Non-Hispanic Black men experience a slightly higher death rate from CHD than do White men. In 2020 the overall age-adjusted CHD death rate was 91.8 per 100,000 population, with death rates of 126.3 for White men and 149.7 per 100,000 for non-Hispanic Black men. The racial gap in CHD mortality is closing. In 2005 the rate for non-Hispanic Whites was 147.3 compared with 175.7 per 100,000 for non-Hispanic Blacks. By 2020 both rates declined, with the age-adjusted CHD mortality rate per 100,000 being 91.5 for non-Hispanic Whites and 111.5 for non-Hispanic Blacks.[1]

Although national data on CHD mortality among Hispanic Americans are limited, existing data suggest that age-adjusted death rates in 2020 for CHD were 75.6 per

100,000 for Hispanics or Latinos/Latinas, 62.3 per 100,000 for American Indians or Alaska Natives, and 56.1 for Asians or Pacific Islanders.[1]

A family history of premature CHD increases the risk of CHD. The clustering of CHD in families is not fully understood but is believed to be a combination of genetics and higher levels of risk factors within these families (e.g., similar dietary patterns).

CHD incidence and mortality rates are higher among people of lower socioeconomic status (SES) than among those in the middle or upper classes.[4] The greatest declines in CHD mortality over time among all races in the United States have been among those with the highest levels of income.[16] Not surprisingly, the gradient of CHD mortality associated with SES is similar to the gradient of risk factors; for example, cigarette smoking, obesity, and high blood pressure are more common among people with lower income and formal education levels.[17]

In addition, neighborhood SES effects may persist above those related to differing distributions of individual-level risk factors. In general, living in a low-SES neighborhood is associated with increased risk of CHD and increased levels of risk factors. However, complex interactions between individual- and neighborhood-level SES on CHD risk factors in Blacks have been observed. For example, one analysis of Black men living in Jackson, Mississippi, found that lower individual SES was associated with increased serum cholesterol in higher-SES neighborhoods and decreased serum cholesterol in lower-SES neighborhoods. Another study of participants also from Jackson, MS, observed an increased risk of CVD associated with increasing neighborhood disadvantage, independent of individual-level SES but only in Black women.[18]

Geographic Distribution

In the United States, age-adjusted CHD death rates show striking variation by geographic region. In 2020 the age-adjusted death rates in the United States varied from a high of 128.7 per 100,000 in Arkansas to a low of 58.4 per 100,000 in Minnesota.[1] The CHD death rate for the United States is approximately midway between those of other industrialized countries. The Global Burden of Disease 2019 study found that between 1990 and 2019, age-adjusted rates of CHD death per 100,000 were highest in parts of northern Africa and the Middle East, Eastern Europe, and Central Asia. Low rates were noted in certain Caribbean and South American countries, western Europe, Japan, and South Korea. In the countries studied, the highest CHD death rate observed was as much as 20 times the lowest rate.[19,20]

Time Trends

Coronary heart disease was the leading cause of death in the United States for most of the 20th century, with death rates peaking in 1963. Since then, CHD mortality has declined substantially, and in recent years the decline has been accelerating, with the largest rate of decline observed between 1999 and 2010, a decreased rate of 39% in both non-Hispanic White and Black men, and 44% in both non-Hispanic White and Black women. Then, from 2010 to 2019 CHD death rates declined by 19.6% in non-Hispanic White men, 26.6% in non-Hispanic White women, 20.6% in non-Hispanic Black men, and 28.1% in non-Hispanic Black women (Figure 16-3).[1] Overall, from 1999 to 2019 the age-adjusted death rates of CHD fell from 251.2 to 122.1 deaths per 100,000 population in non-Hispanic White men, and from 150.5 to 61.5 deaths per 100,000 population in non-Hispanic White women. The corresponding age-adjusted death rates decreased from 278.7 to 134.2 per 100,000 population in non-Hispanic Black men, and 188.0 to 75.4 per 100,000 population in non-Hispanic Black women.[1] In general, declines in age-adjusted mortality since 1999 have been comparable across race/sex subgroups (Figure 16-3). However, in recent years geographic variability in rates of decline have emerged. Most notably, CHD mortality rates have appeared to increase in counties in Oklahoma, Mississippi, East Texas, and New Mexico.[21]

Factors responsible for the decline in CHD mortality are not fully understood, but changes in lifestyle, reductions in risk factor prevalence, and improvements in medical care and treatment of CHD are thought to have contributed. A study by Ford et al. indicates that approximately 47% of the decline in the CHD death rate from 1980 to 2000

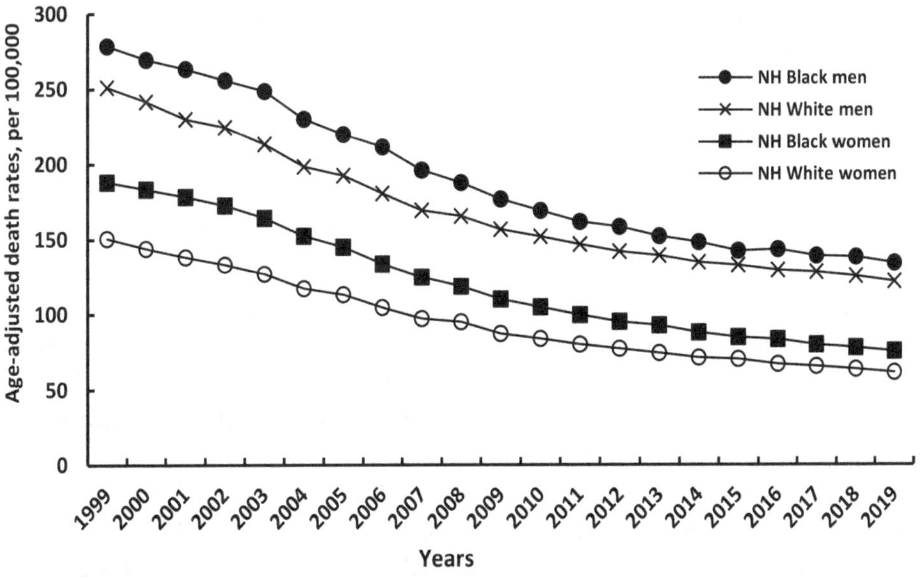

Source: Based on CDC.[1,2]

Note: NH = non-Hispanic. Data are from CDC WONDER multiple cause-of-death files, 1999–2019. Age-adjusted rates were estimated using direct standardization method to the age distribution of the 2000 US standard population. Coronary heart disease is defined as *ICD-10:* I20-I25.

Figure 16-3. Age-Adjusted Death Rates for Coronary Heart Disease by Sex and Race: United States, 1999–2019

was attributed to evidence-based medical treatments, including secondary preventive therapies after or revascularization (11%), initial treatment for acute myocardial infarction or unstable angina (10%), treatments for heart failure (9%), revascularization for chronic angina (5%), and other therapies (12%). Approximately 44% was attributed to changes in major risk factors, including reductions in total cholesterol (24%), systolic blood pressure (20%), smoking prevalence (12%), and physical inactivity (5%). These reductions were partially offset by increases in body mass index (BMI) and prevalence of diabetes, which accounted for an increased number of CHD deaths (8% and 10%, respectively). However, not all groups have benefited equally from these improvements.[22]

Causes

Coronary risk factors can be classified as either modifiable or nonmodifiable. The major independent risk factors for CHD are listed in Figure 16-1 and described in more detail below. Other modifiable risk factors include elevated blood C-reactive protein (CRP), fibrinogen, homocysteine, and secondhand smoke. Alcohol overconsumption and stress may also contribute to CHD risk. Nonmodifiable risk factors are discussed under the previous heading of High-Risk Populations. Note, however, that not all high-risk groups are defined by nonmodifiable factors. Improved SES, for example, although not typically a direct goal of medical or public health intervention, certainly is a legitimate objective for social and economic policy.

Modifiable Risk Factors

High blood pressure (see Chapter 13) is a strong independent risk factor for morbidity and mortality from CHD.[22] People with elevated blood pressure (BP) are two to four times as susceptible to CHD as are people with normal BP. However, it is important to note that risk of CHD generally increases as levels of systolic or diastolic BP rise whether or not one is looking at a population group above or below a particular high BP cut point. Studies indicate that increased BP is clearly associated with an increased risk of lifetime death from CHD.[23] Therefore, BP reduction by individuals labeled normotensive by conventional definitions can also be beneficial.

Studies have shown that most BP-lowering medications are equally effective in preventing risk of fatal and nonfatal cardiovascular events, including CHD in both younger and older patients with high BP, whereas beta blockers, though being equally effective as the other agents in patients younger than 65 years, lose some of their effectiveness at an older age.[24]

Tobacco use (see Chapter 7) is a major cause of CHD among both men and women. People who smoke have twice the risk of heart attack as nonsmokers. Smoking is also the major risk factor for sudden death from heart attack, with people who smoke having risk two to four times that of nonsmokers. The risk increases with the number of cigarettes smoked. Following the first Surgeon General's Report on Smoking in 1964, the prevalence of cigarette smoking rates declined sharply for men from 51.2% in 1965 to 14.1% in 2020, and for women from 33.7% in 1965 to 11.0% in 2020. These decreasing trends in cigarette smoking have made a significant contribution to risk reduction of CVD, cancer, and other diseases. However, cigarette smoking and other types of tobacco use (e.g., e-cigarettes, smokeless tobacco) remain a serious public health issue because of the high associated risk of disease. Overall, people who smoke cigarettes are two to four times more likely to develop CHD compared with nonsmokers. People who smoke heavily (i.e., those who smoke two or more packs per day) die from CHD at a rate two to three times that of nonsmokers. Studies have shown, however, that people who stop smoking experience a rapid and substantial reduction in CHD mortality. For people who have smoked a pack or less per day, within 10 years of quitting, death rates from CHD drop to the level of people who have never smoked.[25,26]

In addition, a number of studies suggest that exposure to environmental tobacco smoking (also called passive smoking or secondhand smoke) increases the risk of CHD. For example, a recent meta-analysis in cohort studies indicated that environmental tobacco smoking was associated with a 12% higher increase in the risk of cardiovascular disease (adjusted hazard ratio [HR] 1.12; 95% CI, 1.06–1.20), with the highest risk of mortality being observed for those who were exposed to environmental tobacco smoking at home, at work, and in public places (adjusted HR 1.26; 95% CI, 1.13–1.40).[27] An estimated 34,000 nonsmokers die from heart disease each year as a result of exposure to secondhand smoke.[28] The association between environmental tobacco smoking and CHD mortality is elevating the importance of this critical public health issue to new heights.

Cholesterol (see Chapter 14) is the blood lipid most strongly associated with CHD. The risk of CHD increases steadily as blood cholesterol levels increase in a population. US population studies suggest that optimal total cholesterol levels are about 150 mg/dL (3.8 mmol/L), which corresponds to a low-density lipoprotein (LDL) cholesterol level of about 100 mg/dL (2.6 mmol/L). Randomized clinical trials of cholesterol-lowering drugs in high-risk patients confirm that cholesterol-lowering (specifically for LDL) produces marked reduction of atherosclerotic cardiovascular disease, including CHD.[29]

Cholesterol is transported in the blood by LDLs, very low-density lipoproteins, and high-density lipoproteins (HDLs). High levels of LDL are a leading factor in the progression of atherosclerosis and in the subsequent development of CHD.[30] The very low-density lipoproteins, which are composed primarily of triglyceride, account for 10% to 15% of the total serum cholesterol. The role of triglycerides in development of CHD has been slower to be confirmed, with recent studies finding a similar pattern of elevated triglycerides in patients with CHD as seen with elevated LDL. More recently, a causal link between high triglycerides and CHD has been reported.[30]

The level of HDL is inversely related to CHD: the lower the level of HDL, the higher the risk of CHD. The HDL level correlates inversely with LDL size and triglyceride level, and this, coupled with the complex metabolic interrelationships of these particles, makes it more difficult to separate the independent contributions of various lipids to CHD. It is quite possible all play a role; one hypothesis is that LDL may be more important in early stage atherogenesis, whereas low HDL and triglyceride elevation develops closer to the clinical onset of CHD. For example, studies show an increased triglycerides-to-HDL ratio is an independent predictor of coronary heart disease.[31]

C-reactive protein is an inflammatory biomarker strongly associated with CHD, inflammation, and the metabolic syndrome. Although CRP, synthesized primarily in the liver, was discovered in 1930,[32] this protein has received substantial attention in recent years as a promising biological predictor of atherosclerotic disease. An evolving body of work suggests even small increases in CRP within the normal range are predictive of future vascular events in apparently healthy, asymptomatic individuals. A number of prospective studies have demonstrated that CRP also predicts recurrent events and increased mortality in patients with acute coronary syndromes, chronic stable angina, ischemic stroke, and peripheral vascular disease.[33,34]

Fibrinogen is a circulating glycoprotein that acts at the final step in the coagulation response to vascular and tissue injury. Epidemiological data support an independent association between elevated levels of fibrinogen and CHD.[34,35] Two meta-analyses involving 18 and 22 prospective, long-term studies demonstrated strong, statistically significant risk for individuals in the upper third of baseline fibrinogen concentration compared with those in the lower third (relative risk 1.8; 95% CI, 1.6–2.0).[35]

Another plasma constituent, homocysteine, is receiving increased attention as a potentially modifiable risk factor for acute CHD events. Plasma homocysteine levels have been found to be positively associated with risk of CHD events.[36] A recent review conducted by Humphrey and colleagues indicated that most studies found elevations of 20% to 50% in CHD risk for each increase of 5 micromoles per liter (μmol/L) in homocysteine level. A meta-analysis yielded a combined risk ratio for coronary events of 1.18 (95% CI, 1.10–1.26) for each increase of 5 μmol/L in homocysteine level.[37]

Although the underlying mechanisms linking diabetes (see Chapter 12) and CHD are complex and still not fully understood, diabetes is generally considered a major CHD risk factor. Among people with diabetes, CHD is the most common cause of morbidity and mortality, and individuals with diabetes experience CHD at rates two to four times greater than those without the disease. Data from national studies show that in 2011–2016 there was a disproportionately high prevalence of diabetes in non-Hispanic Blacks (20.4%) compared with non-Hispanic Whites (12.1%).[38] The 2020 overall death rate per 100,000 population from diabetes was 31.0. Death rates were 35.0 for White men, 45.2 for Black men, 25.3 for White women, and 38.9 for Black women.[1]

Obesity has widely been defined by using BMI (weight [kg]/height [m^2]). A BMI of 25 and higher indicates overweight, and 30 or higher indicates obesity in adults. Obesity and overweight have significant associations with increases in blood pressure, serum total cholesterol, and glucose, and with decreases in serum HDL levels. In addition, obesity has been well documented as an independent risk factor for CVD and diabetes. Recent studies have observed a J-shaped relationship between BMI and CHD mortality and note that even small increases in BMI can result in increased risk of CHD.[39]

Recent studies suggest that the distribution of fat deposits on the body may also affect CHD risk. Upper body or abdominal fat ("central obesity" or "apple shape") appears to increase risk more than lower body fat ("pear shape"). Men and women in the upper quintile of subscapular skinfold as well as men with a waist-to-hip ratio greater than 1.0 and women with a ratio greater than 0.8 experience increased CHD risk. The tendency toward abdominal disposition of body fat seems to increase CHD risk across all levels of BMI.[40]

Physical inactivity (see Chapter 9) is increasingly recognized as a major risk factor for CHD. More than 46% of US adults do not engage in the recommended amount of aerobic physical activity (defined as light-to-moderate sustained activity for 150 min/wk or vigorous activity for 75 min/wk), and more than 76% of US adults do not engage in the recommended amount of both aerobic and strength-training physical activity (defined as moderate intensity involving all muscle groups ≥2 d/wk).[41] Physical activity decreases body weight, decreases blood pressure, and improves insulin sensitivity.[42] Mounting evidence suggests small amounts of physical activity can also have a significant impact on heart disease mortality.[43] The greatest benefits appear to occur with the move from a completely sedentary lifestyle to very modest levels of activity.

Moderate-to-heavy alcohol consumption is known to raise blood pressure levels and to increase CHD mortality. However, in most studies light regular drinking (≤2 drinks/d) has been associated with modest reductions in CHD risk. The pathway for this protection appears to be through changes in HDL-cholesterol, fibrinogen, and hemoglobin A1c.[44] The relationship to other risk factors and the social consequences of alcohol use, however, preclude any public health recommendation for alcohol use (see Chapter 10).

Psychological factors and stress also have been studied in relation to the development of CHD. Perhaps the earliest studied is the type A behavior pattern, characterized by excessive competitiveness, hostility, impatience, fast speech, and quick motor movements, although this is not as widely studied anymore.[45] Considerable attention has been devoted to the exploration of specific psychological factors, including anger, job stress, anxiety, and social support.[46] Causal connections among these specific psychological risk factors and CHD have yet to be clearly established, but evidence supporting a causal role for anger, both as an event trigger and a long-term risk factor, and social support, particularly in extending survival among those with disease, is mounting.[47]

Lastly, risk factors for heart disease tend to cluster; that is, individuals with CHD are likely to have more than one risk factor. The greater the level of any single risk factor, the greater the chance of developing CHD. Moreover, the likelihood of developing CHD increases markedly when risk factors manifest simultaneously. There is at least an additive contribution to CHD risk for the major risk factors of high blood pressure, high LDL-cholesterol, and fibrinogen, as evident in the findings of the Prospective Cardiovascular Münster (PROCAM) study.[48]

Population-Attributable Risk

Coronary heart disease is a multifactorial disease, and precisely quantifying the contribution of each risk factor to overall heart disease is difficult. We can, however, roughly gauge the importance of risk factors by estimating population-attributable risk, which is the percentage of CHD that could be prevented by eliminating a particular risk factor in the population. There are several things that need to be remembered when one is considering population-attributable risks, with the two most important being (1) when there are many factors contributing to a disease, as is the case with CHD, these percentages will sum to more than 100%; and (2) when risk factors are continuous, like blood pressure or cholesterol level, the population-attributable risk estimated depends greatly on the cut point chosen to designate who is at high risk. Table 16-1 shows the proportion of CHD mortality that can be attributed to the risk factors discussed previously.[49–54]

Evidence-Based Interventions

Prevention

Because of the multiple risk factors involved in CHD, modest changes in one or more risk factors can have a large public health impact. Primary prevention of CHD involves controlling the major preventable risk factors: hypertension, high blood cholesterol, tobacco use, diet, and physical inactivity (see the related chapters accordingly). Other effective methods of prevention include diabetes control, weight management, and limitations in alcohol consumption (see Chapters 10–12).

The multifactorial nature of CHD etiology calls for multiple intervention strategies. In addition to the early detection and control of risk factors in adults, prevention approaches may include early and systematic health education regarding the importance of lifestyle behaviors in young people, such as avoiding tobacco, eating a healthy diet, and performing adequate physical activity. Other prevention interventions can include policy-related or environmental changes such as improved food choices in schools, improved food labeling in grocery stores, elimination of cigarette vending machines, and provision of smoke-free environments. (The multifaceted approach to risk reduction is discussed in Chapter 4 on intervention strategies.)

In 2010 AHA created the Life's Simple 7 (LS7) to define ideal cardiovascular health on a collection of seven key modifiable risk factors: blood pressure, cholesterol, blood sugar,

Table 16-1. Modifiable Risk Factors for Coronary Heart Disease in the United States

Magnitude	Risk Factor	Best Estimate (%) of PAR (Range)
Strong (relative risk >4)	None	
Moderate (relative risk 2-4)	High blood pressure (≥140/90 mm Hg)	25 (20-40)
	Cigarette smoking	22 (17-25)
	Elevated cholesterol (≥200 mg/dL)	43 (39-50)
	Diabetes (fasting glucose ≥140 mg/dL)	8 (1-15)
Weak (relative risk <2)	Obesity	17 (7-32)
	Physical inactivity	35 (23-46)
	Secondhand smoke exposure	18 (8-23)
	Elevated C-reactive protein (>3.0 mg/L)	19 (11-25)
	Elevated fibrinogen (>3.74 g/L)	21 (17-25)
	Elevated homocysteine (>15 μmol/L)	5 (2-9)
Possible risk factors	Psychological factors	
	Alcohol use	
	Elevated plasma homocysteine	
	Infectious agents	
	Helicobacter pylori	
	Herpes simplex type 1	
	Chlamydia pneumoniae	
	Cytomegalovirus	
	Trimethylamine-N-oxide (TMAO)	
	Sleep disorders	

Source: Based on Tsao et al.,[4] Danesh et al.,[35] Farmer et al.,[49] Cheng et al.,[50] Fox et al.,[51] Heidrich et al.,[52] Howard et al.,[53] and Li et al.[54]

Note: PAR = population-attributable risk.

physical activity, diet, weight, and smoking. Studies have shown that adherence to LS7 guidelines is associated with a decreased lifetime risk of CHD and heart failure.[55]

When one is considering prevention strategies, it is also important to recognize that CHD is affected by the social and economic characteristics of a community, including levels of income, education, and occupations. Positive changes in public health are, therefore, often the result of general social and economic development policies, rather than public health policies per se. Research has even found that when risk factors are held constant, those individuals with lower SES have higher CHD risk factors and a higher risk of coronary heart disease than do those with higher SES.[56]

Screening

The principal methods of early detection for CHD include screening for high blood pressure and elevated serum cholesterol and assessing behavioral factors such as tobacco use, dietary fat intake, and physical activity level.

Screening electrocardiograms are not recommended for the general population but may be appropriate for individuals at increased risk of CHD. This group includes men older than 40 years of age with two or more CHD risk factors, high-risk sedentary men planning to begin an exercise program, and people who would endanger the safety of others if they were to experience sudden cardiac events.[57] Newer screening technologies include coronary artery calcium scoring and noninvasive angiography with computed tomography. These may be useful tools for screening individuals who are at risk for CHD, specifically those with diabetes. However, some studies argue against using such screening tools, stating that there is insufficient evidence for their effective use on high-risk persons and, moreover, that their use is expensive and potentially harmful in comparison with currently available alternatives.[58]

Treatment

Advances in the treatment of CHD have contributed substantially to major reductions in mortality over the past four decades. Treatment for CHD is tailored to each patient, depending on the cause and severity of the coronary artery disease. Treatment options mainly include (1) healthy lifestyle programs, (2) medications, and (3) surgical and other invasive procedures. Of these, adopting a healthy lifestyle is one of the best treatments for CHD. Either by itself or in combination with medical treatment, a healthy lifestyle can prevent or attenuate disease progression.

When medications and lifestyle adjustments cannot relieve the chest pain symptomatic of CHD, surgery may be necessary to restore adequate function to the heart. Gene therapy is another one of the newest potential treatment modalities, but its effectiveness remains under investigation.[59]

Examples of Evidence-Based Interventions

Two major primary prevention strategies have been used in attempts to reduce cardiovascular mortality rates: the high-risk and the community-based (or population-based) approaches. The high-risk approach aims to identify high-risk individuals through population screening and to refer them for treatment. The Healthy Hearts Program,[60] Emerging Risk Factors Collaboration,[61] and the Multiple Risk Factor Intervention Trial[62] are examples of this approach. Recently a study has focused on using genetic markers to create a CHD risk score to identify who in the population should be directed toward additional screening and intervention programs.[63]

Community-based interventions are a cornerstone of the public health approach to CHD prevention. They are defined as programs that attempt to modify the prevalence of one or more CHD risk factors (e.g., hypertension, smoking, hyperlipidemia, physical inactivity, unhealthy diet), CHD mortality, or both within a specifically identified, circumscribed community. Community-based interventions have typically used education or environmental change to promote and facilitate changes in the lifestyles and other behaviors of a population.[64]

Largely because of a strong favorable but unanticipated secular trend in CHD risk factors in control communities, these interventions tended to have less power to demonstrate overall effectiveness at the community level than originally anticipated. However, within each intervention program, individual components were frequently shown to be successful in analyses of intermediate or process measures, as well as endpoints limited to subpopulations most likely to be exposed to the component (e.g., schoolchildren participating in school-based program with a home component).[65] In addition, success has been found in intervention programs that are designed for specific communities. An example of this is Partnership for an Active Community Environment, whose committee, as a means to improve cardiovascular health, installed a walking path and playground in a low-income neighborhood in New Orleans.[66] A recent review of 21 published major community-based CVD intervention programs worldwide showed positive impact on CHD risk factors within a distinct population.[67]

More recent community-based CHD prevention programs have focused on discrete populations, including the socioeconomically disadvantaged, ethnic minorities, young adults, and rural communities.[68] In 2012 the National Heart, Lung, and Blood Institute directed its efforts at reducing heart health disparities by funding nine strategic champions. This program is aimed at new community health worker projects in African American, American Indian, Filipino American, and Hispanic/Latin American communities. An example of this type of focused community-based program was recently conducted in California and directed toward Latina women. The pilot program for this intervention found that a targeted community-based prevention program was effective at improving cardiac health in the selected population.[69]

It is important to keep in mind that existing community-based interventions may not have the same impact when applied to different at-risk populations. This has been observed with the Exercise and Nutrition Interventions for Cardiovascular Health (ENCORE) study. The ENCORE study was designed to test the effect of two different dietary patterns on risk factors for CHD: the Dietary Approaches to Stop Hypertension (DASH) diet alone and the DASH diet plus weight management.[70] Although the DASH diet has been found to be effective, adherence to the DASH diet is not the same across races, and thus this intervention has different results when applied to different at-risk racial groups.[71]

Community-based interventions have been evolving in recent years to be able to take advantage of the shifting use of technology in our lives and how new technology can be used specifically in health interventions. An example of this is the mobile phone–based health (mHEALTH) intervention. Participants in the intervention received monthly motivational calls and weekly text messages that included diet and exercise information. Evaluations of the mHEALTH intervention found reductions in weight and improvement in healthy eating habits among those in the intervention group compared with those in standard care.[72] Programs such as these have an added benefit of being cost-effective and able to reach many more people than in-person community-based interventions are able to do.[73] However, not all risk factors appear to benefit from technology-based approaches. A recent meta-analysis of studies using digital technology interventions for cardiovascular risk factor modification found that in patients with CVD, digital technology–based interventions were effective at improving cholesterol, physical activity, diet, and medication adherence but failed to demonstrate improvements in BMI, triglycerides, blood pressure, alcohol, and smoking.[74]

Coronary heart disease along with its related mortality is not just an issue in the United States but is also on the rise in low- and middle-income countries. Recently there was an evaluation of the Program of Lifestyle Intervention in Families for Cardiovascular Risk Reduction (PROLIFIC) trial, which targeted families with a history of coronary heart disease in India. Families in the intervention arm received visits from trained health care workers to conduct lifestyle intervention education (diet, physical activity, smoking cessation, etc.), lead support groups, and help link family members to primary care providers. After two years of follow-up it was observed that participants in the intervention group as compared with those undergoing usual care were two times more likely to maintain blood pressure, fasting blood glucose, and LDL within healthy ranges. Over two years those in the intervention group also demonstrated a larger decline in Framingham Risk Score (–3.3%) compared with the usual care group (–0.8%).[75]

A recent example of a successful community-based intervention in China involved utilizing smartphones to deliver health education materials and monitor heart rate as a means of home-based cardiac rehabilitation. Compared with participants receiving a usual standard of care, those in the intervention group experienced significantly lower rates of major adverse cardiac events and hospitalizations during the follow-up period.[76]

In sum, numerous insights have been gained from these pioneering community CVD prevention interventions relating to the following: effective use of mass media; building on existing settings or institutions; creating strategies for making a healthy heart lifestyle doable; developing approaches to support environmental, legislative, and policy changes; and establishing and maintaining community coalitions. One of the most important common threads in the truly exemplary prevention and control programs is their reliance on multiple channels and multiple levels. This strategy appears to be critical in effecting lasting change.

Moving Forward

Epidemiologic research on CHD will likely focus on emerging, yet not completely understood, modifiable factors, including plasma CRP, fibrinogen, homocysteine, and known but complex risk factors such as serum cholesterol and body weight. Studies focusing on subclinical endpoints will be important in revealing undiscovered risk factors potentially significant in primary prevention. For example, further exploration of the importance of infection and inflammation in increasing the risk of atherosclerosis may prove fruitful. Population-based studies devising novel means of using information on known risk factors may also be crucial to advancing secondary prevention strategies.

A new area of CHD research is exploring the genetic factors that can contribute to developing CHD, with specific focus on expanding research and understanding of genetic risk factors for CHD in non-Hispanic Blacks.[77] It is suspected that these unknown genetic risk factors account for 40% to 60% of CHD risk. Although what role genetics will serve in the future of CHD prevention remains unclear, it is already being studied for its potential as a screening tool and the creation of a genetic risk score.[63]

New and important fields of research have developed in response to the novel SARS-CoV-2 virus and global pandemic. A meta-analysis of 40 studies found that CHD diagnosis is a significant risk factor for mortality upon SARS-CoV-2 infection (OR 3.75, 95% CI, 2.91–4.82) as well as severe infection (OR 3.23, 95% CI, 2.19–4.77) and ICU admission (OR 2.25, 95% CI, 1.34–3.79).[78] Patients with SARS-CoV-2 were 63% more likely to suffer a heart attack, and one year post SARS-CoV-2 infection there remains an excess burden for myocardial infarction of 2.91 (95% CI, 2.38–3.49) per 1,000 people.[79] It is not yet fully understood how SARS-CoV-2 will affect long-term cardiovascular health; however, it is believed that infection with SARS-CoV-2 can lead to vascular damage through a series of potential pathways, and SARS-CoV-2 infection has been observed to precede incident myocardial injury in up to 30% of patients.[80] Therefore, areas of interest include outcomes from SARS-CoV-2 infection in people with a history of and at high risk for CHD (increased mortality), long-term effects on cardiovascular health and risk factors for CHD after infection with SARS-CoV-2 (heart valve/vessel damage), and how the period of quarantine has affected the overall cardiovascular health of communities (e.g., increase in unhealthy lifestyle behaviors, lack of access to preventive care/therapies, delaying care).[10]

There is also growing interest in and recognition of the importance of conducting more research and demonstrating efforts involving policy and environmental approaches to reduce CHD risk factors. Collaborations with nontraditional partners will be essential for success. Population-based prevention research should focus on CHD research in special populations such as women, children, older adults, and racial and ethnic minorities, addressing the applicability of current knowledge to these populations and designing population-specific interventions, like the Jackson Heart Study (JHS),[81] Multi-Ethnic

Study of Atherosclerosis (MESA),[82] and the Hispanic Community Health Study/Study of Latinos (HCHS/SOL).[83] The JHS aims to examine genetic and environmental factors on risk factors for CVD in a Black population in Jackson, Mississippi.[77,81] The MESA is designed to study the prevalence, correlation, and progression of subclinical CVD in multiple ethnicities (non-Hispanic White, non-Hispanic Black, Hispanic, and Chinese).[8,84] The HCHS/SOL is a multicenter epidemiologic study in Hispanic/Latino populations to determine the role of acculturation in the prevalence and development of disease and to identify risk factors playing a protective or harmful role in Hispanics/Latinos.[83]

CEREBROVASCULAR DISEASE

Introduction

Cerebrovascular disease (stroke), a disease caused by loss of blood flow to part of the brain resulting in damage to brain tissue, poses a serious public health concern. Stroke is a major cause of serious disability for adults and a leading cause of death in the nation. In 2019 stroke caused almost 150,000 deaths in the United States, with a crude death rate of 45.7 per 100,000 population. More than 795,000 people have a stroke each year in the United States. Of those, the majority are first or new strokes, but nearly one in four is recurrent. About 25% die at the time of the stroke event or soon after, and 15% to 30% remain permanently disabled. Of all strokes, 87% are ischemic, 10% are intracerebral hemorrhage, and 3% are subarachnoid hemorrhage.[22] Worldwide, the burden of stroke has also posed a serious public health problem. In 2010 there were an estimated 11.6 million events of incident ischemic stroke and 5.3 million events of incident hemorrhagic stroke, with 63% and 80% of these, respectively, occurring in low- and middle-income counties.[3] According to the Global Burden of Disease 2016 Lifetime Risk of Stroke Collaborators, the mean global lifetime risk of stroke increased from 22.8% in 1990 to 24.9% in 2016, a relative increase of 8.9% after accounting for the competing risk of death attributable to any cause other than stroke.[22]

Stroke-associated societal costs, including direct costs associated with medical care and indirect costs because of lost productivity, were estimated at $52.8 billion in 2017 to 2018. The estimated direct medical cost of stroke was $33.4 billion. This includes hospital outpatient or office-based health care professional visits, hospital inpatient stays, emergency department visits, prescribed medicines, and home health care.[22] Transport of stroke patients to the hospital results in faster treatment. However, one-third of stroke patients do not call 9-1-1 and use emergency medical services (EMS) to get to the hospital. A total of 30 studies included in a recent systematic review indicate that non-Hispanic White patients with stroke were estimated to use emergency medical services at a greater rate (59.8%) than non-Hispanic Black (55.6%), Asian (54.7%), and Hispanic

(53.2%) patients. A greater proportion of non-Hispanic White patients (37.4%) were estimated to arrive within three hours from onset of stroke symptoms than non-Hispanic Black (26.0%) and Hispanic (28.9%) patients. A greater proportion of non-Hispanic White patients (2.8%) were estimated to receive tPA (tissue-type plasminogen activator) as compared with non-Hispanic Black (2.3%), Hispanic (2.6%), and Asian (2.3%) patients. As shown in this review, racial disparities exist at key points along the continuum of stroke care from onset of stroke symptoms to treatment.[85]

Pathophysiology

Stroke occurs when an artery in the brain is either ruptured or clogged by a blood clot, resulting in an interruption or a severe restriction of blood supply used to provide oxygen and nutrients to brain tissue. Two major types of stroke include ischemic and hemorrhagic. Ischemic strokes account for approximately 87% of all strokes and are caused by blockage attributable to a blood clot (thrombus), a wandering clot (embolus), or narrowing of the artery because of atherosclerotic plaque.[7] The major form of ischemic stroke, cerebral thrombosis, is caused when a blood clot forms and blocks blood flow in the cerebral artery. This is generally the result of atherosclerosis in the cerebral vessels. Cerebral embolism occurs when a clot breaks loose from another part of the body, often the heart, and lodges in a cerebral artery.

Transient ischemic attacks (TIAs), or "ministrokes," exhibit symptoms similar to ischemic strokes but are transient in nature, with a thrombus or embolus quickly dislodging, allowing restored blood flow. Typically, a TIA does not result in lasting neurological impairment or deficits. However, TIAs are important in predicting future strokes, as about 10% of ischemic strokes are preceded by a TIA and about 40% of TIAs lead to stroke.[3]

The other type of stroke, hemorrhagic, is caused by intracerebral or subarachnoid hemorrhaging. The rupturing of blood vessels because of head injury or a burst aneurysm can lead to bleeding into brain tissue (intracerebral hemorrhage) or into the space between the brain and the skull (subarachnoid hemorrhage). The severity of hemorrhagic stroke depends on the location and amount of bleeding. Although subarachnoid hemorrhaging is life-threatening, with mortality averaging 40% within the first month of bleeding, those who survive the initial stroke and the following critical period often make remarkable recoveries. Hemorrhagic strokes account for 13% of all strokes.[7]

Descriptive Epidemiology

High-Risk Populations and Health Disparities

Age is a strong risk factor for stroke. After age 55, the rate of stroke incidence doubles in each successive decade. Stroke mortality also increases sharply with age. In 2019, the stroke death rate ranged from 30.5 per 100,000 in those aged 55 to 64 to 977.3 per 100,000 in people aged 85 and older.[1]

In the United States, distinct differences in stroke incidence, prevalence, and mortality rates exist among racial groups. In the Reasons for Geographic and Racial Differences in Stroke (REGARDS) cohort, the results from 25,789 participants with over 222,120 person-years follow-up indicate stroke incidence rates in non-Hispanic Black women and men were 2.92 and 4.04, respectively, per 1,000 person-years in those aged 45 to 64 and were 6.7 and 7.11, respectively, per 1,000 person-years in those aged 65 to 74. The corresponding stroke incidence rates were 1.72 and 2.52, respectively, per 1,000 person-years in non-Hispanic White women and men aged 45 to 64 and were 4.39 and 6.15, respectively, per 1,000 person-years in those aged 65 to 74. In those aged 75 and older, non-Hispanic White women and men had higher stroke incidence rates than did non-Hispanic Black women and men.[86] Figure 16-4 shows a long-term decreased trend of stroke death rates for non-Hispanic Black and White men and women from 1999 to 2019, although rates have plateaued over the past decade.[1] However, non-Hispanic Blacks have significantly higher stroke death rates than non-Hispanic Whites. Furthermore, non-Hispanic Black men have higher stroke death rates than women, but the sex differences are much smaller in non-Hispanic Whites.[1]

Results from the Brain Attack Surveillance in Corpus Christi (BASIC) study suggest that Mexican Americans have twofold-higher cumulative incidence for stroke (first ever, recurrent, and TIA) compared with non-Hispanic Whites in younger populations aged 42 to 59 years. The crude three-year cumulative incidence (2000–2002) was 16.8 per

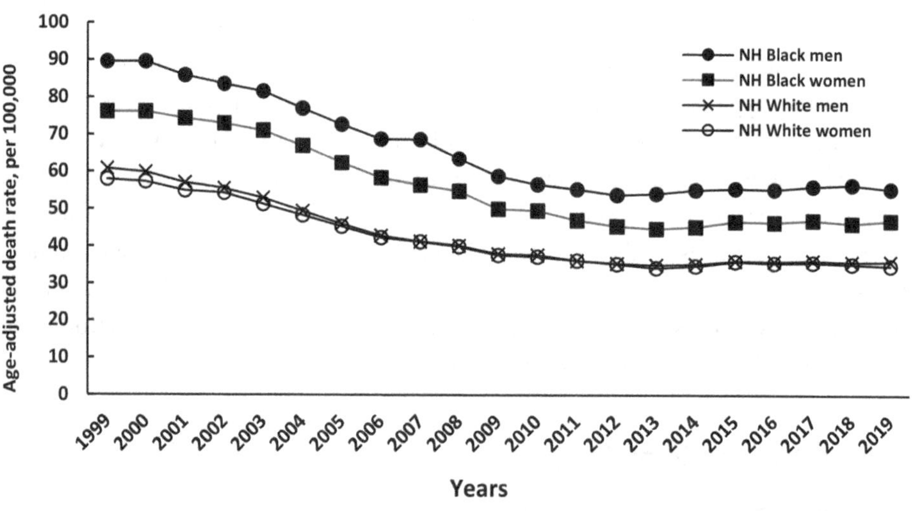

Source: Based on CDC.[1,2]

Note: NH = Non-Hispanic. Age-adjusted rates were estimated using direct standardization method to the age distribution of the 2000 US standard population. Stroke is defined as *ICD-10:* I60-I69.

Figure 16-4. Age-Adjusted Death Rates for Stroke by Sex and Race in the United States, 1999–2019

1,000 in Mexican Americans and 13.6 per 1,000 in non-Hispanic Whites. Specifically, Mexican Americans had a higher cumulative incidence of ischemic stroke at younger ages (45–59 years: rate ratio [RR] 2.04 [95% CI, 1.55–2.69]; 60–74 years: RR 1.58 [95% CI, 1.31–1.91]), but not at older ages (≥75 years: RR 1.12 [95% CI, 0.94–1.32]).[87] Despite the higher incidence rates of stroke for Hispanics compared with non-Hispanic Whites in younger populations, Hispanic stroke survivors tend to live longer, as evidenced by an approximately 15% to 20% decrease in mortality compared with non-Hispanic Whites in 2005.[7,88] However, caution should be taken when interpreting Hispanic mortality rates because of potential reporting inconsistencies on death certificates and surveys.

Risk of stroke is greatly increased among people who have previously had a TIA, sometimes called a ministroke. It is different from the major types of strokes (ischemic stroke and hemorrhagic stroke) because blood flow to the brain is blocked for only a short time, usually no more than five minutes. Approximately one-third to one-half of people who have had one or more TIAs will later have a stroke.[7,22] Risk of TIA increases with age and occurs more often in men. After TIA, the 90-day risk of stroke ranges from 10% to 15%. People who have had TIAs are nearly 10 times more likely to have a stroke than are people of the same age and sex who have not had a TIA. However, only about 15% of all strokes are preceded by TIAs.[7,22]

The risk for stroke is higher for people with a family history of stroke. Positive paternal family history is associated with a doubling of stroke risk, whereas maternal family history increases stroke risk about 40%. The effect of family history appears to be about the same in non-Hispanic Black and non-Hispanic White populations.[89] In the Framingham Heart Study, a documented parental ischemic stroke by the age of 65 years was associated with a threefold increase in ischemic stroke risk in offspring, even after adjustment for other known stroke risk factors. The absolute magnitude of the increased risk was greatest in those in the highest quintile of the Framingham Risk Score. By age 65, people in the highest quintile with an early parental ischemic stroke had a 25% risk of stroke compared with a 7.5% risk of ischemic stroke for those without such a history.[3]

Stroke Belt is a well-known term in the United States. This term was used to describe a group of states clustered in the southeastern part of the country, where 11 states had age-adjusted stroke mortality rates more than 10% or incidence rates more than 18% higher than the national average in early 1980. These states included Alabama, Arkansas, Georgia, Indiana, Kentucky, Louisiana, Mississippi, North Carolina, South Carolina, Tennessee, and Virginia.[90] The burden of stroke death remains a serious public health concern in these states. In 2019 among 50 states and the District of Columbia, Mississippi had the highest age-adjusted stroke mortality (52.1/100,000), followed by Alabama (51.5), Louisiana (42.3), Kentucky (42.5), South Carolina (42.2), Georgia (41.9), Tennessee (41.8), North Carolina (41.5), Indiana (41.4), Arkansas (40.07), and Virginia (38.3). Among these 11 states, the average age-adjusted stroke mortality was 43.5, and for the rest of states it was 34.4 per 100,000 in 2019 (Figure 16-5).[1]

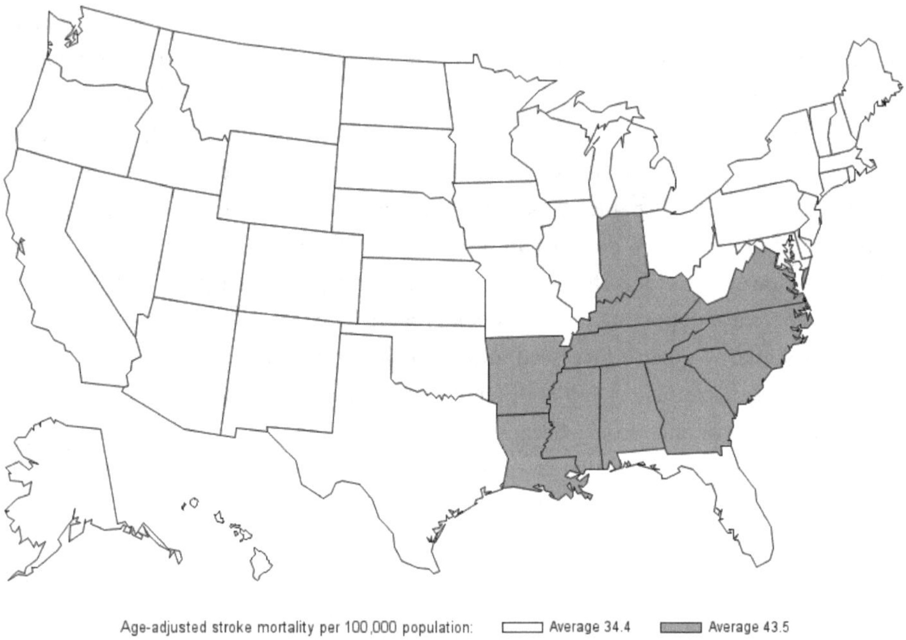

Source: Based on CDC.[1,2]

Note: Data are from CDC WONDER multiple cause-of- death files, 1999-2019 Cooperative Program. Rate is per 100,000 individuals by population.

Figure 16-5. Age-Adjusted Stroke Death Rate by Stroke Belt (Gray) and Non–Stroke Belt (White) States: United States, 2019

Causes

The major modifiable risk factors for stroke include high blood pressure, atrial fibrillation (AF), PAD, cigarette smoking, diabetes, dyslipidemia, obesity, and physical inactivity (Table 16-2), with nutrition, high blood pressure, physical inactivity, diabetes, and AF contributing the highest population-attributable risk percentages in those aged 80 to 89 years.[91–93] As most of the risk factors are also associated with atherosclerotic cerebrovascular disease, treatment, management, and primary and secondary prevention of stroke remain targeted to reduce these factors. Some studies suggest a possible increased risk associated with sleep-disordered breathing and comorbid chronic kidney disease. Other studies show possible increased risk associated with race and genetic factors, including increased risk for stroke in identical twins when one has suffered a stroke.[94]

Modifiable Risk Factors

High blood pressure remains the single most significant modifiable and treatable risk factor for stroke. The risk increases with increasing blood pressure, both systolic and

Table 16-2. Modifiable Risk Factors for Stroke

Relative Magnitude Risk	Risk Factor	Estimated PAR, %
Strong		
4	Hypertension and diabetes	49.5
4	Hypertension (50 y)	40
4	Atrial fibrillation (50–59 y)	1.5
Moderate		
2.0	Peripheral arterial disease	3.0
1.8	Cigarette smoking	12-18
1.8-6	Diabetes	5-27
2.0	Dyslipidemia (high total cholesterol)	15
1.75-2.37	Obesity	12-20
2.7	Physical inactivity	30
Possible		
2.15	Obstructive sleep apnea (OSA)	NA
2.0	Vitamin D deficiency	
1.5-2.5	Dyslipidemia (low HDL-cholesterol)	10
1.4	Postmenopausal hormone therapy	7
1.5	Sodium intake >2,300 mg	NA
1.4	Potassium <4,700 mg	NA

Source: Based on Tsao et al.,[4] Sacco et al.,[91] Wang et al.,[92] and Xie et al.[93]

Note: HDL = high-density lipoprotein; NA = not available; PAR = population-attributable risk.

diastolic. In clinical trials, antihypertensive therapy has been associated with reductions in stroke incidence, with an average 41% reduction in stroke risk with systolic blood pressure reductions of 10 mm Hg.[3] Hypertension is particularly prevalent in non-Hispanic Blacks, affecting 41% of men and 44% of women. High blood pressure occurs much earlier in life in non-Hispanic Blacks than Whites, and the higher systolic blood pressure explains about 50% of excess risk of stroke in non-Hispanic Blacks compared with Whites.[95]

Several studies have shown significantly lower rates of recurrent stroke with lower blood pressure levels. Most recently, the blood pressure reduction component of the Secondary Prevention of Small Subcortical Strokes trial showed that targeting a systolic blood pressure less than 130 mm Hg was likely to reduce recurrent stroke by about 20% ($p = .08$) and significantly reduced intracerebral hemorrhagic stroke by two-thirds.[96]

Because of the recognized significant role of high blood pressure in stroke and other major forms of cardiovascular disease, in 2017 the American Heart Association and American Stroke Association (AHA/ASA) issued updated guidelines for the prevention, detection, evaluation, and management of high blood pressure in adults. The 2017 guidelines define blood pressures as four groups: normal (systolic BP/disastolic BP [SBP/DBP] <120/80 mm Hg), elevated (SBP/DBP 120–129/<80 mm Hg), hypertension Stage 1 (SBP/DBP 130–139/80–89 mm Hg), and hypertension Stage 2 (SBP/DBP ≥140/90 mm Hg). The increased risk of CVD among adults with Stage 2 hypertension is well established. An increasing number of individual studies and meta-analyses of observational data have reported a gradient of progressively higher CVD risk going from normal BP to elevated BP and Stage 1 hypertension.[97] Meanwhile, a scientific statement from AHA identified resistant hypertension, defined as above-goal elevated BP of 130/80 mm Hg in patients despite the concurrent use of three anti-hypertensive drug classes, as being significantly associated with great risks of adverse cardiovascular events, including stroke.[22]

Disorders of glucose metabolism are also major risk factors for stroke,[3] with uncontrolled diabetes leading to arterial damage and increased risk for dyslipidemia, atherosclerosis, and hypertension—all of which confer high risk for stroke. These disorders are highly prevalent in patients with stroke: 28% have prediabetes, and 25% to 45% have diabetes. In addition, diabetes is independently associated with a 60% risk (HR 1.59; 95% CI, 1.07–2.37) for recurrent stroke in the elderly.[95]

Data from the US National Hospital Discharge Surveys revealed that the prevalence rates of hospitalization as a result of stroke stay for men were 23%, 30%, and 27% in the years of 1980 to 1989, 1990 to 1999, and 2000 to 2010, respectively, and were 17.3%, 22%, and 19.34%, respectively, in women. It should be noted that there is a significantly increased trend of stroke hospitalization in younger adults, those aged 18 to 54 years. In addition, there were significantly increased trends of stroke patients with multimorbidity of hypertension, diabetes, arrhythmias, and hyperlipidemia from 1980 to 2010.[98] The rise in the comorbid diseases was more pronounced in individuals who were relatively younger, Black or "other" race, on Medicaid, or admitted to hospitals located in the South. Factors independently associated with higher odds of diabetes in acute ischemic stroke patients were Black or "other" (vs. White) race, congestive heart failure, peripheral vascular disease, and history of myocardial infarction, renal disease, or hypertension.[99]

Atrial fibrillation (AF), defined as a supraventricular tachyarrhythmia with uncoordinated atrial activation and consequently ineffective atrial contraction, is one of the major cardiac rhythm disturbances, responsible for a high rate of cardiovascular and cerebrovascular morbidity and mortality and resulting in a high health care costs and public health burden. In the United States, AF currently affects about three to five million individuals and is expected to affect greater than eight million people by 2050. AF is a well-known risk factor for ischemic stroke, causing a fivefold increased risk of stroke.[3,59] Data from the L'Aquila Stroke Registry (1994–1998) reported a prevalence of AF in patients with ischemic stroke of about 24.6%.[100,101] In addition, the risk of stroke attributable to AF increases with age, from 1.5% in those aged 50 to 59 years to 23.5% in those aged 80 to 89 years.[7] Because AF is often asymptomatic and likely frequently undetected clinically, the stroke risk attributed to AF may be substantially underestimated.

A U-shaped association between body weight and risk of stroke mortality has been observed by several studies. Potential mechanisms include nutritional reserve aiding survival recovery and greater frequency of atherosclerotic than thromboembolic infarcts in individuals with higher body mass index.[102] Several studies have also shown an association between cigarette smoking and an increased risk of stroke. The Framingham Heart Study in 1988 assessed cigarette smoking as a risk factor for stroke and found that the risk increase is dose-dependent. Cigarette smoking has also been shown to be strongly associated with carotid stenosis. Current smokers have a two-to-four-times increased risk of stroke compared with nonsmokers or those who have quit for greater than 10 years.[3] Smoking cessation, but not necessarily reduction, resulted in decreased risk and incidence of strokes and sustained ex-smokers' risk for stroke was not significantly different from never-smokers' risk.[103] In addition, environmental exposure to secondhand smoke has been identified as a risk factor for stroke, increasing risk by as much as 30% among nonsmokers.[95]

Physical activity level is inversely proportional to stroke risk. The Global Burden of Disease 2019 study demonstrated that the burden of stroke attributable to physical inactivity was around 1.68% globally and 2.75% in high-income countries.[20,22] Several other studies, including the Physicians' Health Study,[104] the EPIC-Norfolk study,[105] the Nurses' Health Study,[106] the Northern Manhattan Stroke Study,[91] and the national REGARDS,[107] support this relationship. For example, results from REGARDS found that participants reporting physical activity fewer than four times per week had a 20% increased risk of incident stroke over a mean of 5.7 years compared with those exercising four or more times per week. This relationship, which was more pronounced in men than in women, may be explained in large part by the effect of physical activity on reducing traditional risk factors, such as obesity and diabetes.[107]

A number of studies have demonstrated that a certain diet pattern or nutrients are associated with risk reduction for stroke.[3,108] In a randomized clinical trial conducted in Spain, adherence to a Mediterranean-style diet that was higher in nuts and olive oil was associated with a reduced risk of stroke (HR 0.54; 95% CI, 0.35–0.84). The protective benefit of the Mediterranean diet observed was greater for strokes than for myocardial infarction, but stroke subtype was not available.[109] In the Nurses Health and Health Professionals Follow-up Studies, each one-serving increase in sugar-sweetened soda was associated with a 13% increased risk of ischemic stroke, but not hemorrhagic stroke. Each one-serving increase in low-calorie or diet soda was associated with a 7% increased risk of ischemic stroke and 27% increased risk of hemorrhagic stroke.[110] In the recent decade vitamin D deficiency was observed to predict risk of stroke.[111] Data from the National Health and Nutrition Examination Survey suggests that serum 25(OH)D (a marker of vitamin D intake) less than 30 nmol/L was associated with 2 times higher risk of prevalent stroke (OR 2.0; 95% CI, 1.14–3.48) than those with normal serum 25(OH)D (50–125 nmol/L).[92]

A significant association between elevated serum cholesterol concentration and risk of ischemic stroke has been reported in several studies,[112] but not others.[113,114] In an analysis by the Emerging Risk Factors Collaboration of individual records on 302,430 people without initial vascular disease from 68 long-term prospective studies, hazard ratio (i.e., relative risk) for ischemic stroke was 1.12 (95% CI, 1.04–1.20) with non-HDL cholesterol.[61]

Sleep-disordered breathing is associated with stroke risk. In a 2017 meta-analysis including 16 cohort studies (N = 24,308 individuals), severe obstructive sleep apnea (OSA) was associated with a doubling in stroke risk (RR 2.15; 95% CI, 1.42–3.24).[22,93] OSA may be particularly associated with stroke occurring at the time of waking up. In a meta-analysis of five studies (N = 591 patients), patients with wake-up stroke had more episodes of low oxygen levels while sleeping than those with non-wake-up stroke, and there was an increased incidence of severe OSA in those with wake-up stroke (OR 3.18; 95% CI, 1.27–7.93).[4,115]

Depression is also a potential risk factor for stroke. In the population-based REGARDS cohort study, participants with depressive symptoms had significantly increased stroke risk compared with participants without depressive symptoms, and with no different effect by race.[4,22]

Population-Attributable Risk

As shown in Table 16-2, an estimated 40% (varies by age group) of stroke deaths are attributed to elevated blood pressure and when comorbid with diabetes represent the greatest population-attributable risk percentage (49.5%). Smoking population-attributable risk varies from 12% to 18%, with risk differences varied by age and sex.[116] It is important to note that modifiable risk factors often interact or are accompanied by nonmodifiable risk factors (e.g., age, sex, genetic factors). When individuals have nonmodifiable factors that put them at greater stroke risk, they benefit from targeted prevention screenings and treatment of modifiable risk factors. Although the population-attributable risk for diabetes, ranging from 5% to 27%, is less than that observed for hypertension, the increasing prevalence and incidence of diabetes suggests the rise of future comorbid cases. Effective lifestyle modifications and interventions will be necessary to combat the growing obesity epidemic and the associated sedentary lifestyle (12%–20% and 30% population-attributable risk, respectively).[117]

Evidence-Based Interventions

Prevention

As described earlier, a number of primary risk factors are associated with first and recurrent stroke. Risk assessment tools, such as the Framingham Stroke Profile, can be used to identify and classify individuals on the basis of risk score (Table 16-3). In 2014 the

Table 16-3. Modified Framingham Stroke Risk Profile

Characteristic	Points										
	0	+1	+2	+3	+4	+5	+6	+7	+8	+9	+10
Men											
Age, y	54-56	57-59	60-62	63-65	66-68	69-72	73-75	76-78	79-81	82-84	85
Untreated systolic blood pressure (mm Hg)	97-105	106-115	116-125	126-135	136-145	146-155	156-165	166-175	176-185	186-195	196-205
Treated systolic blood pressure (mm Hg)	97-105	106-112	113-117	118-123	124-129	130-135	136-142	143-150	151-161	162-176	177-205
History of diabetes	No		Yes								
Cigarette smoking	No			Yes							
Cardiovascular disease	No				Yes						
Atrial fibrillation	No				Yes						
Left ventricular hypertrophy on electrocardiogram	No					Yes					
Women											
Age, y	54-56	57-59	60-62	63-64	65-67	68-70	71-73	74-76	77-78	79-81	82-84
Untreated systolic blood pressure (mm Hg)		95-106	107-118	119-130	131-143	144-155	156-167	168-180	181-192	193-204	205-216
Treated systolic blood pressure (mm Hg)		95-106	107-113	114-119	120-125	126-131	132-139	140-148	149-160	161-204	205-216
History of diabetes	No			Yes							
Cigarette smoking	No			Yes							
Cardiovascular disease	No		Yes								
Atrial fibrillation	No						Yes				
Left ventricular hypertrophy on electrocardiogram	No				Yes						

Source: Based on Sacco et al.[91]

AHA/ASA updated guidelines for the primary prevention of stroke to provide comprehensive and timely evidence-based recommendations on the prevention of stroke among individuals who have not previously experienced a stroke or transient ischemic attack. These include evidence-based recommendations to control risk factors, interventional approaches to atherosclerotic disease of the head and neck circulation, and antithrombotic treatments for preventing thrombotic and thromboembolic stroke. Further recommendations are provided for genetic and pharmacogenetic testing and for the prevention of stroke in a variety of other specific circumstances, including sickle cell disease and patent foramen ovale.[118] These prevention strategies are intended to help reach the Healthy People 2030 goal of reducing stroke deaths from 37.1 per 100,000 population in 2019 to 33.4 per 100,000 population in 2030.[119] This new concept of cardiovascular health, characterized by seven metrics (LS7), including health behaviors (diet quality, physical activity, smoking, BMI) and health factors (blood cholesterol, blood pressure, blood glucose), is expected to play a pivotal role in stroke intervention at the population and community levels.[3,120,121] Meanwhile, three major components of a stroke system of care—pre-event, event, and post-event—have been addressed by the US Centers for Disease Control and Prevention's State Heart Disease and Stroke Prevention programs. These programs highlight comprehensive stroke care ranging from primordial prevention to tertiary prevention (Figure 16-6).[122,123]

Since 2008 the National Heart Disease and Stroke Prevention Program has provided funding to 42 State Heart Disease and Stroke Prevention programs. The majority of resources and effort of these programs should be used to address the "ABCS" of heart disease and stroke prevention—aspirin, blood pressure, cholesterol, and smoking—with the main focus on preventing and controlling high blood pressure and reducing sodium intake. These efforts to address the ABCS include the following strategies:

1. **A**spirin: Increase low dose aspirin therapy according to recognized prevention guidelines.
2. **B**lood pressure: Prevent and control high blood pressure; reduce sodium intake.

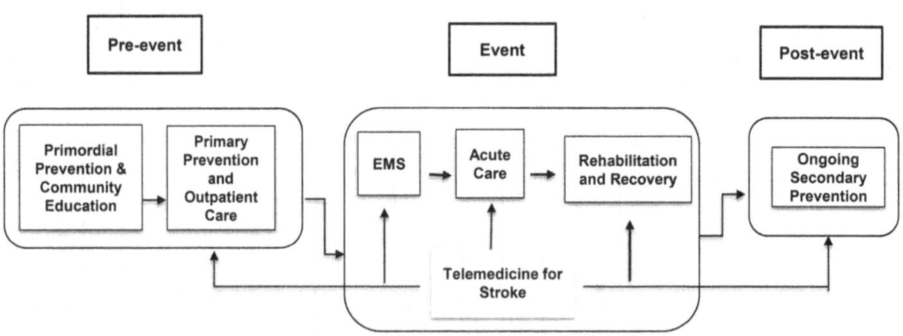

Source: Reprinted from CDC.[122]
Note: EMS = emergency medical services.

Figure 16-6. The Components of a Stroke System of Care

3. **Cholesterol:** Prevent and control high blood cholesterol.
4. **Smoking:** Increase the number of smokers counseled to quit and referred to state quitlines; increase availability of no or low-cost cessation products.[124,125]

On the secondary and tertiary preventions of stroke, states work with EMS agencies to improve care for suspected cases of stroke, the transition from EMS to hospital care, and the transition from the hospital to the next care setting (e.g., long-term care facility, rehabilitation center, primary care provider). Figure 16-6 depicts the components of a stroke system of care.[122]

Screening

Hypertension is a prevalent condition that affects approximately 45% of the adult US population and is a major contributing risk factor for stroke and other forms of CVD. Screening for high blood pressure and controlling Stage 1 (SBP/DBP 130–139/80–89 mm Hg) and Stage 2 hypertension (SBP/DBP ≥140/90 mm Hg) may play a critical role in risk reduction of incident stroke.[126]

Survivors of stroke or TIA are at increased risk for another stroke. All survivors should be routinely monitored for hypertension. In addition to routine monitoring, antihypertensive treatment is recommended for prevention of recurrent stroke and other vascular events.[100] The National Institutes of Health (NIH) developed a scale known as the NIH Stroke Scale (NIHSS) to help diagnose stroke on the basis of the person's level of consciousness, eye muscle and visual impairments, facial muscle deficits, extremity muscle deficits, sensory deficits, and language and speech deficits. There are 11 criteria resulting in a total possible score ranging from 0 to 42. The NIHSS is one of the most widely used and validated scales. Adams et al. found the baseline NIHSS score strongly predicted ischemic stroke outcome at seven days and three months.[127] Previously, Goldstein et al. confirmed the reliability of the NIHSS score for both non-neurologists and neurologists.[128]

Screening for AF (a powerful predictor for stroke) also plays a pivotal role in identifying patients at subclinical stages. The prevalence of AF is expected to rise to nearly 12 million people in the United States by 2030 and to 17.9 million people in the European Union by 2026. Since AF is often asymptomatic, many individuals with AF may be unaware of their condition and do not receive treatment that could prevent a stroke.[129] Studies have shown that use of outpatient telemetry for 21 to 30 days to screen for AF in patients with cryptogenic stroke or TIA has resulted in an AF detection rate of 12% to 23%.[3]

Treatment

Long-term effects of stroke can be devastating; therefore, initial assessment and proper management are crucial to minimizing complications and preventing recurrence. Some common medical complications of stroke include heart attack, heart failure, difficulty swallowing, aspiration pneumonia, deep vein thrombosis or pulmonary embolism, and residual paralysis. Regardless of whether an individual has a history of hypertension, it is important to acknowledge the severity of complications, as approximately half of deaths after strokes are attributable to medical complications.

For survivors with diabetes, particular attention is placed in controlling blood pressure, lipids, glucose, and hemoglobin A1c (>7%). Stroke survivors with comorbid coronary artery disease or elevated cholesterol levels are similarly monitored to ensure proper lipid management following lifestyle modifications, dietary guidelines, and treatment recommendations. Statin agents, in particular, are recommended in lowering cholesterol to reduce the risk of vascular events. Further research is needed to determine the efficacy of lipid management in preventing recurrent stroke or TIA events.

The landmark trial of thrombolytic therapy tissue plasminogen activator (t-PA) conducted by the National Institute of Neurological Disorders and Stroke Recombinant t-PA Stroke Study Group found that sufferers of ischemic stroke treated with t-PA within three hours after the onset of symptoms were at least 30% more likely than patients given placebo to have minimal or no disability at three months and one year. Current guidelines for the management of patients with acute ischemic stroke published by the AHA Stroke Council include specific recommendations for the administration of intravenous recombinant tissue plasminogen activator (rtPA). Despite its effectiveness in improving neurological outcomes, the majority of patients with ischemic stroke are not treated with rtPA, largely because they arrive after the currently approved three-hour time limit for administration of the medication. One of the potential approaches for an increased treatment opportunity has been the designation of a longer time window for treatment. A recent prospective study, the European Cooperative Acute Stroke Study-3, has provided new data on rtPA treatment in the 3- to 4.5-hour window.[130]

Long-term goals include minimizing the physical manifestations of neurological deficits through physical therapy, speech and swallowing therapy, and occupational therapy, in addition to minimizing the risk of recurrence of stroke, including antiplatelet or anticoagulation therapy as necessary, and encouraging strict control or modification of risk factors such as diabetes, dyslipidemia, hypertension, arrhythmias, and smoking cessation. As mentioned, equally important to the individual's recovery and long-term prognosis is addressing and preventing common medical complications.

Moving Forward

Despite decreasing stroke incidence during the second half of the 20th century, stroke continues to be a major cause of death and disability worldwide. There has been increasing recognition that early risk-factor detection and lifestyle modification can prevent or reduce stroke disease burden. Future research to detect surrogate and other potentially modifiable risk factors, including elevated cholesterol, BMI, and specific dietary patterns, is being defined. Further refinement is needed to promote specific interventions to high-risk populations (using risk assessment and other diagnostic tools). Guidelines are needed to tailor interventions to a variety of subpopulations. Creative methods to encourage lifestyle interventions such as diet and occupational and leisure physical activity, along with appropriate treatment to reduce first or recurrent stroke and TIA, is desired to combat the multifactorial nature of the disease. National initiatives partnered with community-based research will provide individual and population-level support to ensure that patients are properly screened, treated, and monitored for primary risk factors. As the world's population ages, development of effective methods of primary and secondary prevention of stroke will be crucial to reduce long-term disability and disease burden.

Since the pandemic of SARS-CoV-2 in early 2020, stroke has risen as a serious health concern for all age groups. History of stroke was observed to be an independent risk factor for severe illness and mortality (mortality OR 1.28; 95% CI, 1.01–1.63) if infected with SARS-CoV-2.[131] In a study of men, an association was observed between infection with SARS-CoV-2 and nearly twice as high a risk of acute stroke after controlling for age, sex, and ethnicity. This increased risk was most remarkable among the younger population (< 50 years).[132] After infection with SARS-CoV-2, an excess burden of stroke of 4.03 (95% CI, 3.32–4.79) per 1,000 persons at 12 months has been observed.[79] The biological mechanism for this increased risk of stroke is still being researched; however, studies have shown that SARS-CoV-2 can result in an increase in blood clots, which can lead to heart damage and stroke.[133]

Management of stroke appears to have remained consistent to pre-pandemic time. A study involving hospitals using the Get With The Guidelines–Stroke registry found data similar in time to tomography, needle, and endovascular therapy between a selected time period of the SARS-CoV-2 pandemic (February–June 2020) and a similar period prior to the virus's emergence (November 2019–February 2020).[134] However, in a study of the same population it was observed that during the SARS-CoV-2 pandemic, stroke patients with SARS-CoV-2 experienced longer times to tomography (median 55 vs. 35 min, $P < 0.001$), needle (median 58.5 vs. 46 min, $P < 0.001$), and endovascular therapy (median 114 vs. 90 min, $P = 0.002$) compared with stroke patients without SARS-CoV-2 diagnosis.[135] This suggests an increase in delay of stroke treatment during the SARS-CoV-2 pandemic was likely attributable to issues relating to the management of the SARS-CoV-2 infection itself.

HEART FAILURE

Introduction

Heart failure (HF) represents a new epidemic of CVD, affecting about six million Americans aged 20 years and older. The prevalence of HF is projected to increase by 46%

from 2012 to 2030, affecting more than eight million US adults aged 18 years and older. The total percentage of the population with HF is projected to reach 3.0% in 2030.[3,4] In 2019 HF as the underlying cause of death was 49.2% higher than in 2010. In 2019, the overall age-adjusted death rate for HF was 24.0 per 100,000 population in men and 18.7 per 100,000 population in women, with variation across race and ethnic groups. In men the age-adjusted death rate was 29.9 for non-Hispanic Blacks, and 24.1 for non-Hispanic Whites. In women the age-adjusted death rate was 21.7 for non-Hispanic Blacks and 18.9 for non-Hispanic Whites.[1]

In addition to the cost in human suffering, care for patients with heart failure places a large economic strain on the health care system, including the Medicare program. In 2020 the total cost for heart failure was estimated to be $43.6 billion. Of this total, 70% was attributable to direct medical costs.[136] Projections show that by 2030 the total cost of heart failure will increase almost 127% to $69.7 billion from 2012. This equals about $244 for every US adult.[3,137]

Pathophysiology

Heart failure is a multisystem disorder characterized by abnormalities of cardiac function, skeletal muscle, renal function, stimulation of the sympathetic nervous system, and a complex pattern of neuro-hormonal changes that impairs the ability of either ventricle to fill with or eject blood.[138] The cardinal manifestations of heart failure are dyspnea (shortness of breath) and fatigue, which may limit exercise tolerance, and fluid retention, which may lead to pulmonary and peripheral edema. Both abnormalities can impair the functional capacity and quality of life of affected individuals, but they may not necessarily dominate the clinical picture at the same time. Three clinical pathophysiological models (hypotheses) for heart failure have been suggested:

- The cardio-renal model, in which heart failure is viewed as a problem of excessive salt and water retention that is caused by abnormalities of renal blood flow.
- The cardio-circulatory, or hemodynamic, model, in which heart failure is thought to arise largely as a result of abnormalities in the pumping capacity of the heart and excessive peripheral vasoconstriction.
- The neuro-hormonal model, in which heart failure progresses as a result of the over-expression of biologically active molecules that are capable of exerting toxic effects on the heart and circulation.

Once measurements of left ventricular function became available, two main subtypes of heart failure were characterized: heart failure with reduced left ventricular (LV) ejection fraction (HFrEF) and heart failure with preserved ejection fraction (HFpEF), with ejection fraction referring to the portion of the total amount of blood ejected with each contraction. HFrEF is frequently caused by coronary artery disease, myocardial infarction, and hypertension, with male predominance. HFpEF is more common among women, and there is more often a background of hypertension and diabetes. HFrEF has been defined as a left ventricular ejection fraction (LVEF) less than 40% to 50%. The reason is that morbidity and mortality increase with lower LVEF. HFpEF has been defined by an LVEF more than 40% to 50%.[8,139] In the latest version of the European Society of Cardiology guidelines for the treatment of heart failure, a grey zone between the two conditions was introduced: heart failure with mid-range ejection fraction (HFmrEF) (LVEF of 40%–50%).[139]

Descriptive Epidemiology

High-Risk Populations and Health Disparities

Heart failure disproportionately affects the older population. The incidence of heart failure approaches 10 per 1,000 population after age 65 years, and approximately 80% of patients hospitalized with heart failure are older than age 65 years.[4,140,141] People with coronary artery disease, hypertension, and diabetes are at particular risk of developing heart failure. About 7 of 10 people with heart failure had high blood pressure before being diagnosed. About 22% of men and 46% of women will develop heart failure within six years of having a heart attack.[142]

Blacks with heart failure are an average of 10 years younger than Whites, have more hospital admissions and readmissions, and suffer a different spectrum of disease that predisposes them to heart failure. Specifically, Blacks have a higher incidence of hypertension, left ventricular hypertrophy, and diabetes. In MESA, Blacks had the highest risk of developing heart failure, followed by Hispanic, Whites, and Chinese Americans (4.6, 3.5, 2.4, and 1.0 cases/1,000 person-years, respectively).[3,143] Data from the ARIC study of the National Heart, Lung, and Blood Institute showed age-adjusted annual hospitalized heart failure incidence was highest for Black men (15.7/1,000), followed by Black women (13.3/1,000), White men (12.3/1,000), and White women (9.9/1,000). This higher risk reflected differences in the prevalence of hypertension, diabetes, and low SES.[143]

Geographic Distribution

Age-adjusted mortality rates for heart failure among all ages vary substantially across the United States. Data from 50 US states show that there were significant variations in age-adjusted heart failure mortality, ranging from the lowest at 5.7 (Vermont) to the highest at 43.7 (Mississippi) per 100,000 population in 2019. A clear east–west gradient was evident, with the highest rates located primarily along the lower Mississippi River Valley and the Ohio River Valley, including parts of the Appalachian region (Figure 16-7).[1]

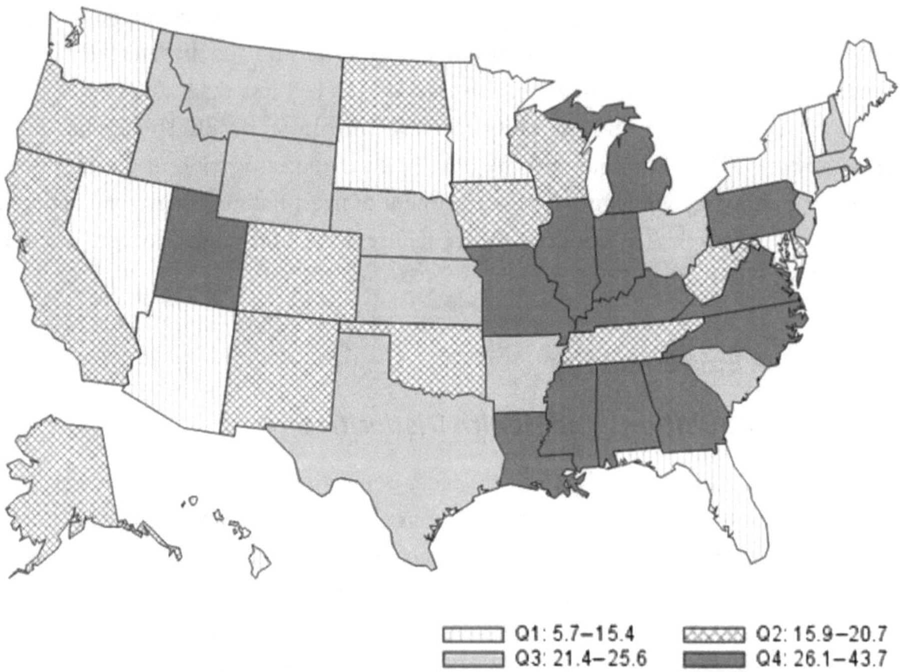

Source: Based on CDC.[1,2]
Note: HF = heart failure. Age-adjusted rates were estimated using direct standardization method to the age distribution of the 2000 US standard population. Heart failure is defined as *ICD-10:* I50.

Figure 16-7. Age-Adjusted Death Rates for HF (per 100,000 Population): United States, 2019

Time Trends

Most current information on the epidemiology of heart failure is derived from several epidemiologic studies in the United States published since 1993.[140,141,144] There have been several consistent findings, including a sharp increase in prevalence with age and strong male preponderance. The prevalence of heart failure has increased in the United States since 1980 in both sexes.[141,144,145]

The aging of the post–World War II baby boom generation is likely to swell the number of patients with heart failure further. Data from the National Hospital Discharge survey between 1980 and 2006 suggested that of three major forms of cardiovascular disease, age-adjusted hospitalization rates in patients aged 65 years and older with primary diagnosis of CHD significantly decreased from the early 1990s, and age-adjusted hospitalization rates in patients aged 65 years and older with a primary diagnosis of stroke significantly decreased from the mid-1980s in both men and women. However, heart failure hospitalization rates have significantly increased, with an estimated annual rate increase of 1.20% in men and 1.55% in women.[141] In contrast to CHD and stroke mortality rates that showed a continued decreased trend over the past decades, an increased trend of HF mortality from 2010 to 2019 was observed in non-Hispanic Whites and non-Hispanic Blacks for both genders (Figure 16-8a).[1] In 2019 non-Hispanic Black men were 24.1% more likely to die from heart failure compared with non-Hispanic Whites, and non-Hispanic Black women were 15% more likely to die than non-Hispanic White women (Figure 16-8b).[1]

Causes

Modifiable Risk Factors

The most common causes of heart failure are coronary artery disease, hypertension, diabetes, heart rhythm disorders (arrhythmias), congenital heart disease, and heart muscle disease (cardiomyopathy). Other risk factors associated with these diseases in general also contribute to heart failure by putting extra stress on the heart, including cardiometabolic syndrome (a clustering of obesity, high blood pressure, increased triglycerides and glucose, and decreased high-density lipoprotein cholesterol), cigarette smoking, alcohol abuse, and a family history of heart failure or other CVDs. Findings from MESA suggest that among a cohort of 6,750 participants within a mean 12-year follow-up, individuals with metabolic syndrome had significantly higher heart failure incidence (6.46/1,000 person-years) than did those without metabolic syndrome (2.73/1,000 person-years).[8]

The odds of developing heart failure are especially high in people who have more than one of these risk factors. For example, a study of the predictors of heart failure among women with CHD found that those with diabetes had the highest risk of developing heart failure. Among diabetic participants with no additional risk factors, the annual incidence of heart failure was 3.0% compared with 8.2% among those with diabetes and at least three additional risk factors. Diabetic persons with fasting glucose greater than 300 mg/dL had a threefold adjusted risk of developing heart failure, compared with diabetic persons with controlled fasting blood sugar levels.[84] Multiple comorbidity in patients with heart failure poses a serious clinical issue. In one study of six selected comorbidities, about 50% of men and 40% of women with heart failure had coexisting CHD, the next common comorbidities being chronic obstructive pulmonary disease, diabetes, renal failure, and pneumonia.[140] Diet-related factors have been suggested as risk factors for heart failure, including low vitamin D and leptin.[146,147]

Population-Attributable Risk

Data from the Framingham Heart Study indicate that myocardial infarction, despite only a 3% to 10% prevalence in the population, accounts for 34% of heart failure in men and 13% in women.[145] Data from a recent pooled cohort of 38,028 participants from six US longitudinal population-based cohorts (ARIC, Coronary Artery Risk Development

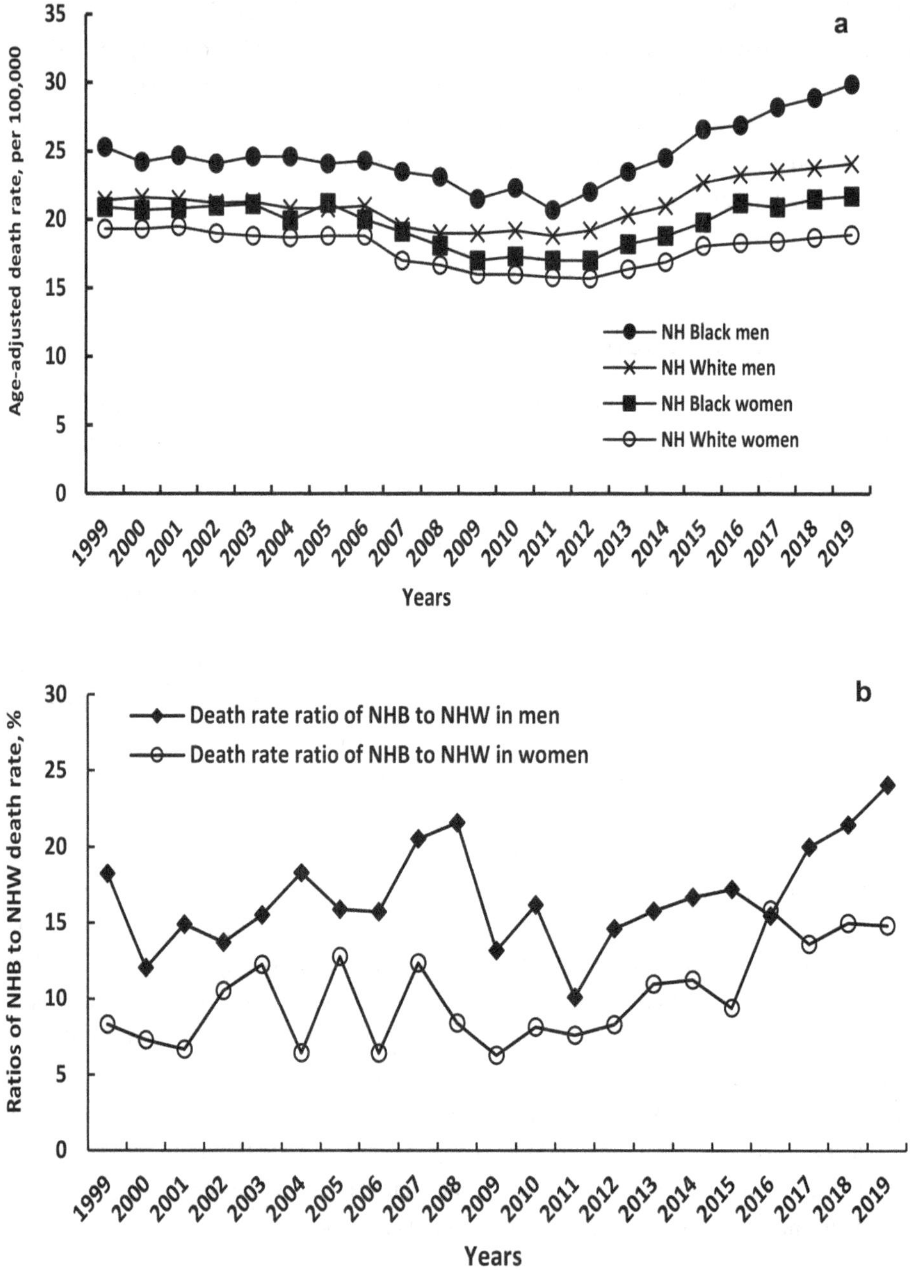

Source: Based on CDC.[1,2]

Note: NH = Non-Hispanic; NHB = Non-Hispanic Black; NHW = Non-Hispanic White. Data are from CDC WONDER multiple cause-of-death files, 1999–2019. Age-adjusted rates were estimated using direct standardization method to the age distribution of the 2000 US standard population. Heart failure is defined as *ICD-10:* I50. Rate is per 100,000 individuals

Figure 16-8. Age-Adjusted Heart Failure Death Rate by (a) Sex and Race, and (b) Death Rate Ratios of Non-Hispanic Black (NHB) to Non-Hispanic White (NHW) in Men and Women: United States, 2019

in Young Adults Study, Cardiovascular Health Study, Framingham Heart Study, Framingham Offspring Study, and MESA) suggest that in non-Hispanic Black men, hypertension has the highest population-attributable fraction (PAF) of 28.3%, followed by obesity (16.2%), diabetes (9.2%), and current smoking (6.8%). However, in non-Hispanic White men, obesity had the highest PAF (21.0%), followed up hypertension (17.3%), diabetes (6.1%), and current smoking (3.8%). In non-Hispanic Black women, the highest PAF was observed with hypertension (25.8%), followed by diabetes (16.4%), obesity (13.15%), and current smoking (6.9%). The corresponding PAF in non-Hispanic White women was obesity (17.9%), followed by hypertension (17.3%), current smoking (6.2%), and diabetes (4.4%), respectively.[148,149]

Evidence-Based Interventions

Early identification of heart failure risk factors and appropriate prevention and treatment will have the greatest impact in reducing progression of the disease. Earlier guidelines for heart failure health care emphasized the functional status and appropriate treatment of patients with heart failure. According to the New York Heart Association Functional Classification, heart failure is classified into four classes that range from patients with asymptomatic left ventricular dysfunction (Class I) to those with severe symptoms at rest or with minimal exertion (Class IV; Table 16-4).[150] This classification helps clinicians assess the severity of a patient's symptoms, guides the choice of therapy, and aids subjective documentation of response or lack of response to therapy.[151]

To emphasize prevention of heart failure, the American College of Cardiology (ACC) and AHA created a new conceptual framework to help health professionals understand the continuum of disease progression in heart failure. Rather than replacing the New York Heart Association classification, the framework defines disease progression in four stages—A, B, C, and D—beginning with patients who have risk factors for developing heart failure all the way to patients with end-stage disease.[152] ACC and AHA addressed

Table 16-4. Heart Failure Classification

Level	Description	Simple Description
I	Cardiac disease without resulting limitations of physical activity.	Asymptomatic
II	Slight limitation of physical activity—comfortable at rest, but ordinary physical activity results in fatigue, dyspnea, or anginal pain.	Symptomatic with moderate exertion
III	Marked limitation in physical activity—comfortable at rest, but less than ordinary physical activity causes fatigue, dyspnea, or anginal pain.	Symptomatic with minimal exertion
IV	Inability to carry on any physical activity without discomfort of symptoms at rest.	Symptomatic at rest

Source: Based on Tsao et al.[4] and Hunt et al.[150]

these four stages in the development of heart failure and recommendations for preventing and treating heart failure by stages.[152,153] In 2017 ACC, AHA, and the Heart Failure Society of America further updated guidelines for the management of heart failure.[151]

Patients in Stage A do not have any diagnosed structural heart disease but do have risk factors that can lead to heart failure. At this stage patient education is key, given that lifestyle modifications that reduce the risk of developing CVD include maintaining an appropriate diet, engaging in regular exercise, maintaining a normal BMI, taking steps to stop smoking, and limiting alcohol consumption.

Like patients in Stage A, those at Stage B are asymptomatic, but they have either structural heart disease or evidence of left ventricular dysfunction. Treatments for Stage B are added to all those mentioned for Stage A in an attempt to prevent the development of overt, symptomatic heart failure. Medications are requested for patients when appropriate.

Patients in Stage C have structural heart disease and current or previous symptoms of heart failure, such as reduced activity tolerance, dyspnea, and fluid retention. Recommended therapies for patients with Stage C are the same as those for patients with Stages A and B. But because these patients are symptomatic, most patients receive medications (such as a diuretic and digoxin, along with angiotensin-converting enzyme inhibitors, angiotensin-receptor blockers, and beta blockers). Other important measures include sodium restriction, administration of the influenza and pneumococcal vaccine, and physical activity, except for patients in an acute decompensated state.

Stage D is reserved for patients with end-stage heart failure. These patients are markedly symptomatic, despite maximal tolerated therapy. In addition to the care outlined for patients in Stages A to C, these patients usually require specialized interventions to control and manage their heart failure, such as mechanical assist devices (biventricular pacemaker or left ventricular assist device).

Because of the clear-cut relationship between preventable difficulties such as coronary heart disease and the tremendous burdens of heart failure medications, comorbidity, and mortality (Stages C and D), a great deal of attention should be focused on preventing the development of ventricular dysfunction in the first place. Clearly, early identification and prevention for patients at risk for heart failure (Stages A and B) are critical to control heart failure.

As an overwhelming majority of heart failure cases are traced to three preventable and treatable conditions—hypertension, coronary heart disease, and diabetes—prevention and treatment of these conditions and risk factors are the focus of efforts to reduce incidence of heart failure. For example, several studies have shown that treating elevated blood pressure can dramatically decrease the risk of developing heart failure. Results from the Swedish Trial in Old Patients with Hypertension indicated that treatment of hypertension reduced the risk of developing heart failure from 4.8% to 2.3%, a 52% relative reduction in those who received active treatment compared with the placebo.[154] A recent meta-analysis suggests that a Mediterranean diet may reduce the risk of incident heart failure, and coenzyme Q10 may reduce the risk of heart failure and all-cause mortality.[155]

Moving Forward

Over the past decade, although there have been many studies on the etiology of heart failure and advances in the care of patients with heart failure, the causes remain poorly understood and the prognosis remains poor. Further research should include the following:

- Continued studies of the mechanisms in the pathophysiology of subtypes of heart failure.
- Studies to identify heart failure risk factors to develop more effective methods of primary prevention, including studies of diet and particular nutrients.
- Continued studies of secondary prevention of heart failure to reduce the mortality of heart failure and to improve quality of life for patients with heart failure.
- Continued studies using multidisciplinary approaches, including pharmacoepidemiology, because patients with heart failure are typically older adults with complex drug regimens for heart failure, multiple concurrent diagnoses, and resulting polypharmacy.
- Community-based studies, along with regional, national, and international cooperative studies, to identify specific prevention and treatment strategies for heart failure among different populations.

In addition, it should be noted that because of the COVID-19 pandemic, SARS-CoV-2 infection has been found to be associated with a 72% increase in risk of heart failure,[79] and infection with SARS-CoV-2 has been observed to increase the immediate risk of heart failure. Even one year after infection, the increased risk of heart failure remains (excess burden 11.61; 95% CI, 10.47–12.78, per 1,000 persons).[79] Inversely, having a history of heart failure appears to increase the risk of severe illness and hospitalization if infected with SARS-CoV-2; in fact, heart failure diagnosis was observed to be the second-largest predictor for SARS-CoV-2 hospitalization (OR 4.43; 95% CI, 2.59–8.04).[156]

The novel SARS-CoV-2 pandemic also affected the management of heart failure. Between January and April 2020, heart failure hospitalizations were observed to decrease by 50% after the first case of SARS-CoV-2. This observation was unique to 2020 and not observed in previous years.[157] A decrease in heart failure hospitalization and delay in admission to urgent care can be seen as a direct consequence of the impact SARS-CoV-2 had on health care access and may have contributed to the increase in heart failure mortality observed during that time.

PERIPHERAL ARTERIAL DISEASE

Introduction

Peripheral arterial disease, or PAD, a disease of blood vessels supplying the arms and legs, causes functional morbidity and increases the risk for other CVD morbidity and mortality. It is associated with intermittent claudication, a classic presentation that involves calf pain and other symptoms.[3,158,159] Approximately 6.5 million (5.8%) US individuals aged 40 and older have PAD.[4] Large numbers of individuals with PAD report different constellations of leg symptoms, and a substantial subgroup (est. 40%) presents without pain.[3] However, when present, the pain of PAD is strongly associated with diminished functional status and quality of life.

Public Health Impact

PAD is a leading cause of lower limb amputation in the United States. Overall, annual Medicare spending for PAD is comparable with annual spending for congestive heart failure and cerebrovascular disease.

The major public health burden of PAD stems from its strong association with CVD mortality—individuals with PAD are more than three times as likely to experience CVD death than like-age non-PAD patients.[160,161] This excess risk of CVD mortality in PAD patients is independent of the effects of other CVD risk factors[162] and represents a very large attributable mortality risk because baseline CVD death rates are high in the older age groups most affected by PAD. The five-year all-cause mortality rate in PAD patients is higher than that among those with either breast cancer or Hodgkin's disease.[163] Finally, in addition to the morbidity associated with lower limb function and the mortality burden, there is a growing body of evidence linking PAD with cognitive decline.[164–166]

Pathophysiology

Peripheral arterial disease is a condition involving atherosclerosis of the arteries in the lower extremities, which is common in older populations. Its pathophysiology is not unique from that of other atherosclerosis-related CVDs. The presence of PAD is, therefore, a strong indication that there are also atherosclerotic manifestations in other vascular territories, particularly the heart or the brain.

In epidemiologic studies, PAD is typically confirmed with the ankle-brachial index (ABI)—a ratio of Doppler-recorded systolic blood pressure in the upper compared with the lower extremities. An ABI below 0.90 is the conventional cut point for PAD case confirmation. Confirmed coronary atherosclerosis is found in very large proportions of patients diagnosed with PAD and also in patients with borderline ABI values. Peripheral arterial disease appears to be more frequently associated with disease at multiple vascular territories than either coronary artery disease or cerebrovascular disease; moreover, the coronary atherosclerosis present in patients with concomitant PAD tends to be more severe than that found in patients with coronary disease alone.[167]

Descriptive Epidemiology

Among individuals aged 40 and older, the annual incidence of PAD and chronic limb-threatening ischemia was 2.69% and 0.35%, respectively, estimated based on nationwide claim data from large employers' health plans and from Medicare and Medicaid programs between 2003 and 2008. Prevalence of ABI-defined PAD in individuals aged 40 or older was estimated between 5.8% and 10.7%.[4] PAD prevalence increases with age, approximately doubling per decade. The prevalence estimates for the US population aged 65 or older range from 12% to 20%. Strong sex differences in PAD prevalence have not been consistently documented. However, data from the Chronic Renal Insufficiency Cohort showed that female chronic kidney disease patients had a higher PAD risk compared with male chronic kidney disease patients at younger ages.[159,168]

Peripheral arterial disease prevalence in Blacks aged 50 or older is at least twofold higher than in non-Hispanic Whites.[169] Prevalence in Hispanic Americans is similar to, or perhaps modestly higher, than that for non-Hispanic Whites.[169,170] Globally, PAD disproportionately affects low- or middle-income countries. It is estimated that 110 million people were living with PAD in 2020, with the highest mortality in Central and Eastern Europe.[4]

Causes

In addition to age and the high-risk groups noted in the previous paragraphs, the constellation of risk factors for PAD is similar to that for other CVDs, including smoking, obesity, unhealthy diet, physical inactivity, elevated glucose, elevated total cholesterol, and hypertension (i.e., LS7 factors). Findings from MESA and ARIC indicate that healthier LS7 scores are associated with a substantially lower risk of PAD.[171,172] Current or former smoking is among the strongest PAD risk factors, with odds ratios (ORs) ranging from 1.3 to 5.4 compared with odds for never-smokers. Diabetes and hypertension are significantly associated with increased risk for PAD, with ORs ranging from 1.38 to 1.84 in individuals with diabetes, and from 1.35 to 1.57 in those with hypertension (SBP/DBP ≥ 140/90 mm Hg).[4] Patients with renal insufficiency also appear to have higher PAD prevalence than do those with normal kidney function, varying from 12% to 38% among people with chronic kidney disease and those receiving dialysis.[173]

A cross-sectional study of patients with PAD in France suggested that isolated systolic hypertension occurred more commonly among patients with PAD than coronary artery disease or CVD—a finding worthy of follow-up in epidemiologic studies.[174] Findings from a recent meta-analysis of 22 studies from high-income countries and 12 from low- or middle-income countries suggest that smoking had the strongest effect on PAD, with meta-odds ratio for current smoking of 2.72 (95% CI, 2.39–3.09) in high-income countries and 1.42 (95% CI, 1.25–1.62) in low- or middle-income countries, followed by diabetes (1.88; 95% CI, 1.66–2.14 vs. 1.47; 95% CI, 1.29–1.68), hypertension (1.55; 95% CI, 1.42–1.71 vs. 1.36; 95% CI, 1.24–1.50), and hypercholesterolemia (1.19; 95% CI, 1.07–1.33 vs. 1.14; 95% CI, 1.03–1.25).[165]

Two less traditional PAD risk factors worth considering as research moves forward are inflammatory biomarkers and genetics. Prospective studies of large cohorts have suggested that CRP, interleukin 6 (IL-6), tumor necrosis factor-alpha (TNF-α), and certain other circulating markers of inflammation are significant predictors of symptomatic PAD incidence.[162,175] In large cross-sectional studies, CRP levels were significantly different in those with and without prevalent PAD.[176] Inflammatory biomarkers also have been significantly associated with all-cause mortality risk through two years of follow-up in a small cohort of PAD patients.[177] While not directly modifiable risk factors, CRP and other inflammatory factors may ultimately prove useful as component biomarkers in the assessment of subclinical PAD, PAD severity, or treatment responsiveness.

As with other CVDs, genetic susceptibility likely plays a role in PAD etiology, but the mechanisms are complex, involving multiple genes and gene–environment interactions. The limited number of family studies of PAD completed to date do support a role for heritable genetics in PAD etiology—it is estimated that heritability of PAD ranges from 20% to 45%—but candidate gene studies have not yielded putative PAD-risk genes.[162] Data from six US community-based cohorts show that non-Hispanic Blacks had the highest lifetime risk of PAD (30%), followed by Hispanics (22%) and non-Hispanic Whites (~19%).[4]

Evidence-Based Interventions

Strategies for primary prevention of PAD do not differ from those for any atherosclerotic chronic disease and will not be discussed here in detail. With respect to treatment, the foundational intervention for the management of symptomatic PAD is exercise. Exercise is hypothesized to improve PAD symptoms via adaptive responses of the muscle or increasing collateral blood flow in the affected limbs.[178] Higher levels of physical activity have been associated with increased survival among PAD patients.[179] Smoking cessation is also advised for the improvement of leg pain symptoms of PAD.[180]

More recently, options for pharmacological therapy of symptomatic PAD have become available, including statins, clopidogrel, and cilostazol.[166]

By far, the single biggest issue related to PAD prevention and control, from a public health perspective, is secondary prevention. Given the high risk of mortality from CVD-related events among patients with PAD, individuals diagnosed with PAD are obvious candidates for interventions designed to reduce CHD and stroke risks. The pursuit of appropriate atherothrombotic risk factor reduction is a cornerstone of PAD treatment guidelines. Smoking cessation, blood pressure control, and cholesterol lowering have been linked with decreased CVD mortality, and blood glucose control and weight loss have been connected with other benefits. Antiplatelet therapy, including aspirin, has been demonstrated in multiple studies to prevent progression of atherosclerosis in patients with PAD, and in some studies to prevent CVD mortality.

Peripheral arterial disease researchers have advocated the use of more formal clinical staging approaches for PAD patients to guide intensity of intervention. However, at the same time studies have shown that physician awareness of the strong link between PAD and future cardiovascular events is low.[181] Also well documented is that PAD patients are less likely to receive CVD risk reduction pharmacotherapy than patients with atherosclerotic disease in other vascular beds.[182] This suggests that patients diagnosed with PAD are not receiving potentially effective interventions as often as indicated.

The REACH Registry, an international, prospective, observational registry of more than 68,000 patients with coronary artery disease, cerebrovascular disease, or PAD, reported that PAD patients had significantly fewer CVD risk factors under control than did the patients in either of the other two diagnostic groups.[183] Moreover, as mentioned earlier, a large proportion of PAD is currently undiagnosed, implying a pressing need to improve disease detection. The ABI measure, though inexpensive and noninvasive, has unfortunately not been found sufficiently sensitive to be used as a population-based screening tool, and secondary prevention in asymptomatic PAD patients is largely still a function of direct recognition of adverse CVD risk-factor profiles. As a consequence, vigilant monitoring of classic CVD risk factors and prompt intervention remain the most promising path for secondary prevention of PAD moving forward.[165]

In instances in which limb pain is severely disabling or the limb is threatened because of ulceration or gangrene, endovascular surgical procedures, such as angioplasty, with and without stents, and arterial bypass surgery are recommended; however, it has been argued that the evidence supporting efficacy of such procedures for PAD is much weaker than that for coronary artery disease.[184] Despite this, endovascular procedures for PAD are one of the fastest-growing surgical procedures in the United States.[159]

It should be also noted that in patients with PAD, infection with SARS-CoV-2 has been found to result in a higher risk of complications from PAD, such as peripheral gangrene. PAD has also been observed to be an independent risk factor for mortality and major cardiac adverse events (MACE) among patients with SARS-CoV-2 infection (mortality OR 1.45; 95% CI, 1.11–1.88; MACE OR 1.48; 95% CI, 1.16–1.87).[185]

As with other chronic diseases, the management of PAD has been affected by the SARS-CoV-2 pandemic. One study noted patients presenting with PAD during the SARS-CoV-2 pandemic were more likely to have advanced or acute PAD than chronic PAD. It is suggested this could be the result of decreased health care access for nonessential services as well as patient reluctance to seek medical care during the early period of the SARS-CoV-2 pandemic.[186]

DISCUSSION QUESTIONS

1. Although cardiovascular disease mortality has declined significantly in the past decades, why do cardiovascular diseases remain a serious public health concern in the United States?
2. What do you think are underlying reasons for any significant health disparities in the burden of cardiovascular disease by sex, by race/ethnicity, and across the US states?
3. What are main modifiable risk factors for cardiovascular disease and how can they be best addressed?
4. What are the potential factors that could explain the increased trend of heart failure mortality in the most recent decade?
5. What are the main strategies to control cardiovascular disease and how are these implemented in states and local jurisdictions?
6. What are the impacts of the SARS-CoV-2 pandemic on patients with cardiovascular disease? How might the pandemic affect future cardiovascular disease prevention and control?

REFERENCES

1. Centers for Disease Control and Prevention, National Center for Health Statistics. CDC WONDER mortality data. 2021. Updated January 11, 2023. Available at: https://wonder.cdc.gov. Accessed January 21, 2023.
2. Centers for Disease Control and Prevention, National Center for Health Statistics. Health, United States, 2019. 2021. Available at: https://www.cdc.gov/nchs/data/hus/hus19-508.pdf. Accessed January 21, 2023.
3. Mozaffarian D, Benjamin EJ, Go AS, et al. Executive summary: heart disease and stroke statistics—2016 update: a report from the American Heart Association. *Circulation.* 2016;133:447–454. doi:10.1161/CIR.0000000000000366
4. Tsao CW, Aday AW, Almarzooq ZI, et al. Heart disease and stroke statistics—2022 update: a report from the American Heart Association. *Circulation.* 2022;145(8):e153–e639. doi:10.1161/CIR.0000000000001052
5. Roser M, Ortiz-Ospina E. Age-adjusted death rate from cardiovascular disease, 2019. Available at: https://ourworldindata.org/grapher/cardiovascular-disease-death-rates. 2022. Accessed January 21, 2023.
6. World Health Organization. Cardiovascular diseases. June 11, 2021. Available at: https://www.who.int/en/news-room/fact-sheets/detail/cardiovascular-diseases-(cvds). Accessed January 21, 2023.

7. Lloyd-Jones D, Adams R, Carnethon M, et al. Heart disease and stroke statistics—2009 update: a report from the American Heart Association Statistics Committee and Stroke Statistics Subcommittee. *Circulation.* 2009;119(3):480–486. doi:10.1161/CIRCULATIONAHA.108.191259
8. Liu L, Lima JA, Post WS, Szklo M. Associations of time-varying obesity and metabolic syndrome with risk of incident heart failure and its subtypes: findings from the Multi-Ethnic Study of Atherosclerosis. *Int J Cardiol.* 2021;338:127–135.
9. Virani SS, Alonso A, Aparicio HJ, et al. Heart disease and stroke statistics—2021 update: a report from the American Heart Association. *Circulation.* 2021;143:e254–e743. doi:10.1161/CIR.0000000000000950
10. American Heart Association. Heart disease likely to remain #1 killer in US indefinitely due to long-term COVID-19 impact. July 21, 2021. Available at: https://newsroom.heart.org/news/heart-disease-likely-to-remain. Accessed January 21, 2023.
11. Ahmad FB, Anderson RN. The leading causes of death in the US for 2020. *JAMA.* 2021;325:1829–1830.
12. Kytömaa S, Hegde S, Claggett B, et al. Association of influenza-like illness activity with hospitalizations for heart failure: the Atherosclerosis Risk in Communities Study. *JAMA Cardiol.* 2019;4:363–369.
13. Ogilvie RP, Lutsey PL, Heiss G, Folsom AR, Steffen LM. Dietary intake and peripheral arterial disease incidence in middle-aged adults: the Atherosclerosis Risk in Communities (ARIC) Study. *Am J Clin Nutr.* 2017;105:651–659.
14. Maas AHEM, Appelman YEA. Gender differences in coronary heart disease. *Neth Heart J.* 2010;18:598–602.
15. Prabakaran S, Schwartz A, Lundberg G. Cardiovascular risk in menopausal women and our evolving understanding of menopausal hormone therapy: risks, benefits, and current guidelines for use. *Ther Adv Endocrinol Metab.* 2021;12:20420188211013917. doi:10.1177/20420188211013917
16. Schultz WM, Kelli HM, Lisko JC, et al. Socioeconomic status and cardiovascular outcomes: challenges and interventions. *Circulation.* 2018;137:2166–2178.
17. Davari M, Maracy MR, Khorasani E. Socioeconomic status, cardiac risk factors, and cardiovascular disease: a novel approach to determination of this association. *ARYA Atheroscler.* 2019;15(6):260. doi:10.22122/arya.v15i6.1595
18. Barber S, Hickson DA, Wang X, Sims M, Nelson C, Diez-Roux AV. Neighborhood disadvantage, poor social conditions, and cardiovascular disease incidence among African American adults in the Jackson Heart Study. *Am J Public Health.* 2016a;106:2219–2226.
19. Finegold JA, Asaria P, Francis DP. Mortality from ischaemic heart disease by country, region, and age: statistics from World Health Organisation and United Nations. *Int J Cardiol.* 2013;168(2):934–945. doi:10.1016/j.ijcard.2012.10.046
20. Vos T, Lim SS, Abbafati C, et al. Global burden of 369 diseases and injuries in 204 countries and territories, 1990–2019: a systematic analysis for the Global Burden of Disease Study 2019. *Lancet.* 2020;396:1204–1222.
21. Vaughan AS, Schieb L, Casper M. Historic and recent trends in county-level coronary heart disease death rates by race, gender, and age group, United States, 1979–2017. *PLoS One.* 2020;15:e0235839.

22. Ford CD, Gray MS, Crowther MR, et al. Depressive symptoms and risk of stroke in a national cohort of Black and White participants from REGARDS. *Neurol Clin Pract* 2021;11(4): e454–e461. doi:10.1212/CPJ.0000000000000983
23. Satoh M, Ohkubo T, Asayama K, et al. Lifetime risk of stroke and coronary heart disease deaths according to blood pressure level: EPOCH-JAPAN (Evidence for Cardiovascular Prevention From Observational Cohorts in Japan). *Hypertension*. 2019;73:52–59.
24. Thomopoulos C, Parati G, Zanchetti A. Effects of blood pressure-lowering treatment on cardiovascular outcomes and mortality: 14–effects of different classes of antihypertensive drugs in older and younger patients: overview and meta-analysis. *J Hypertens*. 2018;36:1637–1647.
25. Oshunbade AA, Kassahun-Yimer W, Valle KA, et al. Cigarette smoking, incident coronary heart disease, and coronary artery calcification in Black adults: the Jackson Heart Study. *J Am Heart Assoc*. 2021;10:e017320.
26. Gallucci G, Tartarone A, Lerose R, Lalinga AV, Capobianco AM. Cardiovascular risk of smoking and benefits of smoking cessation. *J Thorac Dis*. 2020;12:3866.
27. Khoramdad M, Vahedian-azimi A, Karimi L, Rahimi-Bashar F, Amini H, Sahebkar A. Association between passive smoking and cardiovascular disease: a systematic review and meta-analysis. *IUBMB Life*. 2020;72(4):677–686. doi:10.1002/iub.2207
28. Office on Smoking and Health, National Center for Chronic Disease Prevention and Health Promotion. Secondhand smoke general information. September 14, 2022. Available at: https://www.cdc.gov/tobacco/data_statistics/fact_sheets/secondhand_smoke/general_facts/index.htm. Accessed January 21, 2023.
29. Grundy SM, Stone NJ, Bailey AL, et al. AHA/ACC/AACVPR/AAPA/ABC/ACPM/ADA/AGS/APhA/ASPC/NLA/PCNA Guideline on the Management of Blood Cholesterol: a report of the American College of Cardiology/American Heart Association Task Force on Clinical Practice Guidelines. *J Am Coll Cardiol*. 2019;73:e285–e350.
30. Liou L, Kaptoge S. Association of small, dense LDL-cholesterol concentration and lipoprotein particle characteristics with coronary heart disease: a systematic review and meta-analysis. *PLoS One*. 2020;15:e0241993.
31. Dai XY, Zheng YY, Tang JN, et al. Triglyceride to high-density lipoprotein cholesterol ratio as a predictor of long-term mortality in patients with coronary artery disease after undergoing percutaneous coronary intervention: a retrospective cohort study. *Lipids Health Dis*. 2019;18:1–8.
32. Ridker PM, Rifai N. *C-reactive Protein and Cardiovascular Disease*. St. Laurent, Canada: MediEdition; 2006.
33. Shrivastava AK, Singh HV, Raizada A, Singh SK. C-reactive protein, inflammation and coronary heart disease. *Egyptian Heart J*. 2015;67:89–97.
34. Surma S, Banach M. Fibrinogen and atherosclerotic cardiovascular diseases—review of the literature and clinical studies. *Int J Mol Sci*. 2021;23:193.
35. Danesh J, Lewington S, Thompson SG, et al.; Fibrinogen Studies C. Plasma fibrinogen level and the risk of major cardiovascular diseases and nonvascular mortality: an individual participant meta-analysis. *JAMA*. 2005;294(14):1799–1809. doi:10.1001/jama.294.14.1799
36. Wang B, Mo X, Wu Z, Guan X. Systematic review and meta-analysis of the correlation between plasma homocysteine levels and coronary heart disease. *J Thorac Dis*. 2022;14:647.

37. Humphrey LL, Fu R, Rogers K, Freeman M, Helfand M. Homocysteine level and coronary heart disease incidence: a systematic review and meta-analysis. *Mayo Clin Proc.* 2008;83(11):1203–1212. doi: 10.4065/83.11.1203
38. Cheng YJ, Kanaya AM, Araneta MRG, et al. Prevalence of diabetes by race and ethnicity in the United States, 2011–2016. *JAMA.* 2019;322:2389–2398.
39. Kjøllesdal MK, Smith GD, Ariansen I, et al. The association between BMI and mortality using early adulthood BMI as an instrumental variable for midlife BMI. *Sci Rep.* 2018;8:1–9.
40. Piché M-E, Tchernof A, Després J-P. Obesity phenotypes, diabetes, and cardiovascular diseases. *Circ Res.* 2020;126:1477–1500.
41. Piercy KL, Troiano RP. Physical activity guidelines for Americans from the US Department of Health and Human Services: cardiovascular benefits and recommendations. *Circ Cardiovasc Qual Outcomes.* 2018;11:e005263.
42. Balkau B, Mhamdi L, Oppert J M, et al. Physical activity and insulin sensitivity. *Diabetes.* 2008;57:2613–2618.
43. Vasankari V, Halonen J, Vasankari T, et al. Physical activity and sedentary behaviour in secondary prevention of coronary artery disease: a review. *Am J Prev Cardiol.* 2021;5:100146.
44. Ruidavets JB, Ducimetiere P, Evans A, et al. Patterns of alcohol consumption and ischaemic heart disease in culturally divergent countries: the Prospective Epidemiological Study of Myocardial Infarction (PRIME). *BMJ.* 2010;341:c6077.
45. Ikeda A, Iso H, Kawachi I, Inoue M, Tsugane S. Type A behaviour and risk of coronary heart disease: the JPHC Study. *Int J Epidemiol.* 2008;37:1395–1405.
46. Richardson S, Shaffer JA, Falzon L, Krupka D, Davidson KW, Edmondson D. Meta-analysis of perceived stress and its association with incident coronary heart disease. *Am J Cardiol.* 2012;110:1711–1716.
47. Smaardijk VR, Lodder P, Kop WJ, van Gennep B, Maas AH, Mommersteeg PM. Sex- and gender-stratified risks of psychological factors for incident ischemic heart disease: systematic review and meta-analysis. *J Am Heart Assoc.* 2019;(9)8:e010859. doi:10.1161/JAHA.118.010859
48. Assmann G, Schulte H, von Eckardstein A, Huang Y. High-density lipoprotein cholesterol as a predictor of coronary heart disease risk. The PROCAM experience and pathophysiological implications for reverse cholesterol transport. *Atherosclerosis.* 1996;124 Suppl:S11–S20. doi:10.1016/0021-9150(96)05852-2.
49. Farmer ME, White LR, Abbott RD, et al. Blood pressure and cognitive performance: the Framingham Study. *Am J Epidemiol.* 1987;126:1103–1114.
50. Cheng S, Claggett B, Correia A, et al. Temporal trends in the population attributable risk for coronary heart disease: Atherosclerosis Risk in Communities Study. *J Am Coll Cardiol.* 2014;130(10):820–828. doi:10.1161/CIRCULATIONAHA.113.008506
51. Fox ER, Benjamin EJ, Sarpong DF, et al. The relation of C-reactive protein to chronic kidney disease in African Americans: the Jackson Heart Study. *BMC Nephrol.* 2010;11:1. doi:10.1186/1471-2369-11-1
52. Heidrich J, Wellmann J, Heuschmann PU, Kraywinkel K, Keil U. Mortality and morbidity from coronary heart disease attributable to passive smoking. *Eur Heart J.* 2007;28: 2498–2502.

53. Howard G, Wagenknecht LE, Burke GL, et al. Cigarette smoking and progression of atherosclerosis: the Atherosclerosis Risk in Communities (ARIC) Study. *JAMA*. 1998;279(2): 119–124. doi:10.1001/jama.279.2.119
54. Li C, Ma R, Zhang X, et al. Risk of coronary heart disease in the rural population in Xinjiang: a nested case-control study in China. *PLoS One*. 2020;15:e0229598.
55. Hasbani NR, Ligthart S, Brown MR, et al. American Heart Association's Life's Simple 7: lifestyle recommendations, polygenic risk, and lifetime risk of coronary heart disease. *Circulation*. 2022;145:808–818.
56. Safford MM, Reshetnyak E, Sterling MR, et al. Number of social determinants of health and fatal and nonfatal incident coronary heart disease in the REGARDS study. *Circulation*. 2021;143(3):244–253. doi:10.1161/CIRCULATIONAHA.120.048026
57. Moyer VA, Force UPST. Screening for coronary heart disease with electrocardiography: US Preventive Services Task Force recommendation statement. *Ann Intern Med*. 2012;157:512–518.
58. Obisesan OH, Osei AD, Uddin SI, Dzaye O, Blaha MJ. An update on coronary artery calcium interpretation at chest and cardiac CT. *Radiol Cardiothorac Imaging*. 2021;3(1): e200484. doi:10.1148/ryct.2021200484
59. Ylä-Herttuala S, Baker AH. Cardiovascular gene therapy: past, present, and future. *Mol Ther*. 2017;25:1095–1106.
60. Richardson G, Woerden HCv, Morgan L, et al. Healthy Hearts—a community-based primary prevention programme to reduce coronary heart disease. *BMC Cardiovasc Disord*. 2008;8:18. doi:10.1186/1471-2261-8-18
61. Emerging Risk Factors Collaboration. Lipoprotein (a) concentration and the risk of coronary heart disease, stroke, and nonvascular mortality. *JAMA*. 2009;302:412.
62. Stamler J, Vaccaro O, Neaton JD, Wentworth D. Diabetes, other risk factors, and 12-yr cardiovascular mortality for men screened in the Multiple Risk Factor Intervention Trial. *Diabetes Care*. 1993;16:434–444.
63. Tikkanen E, Havulinna AS, Palotie A, Salomaa V, Ripatti S. Genetic risk prediction and a 2-stage risk screening strategy for coronary heart disease. *Atheroscler, Thromb, Vasc Biol*. 2013;33(9):2261–2266. doi: 0.1161/ATVBAHA.112.301120
64. Hassen HY, Ndejjo R, Musinguzi G, Van Geertruyden JP, Abrams S, Bastiaens H. Effectiveness of community-based cardiovascular disease prevention interventions to improve physical activity: a systematic review and meta-regression. *Prev Med*. 2021;153:106797.
65. Simon C, Schweitzer B, Oujaa M, et al. Successful overweight prevention in adolescents by increasing physical activity: a 4-year randomized controlled intervention. *Int J Obes*. 2008;32:1489–1498.
66. Gustat J, Rice J, Parker KM, Becker AB, Farley TA. Effect of changes to the neighborhood built environment on physical activity in a low-income African American neighborhood. *Prev Chronic Dis*. 2012;9:110165.
67. Papadakis S, Moroz I. Population-level interventions for coronary heart disease prevention: what have we learned since the North Karelia project? *Curr Opin Cardiol*. 2008;23:452–461.
68. Gooding HC, Gidding SS, Moran AE, et al. Challenges and opportunities for the prevention and treatment of cardiovascular disease among young adults: report from a National Heart, Lung, and Blood Institute Working Group. *J Am Heart Assoc*. 2020;9:e016115.

69. Altman R, Ybarra JNd, Villablanca AC. Community-based cardiovascular disease prevention to reduce cardiometabolic risk in Latina women: a pilot program. *J Womens Health (Larchmt)*. 2014;23(4):350–357.
70. Hinderliter AL, Sherwood A, Craighead LW, et al. The long-term effects of lifestyle change on blood pressure: one-year follow-up of the ENCORE study. *Am J Hypertens*. 2014;27(5): 734–741. doi:10.1093/ajh/hpt183
71. Lou SP, Han D, Kuczmarski MF, Evans MK, Zonderman AB, Crews DC. Health literacy, numeracy, and Dietary Approaches to Stop Hypertension accordance among hypertensive adults. *Health Educ Behav*. 2023;50(1):49–57. doi:10.1177/10901981221079742
72. Rubinstein A, Miranda JJ, Beratarrechea A, et al. Effectiveness of an mHealth intervention to improve the cardiometabolic profile of people with prehypertension in low-resource urban settings in Latin America: a randomised controlled trial. *Lancet Diabetes Endocrinol*. 2016;4: 52–63.
73. Ni Z, Wu B, Yang Q, Yan LL, Liu C, Shaw RJ. An mHealth intervention to improve medication adherence and health outcomes among patients with coronary heart disease: randomized controlled trial. *J Med Internet Res*. 2022;24:e27202.
74. Akinosun AS, Polson R, Diaz-Skeete Y, et al. Digital technology interventions for risk factor modification in patients with cardiovascular disease: systematic review and meta-analysis. *JMIR mHealth uHealth*. 2021;9(3):e21061.
75. Jeemon P, Harikrishnan S, Ganapathi S, et al. Efficacy of a family-based cardiovascular risk reduction intervention in individuals with a family history of premature coronary heart disease in India (PROLIFIC): an open-label, single-centre, cluster randomised controlled trial. *Lancet Global Health*. 2021;9:e1442–e1450.
76. Ma J, Ge C, Shi Y, et al. Chinese home-based cardiac rehabilitation model delivered by smartphone interaction improves clinical outcomes in patients with coronary heart disease. *Front Cardiovasc Med*. 2021;8:731557. doi:10.3389/fcvm.2021.731557
77. National Heart Lung and Blood Institute. Coronary heart disease research. 2022a. Available at: https://www.nhlbi.nih.gov/research/coronary-heart-disease. Accessed April 8, 2023.
78. Liang C, Zhang W, Li S, Qin G. Coronary heart disease and COVID-19: A meta-analysis. *Medicina Clínica (English ed.)*. 2021;156:547–554.
79. Xie Y, Xu E, Bowe B, Al-Aly Z. Long-term cardiovascular outcomes of COVID-19. *Nat Med*. 2022;28:583–590.
80. Ganatra S, Dani SS, Shah S, et al. Management of cardiovascular disease during coronavirus disease (COVID-19) pandemic. *Trends Cardiovasc Med*. 2020;30:315–325.
81. Jackson Heart Study. About us. 2019. Available at: https://www.jacksonheartstudy.org/About/About-The-JHS. Accessed January 21, 2023.
82. Bild DE, Bluemke DA, Burke GL, et al. Multi-Ethnic Study of Atherosclerosis: objectives and design. *Am J Epidemiol*. 2002;156(9):871–881. doi:10.1093/aje/kwf113
83. Sorlie PD, Avilés-Santa LM, Wassertheil-Smoller S, et al. Design and implementation of the Hispanic Community Health Study/Study of Latinos. *Ann Epidemiol*. 2010;20:629–641.
84. Liu L, Nettleton JA, Bertoni AG, Bluemke DA, Lima JA, Szklo M. Dietary pattern, the metabolic syndrome, and left ventricular mass and systolic function: the Multi-Ethnic Study of Atherosclerosis. *Am J Clin Nutr*. 2009;90:362–368.

85. Ikeme S, Kottenmeier E, Uzochukwu G, Brinjikji W. Evidence-based disparities in stroke care metrics and outcomes in the United States: a systematic review. *Stroke*. 2022;29:670–679.
86. Howard VJ, Madsen TE, Kleindorfer DO, et al. Sex and race differences in the association of incident ischemic stroke with risk factors. *JAMA Neurol*. 2019;76:179–186.
87. Morgenstern LB, Smith MA, Lisabeth LD, et al. Excess stroke in Mexican Americans compared with non-Hispanic Whites: the Brain Attack Surveillance in Corpus Christi Project. *Am J Epidemiol*. 2004;160(4):376–383. doi:10.1093/aje/kwh225
88. Kung HC, Hoyert DL, Xu J, Murphy SL. Deaths: final data for 2005. *Natl Vital Stat Rep*. 2008;56:1–120.
89. Kim H, Friedlander Y, Longstreth WT Jr., Edwards KL, Schwartz SM, Siscovick DS. Family history as a risk factor for stroke in young women. *Am J Prev Med*. 2004;(5)27:391–396. doi:10.1016/j.amepre.2004.08.008
90. Howard G, Howard VJ. Twenty years of progress toward understanding the Stroke Belt. *Stroke*. 2020;51(3):742–750. doi: 10.1161/STROKEAHA.119.024155
91. Sacco RL, Adams R, Albers G, et al. Guidelines for Prevention of Stroke in Patients with Ischemic Stroke or Transient Ischemic Attack: a statement for healthcare professionals from the American Heart Association/American Stroke Association Council on Stroke: co-sponsored by the Council on Cardiovascular Radiology and Intervention: the American Academy of Neurology affirms the value of this guideline. *Circulation*. 2006;113:e409–e449.
92. Wang L, Li S, Sanika G, et al. Association between serum 25-hydroxyvitamin D level and stroke risk: an analysis based on the National Health and Nutrition Examination Survey. *Behav Neurol*. 2021;2021:5457881. doi:10.1155/2021/5457881
93. Xie C, Zhu R, Tian Y, Wang K. Association of obstructive sleep apnoea with the risk of vascular outcomes and all-cause mortality: a meta-analysis. *BMJ Open*. 2017;7:e013983.
94. Baillieul S, Dekkers M, Brill AK, et al. Sleep apnoea and ischaemic stroke: current knowledge and future directions. *Lancet Neurol*. 2022;21:78–88.
95. Guzik A, Bushnell C. Stroke epidemiology and risk factor management. *CONTINUUM (Minneap, Min)*. 2017;23(1, Cerebrovascular Disease):15–39. doi:10.1212/CON.0000000000000416
96. SPS3 Study Group. Blood-pressure targets in patients with recent lacunar stroke: the SPS3 randomised trial. *Lancet*. 2013;382:507–515.
97. Whelton PK, Carey RM, Aronow WS, et al. ACC/AHA/AAPA/ABC/ACPM/AGS/APhA/ASH/ASPC/NMA/PCNA guideline for the prevention, detection, evaluation, and management of high blood pressure in adults: a report of the American College of Cardiology/American Heart Association Task Force on Clinical Practice Guidelines. *J Am Coll Cardiol*. 2018;71(19):e127–e248. doi:10.1016/j.jacc.2017.11.006
98. Liu L, Yang X, Long Y, et al. Changes in the prevalence of hospitalization and comorbidity in US adults with stroke: a three decade cross-sectional and birth cohort analysis. *Int J Stroke*. 2016;11:987–998. doi: 10.1177/1747493016660107
99. Towfighi A, Markovic D, Ovbiagele B. Current national patterns of comorbid diabetes among acute ischemic stroke patients. *Cerebrovasc Dis*. 2012;33:411–418.
100. Pistoia F, Sacco S, Tiseo C, Degan D, Ornello R, Carolei A. The epidemiology of atrial fibrillation and stroke. *Cardiol Clin*. 2016;34:255–268.

101. Marini C, De Santis F, Sacco S, et al. Contribution of atrial fibrillation to incidence and outcome of ischemic stroke: results from a population-based study. *Stroke*. 2005;36:1115–1119.
102. Liu Z, Sanossian N, Starkman S, et al. Adiposity and outcome after ischemic stroke: obesity paradox for mortality and obesity parabola for favorable functional outcomes. *Stroke*. 2021;52:144–151.
103. Pan B, Jin X, Jun L, Qiu S, Zheng Q, Pan M. The relationship between smoking and stroke: a meta-analysis. *Medicine (Baltimore)*. 2019; 98(12):e14872. doi: 10.1097/MD.0000000000014872
104. Lee IM, Hennekens CH, Berger K, Buring JE, Manson JE. Exercise and risk of stroke in male physicians. *Stroke*. 1999;30:1–6.
105. Myint PK, Luben RN, Wareham NJ, Bingham SA, Khaw KT. Combined effect of health behaviours and risk of first ever stroke in 20 040 men and women over 11 years' follow-up in Norfolk cohort of European Prospective Investigation of Cancer (EPIC Norfolk): prospective population study. *BMJ*. 2009;338:b349. doi:10.1136/bmj.b349
106. Hu FB, Stampfer MJ, Colditz GA, et al. Physical activity and risk of stroke in women. *JAMA*. 2000;283:2961–2967.
107. McDonnell MN, Hillier SL, Hooker SP, Le A, Judd SE, Howard VJ. Physical activity frequency and risk of incident stroke in a national US study of Blacks and Whites. *Stroke*. 2013;44:2519–2524.
108. Kernan WN, Ovbiagele B, Black HR, et al. Guidelines for the Prevention of Stroke in Patients with Stroke and Transient Ischemic Attack: a guideline for healthcare professionals from the American Heart Association/American Stroke Association. *Stroke*. 2014;45:2160–2236.
109. Estruch R, Ros E, Salas-Salvadó J, et al. Primary prevention of cardiovascular disease with a Mediterranean diet. *N Engl J Med*. 2013;368:1279–1290.
110. Bernstein AM, de Koning L, Flint AJ, Rexrode KM, Willett WC. Soda consumption and the risk of stroke in men and women. *Am J Clin Nutr*. 2012;95(5):1190–1199. doi:10.3945/ajcn.111.030205
111. Zhou R, Wang M, Huang H, Li W, Hu Y, Wu T. Lower vitamin D status is associated with an increased risk of ischemic stroke: a systematic review and meta-analysis. *Nutrients*. 2018;10:277.
112. Amarenco P, Labreuche J. Lipid management in the prevention of stroke: review and updated meta-analysis of statins for stroke prevention. *Lancet Neurol*. 2009;8:453–463.
113. Prospective Studies Collaboration. Cholesterol, diastolic blood pressure, and stroke: 13 000 strokes in 450 000 people in 45 prospective cohorts. *Lancet*. 1995;346:1647–1653.
114. Yamori Y, Liu L, Mizushima S, Ikeda K, Nara Y; Group CS. Male cardiovascular mortality and dietary markers in 25 population samples of 16 countries. *J Hypertens*. 2006;24: 1499–1505. doi:10.1097/01.hjh.0000239284.12691.2e
115. Xiao Z, Xie M, You Y, Wu H, Zhou G, Li M. Wake-up stroke and sleep-disordered breathing: a meta-analysis of current studies. *J Neurol*. 2018;265:1288–1294.
116. Goldstein LB, Adams R, Alberts MJ, et al. Primary prevention of ischemic stroke: a guideline from the American Heart Association/American Stroke Association Stroke Council: cosponsored by the Atherosclerotic Peripheral Vascular Disease Interdisciplinary Working Group; Cardiovascular Nursing Council; Clinical Cardiology Council; Nutrition, Physical Activity, and Metabolism Council; and the Quality of Care and Outcomes Research Interdisciplinary Working Group: the American Academy of Neurology affirms

the value of this guideline. *Stroke*. 2006;37(6):1583–1633. doi:10.1161/01.STR.0000223048.70103.F1

117. Diener HC, Hankey GJ. Primary and secondary prevention of ischemic stroke and cerebral hemorrhage: JACC focus seminar. *J Am Coll Cardiol*. 2020;75:1804–1818.
118. Meschia JF, Bushnell C, Boden-Albala B, et al. Guidelines for the Primary Prevention of Stroke: a statement for healthcare professionals from the American Heart Association/American Stroke Association. *Stroke*. 2014;45:3754–3832.
119. US Department of Health and Human Services. Reduce stroke deaths—HDS-03. Healthy People 2030. 2019. Available at: https://health.gov/healthypeople/objectives-and-data/browse-objectives/heart-disease-and-stroke/reduce-stroke-deaths-hds-03. Accessed January 21, 2023.
120. Willey JZ, Moon YP, Kahn E, et al. Population attributable risks of hypertension and diabetes for cardiovascular disease and stroke in the Northern Manhattan Study. *J Am Heart Assoc*. 2014;3:e001106.
121. Lin MP, Ovbiagele B, Markovic D, Towfighi A. "Life's Simple 7" and long-term mortality after stroke. *J Am Heart Assoc*. 2015;4:e001470.
122. Centers for Disease Control and Prevention, National Center for Chronic Disease Prevention and Health Promotion, Division for Heart Disease and Stroke Prevention. CDC Stroke Registry. CDC state heart disease and stroke prevention programs. 2016. Updated September 30, 2020. Available at: http://www.cdc.gov/dhdsp/programs/stroke_registry.htm. Accessed January 21, 2023.
123. Schwamm LH, Pancioli A, Acker JE, et al. Recommendations for the establishment of stroke systems of care recommendations from the American Stroke Association's Task Force on the Development of Stroke Systems. *Stroke*. 2005;36:690–703.
124. Centers for Disease Control and Prevention. National Heart Disease and Stroke Prevention Program: staff orientation guide. September 2011, Available at: http://www.cdc.gov/dhdsp/programs/spha/docs/orientation_manual.pdf. Accessed Accessed Januaey 21, 2023.
125. Centers for Disease Control and Prevention. National Heart Disease and Stroke Prevention Program: strategies for states to address the "ABCS" of heart disease and stroke prevention. 2010. Available at: https://www.cdc.gov/dhdsp/programs/spha/docs/abcs_guide.pdf. Accessed June 6, 2022.
126. Guirguis-Blake JM, Evans CV, Webber EM, Coppola EL, Perdue LA, Weyrich MS. Screening for hypertension in adults: updated evidence report and systematic review for the US Preventive Services Task Force. *JAMA*. 2021;325:1657–1669.
127. Adams H, Davis P, Leira E, et al. Baseline NIH Stroke Scale score strongly predicts outcome after stroke: a report of the Trial of Org 10172 in Acute Stroke Treatment (TOAST). *Neurology*. 1999;53:126–126.
128. Goldstein LB, Samsa GP. Reliability of the National Institutes of Health Stroke Scale extension to non-neurologists in the context of a clinical trial. *Stroke*. 1997;28:307–310.
129. Khurshid S, Healey JS, McIntyre WF, Lubitz SA. Population-based screening for atrial fibrillation. *Circ Res*. 2020;127:143–154.
130. Hacke W, Kaste M, Bluhmki E, et al. Thrombolysis with alteplase 3 to 4.5 hours after acute ischemic stroke. *N Engl J Med*. 2008;359:1317–1329. doi: 10.1056/NEJMoa0804656

131. Kummer BR, Klang E, Stein LK, Dhamoon MS, Jetté N. History of stroke is independently associated with in-hospital death in patients with COVID-19. *Stroke*. 2020;51:3112–3114.
132. Tu TM, Seet CYH, Koh JS, et al. Acute ischemic stroke during the convalescent phase of asymptomatic COVID-2019 infection in men. *JAMA Netw open*. 2021;4:e217498–e217498.
133. Mayo Clinic. COVID-19: long-term effects. 2021. Updated June 26, 2022. Available at: https://www.mayoclinic.org/diseases-conditions/coronavirus/in-depth/coronavirus-long-term-effects/art-20490351. Accessed January 21, 2023.
134. Srivastava PK, Zhang S, Xian Y, et al. Treatment and outcomes of patients with ischemic stroke during COVID-19: an analysis from Get With The Guidelines–Stroke. *Stroke*. 2021;52(10):3225–3232. doi:10.1161/STROKEAHA.120.034414
135. Srivastava PK, Zhang S, Xian Y, et al. Acute ischemic stroke in patients with COVID-19: an analysis from Get With The Guidelines–Stroke. *Stroke*. 2021;52(5):1826–1829. doi:10.1161/STROKEAHA.121.034301
136. Urbich M, Globe G, Pantiri K, et al. A systematic review of medical costs associated with heart failure in the USA (2014–2020). *Pharmacoeconomics*. 2020;38:1219–1236.
137. Heidenreich PA, Albert NM, Allen LA, et al. Forecasting the impact of heart failure in the United States: a policy statement from the American Heart Association. *Circ Heart Fail*. 2013;6:606–619.
138. Chioncel O, Parissis J, Mebazaa A, et al. Epidemiology, pathophysiology and contemporary management of cardiogenic shock—a position statement from the Heart Failure Association of the European Society of Cardiology. *Eur J Heart Fail*. 2020;22:1315–1341.
139. Swedberg K. Heart failure subtypes: pathophysiology and definitions. *Diabetes Res Clin Pract*. 2021;175:108815.
140. Liu L. Changes in cardiovascular hospitalization and comorbidity of heart failure in the United States: findings from the National Hospital Discharge Surveys 1980–2006. *Int J Cardiol*. 2011;149:39–45. doi: 10.1016/j.ijcard.2009.11.037
141. Liu L, Eisen HJ. Epidemiology of heart failure and scope of the problem. *Cardiol Clin*. 2014;32:1–8. doi: 10.1016/j.ccl.2013.09.009
142. Thom T, Haase N, Rosamond W, et al. Heart disease and stroke statistics—2006 update: a report from the American Heart Association Statistics Committee and Stroke Statistics Subcommittee. *Circulation*. 2006;113:e85–e151.
143. Bahrami H, Bluemke DA, Kronmal R, et al. Novel metabolic risk factors for incident heart failure and their relationship with obesity: the MESA (Multi-Ethnic Study of Atherosclerosis) study. *J Am Coll Cardiol*. 2008;51:1775–1783.
144. Kannel WB. Vital epidemiologic clues in heart failure. *J Clin Epidemiol*. 2000;53(3):229–235. doi:10.1016/s0895-4356(99)00135-3
145. Kannel WB. Incidence and epidemiology of heart failure. *Heart Fail Rev*. 2000;5(2):167–173. doi: 10.1023/A:1009884820941
146. Packer M. Leptin-aldosterone-neprilysin axis: identification of its distinctive role in the pathogenesis of the three phenotypes of heart failure in people with obesity. *Circulation*. 2018;137:1614–1631.
147. Liu L, Chen M, Hankins SR, et al.; Drexel Cardiovascular Health Collaborative Education, Research, and Evaluation Group. Serum 25-hydroxyvitamin D concentration and

mortality from heart failure and cardiovascular disease, and premature mortality from all-cause in United States adults. *Am J Cardiol.* 2012;110(6):834–839. doi:10.1016/j.amjcard.2012.05.013

148. Sinha A, Ning H, Carnethon MR, et al. Race-and sex-specific population attributable fractions of incident heart failure: a population-based cohort study from the lifetime risk pooling project. *Circ Heart Fail.* 2021;14:e008113.
149. Sinha A, Ning H, Ahmad FS, et al. Association of fasting glucose with lifetime risk of incident heart failure: the Lifetime Risk Pooling Project. *Cardiovasc Diabetol.* 2021;20(1):6. doi:10.1186/s12933-021-01265-y
150. Hunt SA, Abraham WT, Chin MH, et al. ACC/AHA 2005 Guideline Update for the Diagnosis and Management of Chronic Heart Failure in the Adult: a report of the American College of Cardiology/American Heart Association Task Force on Practice Guidelines (Writing Committee to Update the 2001 Guidelines for the Evaluation and Management of Heart Failure): developed in collaboration with the American College of Chest Physicians and the International Society for Heart and Lung Transplantation: endorsed by the Heart Rhythm Society. *Circulation.* 2005;112(12):e154–e235. doi:10.1161/CIRCULATIONAHA.105.167586
151. Yancy CW, Jessup M, Bozkurt B, et al. 2017 ACC/AHA/HFSA focused update of the 2013 ACCF/AHA Guideline for the Management of Heart Failure: a report of the American College of Cardiology/American Heart Association Task Force on Clinical Practice Guidelines and the Heart Failure Society of America. *J Am Coll Cardiol.* 2017;70:776–803.
152. Hunt SA, Abraham WT, Chin MH, et al. 2009 focused update incorporated into the ACC/AHA 2005 Guidelines for the Diagnosis and Management of Heart Failure in Adults: a report of the American College of Cardiology Foundation/American Heart Association Task Force on Practice Guidelines: developed in collaboration with the International Society for Heart and Lung Transplantation. *Circulation.* 2009;119:e391–e479. doi:10.1161/CIRCULATIONAHA.109.192065
153. Rasmusson KD, Hall JA, Renlund DG. The intricacies of heart failure. *Nurs Manage.* 2007;38(5):33–40; quiz 40–41. doi:10.1097/01.LPN.0000269818.97048.a4
154. Maddox TM, Januzzi JL Jr., Allen LA, et al. 2021 update to the 2017 ACC Expert Consensus Decision Pathway for Optimization of Heart Failure Treatment: answers to 10 pivotal issues about heart failure with reduced ejection fraction: a report of the American College of Cardiology Solution Set Oversight Committee. *J Am Coll Cardiol.* 2021;77:772–810.
155. Khan MS, Khan F, Fonarow GC, et al. Dietary interventions and nutritional supplements for heart failure: a systematic appraisal and evidence map. *Eur J Heart Fail.* 2021;23:1468–1476.
156. Italia L, Tomasoni D, Bisegna S, et al. COVID-19 and heart failure: from epidemiology during the pandemic to myocardial injury, myocarditis, and heart failure sequelae. *Front Cardiovasc Med.* 2021;8:713560. doi:10.3389/fcvm.2021.713560.
157. Hall ME, Vaduganathan M, Khan MS, et al. Reductions in heart failure hospitalizations during the COVID-19 pandemic. *J Card Fail.* 2020;26:462.
158. Herrington W, Lacey B, Sherliker P, Armitage J, Lewington S. Epidemiology of atherosclerosis and the potential to reduce the global burden of atherothrombotic disease. *Circ Res.* 2016;118:535–546.

159. Leeper NJ, Hamburg NM. Peripheral vascular disease in 2021. *Circ Res.* 2021;128: 1803–1804.
160. Heald C, Fowkes F, Murray G, Price J; Collaboration ABI. Risk of mortality and cardiovascular disease associated with the ankle-brachial index: systematic review. *Atherosclerosis.* 2006;189:61–69.
161. Berkovitch A, Iakobishvili Z, Fuchs S, et al. Peripheral artery disease, abnormal ankle-brachial index and prognosis after acute coronary syndrome. *Front Cardiovasc Med.* 2022;9:902615. doi:10.3389/fcvm.2022.902615
162. McDermott M, Lloyd-Jones D. The role of biomarkers and genetics in peripheral arterial disease. *J Am Coll Cardiol.* 2009;54:1228–1237.
163. Criqui MH, Vargas V, Denenberg JO, et al. Ethnicity and peripheral arterial disease the San Diego Population Study. *Circulation.* 2005;112:2703–2707.
164. Rafnsson SB, Deary IJ, Fowkes F. Peripheral arterial disease and cognitive function. *Vasc Med.* 2009;14:51–61.
165. Fowkes FGR, Rudan D, Rudan I, et al. Comparison of global estimates of prevalence and risk factors for peripheral artery disease in 2000 and 2010: a systematic review and analysis. *Lancet.* 2013;382:1329–1340.
166. Criqui MH, Matsushita K, Aboyans V, et al. Lower extremity peripheral artery disease: contemporary epidemiology, management gaps, and future directions: a scientific statement from the American Heart Association. *Circulation.* 2021;144:e171–e191.
167. Brevetti G, Sirico G, Giugliano G, et al. Prevalence of hypoechoic carotid plaques in coronary artery disease: relationship with coexistent peripheral arterial disease and leukocyte number. *Vasc Med.* 2009;14:13–19.
168. Pouncey AL, Woodward M. Sex-specific differences in cardiovascular risk, risk factors and risk management in the peripheral arterial disease population. *Diagnostics.* 2022;12:808.
169. Allison MA, Ho E, Denenberg JO, et al. Ethnic-specific prevalence of peripheral arterial disease in the United States. *Am J Prev Med.* 2007;32:328–333.
170. Kalbaugh CA, Witrick B, Sivaraj LB, et al. Non-Hispanic Black and Hispanic patients have worse outcomes than White patients within similar stages of peripheral artery disease. *J Am Heart Assoc.* 2022;11:e023396.
171. Unkart JT, Allison MA, Criqui MH, et al. Life's Simple 7 and peripheral artery disease: the Multi-Ethnic Study of Atherosclerosis. *Am J Prev Med.* 2019;56:262–270.
172. Garg PK, O'Neal WT, Mok Y, Heiss G, Coresh J, Matsushita K. Life's Simple 7 and peripheral artery disease risk: the Atherosclerosis Risk in Communities Study. *Am J Prev Med.* 2018;55:642–649.
173. Johansen KL, Garimella PS, Hicks CW, et al. Central and peripheral arterial diseases in chronic kidney disease: conclusions from a Kidney Disease: Improving Global Outcomes (KDIGO) controversies conference. *Kidney Int.* 2021;100:35–48.
174. Safar M, Priollet P, Luizy F, et al. Peripheral arterial disease and isolated systolic hypertension: the ATTEST study. *J Hum Hypertens.* 2009;23:182–187.
175. Pradhan AD, Shrivastava S, Cook NR, Rifai N, Creager MA, Ridker PM. Symptomatic peripheral arterial disease in women: nontraditional biomarkers of elevated risk. *Circulation.* 2008;117:823–831.

176. Selvin E, Erlinger TP. Prevalence of and risk factors for peripheral arterial disease in the United States results from the National Health and Nutrition Examination Survey, 1999–2000. *Circulation*. 2004;110:738–743.
177. Vidula H, Tian L, Liu K, et al. Biomarkers of inflammation and thrombosis as predictors of near-term mortality in patients with peripheral arterial disease: a cohort study. *Ann Intern Med*. 2008;148:85–93.
178. Carman TL, Fernandez B Jr. Contemporary management of peripheral arterial disease: II. Improving walking distance and quality of life. *Cleve Clin J Med*. 2006;73:S38– S44.
179. Paredes H, Paulino D, Barroso J, Abrantes C, Machado I, Silva I. Supervised physical exercise therapy of peripheral artery disease patients: m-health challenges and opportunities. Paper/Poster presented at: Proceedings of the 54th Hawaii International Conference on System Sciences; January 5, 2021; Kauai, Hawaii.
180. Hankey GJ, Norman PE, Eikelboom JW. Medical treatment of peripheral arterial disease. *JAMA*. 2006;295:547–553.
181. Banerjee A, Fowkes FG, Rothwell PM. Associations between peripheral artery disease and ischemic stroke implications for primary and secondary prevention. *Stroke*. 2010;41: 2102–2107.
182. Bennett P, Silverman S, Gill P. Hypertension and peripheral arterial disease. *J Hum Hypertens*. 2009;23:213–215.
183. Cacoub PP, Abola MTB, Baumgartner I, et al. Cardiovascular risk factor control and outcomes in peripheral artery disease patients in the Reduction of Atherothrombosis for Continued Health (REACH) Registry. *Atherosclerosis*. 2009;204:e86–e92.
184. Cao P, De Rango P. Endovascular treatment of peripheral artery disease (PAD): so old yet so far from evidence! *Eur J Vasc Endovasc Surg*. 2009;37:501–503.
185. Smolderen KG, Lee M, Arora T, Simonov M, Mena-Hurtado C. Peripheral artery disease and COVID-19 outcomes: insights from the Yale DOM-CovX Registry. *Curr Probl Cardiol*. 2021;47(12):101007. doi: 10.1016/j.cpcardiol.2021.10
186. Trunfio R, Deslarzes-Dubuis C, Buso G, et al. The effects of COVID-19 pandemic on patients with lower extremity peripheral arterial disease: a near miss disaster. *Ann Vasc Surg*. 2021;77:71–78.

17

Cancer

Mara Meyer Epstein, ScD, ScM, Kathryn L. Penney, ScD,
and Corinne Joshu, PhD, MPH, MA

LEARNING OBJECTIVES

After completing this chapter, readers should be able to

1. Identify the primary risk factors for major cancers in the United States.
2. Become familiar with current cancer screening opportunities and guidelines in the United States.
3. Understand the public health burden of cancer in the United States.

INTRODUCTION

Cancer is the second leading cause of death in the United States, accounting for an estimated 1.9 million new cases and 609,360 deaths in 2022 (Table 17-1).[1,2]

The most recent US data (2009–2018) show declines in age-adjusted overall incidence (1%/year) and mortality (1.8%/year) rates, with variations by sex and type of cancer. Men have a 40.5% lifetime probability of developing cancer, and women have a 39% lifetime probability.[3] The five-year relative survival across all cancers has also increased, from 49% for those diagnosed between 1975 and 1977 to 68% for those diagnosed between 2011 and 2017.[1,4] However, survival rates vary by cancer type, stage at diagnosis, sex, race/ethnicity, and other factors, including social determinants of health.

Cancer death rates increased steadily from 1930 (when nationwide mortality was first compiled) to 1990, mainly because of a sharp rise in lung cancer. However, overall cancer death rates began to decline in the early 1990s and decreased 1.8% per year between 2010 and 2019. Among men, there was a decreasing annual percentage change (APC) of 1.8% per year from 2001 to 2015 and 2.3% from 2015 to 2018. Among women, there was a decreasing APC of 1.4% per year from 2001 to 2016, and 2.1% from 2016 to 2018.[3] The mortality rate from cancer among men in the United States is now nearly equivalent to that from heart disease among men aged 45 to 64 years (Figure 17-1).[5]

Table 17-1. Public Health Impact of Selected Cancers: United States, 2022

Cancer Type	No. New Cases[a]	No. Deaths	5-Year Survival[b]
All Sites	1,918,030	609,360	68.10%
Breast	287,850	43,250	90.6%
Prostate	268,490	34,500	96.8%
Lung	236,740	130,180	22.9%
Colon and rectum	151,030	52,580	65.1%
Melanoma (skin)	99,780	7,650	93.7%
Bladder	81,180	17,100	77.1%
Non-Hodgkin lymphoma	80,470	20,250	73.8%
Uterus	65,950	12,550	81.3%
Pancreas	62,210	49,830	11.5%
Leukemia	60,650	24,000	65.7%
Oral cavity and pharynx	54,000	11,230	68%
Liver and intrahepatic bile duct	41,260	30,520	20.8%
Stomach	26,380	11,090	33.3%
Ovarian	19,880	12,810	49.7%
Cervix	14,100	4,280	66.7%
Hodgkin lymphoma	8,540	920	89.1%

Source: Based on NCI[1] and ACS.[2]

[a]New cases and deaths estimates for 2022 from the National Cancer Institute's (NCI's) Surveillance, Epidemiology, and End Results (SEER) Program.

[b]Five-year relative survival rates were calculated using data from 2012–2018 from the NCI SEER Program.

Significance

Although cancer occurs more frequently with advancing age, it is also a leading cause of disease-attributable death among US children aged 1 to 19 years.[3] Similarly, racial and ethnic groups are not affected equally by cancer (Figure 17-2).[6,7] As stated by the American Cancer Society (ACS), "although racial classification is a social construct based on appearance, it remains useful for describing health patterns in the United States because long-standing structural racism has contributed to inequalities in the social determinants of health."[8] Black men have the highest overall cancer incidence and mortality rate for most cancers, followed by non-Hispanic White men.[1] The higher overall cancer death rate in Black people is attributable to breast and colorectal cancer in women, and prostate, lung, and colorectal cancer in men.[8]

The causes of these inequalities are not related to race per se but are, rather, a reflection of disparities in and unequal access to income, housing, education, and health care, in addition to differences in cigarette smoking and poor nutrition, which can delay cancer

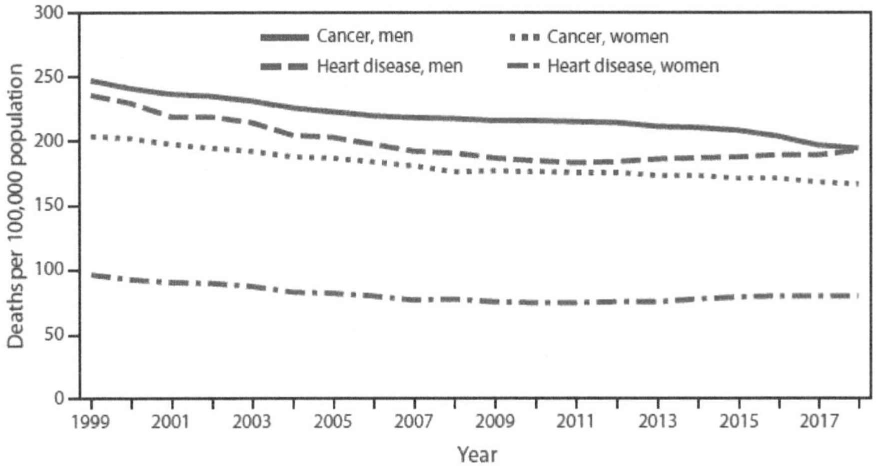

Source: Reprinted from CDC.[5]

Figure 17-1. Age-Adjusted Death Rates per 100,000 From Heart Disease and Cancer for Men and Women Aged 45–64 Years: United States, 1999–2018

diagnosis and treatment,[8,9] resulting in more advanced stages at diagnosis. For example, in 2019 in the United States, 12% of Black people were uninsured and 19.5% lived in poverty, compared with 9% of White people who were uninsured and 8.2% who lived in poverty.[8,10]

In the United States, people of Hispanic origin have overall lower incidence of cancer than non-Hispanic White and non-Hispanic Black people.[1,11] Cancers that may be more common among the Hispanic population than other race/ethnic groups include cancers associated with infection, such as stomach (i.e., *Helicobacter pylori*), liver (i.e., hepatitis B and C viruses), and cervical (i.e., human papillomavirus) cancers, as well as gallbladder cancer.[12] However, Hispanics in the United States represent a diverse group, and cancer rates vary by country of origin.[2,12]

Hispanics are the most likely of all US racial/ethnic groups to be uninsured, even following the enactment of the Affordable Care Act, with variation in insurance rates by country of origin and nativity. In addition, 16% of all Hispanics lived in poverty in 2019.[12] Hispanic people are less likely than non-Hispanic White people to be screened for breast, cervical, colorectal, and prostate cancers and less likely to be diagnosed at an early stage for many cancers.[12] Cancer risk among Hispanics also varies by country of origin, acculturation, and place of birth: US-born Hispanic men have higher cancer death rates than non-US–born Hispanic men.[12,13] Thus, future prevention efforts may need to target population by country of origin rather than generalizing to the entire Hispanic population.

The estimated costs of cancer-related health care in 2015 were $183 billion, with $5.6 billion paid out of pocket by patients in 2018.[14,15] Costs are predicted to increase by 34% by 2030. Indirect costs, such as lost work productivity, were estimated at $115.8 billion in 2000 and then $147.6 billion in 2020 because of population growth and aging.[16]

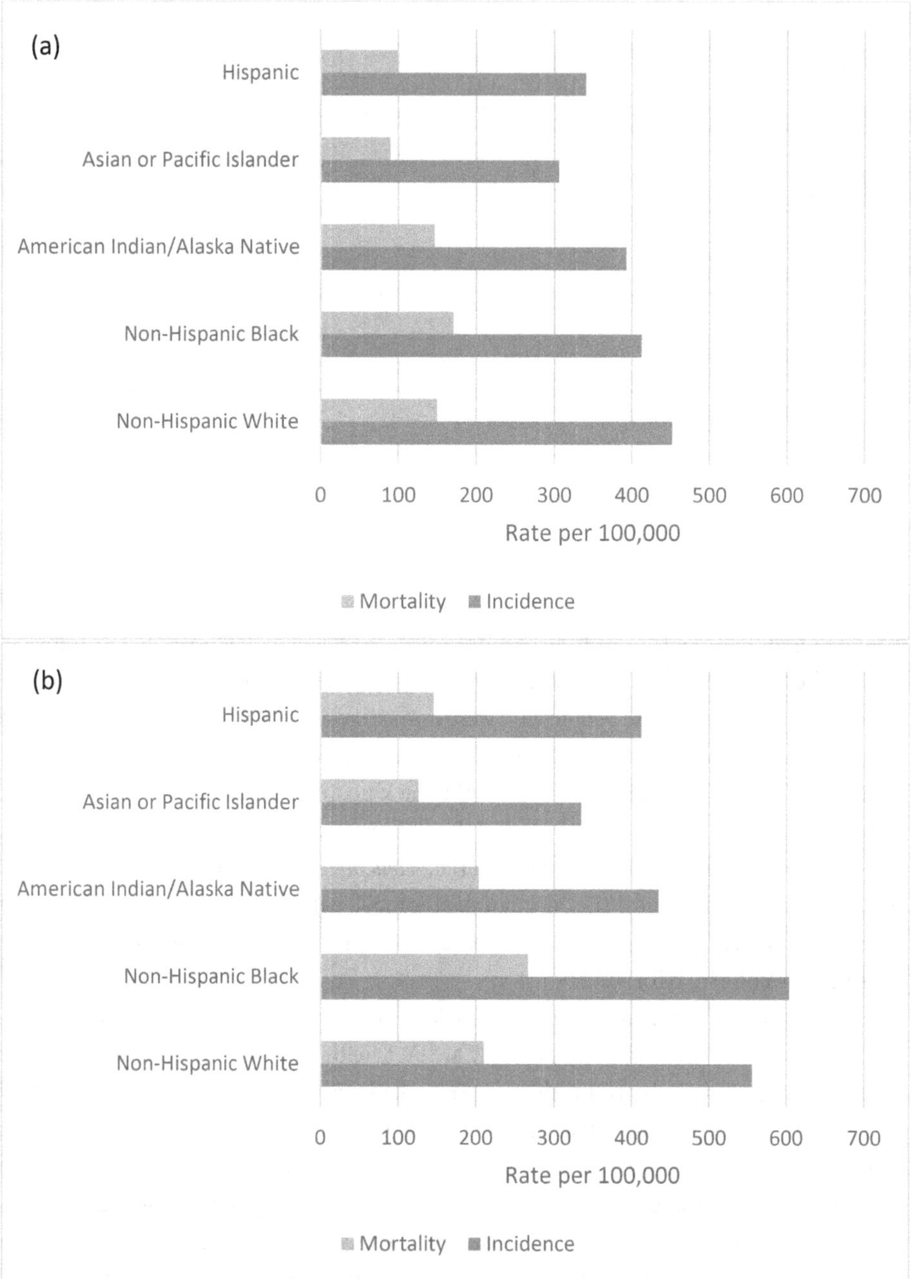

Source: Based on NCI.[6,7]

Note: Incidence rates were adapted from the SEER 22 Incidence Database (where years of diagnosis were 2000–2019); mortality rates were adapted from the US Mortality (Total US) Database through SEER, referencing deaths from all malignant cancers (where years of death were 2000–2019). Rates are per 100,000.

Figure 17-2. Cancer Incidence and Mortality Age-Adjusted Rates in (a) Women and (b) Men, by Race and Ethnic Group: United States, 2000–2019

In contrast to the huge cost of cancer treatment, the total national resources dedicated to early detection activities, such as screening for breast, cervical, and colorectal cancer, are considerably smaller. The allocation of national resources to the primary prevention of cancer (e.g., tobacco control, dietary intervention) is even smaller.

Pathophysiology

Cancer has a complex set of upstream causes and downstream consequences (Figure 17-3). Occurring as a result of alterations in the mechanisms that control normal cell behavior, cancer cells are different than normal cells, as they (1) acquire inappropriate growth properties and (2) generally lose their ability to serve the functions they normally have in a given tissue. Cancer comprises a diverse group of diseases characterized by uncontrolled growth and spread of these abnormal cells. Tumors, or abnormal growth of tissue, may be either benign or malignant. Benign tumors are generally innocuous and slow-growing, although they can cause morbidity and mortality through their impact on normal surrounding tissues and organs. In contrast, malignant tumors (commonly called cancers) contain abnormal genetic material and may grow more rapidly. The principal danger of a cancer is its tendency to invade neighboring tissues or organs, or to metastasize and to grow in other areas of the body. If this spread remains untreated, cancer cells invade vital organs or cause dysfunction by displacing normal tissue.

Different cancer types have widely varying induction periods—that is, the time between exposure to cancer-causing agents and cancer occurrence. For example, the induction period for some types of leukemia may be as short as a few years, compared with induction periods as long as four or five decades for some types of bladder cancer.

Cancers are classified according to their organ or tissue of origin (site code) and according to their histologic features (morphology code). The most widely used classification schemes are the World Health Organization's 2005 *International Statistical Classification of Disease and Related Health Problems, Tenth Revision* (*ICD-10*) and its

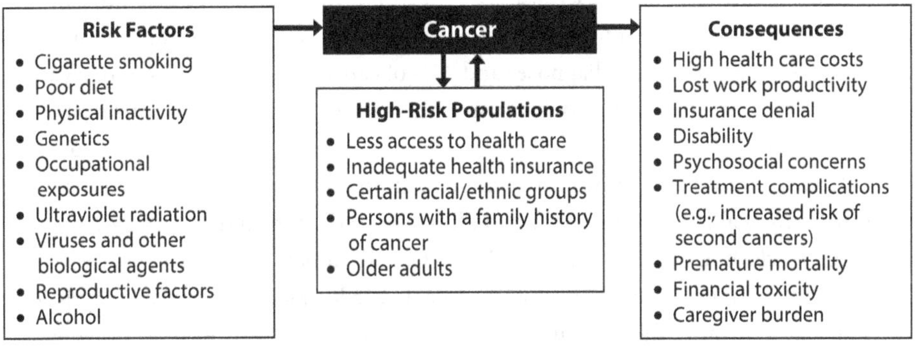

Figure 17-3. Cancer: Risk Factors, Consequences, and High-Risk Populations

2000 *International Classification of Diseases for Oncology*, Third Edition (*ICD-O-3*). The existence of hundreds of cancer varieties is readily apparent with 43 organs of origin and multiple histologic types for each organ.[17]

In addition to being grouped by site and histologic features, cancers are classified according to their stage at diagnosis, or the extent to which the cancer has grown locally or invaded other tissues or organs. Cancer cells may remain at their original site (local stage), spread to an adjacent area of the body (regional stage), or spread (metastasize) throughout the body (distant stage).

Cancer registries collect detailed information on patients with cancer through reports from hospitals and medical clinics (see also Chapter 3 on surveillance). Cancer registry data have many valuable uses, such as evaluation of cancer incidence patterns, cancer risk factors, effects of prevention and early detection efforts, survival patterns, and treatment effects. In the United States, the National Cancer Institute's Surveillance, Epidemiology, and End Results (SEER) Program has collected population-based data on newly diagnosed cancers since 1973, covering approximately 48% of the US population.[18] SEER is designed to assemble and periodically report estimates of cancer incidence, mortality, survival, and prevalence in the United States and monitor trends in cancer over time, among other important functions.[18]

The US Centers for Disease Control and Prevention established the National Program of Cancer Registries (NPCR; Public Law 102-515) and has funded 45 states, the District of Columbia, and three US territories to develop registries or to enhance current registries. The NPCR provides cancer incidence information on 96% of the US population, and the data are designed to monitor cancer trends and patterns over time in various populations, guide planning and evaluation of cancer control programs, and help set priorities for allocating health resources.[19]

Prevention

Several studies have been conducted to estimate the proportion of overall cancer deaths attributable to various modifiable causes.[20–23] The Harvard Center for Cancer Prevention[24] and Danaei et al.[25] provide a useful benchmark on which to base preventive efforts. It is estimated that 19% of cancer diagnoses and 29% of cancer deaths are a result of cigarette smoking.[20] Cancer cases and deaths in the United States are also largely attributable to excess body weight (7.8% and 6.5%, respectively) and alcohol use (5.6% and 4.0%, respectively). Other factors toward which prevention efforts should be directed include poor diet, physical inactivity, exposure to ultraviolet radiation, and certain carcinogenic infections, including *H. pylori*, hepatitis B and C, and human papillomavirus.[20]

In 1985 the National Cancer Institute set a goal of reducing cancer mortality by 50% by the year 2000 through the systematic application of existing cancer control technologies.[26] Although this 50% goal proved to be overly ambitious and was not achieved, it was extremely beneficial in focusing cancer control efforts at all levels of public health practice. The National Cancer Moonshot Initiative, launched in January 2016 to accelerate cancer research, aims to make more therapies available to more patients while also improving our ability to prevent cancer and detect it at an early stage.[27] The renewed Cancer Moonshot Initiative, announced in February 2022, set an ambitious goal of reducing cancer deaths by at least 50% over the next 25 years. To achieve this goal, in addition to increasing research funds, the government and its associated health agencies will need to address the social determinants of health, including access to care and adequate insurance coverage.

In addition to setting these National Cancer Institute goals, the US Public Health Service has established a variety of objectives related to cancer prevention and control through the use of evidence-based measures in Healthy People 2030.[28] It has been noted that without a stronger US commitment to cancer prevention, public health goals for reducing cancer mortality are unlikely to be achieved.[29,30]

Screening

Primary and secondary prevention through population-based screening programs are available for some, but not all, cancer types. Following a comprehensive review of the literature, the US Preventive Services Task Force (USPSTF) issues evidence-based recommendations. These guidelines are revisited at regular intervals and include a period for public comment on draft recommendation statements. Screening recommendations are graded from A (recommends the service with high certainty that the net benefit is substantial) to D (recommends against the service).[31] Other organizations, including ACS, the National Comprehensive Cancer Network, and professional organizations like the American Urological Association, publish their own screening recommendations, which may not agree with USPSTF recommendations. Nonetheless, this section summarizes only the current USPSTF recommendations, as they may be used to determine insurance coverage for services, and includes only cancers detailed in this chapter (Table 17-2).[31] Screening modalities are not currently available for leukemia and lymphoma.

Treatment

A cancer treatment plan will vary according to cancer subtype, available treatment options, and patient preferences and goals. Discussions of plans should take place between care provider teams, patients, and when appropriate, patients' families and caregivers. Patients may wish to communicate with their provider team about their priorities, including attempting a cure, alleviating symptoms, maintaining quality of life, or seeking palliation. Most cancers are treated with either surgery, radiation therapy, chemotherapy,

Table 17-2. Summary of Current US Preventive Services Task Force Recommendations for Cancer Screening

Cancer	Year of Most Recent Publication	Grade	Summary of Recommendations
Bladder	2011 (updated 2021)	I	Current evidence is deemed insufficient to assess the balance of benefits and harms of screening for bladder cancer in asymptomatic adults.
Breast	2016	B, C	**Grade B:** Biennial screening mammography is recommended for women aged 50–74 years. **Grade C:** The decision to start screening mammography in women prior to 50 years of age should be an individual one; women may choose to begin biennial screening between the ages of 40 and 49 years.
Cervical	2018	A, D	**Grade A:** Screening for cervical cancer should take place every three years with cervical cytology in women aged 21–29 years. For women aged 30–65 years, screening should take place every three years with cervical cytology alone, every 5 years with high-risk human papillomavirus (hrHPV) testing alone, or every 5 years with hrHPV testing in combination with cytology (co-testing). **Grade D:** The task force recommends against screening for cervical cancer in women aged <21 years; in women who have had a hysterectomy with removal of the cervix; and in women aged >65 years who are not at high risk.
Colorectal	2021	A, B, C	**Grade A:** Screening for colorectal cancer is recommended for all adults aged 50–75 years. **Grade B:** Screening for colorectal cancer is recommended for adults aged 45–49 years. **Grade C:** Clinicians should selectively offer screening for colorectal cancer in adults aged 76–85 years.
Lung	2021	B	Annual screening for lung cancer with low-dose computed tomography (LDCT) is recommended for adults aged 50–80 years who have a 20-pack-year smoking history and currently smoke or have quit within the past 15 years. Screening should be discontinued once a person has not smoked for 15 years or develops a health problem that substantially limits life expectancy or the ability or willingness to have curative lung surgery.
Skin	2016	I	Current evidence is insufficient to assess the balance of benefits and harms of visual skin examination by a clinician to screen for skin cancer in adults.
Oral	2013	I	Current evidence is insufficient to assess the balance of benefits and harms of screening for oral cancer in asymptomatic adults.
Prostate	2018	C, D	**Grade C:** For men aged 55–69 years, the decision to undergo periodic prostate-specific antigen (PSA)-based screening for prostate cancer should be an individual one. Before deciding whether to be screened, men should have an opportunity to discuss the potential benefits and harms of screening with their clinician and to incorporate their values and preferences in the decision. **Grade D:** The task force recommends against PSA-based screening for prostate cancer in men aged >70 years.

Source: Based on US Preventive Services Task Force.[31]

Note: hrHPV = high-risk human papillomavirus; LDCT = low-dose computed tomography; PSA = prostate-specific antigen.

or a combination of these approaches. More recently, immunotherapy—that is, treatment that uses a patient's immune system to help fight the cancer—has emerged as a "fourth pillar" of cancer treatment for patients diagnosed with both solid and hematologic cancers.[32,33] Current developments in the areas of personalized medicine and targeted therapies continue to add new tools to the cancer-fighting arsenal, with the hope of reducing morbidity and mortality across cancer types.

Summary

Describing each cancer site in detail in this chapter would be impractical. Therefore, we have limited this discussion to cancers that have one or more of the following characteristics: (1) they account for a major proportion of all cancer cases, or (2) they can be reduced through scientifically proven prevention and control measures.

Cancer is a disease of aging, with rates of new diagnoses increasing with age. As the US population ages, cancer incidence is expected to rise, along with the need for improved access to care, innovative treatments, support for patients and their caregivers, and care for survivors. However, through reduction in risk factors and adherence to national screening recommendations, people may prevent cancer or catch the disease at earlier stages. Furthermore, the development of new and effective treatment options, including those tailored to specific molecular subtypes of cancer, will continue to reduce morbidity and mortality from this disease.

LUNG CANCER

Significance

Lung cancer is the leading cause of cancer deaths in the United States and accounted for an estimated 130,180 deaths in 2022.[34] Lung cancer is also the most common cause of cancer death worldwide. This high mortality rate results from both a high incidence rate and a low survival: only 22% of US lung cancer patients survive five years after diagnosis.[34] There has been some improvement in lung cancer survival recently with the three-year survival increasing from 19% in 2001 to 31% in 2017.[34]

Pathophysiology

Lung cancers often arise from the cells lining the bronchi or in other parts of the lung, including the bronchioles, which are smaller branches of the bronchi, or the alveoli, which are air sacs that absorb oxygen into the blood and remove carbon dioxide from the blood.[35] There are two main types of lung cancer: non-small cell and small cell. The major types of non-small cell lung cancer are adenocarcinoma (~ 44% of all lung cancers), squamous cell cancer (~20% of all lung cancers), and large-cell cancer (~1% of all lung cancers).[36] Small-cell lung cancer (~11% of all lung cancers) appears to grow and spread the most rapidly.[35,36] Numerous genetic factors have been associated with an increased risk of lung cancer; these are likely to involve a variety of cellular pathways, including DNA repair, cell cycle, and detoxification.[37,38]

Descriptive Epidemiology

Lung cancer incidence trends largely reflect smoking prevalence trends, as smoking is the cause of the vast majority of lung cancer in the United States. Thus, its descriptive epidemiology mirrors smoking patterns and trends (see Chapter 7). Among males, lung cancer mortality is highest among Black males, followed by White males and American Indian/Alaska Native males.[34] Among females, lung cancer mortality is highest among White females, followed by American Indian/Alaska Native females and Black females. Lung cancer incidence and mortality are also highest in states with the highest smoking prevalence, including Kentucky.[34] Lung cancer incidence decreased between 2009 and 2018 by almost 3% annually in men and 1% annually in women. In women, the decline started after men and has been slower, as women began smoking later than men and were slower to quit smoking.[34] In men, lung cancer mortality has declined by 56% between 1990 and 2019. In women, lung cancer mortality has declined by 32% between 2002 and 2019.[34] Three-year survival has increased in recent years, from 19% in 2001 to 31% in 2017, largely as a result of improvements in diagnostic procedures and treatments.[34]

Risk Factors and Prevention

The strongest risk factor for lung cancer is cigarette smoking (Figure 17-3). Approximately 81% of lung cancer deaths in 2020 were attributed to smoking and another 2% to secondhand smoke exposure. The association between smoking and lung cancer is one of the most widely studied and clearly defined relationships in chronic disease epidemiology. People who currently smoke cigarettes have a sevenfold or higher risk of lung cancer than people who never smoke, and risk increases with increased smoking intensity and/or duration.[39,40] Exposure to radon gas increases the risk of lung cancer.[40] Radon is naturally occurring and can become more concentrated indoors. The Environmental Protection Agency lists radon as the second-most common cause of lung cancer in the United States and the leading cause among nonsmokers. People exposed to asbestos also have several times' higher risk of lung cancer; risk is further increased among those who also smoke. Among dietary factors, convincing evidence shows that arsenic in drinking water and intake of high-dose supplements of beta-carotene increases the risk of lung cancer.[41]

USPSTF recommends annual screening for lung cancer with low-dose computed tomography (LDCT) in adults aged 50 to 80 years who have a 20-pack-year smoking history and currently smoke or have quit within the past 15 years (Table 17-2).[42] Once a person reaches 15 years since smoking cessation or develops a health problem that limits life expectancy or the ability to have curative surgery, screening should be discontinued. Lung cancer screening has been low overall, with just 5% among eligible individuals in 2018. However, screening prevalence was as high as 10% to 15% in some states, including Kentucky, where lung cancer incidence is high.[34]

Areas of Future Research

Smoking remains a major cause of lung cancer. Continued research into the most effective methods to increase smoking cessation and prevent smoking initiation are still needed. In addition, strategies to improve access to and uptake of lung cancer screening among those at highest risk could improve outcomes. Additional research is also needed to better understand the descriptive epidemiology of lung cancer among never-smokers and associated risk factors; this research may be aided by the addition of smoking status to some cancer registries.[34]

COLORECTAL CANCER

Significance

Cancer of the colon and rectum, also known as colorectal cancer, is the third-most commonly diagnosed cancer and the third leading cause of cancer death in men and women in the United States.[34] In 2022 it was estimated that approximately 80,690 new cases of colon and rectum cancer would be diagnosed in men and 70,340 new cases would be diagnosed in women. The overall five-year survival rate for colorectal cancer is 65%, with a rate of 91% for cancers identified in the local stage.[34] However, only 34% of cases are diagnosed at local stage.[34] Early colorectal cancers often have no symptoms, and thus they are not detected without screening.[43]

Pathophysiology

Colorectal cancers typically begin as a growth, or polyp, on the inner lining, or mucosal layer, of the colon or rectum.[43] Polyps can be broadly grouped into three categories: adenomas, sessile polyps, and hyperplastic polyps. Some, but not all, polyps can become cancer, usually over the course of many years. Most colorectal cancers are sporadic or occur among those without a family history or inherited syndrome.[44] More than 90% of colorectal cancers are adenocarcinomas. Adenomas are the precursors for 85% to 90% of sporadic colorectal cancers.[44] Although only around 10% of adenomas develop into cancer, several factors increase the likelihood, including larger size (≥1 cm in surface diameter), multiplicity, degree of dysplasia, and villous histology.[44] Sessile polyps are a heterogeneous group of lesions, including traditional and sessile serrated adenomas, which are precursors for 10% to 15% of sporadic colorectal cancers.[44] Hyperplastic polyps, previously thought to lack malignant potential, are the most prevalent type of sessile polyp, and a subset of such polyps can progress into colorectal cancer.[44]

Descriptive Epidemiology

Colorectal cancer incidence and mortality increase steeply with age and are higher in men than in women. Colorectal cancer incidence is highest among those who are non-Hispanic Black and American Indian/Alaska Native and lowest among Asians/Pacific Islanders. Of note, colorectal cancer mortality between 2013 and 2017 was 50% higher among non-Hispanic Blacks than among non-Hispanic Whites.[45] Colorectal cancer also varies within widely defined racial/ethnic groups; Alaska Natives have the highest incidence and mortality in the United States, with rates nearly twice those of non-Hispanic Blacks. Since the mid-1980s colorectal cancer incidence has declined overall, with steeper declines in the 2000s, which has been attributed to changes in risk factors, such as a decrease in smoking and increases in colorectal cancer screening. However, among those younger than 50 years of age, incidence rates have been increasing by 1.5% per year, and the reasons for this increase are unknown.[34] Like incidence rates overall, colorectal cancer mortality rates have also been decreasing over time, 1.8% per year between 2012 and 2017.[46]

Risk Factors and Prevention

Nonmodifiable risk factors include family history and certain health conditions. Approximately 25% of colorectal cancers occur among those with family history of colorectal cancer or adenomas.[44] Hereditary syndromes, including familial adenomatous polyposis and hereditary nonpolyposis colorectal cancer, account for approximately 5% of colorectal cancer.[44] Inflammatory bowel disease also increases risk of colorectal cancer through chronic inflammation, though it explains less than 2% of colorectal cancer.[44] People with type 2 diabetes also have an increased risk of colorectal cancer.[43]

There is now considerable evidence that several lifestyle factors influence colorectal cancer risk. Smoking is a risk factor for colorectal cancer.[47] Body fatness increases risk, whereas physical activity decreases risk.[41] With regard to diet, consuming whole grains, dairy, and foods high in dietary fiber decreases risk, whereas consuming alcohol, red meat, and processed meat increases risk.[41] The International Agency for Research on Cancer classified red meat as a probable carcinogen to humans and processed meat as a carcinogen to humans largely on the basis of the associations with colorectal cancer.[48]

Current evidence suggests that a substantial proportion of colorectal cancer incidence and death can be potentially prevented through lifestyle modification.[49]

The principal screening tests for early detection of colorectal cancer are colonoscopy, sigmoidoscopy, stool tests for occult blood, CT colonography, and multi-targeted stool DNA tests. Colorectal cancer screening via colonoscopy not only can prevent cancer through the detection and removal of precancerous polyps but also can detect cancer at an earlier stage, when survival is higher. Thus, it decreases colorectal cancer mortality by reducing incidence and improving survival. USPSTF recommends colorectal screening for average-risk adults aged 45 to 75 years (Table 17-2).[50] Follow-up screens are determined on the basis of screening results and methodology. Colonoscopies are performed every 10 years for average-risk adults and at more frequent intervals for people who have had precancerous polyps previously detected. Stool-based tests are performed every one to three years and require a follow-up colonoscopy if positive. Despite the benefit of screening, only 67% of those between ages 50 and 75 years in the United States report having had a recent colorectal cancer screening test; rates are particularly low (30%) for those individuals without insurance.[46] Improving access to colorectal cancer screening across all populations could have an important impact on colorectal cancer burden in the United States.[46]

Areas of Future Research

Colorectal cancer has been increasing among those less than 50 years of age. Additional research into whether the colorectal cancer risk factors among younger adults are similar to or distinct from those among older adults will lead to increased opportunities for primary prevention and help to further optimize screening strategies. In addition, given the pronounced difference in mortality among Black or Native American/Alaska Native individuals as compared with those who are non-Hispanic White, additional work is needed to address disparities in the social determinants of health and access to care that contribute to colorectal cancer incidence and mortality.

BREAST CANCER

Significance

Breast cancer is the most common cancer type among women in the United States and the second leading cause of cancer death.[2] It was estimated that in 2022 there would be 287,850 new cases of invasive cancer and 43,250 deaths among females.[2] Breast cancer rarely occurs in men, accounting for less than 1% of breast cancer cases in the United States.[2] Approximately one of every eight women will develop breast cancer during her lifetime, with an overall five-year survival rate of 90%.[51] However, survival can range from 29% for distant-stage cancer to 99% for local-stage cancer.[51]

Pathophysiology

Noninvasive breast lesions can be confined to the duct (ductal carcinoma in situ) or to the lobule (lobular carcinoma in situ), and some of their forms can be considered precursor lesions of invasive carcinoma.[52] The predominant cell type of breast cancer is adenocarcinoma (~95% of cases). Hormones, both endogenous and exogenous, play a role in breast cancer pathogenesis, as they increase cell proliferation in the breast and the opportunity for random genetic errors during cell division deaths.[53] Proliferation is mediated by hormone receptors. Estrogen and progesterone receptors are often present in breast cancer tumors. When receptors are present above a certain threshold value, the tumor is considered receptor positive. Women with receptor-positive tumors respond better to hormonal therapy and show increased survival rates; they may also have different risk factors than women with receptor-negative disease.

Descriptive Epidemiology

Incidence and mortality increase with age, with the risk of being diagnosed ranging from 1 in 204 (0.5%) at age 30 to 1 in 24 (4.1%) at age 70.[51] Although the incidence of breast cancer is higher in Whites, mortality rates are 35% higher among Black women than among White women.[54] Disparities in health outcomes are attributed to tumor behavior, psychosocial or behavioral factors, socioeconomic status, variation in access to care, and screening and treatment differences.[55]

Breast cancer incidence rates in the United States rose sharply throughout the 1980s, in part because of the increase in use of mammography screening. Later, incidence rates decreased slightly from 132 per 100,000 in 1990 to 124 per 100,000 in 2004, remaining relatively stable since 2004 for White women (119/100,000 in 1990 to 118/100,000 in 2004) but slightly increased for Black women.[56] Between 1973 and 1990, breast cancer mortality rates increased 2% among US women overall and 21% among Black women.[57] Since 1990 the overall breast cancer mortality rate has decreased by 36%, with data from 2003 to 2010 establishing the decrease at a rate of 1.9% per year among White women and 1.4% among Black women.[58] Overall age-adjusted death rates have decreased 1.3% per year on average between 2010 and 2019.[51]

Risk Factors and Prevention

Nonmodifiable risk factors are family history of breast cancer, genetic predispositions (*BRCA1*, *BRCA2*, and other genes), history of radiation exposure, early menarche, late menopause, nulliparity, and race.[59] Women with a first-degree relative with breast cancer have up to a threefold increased risk of developing the disease.[60] Mutations in *BRCA1* (breast cancer 1) or *BRCA2* (breast cancer 2) genes correspond with a 72% and 69%

(respectively) risk of developing breast cancer by age 80.[61] These germline mutations likely account for 2% to 5% of all breast cancers, while hundreds of common genetic variants also have been shown to increase risk.[62] Previous diagnosis of high-risk breast lesions is also associated with significant increased risk of incident breast cancer. Higher mammographic density—that is, the percentage of breast tissue that appears dense on a mammogram—is also a strong risk factor for breast cancer.[63]

Through numerous epidemiologic studies, an array of modifiable breast cancer risk factors has been established. Despite the large number of risk factors, few are strongly associated with the development of breast cancer, and no single factor or combination of factors can predict the occurrence of breast cancer in any one individual.

The risk associated with reproductive variables—never having children, being of a late age at first birth, having an early menarche, having a late menopause—is related to the hormonal environment to which the breast tissue is exposed (e.g., during pregnancy, during a long menstrual history).[53,57] Conversely, lactation is associated with a 4.3% decrease in risk for every 12 months of breast-feeding.[64]

Increased body fat is associated with an increased risk among postmenopausal women and decreased risk among premenopausal women.[53] Physical activity has an inverse, dose–response effect on breast cancer risk.

Investigation of endogenous hormones has shown an increased risk of breast cancer among premenopausal women with high blood levels of insulin-like growth factor 1 and among postmenopausal women with high blood estrogens. Exogenous hormones, such as oral contraceptive and postmenopausal hormones, have been associated with an increased risk of breast cancer.[65,66] Although current and recent users of oral contraceptives may have a slight elevation in risk, these women tend to be younger with a low absolute risk. Likewise, current users of postmenopausal hormones and those with the longest duration of use are also at an increased risk of breast cancer, though this risk is mitigated if hormone use has stopped for five or more years, regardless of previous duration.

Several dietary factors have also been examined in relation to breast cancer risk. Current evidence regarding fat and fruit and vegetable intake has been inconclusive or unsupportive of a relationship to breast cancer risk.[53] However, beta-carotene and folate intake do appear to be protective against breast cancer. Moderate-to-heavy alcohol consumption is associated with an increased risk of breast cancer.[67] High intake of folic acid may protect against the risk associated with alcohol intake.[68]

Areas of Future Research

Although several possible risk factors for breast cancer—diet, alcohol use, physical inactivity—are amenable to primary prevention, more research is required to identify the best policies or interventions at a population level.[69] Another ongoing area of research is identifying risk factors for specific molecular subtypes (often defined by estrogen and progesterone receptor status, but also using other methods). Many well-known risk factors have been differentially associated with different subtypes,[70] and future epidemiologic studies considering these subtypes may identify new risk factors.

CERVICAL CANCER

Significance

Invasive cancer of the uterine cervix, commonly known as cervical cancer, had an estimated 14,100 new cases diagnosed and 4,280 deaths in the United States in 2022.[34] In situ cervical cancer—that is, cervical cancer detected in the earliest, premalignant stage—is much more common, accounting for about 60,000 US cases per year. Cervical cancer is the 21st most common cancer in the United States, yet it is the fourth most common cancer among women worldwide, with an estimated 604,127 incident cases in 2020.[71] The overall five-year survival rate for cervical cancer is 66% in the United States; however, this ranges from 92% for localized disease to 18% for distant stage disease.[2]

Pathophysiology

Nearly all cases of cervical cancer are believed to result from persistent infection with one of about 15 genotypes of carcinogenic human papilloma virus (HPV).[72] There are four major steps in cervical cancer development: (1) infection of metaplastic epithelium at the cervical transformation zone, (2) viral persistence, (3) progression of persistently infected epithelium to cervical precancer, and (4) invasion through the basement membrane of the epithelium. Early stages of cervical cancer are characterized by dysplasia, or the presence of cells that are altered in size, shape, and organization. Preclinical, preinvasive changes in the cervix are called cervical intraepithelial neoplasia. These early cervical cancer changes can easily be detected through the Papanicolaou (Pap) test, which involves collecting and analyzing a small sample of cells from the cervix. The major cell types observed for invasive cervical cancer are squamous cell cancer (~65% of cases) and adenocarcinoma (~28% of cases).[73]

Descriptive Epidemiology

Cervical cancer incidence increases sharply until age 45 and peaks around that age. The incidence of cervical cancer is higher among Black women (8.8/100,000) than among Whites (7.2/100,000), with mortality rates significantly higher among Black women than White women (3.4 vs. 2.0/100,000).[34] Elevated cervical cancer rates are also observed for Hispanics, American Indians, and Hawaiian natives. Women of lower socioeconomic status are at higher risk of cervical cancer.

Between 1975 and 2012, invasive cervical cancer incidence has decreased by half (14.8/100,000 to 6.7/100,000).[4] In women younger than 50 years, these rates remained steady from 2008 to 2012, but then declined through 2017.[74] Survival for cervical cancer patients has not improved over the last few decades, likely because of a lack of treatment advances and an increasing proportion of diagnosed adenocarcinoma, which is not easily detected by current screening methods.[34] Cervical cancer remains the second leading cause of cancer death (after breast cancer) among women aged 20 to 39 years.[34]

Risk Factors and Prevention

The primary risk factor for cervical cancer is infection with HPV. This virus is now accepted to be the central, necessary cause of virtually all cases of cervical cancer.[75] There are likely more than 100 types of HPV, with about 30 of these transmitted by sexual contact, and approximately 20 causally related to cervical cancer. The relative risk for HPV-DNA and cervical cancer was estimated at 158 (95% CI, 113–221) in the International Agency for Research on Cancer multicenter study,[76] among the highest effect sizes observed for any human cancer.[77] Estimates of attributable risk for HPV infection and cervical cancer range from 90% to 98%, suggesting that nearly all cases of cervical cancer are attributable to HPV infection.

Given that HPV infection is a necessary cause, many risk factors relate to the likelihood of HPV infection. Furthermore, while HPV infection is common, most infections do not lead to invasive cancer, suggesting the presence of other risk factors. Other established risk factors for cervical cancer include long-term use of hormonal contraceptives, cigarette smoking, five or more pregnancies, and sexual risk factors: partners with greater than six other sexual partners and HPV infection in a male partner.[77] Several behavioral changes may reduce the risk of cervical cancer, including limiting the number of sexual partners, delaying intercourse until a later age, using protection or choosing abstinence to avoid sexually transmitted infections, and eliminating cigarette smoking.

Three vaccines have been approved by the US Food and Drug Administration for the prevention of the HPV infection, with Gardasil 9 being the only vaccine used in the United States since 2016. It is recommended that individuals receive the vaccine between 9 and 26 years of age. If given before individuals engage in sexual activity, the vaccines are considered highly effective in preventing the HPV infection. The approved vaccine provides protection against infection with these HPV types for at least 10 years.

Areas of Future Research

Further research into the causes of cervical cancer will lead to increased opportunities for primary prevention. A better understanding of the interaction among multiple risk factors is also needed. Given the high rates of cervical cancer mortality among minority and economically disadvantaged women, better targeting of proven cervical cancer control measures is clearly needed.

PROSTATE CANCER

Significance

Prostate cancer is the most common cancer diagnosed among men and the second most common cause of cancer death among men in the United States. In 2022 it was estimated that approximately 268,490 new prostate cancer cases would be diagnosed and that 34,500 prostate cancer deaths would occur.[34] Approximately 12.5% of men will be diagnosed with prostate cancer during their lifetime. The five-year survival of prostate cancer is 97.5%.[78]

Descriptive Epidemiology

Prostate cancer incidence rates increased dramatically in the early 1990s with the detection of asymptomatic prostate cancer via the widespread use of prostate-specific antigen (PSA) screening.[79] While mortality rates decreased and five-year survival increased overall since this time, primarily as a result of a combination of better treatments, early detection, and overdiagnosis of PSA-detected indolent cancers, there has more recently been an increase in prostate cancer deaths likely as a consequence of recent past changes in screening recommendations. It is important to note that the risk of prostate cancer is 73% higher in Black men than in non-Hispanic White men.[2] Furthermore, Black men are at least two times more likely to die of prostate cancer than any other group.[73] While there are many hypotheses, including genetics, the prevalence of risk factors, and screening and treatment disparities, the reasons underlying these differences are not well understood.

Risk Factors and Prevention

The causes of prostate cancer are largely unknown. The only conclusive risk factors are not modifiable, and these include older age, African ancestry, and family history of prostate cancer,[80] as well as common and rare genetic variants.[81,82] Although obesity and smoking do not appear to increase risk overall, both increase the risk of aggressive or fatal disease.[47,83]

Areas of Future Research

Prostate cancer is extremely common, as autopsy studies show that approximately 35% of White men and 51% of Black men aged 70 to 79 years had detectable prostate cancer.[84] However, most men with prostate cancer die with their disease and not from it. A current and future direction of prostate cancer epidemiologic research is to focus more on identifying risk factors specifically for aggressive and fatal prostate cancer.[85]

LYMPHOMA

Significance

Lymphomas are cancers that affect a type of white blood cell called lymphocytes, primarily in the lymph nodes, spleen, and thymus. Lymphomas are generally classified as either Hodgkin lymphoma or non-Hodgkin lymphoma. If an abnormal cell type called a Reed-Sternberg cell is detected in a patient's cancer cells, then the lymphoma is classified as Hodgkin lymphoma. Otherwise, the lymphoma is classified as non-Hodgkin lymphoma.[61]

Hodgkin Lymphoma

In 2021 an estimated 8,830 cases of Hodgkin lymphoma were reported, and 960 deaths occurred.[86] The overall risk of being diagnosed with Hodgkin lymphoma over a lifetime is 0.2%, as deducted on the basis of data from 2016 to 2018.[86] Hodgkin lymphoma has two main subtypes: classical Hodgkin lymphoma and nodular lymphocyte-predominant Hodgkin lymphoma. Classical Hodgkin lymphoma is further divided into four subtypes that together account for approximately 95% of all Hodgkin lymphoma cases.

Non-Hodgkin Lymphoma

In 2021 there were an estimated 81,560 new diagnoses of non-Hodgkin lymphoma and 20,720 deaths.[87] Approximately 2.1% of men and women will be diagnosed with non-Hodgkin's lymphoma at some point during their lifetime, given the 2016 to 2018 data.[87] Non-Hodgkin lymphoma has over 60 histologic subtypes, with the two most common subtypes—diffuse large B-cell lymphoma (DLBCL) and follicular lymphoma—accounting for about half of all non-Hodgkin lymphoma cases.

Descriptive Epidemiology

Hodgkin Lymphoma

The age distribution of Hodgkin lymphoma incidence is bimodal, with one peak in young adulthood and a second after ages 55 to 60 years. Known risk factors for Hodgkin lymphoma include family history of lymphoma, male sex, and past infection with Epstein-Barr virus. The risk of Hodgkin lymphoma is also higher in immunosuppressed people, including those infected with HIV.[2] Incidence rates are slightly higher in White populations than other race/ethnic groups.[86] However, patients with lower socioeconomic status, as well as Black and Hispanic patients, had an increased risk of Hodgkin lymphoma–specific mortality compared with patients having highest socioeconomic status and with White patients, respectively.[88–90] Across subtypes, the five-year relative survival rate is 89.1%, calculated on the basis of data from 2012 to 2018.[86]

Non-Hodgkin Lymphoma

The incidence of non-Hodgkin lymphoma overall is higher among men compared with women and is higher among Whites compared with other race/ethnic groups.[87] Non-Hodgkin lymphoma risk factors include increasing age, family history of non-Hodgkin lymphoma, and having a weakened immune system (e.g. organ transplant recipients), certain autoimmune diseases, and certain infections. Exposure to radiation, specific chemicals, or drugs, including prior chemotherapy, may also increase the risk of developing non-Hodgkin lymphoma later in life.[2,91,92] The US incidence rate of non-Hodgkin lymphoma has decreased by 0.9% each year, and death rates have been falling on average 2.2% each year between 2010 and 2019.[87]

The five-year relative survival rate across all subtypes of non-Hodgkin lymphoma is 73.8%, according to data from 2012 to 2018; however, this rate varies between aggressive and indolent histological subtypes.[87]

Risk Factors and Prevention

The causes of lymphoma are not well understood, in part because of the diversity of histologic forms of cancer in these diagnoses. Immune system disorders, infection with HIV or Epstein-Barr virus, and treatment with immunosuppressive drugs (e.g., in transplant patients) increase risk of non-Hodgkin lymphoma.[93] There is also some evidence that exposure to certain herbicides and pesticides elevates non-Hodgkin lymphoma risk, including phenoxy acid–based herbicides (such as 2,4-dichloro-phenoxyacetic acid) and chlorophenols.

Current evidence indicates the Epstein-Barr virus may play a role in the development of a subset of classical Hodgkin lymphoma cases on the basis of its epidemiologic features, age at onset, and spatial clustering.[62,94]

Because the causes of lymphoma are not fully understood, clear prevention strategies are unavailable. Given the growing evidence of an association between pesticide use and non-Hodgkin lymphoma, however, prudent use of these chemicals is warranted. No screening tests are yet available for the early detection of lymphoma. More research is needed to clarify the role of obesity, physical activity, and diet in the development of non-Hodgkin lymphoma.

Although the five-year survival for Hodgkin lymphoma is high, treatment for Hodgkin lymphoma appears to result in a high rate of secondary malignancies later in life.[62,95]

Recent years have seen a gradual shift in treatment regimens to minimize late complications and toxicities of therapy.

Areas of Future Research

Recently, molecular subtypes of DLBCL, a common and aggressive form of non-Hodgkin lymphoma, have been identified: germinal center B-cell (GCB) and activated B-cell (ABC). Research has shown that patients with different subtypes of DLBCL may respond differently to treatment. Further research could continue to investigate the differences in molecular subtypes of lymphoma with regard to risk factors, treatment response, and patient outcome. In addition, several subtypes of lymphoma tend to recur (e.g., follicular lymphoma). More research is needed to identify factors that predict recurrence and to identify patients at high risk for disease recurrence.

LEUKEMIA

Significance

Leukemia comprises a variety of cancers that arise in the bone marrow, lymph nodes, or other lymphoid tissue with immune function. Leukemia affects both children and adults and accounts for about 25% of cancers among children and 2% of newly diagnosed adult cancer cases per year.[54,96] There are four main types of leukemia: acute myeloid (including acute monocytic) leukemia, acute lymphocytic leukemia, chronic lymphocytic leukemia, and chronic myeloid leukemia. In the United States, acute lymphocytic leukemia accounts for 75% of leukemia cases among children.[2] The most common leukemia types among adults are chronic lymphocytic leukemia (38%) and acute myeloid leukemia (31%).

Descriptive Epidemiology

Leukemia is 61% more common among men in the United States than among women and is more common in White than in Black or Hispanic populations.[97] Across all ages, leukemia mortality has declined over the past 50 years. In 1975 the five-year survival rate for leukemia was just 33%. The five-year survival rate increased to 59% in 2005 and 65% from 2011 to 2017.[97] In particular, over the past few decades survival among children with acute lymphocytic leukemia has increased dramatically (from just 10% in the 1960s to 76% in children aged 0–14 years and 92% in adolescents aged 15–19 years in 2011–2017) as the result of improvements in therapy.[2,98] Across all subtypes, leukemia incidence among children and adolescents increased by about 1% per year from 2009 to 2018, although rates in adults remained stable. From 2010 to 2019, the mortality rate from leukemia declined by 3% per year in children and 2% per year in adults, although rates vary by subtype.[2]

Risk Factors and Prevention

The major causes of leukemia are unknown; however, several risk factors have been identified, including genetic abnormalities such as Down syndrome, exposure to ionizing radiation, including treatments for prior cancers, and workplace exposure to benzene and other related solvents.[2] Adult T-cell leukemia is strongly associated with infection by human T-lymphotrophic virus, type 1, in endemic areas.[99] Increasing evidence suggests that cigarette smoking is a causative risk factor for some forms of leukemia, including acute myeloid leukemia, in adults.[47] Some evidence suggests parental smoking in the pre- and postnatal periods may increase the risk of acute leukemia in children, but further research is needed to clarify this association.[100] Earlier hypotheses that residential exposure to magnetic fields may increase leukemia risk among children have not been consistent, and overall evidence is weak.[101]

Because the causes of leukemia are largely undetermined, primary prevention is difficult. Reducing occupational and environmental exposures to radiation and leukemogenic chemicals and eliminating cigarette smoking may reduce leukemia incidence. Because symptoms often appear late, diagnosing leukemia early is difficult and no routine screening test exists.

BLADDER CANCER

Significance

Bladder cancer is the most common cancer of the urinary tract, estimated to account for 81,180 new cases and 17,100 deaths in the United States in 2022.[2]

Pathophysiology

Bladder carcinoma in situ is the only in situ disease that is required to be reported to registries. In situ means that the cancer is confined to where it began growing and has not spread beyond this layer of tissue. Despite being noninvasive, bladder carcinoma in situ has a high rate of recurrence after treatment and can progress to invasive disease, though five-year survival is high in this group (96%).[2] Most bladder cancers are urothelial carcinomas (90%), and squamous cell carcinoma, a more aggressive form of the disease, is the second most common histological subtype (~5%).

Descriptive Epidemiology

The incidence rate of bladder cancer is almost four times higher among men than women, and about two times higher among Whites than Blacks.[4,102] However, five-year survival is higher among Whites (78%) than Blacks (65%)[2] in recent years. In addition, the mortality rate in both men and women is 4.2 per 100,000, but this is notable because the incidence of bladder cancer is significantly higher in men than women.[102] The reasons for the striking differences in incidence and survival by sex and race are not well established. After decades of slight increases, incidence rates of bladder cancer declined by about 1% from 2009 to 2018.[2] Furthermore, the mortality rate decreased 1.7% per year from 2015 to 2017 after years of stable mortality.[2]

Risk Factors and Prevention

Cigarette smoking is the best-established cause of bladder cancer. Bladder cancer risk for someone who currently smokes is approximately three times that for a nonsmoker, and smoking is estimated to account for 50% to 65% of cases in men and 20% to 30% of cases in women.[103,104] More than 40 occupational groups and exposures have been associated with bladder cancer, yet only a few of these are well established.[101] Among these, bladder cancer incidence was highest for workers exposed to aromatic amines and polycyclic aromatic hydrocarbons, including tobacco and dye workers, and chimney sweeps.[105] Bladder cancer mortality was highest for workers exposed to heavy metals and polycyclic aromatic hydrocarbons, including chemical and metal workers.[105]

Areas of Future Research

Understanding the biological reasons for the sex disparities in bladder cancer—with much higher incidence in men but higher mortality in women—is an area of current and future research. A recent study performing molecular subtyping using transcriptomics data observed that the rates of basal/squamous subtype tumors were higher in females, while luminal papillary and neuroendocrine-like subtypes were more common in males.[106] These latter subtypes are thought to be less aggressive, which may suggest a potential reason for the difference in mortality. More research in this area may provide insight into future prevention and treatment strategies.

ORAL AND PHARYNGEAL CANCER

Significance

Cancer of the oral cavity—that is, lip, salivary gland, mouth, and pharynx—accounted for an estimated 54,010 new cases and 10,850 US deaths in 2021.[107]

Descriptive Epidemiology

In the United States, according to data from 2015 to 2019, men are twice as likely to be diagnosed with cancer of the oral cavity and pharynx and have an age-adjusted mortality rate that is 2.8 times higher than that of women. While incidence rates are higher in Whites than other race/ethnic groups, Black persons have the highest age-adjusted mortality rate from oral and pharyngeal cancers. The median age at diagnosis is 64 years. On average, diagnosis rates have increased by 0.9% per year between 2009 and 2018, while mortality rates have increased by 0.4% per year between 2010 and 2019.[107] The overall five-year survival rate for oral cancer in the United States is 67%, although survival for cancer diagnosed in the local stage is 85%.[107]

Risk Factors and Prevention

The use of tobacco in any form—cigarettes, cigars, and pipes, as well as the use of chewing tobacco and snuff—substantially elevates the risk of cancer of the tongue, mouth, and pharynx, and is responsible for up to 30% of oral cancer cases.[108,109] Cigarette smokers have a risk of developing oral cancer that is three times greater than that of nonsmokers.[110] Excessive alcohol consumption is also associated with cancer of the oral cavity. Smoking and drinking are independent risk factors for oral cancer and also interact synergistically to multiply risk.[111] Fruit and vegetable intake, as well as certain nutrients including vitamin C and carotene and other carotenoids, have been shown to have an inverse relationship with oral cancer risk.[112]

Infection with human papillomavirus (HPV) has been associated with oropharyngeal cancer and may cause 73% to 90% of these cancers worldwide.[113] Patients with HPV-positive oropharyngeal tumors may also have better overall survival than patients with HPV-negative tumors.[114] HPV-positive tumors are more often diagnosed among patients who are male, White, or of a younger age, which is likely related to an increase in high-risk oral HPV infection and sexual behaviors among these populations, according to Gillison et al.[115]

Oral and pharyngeal cancers are largely preventable. Oral cancer death rates could be reduced significantly through primary prevention and early detection. Eliminating smoking and smokeless tobacco use and reducing heavy alcohol consumption would substantially reduce oral cancer incidence. In addition, HPV vaccination could help reduce rates of HPV-positive subtypes of oropharyngeal cancer. Recent data provided evidence of herd protection from increasing HPV vaccination rates, with a declining prevalence of vaccine-type oral HPV infection among unvaccinated males.[116]

USPSTF concluded that there is insufficient evidence to recommend screening of the general or high-risk population for oral cancer in the United States, as reported by Olson et al.[110] New techniques to detect precursor lesions, along with additional studies addressing the association between screening and cancer outcomes, are needed before these guidelines could be changed.[115] There currently exists no approved test for HPV in the oral cavity.

In contrast to USPSTF, ACS recommends monthly self-examination of the oral cavity for abnormal lesions, in addition to examination by a dentist or doctor as part of periodic health checkup.[54,117]

Areas of Future Research

Current research is focused on learning about mutations in the DNA of oral and pharyngeal cells that lead to cancer. Genes that are frequently mutated in oropharyngeal cancers include *PIK3CA* and *TP53*. Some studies suggest that testing for mutations in these genes may help identify cancer cases earlier in the disease process. In addition, clinical trials and other studies of treatment for oropharyngeal cancers seek to test and refine new therapies, including targeted drug therapies and immunotherapy.

MELANOMA OF THE SKIN

Significance

Melanoma is a common diagnosis and was expected to be the fifth most common cancer in 2022, with an estimate of 99,780 new cases and 7,650 deaths.[34]

Descriptive Epidemiology

The lifetime probability of developing melanoma is 3.7% for men and 2.5% for women.[34] Melanoma incidence has been increasing for decades, though recent evidence suggests that it has begun to stabilize, with only a 1% increase among those under 50 years of age. The overall five-year survival for melanoma is 93%. However, melanoma has the largest Black-White absolute survival difference (22%). Mortality has been declining, in part as a result of improvements in treatments for metastatic melanoma.

Risk Factors and Prevention

Globally, ultraviolet radiation, from the sun and artificial sources, accounts for an estimated 75% of melanoma cases.[118] Recreational sun exposure, especially intense, repeated, and blistering overdoses during childhood, increases risk for melanoma. Risk is highest among fair-skinned people who sunburn easily. Indoor tanning and artificial sunlamps have also been associated with an increased melanoma risk.[119] A family history of melanoma increases the risk by two to eight times. Both benign acquired nevi (e.g., moles) and atypical nevi (e.g., moles with irregular pigmentation and borders) are markers of increased melanoma risk and precursors of melanoma in some cases.

Although there is currently insufficient evidence to support screening for skin cancer (Table 17-2), USPSTF recommends counseling parents of young children and young people up to age 24 years with fair skin types about minimizing exposure to ultraviolet radiation to reduce their risk of skin cancer.[120]

DISCUSSION QUESTIONS

1. Which risk factors are shared across several cancers? Are they modifiable?
2. Given limited resources, which areas of future research should be prioritized? Which do you think will have the biggest impacts on public health?
3. What efforts related to cancer prevention would you prioritize as a public health official and why? What factors go into making those decisions?

REFERENCES

1. National Cancer Institute. SEER Cancer Stat Facts: cancer of any site. Available at: https://seer.cancer.gov/statfacts/html/all.html. Accessed January 23, 2023.
2. American Cancer Society. *Cancer Facts & Figures 2022*. Atlanta, GA: American Cancer Society; 2022.
3. Siegel RL, Miller KD, Fuchs HE, Jemal A. Cancer statistics, 2021. *CA Cancer J Clin.* 2021;71(1):7–33.
4. American Cancer Society. *Cancer Facts & Figures 2016*. Atlanta, GA: American Cancer Society; 2016.
5. Cancer and heart disease death rates, among men and women aged 45–64 Years—United States, 1999–2018. *MMWR Morb Mortal Wkly Rep*. 2020;69(21):658. doi:10.15585/mmwr.mm6921a46.
6. National Cancer Institute, Surveillance, Epidemiology, and End Results Program. Adjustments for Areas Impacted by Hurricanes Katrina and Rita. November 2021. Available at: https://seer.cancer.gov/data/hurricane.html. Accessed January 24, 2023.
7. National Cancer Institute. SEER Program. SEER*Stat Database: mortality—all COD, aggregated with state, total US (1990–2019). DCCPS, Surveillance Research Program, Surveillance Systems Branch, released April 2022. Underlying mortality data provided by NCHS. Available at: www.cdc.gov/nchs. Accessed January 27, 2023.
8. American Cancer Society. *Cancer Facts & Figures for African American/Black People 2022–2024.* Atlanta, GA: American Cancer Society, 2022.
9. Ghafoor A, Jemal A, Cokkinides V, et al. Cancer statistics for African Americans. *CA Cancer J Clin*. 2002;52(6):326–341.
10. Finegold K, Conmy A, Chu RC, Bosworth A, Sommers BD. *Trends in the US Uninsured Population, 2010–2020*. Issue brief HP-2021-02. Washington, DC: Office of the Assistant Secretary for Planning and Evaluation, US Department of Health and Human Services. February 11, 2021.

11. American Cancer Society. *Cancer Facts & Figures for Hispanics/Latinos 2015–2017*. Atlanta, GA: American Cancer Society; 2015.
12. American Cancer Society. *Cancer Facts & Figures for Hispanic/Latino People 2021–2023*. Atlanta, GA: American Cancer Society; 2021.
13. Howe HL, Wu X, Ries LA, et al. Annual report to the nation on the status of cancer, 1975–2003, featuring cancer among US Hispanic/Latino populations. *Cancer*. 2006;107(8): 1711–1742.
14. American Cancer Society Cancer Action Network. The costs of cancer: 2020 edition. October 2020. Available at: https://www.fightcancer.org/sites/default/files/National%20Documents/Costs-of-Cancer-2020-10222020.pdf. Accessed January 23, 2023.
15. Agency for Healthcare Research and Quality. Medical expenditure panel survey. Available at: https://meps.ahrq.gov/mepsweb/index.jsp. Accessed January 23, 2023.
16. Yabroff KR, Lund J, Kepka D, Mariotto A. Economic burden of cancer in the United States: estimates, projections, and future research. *Cancer Epidemiol Biomarkers Prev*. 2011;20(10): 2006–2014.
17. Giordano TJ. Morphologic and molecular classification of human cancer. In: Schottenfeld D, Fraumeni JF Jr., eds. Cancer *Epidemiology and Prevention*. 3rd ed. New York, NY: Oxford University Press; 2006:10–20.
18. National Cancer Institute. Goals of the SEER Program. Available at: http://seer.cancer.gov/about/goals.html. Accessed January 23, 2023.
19. Centers for Disease Control and Prevention. National Program of Cancer Registries: about the program. 2018. Updated August 31, 2022. Available at: http://www.cdc.gov/cancer/npcr/about.htm. Accessed January 23, 2023.
20. Islami F, Goding Sauer A, Miller KD, et al. Proportion and number of cancer cases and deaths attributable to potentially modifiable risk factors in the United States. *CA Cancer J Clin*. 2018;68(1):31–54.
21. Danaei G, Vander Hoorn S, Lopez AD, Murray CJ, Ezzati M; Comparative Risk Assessment Collaborating Group. Causes of cancer in the world: comparative risk assessment of nine behavioural and environmental risk factors. *Lancet*. 2005;366(9499):1784–1793.
22. Doll R, Peto R. *The Causes of Cancer. Quantitative Estimates of Avoidable Risks of Cancer in the United States Today*. New York, NY: Oxford University Press; 1981.
23. Miller A. Planning cancer control strategies. *Chronic Dis Can*. 1992;13(1):S1–S40.
24. Harvard Report on Cancer Prevention. Vol. 1: causes of human cancer. *Cancer Causes Control*. 1996;7(suppl 1):S3–S59.
25. Danaei G, Ding EL, Mozaffarian D, et al. The preventable causes of death in the United States: comparative risk assessment of dietary, lifestyle, and metabolic risk factors. *PLoS Med*. 2009;6(4):e1000058.
26. Greenwald P, Sondik E. *Cancer Control Objectives for the Nation: 1985–2000*. NIH publication 86-2880. Bethesda, MD: US Dept of Health and Human Services, National Institutes of Health; 1986.
27. National Cancer Institute. Vice President Biden's cancer initiative: Cancer Moonshot. 2016. Available at: http://www.cancer.gov/research/key-initiatives/moonshot-cancer-initiative. Accessed January 23, 2023.

28. US Department of Health and Human Services. Cancer, Healthy People 2030. 2021. Available at: https://health.gov/healthypeople/objectives-and-data/browse-objectives/cancer. Accessed January 23, 2023.
29. Bailar JC III, Gornik HL. Cancer undefeated. *N Engl J Med.* 1997;336(22):1569–1574.
30. Byers T, Mouchawar J, Marks J, et al. The American Cancer Society challenge goals. How far can cancer rates decline in the US by the year 2015? *Cancer.* 1999;86(4):715–727.
31. US Preventive Services Task Force. Grade definitions. October 2018. Available at: https://www.uspreventiveservicestaskforce.org/uspstf/about-uspstf/methods-and-processes/grade-definitions. Accessed January 23, 2023.
32. Singh AK, McGuirk JP. CAR T cells: continuation in a revolution of immunotherapy. *Lancet Oncol.* 2020;21(3):e168–e178.
33. McCune JS. Rapid advances in immunotherapy to treat cancer. *Clin Pharmacol Ther.* 2018;103(4):540–544.
34. Siegel RL, Miller KD, Fuchs HE, Jemal A. Cancer statistics, 2022. *CA Cancer J Clin.* 2022;72(1):7–33.
35. American Cancer Society. What is lung cancer? Updated January 12, 2023. Available at: https://www.cancer.org/cancer/lung-cancer/about/what-is.html. Accessed January 23, 2023.
36. National Cancer Institute. SEER*Explorer: an interactive website for SEER cancer statistics. Available at: https://seer.cancer.gov/explorer. Accessed January 23, 2023.
37. Wang J, Liu Q, Yuan S, et al. Genetic predisposition to lung cancer: comprehensive literature integration, meta-analysis, and multiple evidence assessment of candidate-gene association studies. *Sci Rep.* 2017;7(1):8371.
38. Liu C, Cui H, Gu D, et al. Genetic polymorphisms and lung cancer risk: evidence from meta-analyses and genome-wide association studies. *Lung Cancer.* 2017;113:18–29.
39. O'Keeffe LM, Taylor G, Huxley RR, Mitchell P, Woodward M, Peters SAE. Smoking as a risk factor for lung cancer in women and men: a systematic review and meta-analysis. *BMJ Open.* 2018;8(10):e021611.
40. American Cancer Society. Lung cancer risk factors. Updated January 12, 2023. Available at: https://www.cancer.org/cancer/lung-cancer/causes-risks-prevention/risk-factors.html. Accessed January 23, 2023.
41. World Cancer Research Fund; American Institute for Cancer Research. *Diet, Nutrition, Physical Activity and Cancer: A Global Perspective.* Continuous Update Project Expert Report 2018. Available at: www.wcrf.org/wp-content/uploads/2021/02/Summary-of-Third-Expert-Report-2018.pdf. Accessed January 23, 2023.
42. US Preventive Services Task Force. Final Recommendation Statement. Lung cancer: screening. March 9, 2021. Available at: https://www.uspreventiveservicestaskforce.org/uspstf/recommendation/lung-cancer-screening. Accessed January 23, 2023.
43. American Cancer Society. *Colorectal Cancer Facts & Figures 2020–2022.* Atlanta, GA: American Cancer Society; 2020.
44. Keum N, Giovannucci E. Global burden of colorectal cancer: emerging trends, risk factors and prevention strategies. *Nat Rev Gastroenterol Hepatol.* 2019;16(12):713–732.
45. Siegel R, Desantis C, Jemal A. Colorectal cancer statistics, 2014. *CA Cancer J Clin.* 2014;64(2):104–117.

46. Siegel RL, Miller KD, Goding Sauer A, et al. Colorectal cancer statistics, 2020. *CA Cancer J Clin.* 2020;70(3):145–164.
47. US Department of Health and Human Services. *The Health Consequences of Smoking—50 Years of Progress: A Report of the Surgeon General.* Atlanta, GA: US Dept of Health and Human Services, Centers for Disease Control and Prevention, National Center for Chronic Disease Prevention and Health Promotion, Office on Smoking and Health; 2014.
48. World Health Organization, International Agency for Research on Cancer. IARC Monographs evaluate consumption of red meat and processed meat. Lyon, France: International Agency for Research on Cancer; 2015.
49. Song M, Giovannucci E. Preventable incidence and mortality of carcinoma associated with lifestyle factors among White adults in the United States. *JAMA Oncol.* 2016;2(9):1154–1161.
50. US Preventive Services Task Force. Final Recommendation Statement. Colorectal cancer: screening. May 18, 2021. Available at: https://www.uspreventiveservicestaskforce.org/uspstf/recommendation/colorectal-cancer-screening. Accessed January 23, 2023.
51. National Cancer Institute. SEER Cancer Stat Facts: female breast cancer. Available at: https://seer.cancer.gov/statfacts/html/breast.html. Accessed January 23, 2023.
52. Houghton J, George WD, Cuzick J, et al. Radiotherapy and tamoxifen in women with completely excised ductal carcinoma in situ of the breast in the UK, Australia, and New Zealand: randomised controlled trial. *Lancet.* 2003;362(9378):95–102.
53. Colditz GA, Baer HJ, Tamimi RM. Breast cancer. In: Schottenfeld D, Fraumeni JF Jr., eds. *Cancer Epidemiology and Prevention.* 3rd ed. New York, NY: Oxford University Press; 2006:995–1012.
54. American Cancer Society. *Cancer Facts & Figures 2014.* Atlanta, GA: American Cancer Society, 2014.
55. Wheeler SB, Reeder-Hayes KE, Carey LA. Disparities in breast cancer treatment and outcomes: biological, social, and health system determinants and opportunities for research. *Oncologist.* 2013;18(9):986–993.
56. American Cancer Society. *Breast Cancer Facts & Figures 2015–2016.* Atlanta, GA: American Cancer Society; 2015.
57. US Department of Health and Human Services. *Cancer Rates and Risks.* 4th ed. USDHHS publication 96-691. Washington, DC: US Dept of Health and Human Services; 1996.
58. American Cancer Society. *Cancer Facts & Figures for African Americans 2016–2018.* Atlanta, GA: American Cancer Society; 2016.
59. Hunt K, Green M, Buchholz T. Diseases of the breast. In: Townsend C, Beauchamp R, Evers B, Mattox K, eds. *Sabiston Textbook of Surgery.* 19th ed. Philadelphia, PA: Saunders; 2012:824–869.
60. Yang Q, Khoury MJ, Rodriguez C, Calle EE, Tatham LM, Flanders WD. Family history score as a predictor of breast cancer mortality: prospective data from the Cancer Prevention Study II, United States, 1982–1991. *Am J Epidemiol.* 1998;147(7):652–659.
61. Kuchenbaecker KB, Hopper JL, Barnes DR, et al. Risks of breast, ovarian, and contralateral breast cancer for *BRCA1* and *BRCA2* mutation carriers. *JAMA.* 2017;317(23):2402–2416.

62. Mueller NE, Grufferman S. Hodgkin's lymphoma. In: Schottenfeld D, Fraumeni JF Jr., eds. *Cancer Epidemiology and Prevention*. 3rd ed. New York, NY: Oxford University Press; 2006:872–897.
63. Pettersson A, Graff RE, Ursin G, et al. Mammographic density phenotypes and risk of breast cancer: a meta-analysis. *J Natl Cancer Inst*. 2014;106(5).
64. Collaborative Group on Hormonal Factors in Breast Cancer. Breast cancer and breastfeeding: collaborative reanalysis of individual data from 47 epidemiological studies in 30 countries, including 50,302 women with breast cancer and 96,973 women without the disease. *Lancet*. 2002:360(9328):187–195.
65. Beral V; Million Women Study Collaborators. Breast cancer and hormone-replacement therapy in the Million Women Study [erratum in: *Lancet*. 2003;362(9390):1160]. *Lancet*. 2003;362(9382):419–427.
66. Chen C, Weiss NS, Newcomb P, Barlow W, White E. Hormone replacement therapy in relation to breast cancer. *JAMA*. 2002;287(6):734–741.
67. Longnecker MP. Alcoholic beverage consumption in relation to risk of breast cancer: meta-analysis and review. *Cancer Causes Control*. 1994;5(1):73–82.
68. Zhang SM, Willett WC, Selhub J, et al. Plasma folate, vitamin B6, vitamin B12, homocysteine, and risk of breast cancer. *J Natl Cancer Inst*. 2003;95(5):373–380.
69. Ferrini K, Ghelfi F, Mannucci R, Titta L. Lifestyle, nutrition and breast cancer: facts and presumptions for consideration. *Ecancermedicalscience*. 2015;23(9):557.
70. Oh H, Eliassen AH, Beck AH, et al. Breast cancer risk factors in relation to estrogen receptor, progesterone receptor, insulin-like growth factor-1 receptor, and Ki67 expression in normal breast tissue. *NPJ Breast Cancer*. 2017;3:39.
71. Sung H, Ferlay J, Siegel RL, et al. Global Cancer Statistics 2020: GLOBOCAN estimates of incidence and mortality worldwide for 36 cancers in 185 countries. *CA Cancer J Clin*. 2021;71(3):209–249.
72. Schiffman M, Castle PE, Jeronimo J, Rodriguez AC, Wacholder S. Human papillomavirus and cervical cancer. *Lancet*. (2007):370(9590):890–907.
73. Howlader N, Noone AM, Krapcho M, et al., eds. SEER cancer statistics review, 1975–2012. National Cancer Institute. Updated November 18, 2015. Available at: http://seer.cancer.gov/csr/1975_2012. Accessed January 23, 2023.
74. Mix JM, Van Dyne EA, Saraiya M, Hallowell BD, Thomas CC. Assessing impact of HPV vaccination on cervical cancer incidence among women aged 15–29 years in the United States, 1999–2017: an ecologic study. *Cancer Epidemiol Biomarkers Prev*. 2021;30(1):30–37.
75. Schiffman M, Hildesheim A. Cervical cancer. In: Schottenfeld D, Fraumeni JF Jr., eds. *Cancer Epidemiology and Prevention*. 3rd ed. New York, NY: Oxford University Press; 2006:1044–1067.
76. Munoz N, Bosch FX, de Sanjose S, et al. Epidemiologic classification of human papillomavirus types associated with cervical cancer. *N Engl J Med*. 2003;348(6):518–527.
77. Bosch FX, de Sanjose S. Chapter 1: human papillomavirus and cervical cancer—burden and assessment of causality. *J Natl Cancer Inst Monogr*. 2003(31):3–13.
78. National Cancer Institute. SEER Cancer Stat Facts: prostate cancer. Available at: https://seer.cancer.gov/statfacts/html/prost.html. Accessed January 23, 2023.

79. Siegel RL, Miller KD, Jemal A. Cancer statistics, 2016. *CA Cancer J Clin.* 2016;66(1):7-30.
80. Platz EA, Giovannucci E. Prostate cancer. In: Schottenfeld D, Fraumeni JF Jr., eds. *Cancer Epidemiology and Prevention.* 3rd ed. New York, NY: Oxford University Press; 2006: 1128–1150.
81. Conti DV, Darst BF, Moss LC, et al. Trans-ancestry genome-wide association meta-analysis of prostate cancer identifies new susceptibility loci and informs genetic risk prediction. *Nat Genet.* 2021;53(1):65–75.
82. Darst BF, Sheng X, Eeles RA, Kote-Jarai Z, Conti DV, Haiman CA. Combined effect of a polygenic risk score and rare genetic variants on prostate cancer risk. *Eur Urol.* 2021;80(2): 134–138.
83. Cao Y, Ma J. Body mass index, prostate cancer-specific mortality, and biochemical recurrence: a systematic review and meta-analysis. *Cancer Prev Res (Phila).* 2011;4(4):486–501.
84. Jahn JL, Giovannucci EL, Stampfer MJ. The high prevalence of undiagnosed prostate cancer at autopsy: implications for epidemiology and treatment of prostate cancer in the prostate-specific antigen-era. *Int J Cancer.* 2015;137(12):2795–2802.
85. Hurwitz LM, Agalliu I, Albanes D, et al. Recommended definitions of aggressive prostate cancer for etiologic epidemiologic research. *J Natl Cancer Inst.* 2021;113(6):727–734.
86. National Cancer Institute. SEER Cancer Stat Facts: Hodgkin lymphoma. Available at: https://seer.cancer.gov/statfacts/html/hodg.html. Accessed January 23, 2023.
87. National Cancer Institute. SEER Cancer Stat Facts: non-Hodgkin lymphoma. Available at: https://seer.cancer.gov/statfacts/html/nhl.html. Accessed January 23, 2023.
88. Keegan TH, Clarke CA, Chang ET, Shema SJ, Glaser SL. Disparities in survival after Hodgkin lymphoma: a population-based study. *Cancer Causes Control.* 2009;20(10):1881–1892.
89. Keegan TH, DeRouen MC, Parsons HM, et al. Impact of treatment and insurance on socioeconomic disparities in survival after adolescent and young adult Hodgkin lymphoma: a population-based study. *Cancer Epidemiol Biomarkers Prev.* 2016;25(2):264–273.
90. Evens AM, Antillon M, Aschebrook-Kilfoy B, Chiu BC. Racial disparities in Hodgkin's lymphoma: a comprehensive population-based analysis. *Ann Oncol.* 2012;23(8):2128–2137.
91. Morton LM, Wang SS, Cozen W, et al. Etiologic heterogeneity among non-Hodgkin lymphoma subtypes. *Blood.* 2008;112(13):5150–5160.
92. Alexander DD, Mink PJ, Adami HO, et al. The non-Hodgkin lymphomas: a review of the epidemiologic literature. *Int J Cancer.* 2007;120(suppl 12):1–39.
93. Hartge P, Bracci PM, Wang SS, et al. Non-Hodgkin's lymphoma. In: Schottenfeld D, Fraumeni JF Jr., eds. *Cancer Epidemiology and Prevention.* 3rd ed. New York, NY: Oxford University Press; 2006:898–918.
94. Murray PG, Young LS. An etiological role for the Epstein-Barr virus in the pathogenesis of classical Hodgkin lymphoma. *Blood.* 2019;134(7):591–596.
95. Schaapveld M, Aleman BM, van Eggermond AM, et al. Second cancer risk up to 40 years after treatment for Hodgkin's lymphoma. *N Engl J Med.* 2015;373(26):2499–2511.
96. National Cancer Institute. SEER Cancer Stat Facts: childhood leukemia. Available at: https://seer.cancer.gov/statfacts/html/childleuk.html. Accessed January 23, 2023.
97. National Cancer Institute. SEER Cancer Stat Facts: leukemia. Available at: https://seer.cancer.gov/statfacts/html/leuks.html. Accessed January 23, 2023.

98. Dixon SB, Chen Y, Yasui Y, et al. Reduced morbidity and mortality in survivors of childhood acute lymphoblastic leukemia: a report from the Childhood Cancer Survivor Study. *J Clin Oncol.* 2020;38(29):3418–3429.
99. Blattner W. T-cell lymphotrophic viruses and cancer causation. In: deVita VT, Hellman S, Rosenberg SA, eds. *Cancer: Principles and Practice of Oncology.* Philadelphia, PA: Lippincott; 1993.
100. Frederiksen LE, Erdmann F, Wesseling C, Winther JF, Mora AM. Parental tobacco smoking and risk of childhood leukemia in Costa Rica: a population-based case-control study. *Environ Res.* 2020;180:108827.
101. Linet MS, Taggart T, Severson RK, et al. Cellular telephones and non-Hodgkin lymphoma. *Int J Cancer.* 2006;119(10):2382–2388.
102. National Cancer Institute. SEER Cancer Stat Facts: bladder cancer. Available at: https://seer.cancer.gov/statfacts/html/urinb.html. Accessed January 23, 2023.
103. Al-Zalabani AH, Stewart KF, Wesselius A, Schols AM, Zeegers MP. Modifiable risk factors for the prevention of bladder cancer: a systematic review of meta-analyses. *Eur J Epidemiol.* 2016;31(9):811–851.
104. Silverman D, Devesa S, Moore L, Rothman N. Bladder cancer. In: Schottenfeld D, Fraumeni JF Jr., eds. *Cancer Epidemiology and Prevention.* 3rd ed. New York, NY: Oxford University Press; 2006:1101–1127.
105. Cumberbatch MG, Cox A, Teare D, Catto JW. Contemporary occupational carcinogen exposure and bladder cancer: a systematic review and meta-analysis. *JAMA Oncol.* 2015;1(9):1282–1290.
106. de Jong JJ, Boormans JL, van Rhijn BWG, et al. Distribution of molecular subtypes in muscle-invasive bladder cancer is driven by sex-specific differences. *Eur Urol Oncol.* 2020;3(4):420–423.
107. National Cancer Institute. SEER Cancer Stat Facts: oral cavity and pharynx cancer. Available at: https://seer.cancer.gov/statfacts/html/oralcav.html. Accessed January 23, 2023.
108. Mayne ST, Morse DE, Winn DM. Cancers of the oral cavity and pharynx. In: Schottenfeld D, Fraumeni JF Jr., eds. *Cancer Epidemiology and Prevention.* 3rd ed. New York, NY: Oxford University Press; 2006:674–696.
109. Petti S. Lifestyle risk factors for oral cancer. *Oral Oncol.* 2009;45(4–5):340–350.
110. Olson CM, Burda BU, Beil T, Whitlock EP. *Screening for Oral Cancer: A Targeted Evidence Update for the US Preventive Services Task Force.* Evidence Synthesis 102. AHRQ publication 13-05186-EF-1. Rockville, MD: Agency for Healthcare Research and Quality; 2013.
111. Blot WJ, McLaughlin JK, Winn DM, et al. Smoking and drinking in relation to oral and pharyngeal cancer. *Cancer Res.* 1988;48(11):3282–3287.
112. Leoncini E, Nedovic D, Panic N, Pastorino R, Edefonti V, Boccia S. Carotenoid intake from natural sources and head and neck cancer: a systematic review and meta-analysis of epidemiological studies. *Cancer Epidemiol Biomarkers Prev.* 2015;24(7):1003–1011.
113. de Martel C, Plummer M, Vignat J, Franceschi S. Worldwide burden of cancer attributable to HPV by site, country and HPV type. *Int J Cancer.* 2017;141(4):664–670.
114. Ang KK, Harris J, Wheeler R, et al. Human papillomavirus and survival of patients with oropharyngeal cancer. *N Engl J Med.* 2010;363(1):24–35.

115. Gillison ML, Chaturvedi AK, Anderson WF, Fakhry C. Epidemiology of human papillomavirus-positive head and neck squamous cell carcinoma. *J Clin Oncol.* 2015;33(29):3235–3242.
116. Chaturvedi AK, Graubard BI, Broutian T, et al. Prevalence of oral HPV infection in unvaccinated men and women in the United States, 2009–2016. *JAMA*. 2019;322(10):977–979.
117. American Cancer Society. Can oral cavity and oropharyngeal cancers be found early? 2014. Updated March 23, 2021. Available at: https://www.cancer.org/cancer/types/oral-cavity-and-oropharyngeal-cancer/detection-diagnosis-staging/detection.html. Accessed January 23, 2023.
118. Arnold M, de Vries E, Whiteman DC, et al. Global burden of cutaneous melanoma attributable to ultraviolet radiation in 2012. *Int J Cancer*. 2018;143(6):1305–1314.
119. Colantonio S, Bracken MB, Beecker J. The association of indoor tanning and melanoma in adults: systematic review and meta-analysis. *J Am Acad Dermatol.* 2014;70(5):847–857 e841–818.
120. US Preventive Services Task Force; Grossman DC, Curry SJ, et al. Behavioral counseling to prevent skin cancer: US Preventive Services Task Force recommendation statement. *JAMA*. 2018;319(11):1134–1142.

18

Chronic Respiratory Diseases

Donita R. Croft, MD, MS, and Henry A. Anderson, MD

LEARNING OBJECTIVES

After completing this chapter, readers should be able to

1. Describe the burden of chronic respiratory diseases in the United States.
2. Identify who is affected by chronic respiratory disease.
3. Describe approaches to mitigate the effects of chronic respiratory disease in the United States.

INTRODUCTION

Chronic respiratory diseases include a broad range of conditions that can be categorized as airway diseases, interstitial diseases, pulmonary vascular diseases, occupational and environmental lung diseases, and chest wall diseases. The causes and consequences of chronic respiratory diseases are complex and related to the specific type of disease (Figure 18-1). Chronic lower respiratory diseases were the sixth leading cause of death in the United States in 2020, responsible for 4.5% of US deaths. This was down from the third leading cause and 5.7% of US deaths in 2013, with deaths from COVID-19, unintentional illness, and strokes surpassing chronic lower respiratory diseases by 2020.[1] Hospitalizations and the need for emergency care and frequent outpatient visits are adverse outcomes of chronic respiratory diseases.

Significance

The primary consequence of chronic respiratory diseases that causes morbidity is dyspnea, or pathologic breathlessness. Depending on the severity, dyspnea may result in restrictions ranging from inability to climb stairs to constant breathlessness and difficulty performing activities of daily living. This may have serious repercussions on quality of life. Chronic respiratory disease causes impaired respiratory tract clearance mechanisms, excessive mucus production, and reduced lung capacity, which can contribute to more frequent, severe, and prolonged acute viral and bacterial respiratory infections.

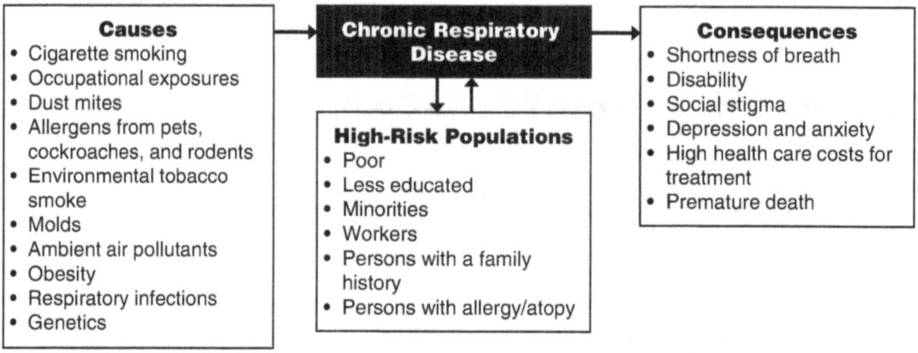

Figure 18-1. Chronic Respiratory Diseases: Causes, Consequences, and High-Risk Populations

Cough, chest pain, excessive sputum production, wheezing, and coughing of blood are other commonly observed symptoms of respiratory disease. As is the case for dyspnea, these symptoms can manifest in different respiratory and nonrespiratory disorders.

Among the challenges of describing symptoms commonly observed in respiratory disease is that terminology can differ greatly among clinicians describing similar patterns of respiratory impairment. The use of the term *chronic obstructive pulmonary disease* (COPD) can describe sets of symptoms that are alternatively described as chronic bronchitis, emphysema, or asthma; as such, assigning a definition on the basis of clinical, physiologic, or pathologic criteria may be problematic (Figure 18-2). Clinicians may also

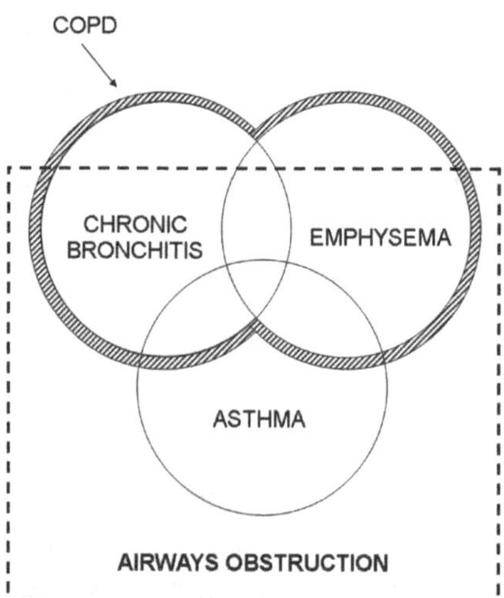

Note: COPD = chronic obstructive pulmonary disease. COPD includes patients with chronic bronchitis and emphysema and a subset of patients with asthma. Patients with COPD found outside the box for airways obstruction would have clinical or radiographic features of chronic bronchitis or emphysema.

Figure 18-2. Schema of Chronic Obstructive Pulmonary Disease

Table 18-1. Respiratory Diseases in the United States

Disease	*ICD-10* Code	Definition	No. Deaths, 2020
Asthma	J45–J46	A heterogeneous disease with chronic airway inflammation, a history of respiratory symptoms that vary in intensity over time, and variable expiratory airflow limitation.	4,145
Bronchitis	J40–J42	Excessive tracheobronchial mucus production associated with narrowing of the bronchial airways and cough.	457
Emphysema	J43	Alveolar destruction and associated airspace enlargement.	7,425
Other chronic obstructive pulmonary diseases (COPD)	J44	Asthma with chronic obstructive pulmonary disease and other chronic airway obstruction.	139,633
Cystic fibrosis	E84	Genetic disease with exocrine gland dysfunction resulting in pancreatic insufficiency, chronic progressive lung disease, and elevated sweat chloride production.	269
Bronchiectasis	J47	Bronchial wall destruction.	997
Pneumoconioses (and other externally induced alveolar diseases)	J60–J67	Dust-, fume- or mist-induced pneumoconiosis or lung injury (not immunologically mediated).	746
Sarcoidosis	D86	An interstitial lung disease characterized by non-necrotizing granulomas and enlarged lymph nodes.	1,138

Source: Based on CDC NCHS.[2]

Note: ICD-10 = *International Classification of Diseases*, Tenth Revision. Data are from the Multiple Cause of Death Files, 1999–2020, as compiled from data provided by the 57 vital statistics jurisdictions through the Vital Statistics Cooperative Program.

use the term *COPD* to describe nonspecific respiratory symptoms in cases in which airflow impairment may be either absent or present. The *International Classification of Diseases*, Tenth Revision (*ICD-10*) codes and the definitions used in this chapter are presented in Table 18-1.[2]

Pathophysiology

The diagnostic tests and associated criteria for definition differ among various chronic respiratory diseases. Chronic bronchitis is diagnosed by clinical signs and reported symptom history, whereas other forms of COPD and asthma are diagnosed by clinical evaluation and spirometric tests of lung function. Emphysema is defined in histopathologic terms (i.e., study of lung tissue) and is diagnosed with certainty only with lung biopsy or autopsy, although for practical purposes computerized axial tomography (CT) scanning of the chest is relied on to visualize the anatomic changes caused by emphysema. One manifestation of the occupation-related pneumoconioses, or dust-induced lung conditions, is a fibrotic response to deposition of inorganic material. Diagnosis requires an exposure history and X-ray assessment. In a heterogeneous group of lung disorders, interstitial lung diseases, the chest X-ray, chest CT, and pulmonary function tests are used for evaluation and monitoring of disease activity.

Spirometric testing is simple and inexpensive and is a sensitive and noninvasive method of assessing obstructive lung diseases as well as different fibrotic or restrictive lung diseases. Spirometry measures the exhaled volume of air as a function of time, including the forced expiratory volume in the first one second (FEV1) and forced vital capacity (FVC). Using the FVC and FEV1, lung disorders can be categorized into those with airflow obstruction (ratio of FEV1:FVC less than predicted) or restriction (FVC < 80% predicted).

In addition to spirometry, other lung function tests can include measurement of total lung capacity, functional residual capacity, carbon monoxide diffusing capacity, and cardiopulmonary exercise testing. Assessment of lung function following bronchoprovocation with methacholine or histamine may indicate airway hyperreactivity and is sometimes performed if asthma is suspected but spirometry is inconclusive.

The chest radiograph is helpful in the clinical evaluation of chronic lung diseases. However, its role in the screening or epidemiologic study is limited by expense, feasibility, and technical considerations. A uniform method of chest radiograph interpretation has been developed by the International Labour Office (ILO) for use in selected clinical settings (e.g., disability assessment for occupational lung disease) and for research purposes. The system categorizes opacities and pleural changes on the chest radiograph by their shape, size, location, and density.[3,4] Physicians who obtain additional training in ILO chest X-ray interpretation and pass an examination are called B readers. Methods similar to the ILO chest X-ray interpretation have also been developed for standardized interpretation of CT images of the chest.[5]

This chapter not only discusses two major chronic lung diseases—asthma and COPD—but also includes shorter descriptions of a variety of other chronic respiratory diseases.

CHRONIC OBSTRUCTIVE PULMONARY DISEASE

Chronic obstructive pulmonary disease (COPD) has been defined as a disease chiefly marked by airway obstruction that is not fully reversible. The condition is usually progressive in nature and is associated with an abnormal inflammatory response of the lungs to noxious particles and gases. The obstructive conditions chronic bronchitis and emphysema are grouped together under the broader heading of COPD and can be difficult to distinguish from each other clinically. COPD can also overlap with asthma.

Significance

In the Interactive Summary Health Statistics for Adults from 2019 to 2020, the self-reported prevalence of adults who had ever been diagnosed with COPD, emphysema, or chronic bronchitis was 5.0%.[6] For adults aged 40 to 79 years, population projections based on spirometry data from physical examinations from the National Health and Nutrition Examination Survey (NHANES) from 2007 to 2010 place the prevalence of mild and moderate obstructive pulmonary disease between 10.2% and 20.9%.[7] These findings suggest that prevalence estimates made on the basis of self-reported data may significantly underestimate actual COPD prevalence. In 2018 there were 873,000 emergency department visits for COPD in the United States and a national mortality rate of 42.7 per 100,000 population.[8] The inpatient hospitalization rates in the United States for COPD were 33.4 (women) and 31.6 (men) per 10,000 population in 2010.[9] For all health end-points related to COPD, however, imprecise and variable definitions make the quantification of prevalence, morbidity, and mortality difficult.

An estimate of the economic costs of COPD in the United States was placed at $36 billion—including $32.1 billion for direct medical costs and $3.9 billion for absenteeism.[9] Primary payers of direct costs included Medicare (51%), Medicaid (25%), and private insurance (18%).

Pathophysiology

Pathologic changes of COPD occur mostly in the proximal and peripheral airways, lung parenchyma, and pulmonary vasculature. These changes consist of inflammatory responses and increases in goblet cell number and mucous gland size. This inflammation is an amplification of normal inflammatory responses to toxic gases and particulates, although the mechanism of this is not well understood. This response is most observed with ongoing exposure to tobacco smoke.[10,11] There is evidence that oxidative stress, fibrotic changes of the peripheral airways, and an imbalance between protease, which breaks down the structure of lung tissue, and antiprotease also lead to the changes seen with COPD. The result is the destruction of the bronchioles, alveolar ducts, and alveoli that constitute gas exchange air spaces.

The chief physiological result is obstructed expiratory airflow, reduced gas transfer capacity, hypersecretion of mucus, and eventually pulmonary hypertension.

In adults, the onset of COPD often begins with a moderate decline in lung function capacity before age 50. In many cases COPD would be observable by spirometry, but medical attention may not be sought until symptoms such as dyspnea are observed. Among smokers, a cough may provide early evidence of the onset of COPD. In the typical case, the decline in lung function accelerates after the age of 50.[10] As the disease progresses, the damage to the lungs ultimately results in inadequate oxygen delivery. COPD is a common comorbid condition among patients presenting with cardiovascular disease and other systemic conditions.

Descriptive Epidemiology

High-Risk Populations

Cigarette smoking is the main risk factor for COPD, but exposure to biomass fuel, air pollution, dust, and particulate matter are other factors that cause COPD. The prevalence of COPD also increases with age, especially after 40 years.[10] This increase in risk with age is attributable to both increased cumulative tobacco smoke exposure among smokers and a generally observed decline in lung function with age across populations. Women appear to be more susceptible to COPD than men. In pooled data of 17,139 patients from 22 COPD cohorts internationally, women were younger and had lower pack-year histories than men. Although women had more exacerbations and more dyspnea, they had relatively greater lung function when measured by FEV1% and a higher five-year survival.[12] Improvements in lung function upon tobacco cessation also appear to be greater among women than among men.

There are genetic risk factors for COPD. A small number of patients with COPD have a deficiency of the protein alpha-1 antitrypsin, which occurs most commonly in Whites of Scandinavian descent. This protein acts to inhibit the destructive capabilities of the white blood cell elastase responsible for degradation of lung tissue, and deficiencies of alpha-1 antitrypsin have been associated with emphysema. In addition, there are single gene variations that have been associated with COPD. Smokers who have a sibling with severe COPD are at higher risk of airway obstruction, which suggests a genetic component. Abnormal lung development is also a risk factor for COPD, including processes that occur during gestation, at birth, and throughout childhood and adolescence such as low birth weight or recurrent infections.[10]

Geographic Distribution

By state, COPD mortality rates tend to be higher in some parts of the West and South, including Appalachia. Mortality data from 2010 showed the highest age-adjusted COPD mortality rates among adults aged 25 years and older in Oklahoma (102.6/100,000 population), West Virginia (95.1), Kentucky (90.7), and Wyoming (89.6), whereas the lowest rates were found in Hawaii (24.8/100,000) and the District of Columbia (37.7).[13] This geographic pattern was unchanged in 2019, with the highest age-adjusted COPD mortality rates among adults age 45 years and older in Oklahoma, West Virginia, and Kentucky (174.2–174.6/100,000), and the lowest rates in Hawaii (44.5/100,000) and the District of Columbia (50.8; Figure 18-3).[14] Although theories regarding population

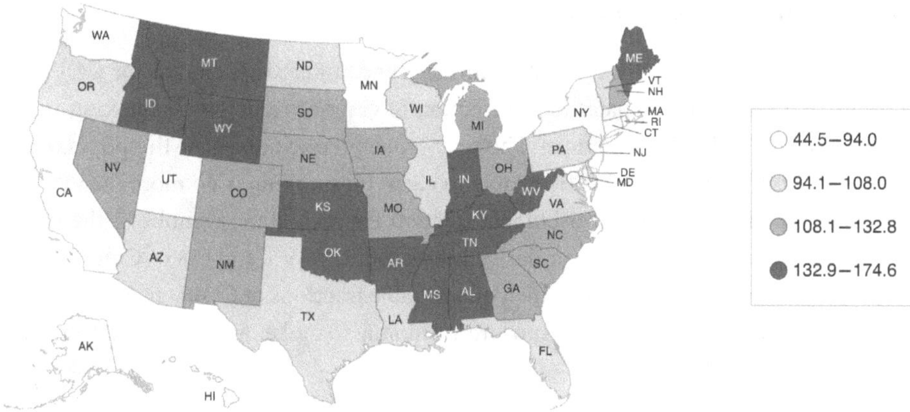

Source: Based on CDC.[14]

Note: ICD-10 = International Classification of Diseases, Tenth Revision. Underlying cause of death *ICD-10* codes: J40–J44. Death rates (per 100,000 population) age-standardized to the 2000 US projected population.

Figure 18-3. Age-Adjusted Death Rate for COPD Among US Adults Aged 45 Years and Older: National Vital Statistics System, 2019

migration, ambient air pollutants, and diagnostic differences have been postulated, this discrepancy has yet to be fully explained.

Time Trends

In 2010 there was a national mortality rate for COPD of 63.1 per 100,000 population.[13] By 2018 this had decreased to 42.7 per 100,000 population.[15]

Causes

Modifiable Risk Factors

The most commonly encountered risk factor for the development of COPD is cigarette smoking. This risk is dose-related, and factors such as age of starting to smoke, total pack-years smoked, and current smoking status are all predictive of COPD mortality.[10] Exposure to secondhand smoke also contributes to the risk of developing COPD, and exposure during childhood is associated with COPD and related respiratory symptoms in adulthood.[16]

Occupational exposure to organic and inorganic dusts and fumes may contribute to the development of COPD.[17] In addition, indoor pollution from the burning of biomass in poorly ventilated dwellings can contribute to the development of COPD, especially in developing countries.[18] Although outdoor air pollution can contribute to COPD exacerbations, its role in the development of COPD remains unclear.

Population-Attributable Risk

Cigarette smoking is by far the most commonly encountered risk factor for COPD in the United States, and estimates of the fraction of cases attributable to smoking range from 45% to 90%.[19] The American Thoracic Society concluded that the population-attributable fraction of COPD attributable to cigarette smoking is no more than 80%.[20] Estimates for the population-attributable fraction for secondhand smoke in the home and work environments have been derived to account for 9% and 7% of COPD cases, respectively.[21] Other factors from which quantifiable fractions of COPD may be derived include occupational exposures, exposure to biomass smoke, and exposure to traffic and outdoor air pollutants.[20]

Evidence-Based Interventions

Prevention

Because of the primacy of tobacco smoking as a risk factor for COPD, prevention of tobacco smoking is the single most important preventive activity to reduce the burden of COPD. Because the effect of tobacco smoking on COPD is dose-related, any reduction in smoking may bring about a reduction in related COPD morbidity. When a smoker quits, the age-related rate of decline in FEV1 can approach the rate of lung function decline in never-smokers, but it does not return to the level of lung function seen in never-smokers.

For individuals exposed to multiple risk factors, the effect of the collective set of risk factors appears to be additive. As such, identifying individuals with multiple risk factors, such as smoking and occupational exposures, may provide an important avenue for COPD prevention.

Screening

Because interventions aimed at reducing harmful exposures can be effective in slowing the progression of COPD, early detection of disease is beneficial for patients. The primary mode of screening for COPD is to measure airflow obstruction with spirometry or peak airflow measurement. Because there is a large population that may be in the early stages of COPD without being aware of it, increasing awareness of the relationship between symptoms such as chronic cough and excessive sputum production and COPD may increase the fraction of patients who are appropriately diagnosed with COPD. Broad population-based screening should be limited to individuals at high risk for developing COPD, such as cigarette smokers. Screening for genetic markers for alpha-1 antitrypsin deficiency is available for individuals for whom a genetic predisposition to the deficiency is suspected.

Treatment

The most effective treatment for COPD is to avoid exposure to agents that cause or exacerbate COPD, such as cigarette smoke, workplace dusts, and ambient air pollutants. Once COPD has been diagnosed, the objectives of disease management are to relieve symptoms, improve exercise tolerance and health status, and prevent and treat complications and exacerbations.[10] Medications, such as inhaled bronchodilators and corticosteroids, can help reduce the symptoms of COPD. When the progression of disease results in decreased blood oxygen, supplemental oxygen therapy has been shown to increase survival.[22] Pulmonary rehabilitation such as exercise training and breathing retraining have been shown to decrease dyspnea, increase exercise tolerance, and improve patients' quality of life. Surgical approaches, such as valves placed within the airway or removal of emphysematous portions of lung or lung transplantation, can be effective in increasing survival in selected circumstances. Pneumococcal and influenza vaccination are recommended for people diagnosed with COPD.[10]

Moving Forward

Although the primary risk factors for COPD are well established, differences in regional COPD mortality rates that remain unexplained by tobacco smoking patterns may offer an opportunity to better understand the epidemiology of COPD. Additional studies of the cellular basis of COPD and identification of more sensitive and specific biochemical, genetic, and molecular markers of COPD may lead to better approaches for the diagnosis and control of COPD. Additional epidemiologic studies assessing the interaction between cigarette smoking and exposures from environmental and occupational sources may aid in assessing the relative efficacy of various avenues for intervention. Longitudinal epidemiology studies may help identify and quantify risk factors that contribute to the development of COPD, either independently or in tandem with established COPD risk factors.

ASTHMA

Asthma is characterized by chronic airway inflammation, airway hyperresponsiveness, and a history of respiratory symptoms and expiratory airflow obstruction that vary in intensity over time. The symptoms most commonly occurring with asthma are wheezing, dyspnea, chest tightness, and coughing. Asthma is a heterogeneous illness with some recognizable clusters based on demographics and clinical characteristics that are referred to as asthma phenotypes. These can be helpful in determining treatment plans.[23] According to the Behavioral Risk Factor Surveillance System, the lifetime asthma prevalence of American adults in 2020 was 13.9%.[24] Although much effort has been made to develop standardized diagnostic criteria for asthma, estimates of asthma prevalence continue to vary with different data collection approaches, which can make comparison of data difficult.

Significance

In 2020, 8.4% of adults and 5.8% of children under 18 years of age were reported to currently have asthma. Of those with asthma, 60% of adults and 44% of children had poorly controlled asthma, which can lead to high work and school absenteeism.[25] In 2018, asthma accounted for 5.8 million outpatient office visits.[26]

Pathophysiology

Historically, asthma has been classified into two categories: allergic or atopic and nonallergic or nonatopic asthma. People with atopy produce abnormal amounts of immunoglobulin E (IgE) and eosinophils in response to antigens. Genetic and environmental factors appear to affect whether susceptible people progress to having asthma.

Patients with asthma show evidence of mucosal edema, epithelial disruption, infiltration with inflammatory cells, and excessive amounts of mucus in airways. The development of the changes responsible for airway obstruction and hyperresponsiveness is primarily attributable to inflammatory responses in the airways of patients. In allergic asthma, IgE–antigen complexes bind to the membranes of various connective tissue cells, causing the release of signaling chemical agents responsible for an asthmatic response. Positive responses to skin tests for common allergens are more common among atopic people than those without atopy and among people with asthma than those without asthma.[27]

Symptoms of asthma, such as intermittent wheezing or shortness of breath triggered by specific environmental exposures, cold air, strong scents, or exercise, frequently appear in children before the age of five years.[23] About 50% of adults who were diagnosed with asthma as children no longer have the condition, with about half of these becoming totally symptom-free.[28] Conversely, about one-fourth of childhood asthma cases persist with a similar degree of severity into adulthood, and the remaining one-fourth may experience a temporary cessation in symptoms, with symptoms returning in adulthood.[29] Approximately 16% of adults have a remission, at least a one-year symptom-free period, within five years of their asthma diagnosis.[23]

Descriptive Epidemiology

High-Risk Populations

Although there is a range of factors that are useful for describing the distribution of asthma and asthma-related adverse health outcomes among populations, the most important determinants of asthma and related morbidity and mortality are race/ethnicity, poverty level, age, and sex. Racial disparities for asthma are found for a range of endpoints, most notably prevalence, mortality, and hospitalizations. It is important to note that there is no evidence that these racial disparities are caused by an intrinsic difference between racial groups; these are very likely attributable to the health effects of systemic racism. Data from the 2018 to 2020 National Health Interview Survey found significantly higher values of current asthma prevalence for non-Hispanic African Americans than for non-Hispanic Whites (10.3% vs. 8.1%). When the data were limited to children, the disparity was even more striking (12.3% vs. 5.5%). Across all racial groups, Hispanic ethnicity was not associated with higher asthma prevalence. Non-Hispanic Asians had the lowest prevalence at 3.5%, and non-Hispanic American Indian/Alaska Native adults had high prevalence at 11.3%. The asthma prevalence for females was higher than for males in both children and adults, with an overall prevalence of 9.5% for females and 6.1% for males.[25]

Differences in asthma health care utilization for persons with current asthma by age, sex, and race are depicted in Figure 18-4.[30] In 2020 the asthma mortality rate for non-Hispanic African Americans was nearly three times higher compared with that for non-Hispanic Whites (28.7 vs. 10.8/1,000,000 population, respectively).[25]

Time Trends

Data sources available for asthma surveillance have changed over time. Based on survey responses regarding whether a family member had asthma in the past

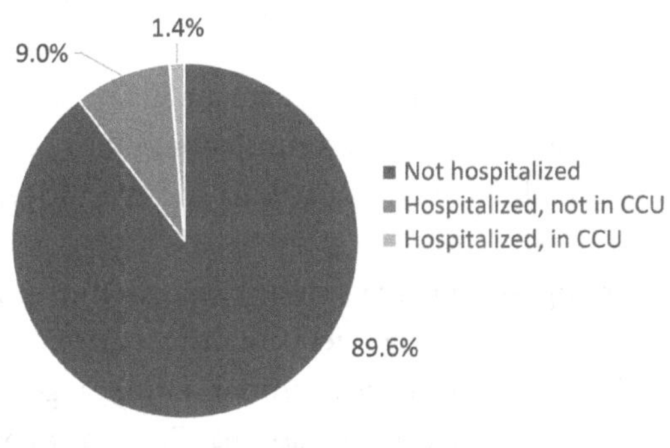

Source: Based on Qin X et al.[30]

Note: CCU = critical care unit; ED = emergency department. Percentage of ED visits with asthma as the primary diagnosis that were admitted to a CCU. Based on a sample of visits to EDs in noninstitutional general and short-stay hospitals, exclusive of federal, military, and Veterans administration hospitals, located in the 50 states and the District of Columbia. Defined as ED visits with a diagnosis of asthma (ICD-9-CM 493.0) as the primary diagnosis for the current visit.

Figure 18-4. Percentage of Emergency Department Visits for Asthma Admitted to a Critical Care Unit: National Hospital Ambulatory Medical Care Survey, United States, 2010–2015

12 months, asthma prevalence increased from 3.1% in 1980 to 5.5% in 1996, an increase of 3.8% per year. This increase occurred among all age, sex, and race subgroups. Although changes in survey questions make comparisons from 1997 to 2000 with newer national prevalence data problematic, current asthma prevalence was relatively unchanged from 2001 to 2020, with 7.3% in 2001, 8.4% in 2010, and 7.8% in 2020.[25,30] Data on asthma mortality suggest that death rates increased from 1980 through 1989, remained stable from 1989 to 1998, and have declined by 4.9% per year from 1999 to 2009.[30] The mortality rate in 2020 was 12.6 asthma deaths per million Americans.[25]

Seasonal trends have been consistently exhibited for both asthma morbidity and mortality. Asthma hospitalization rates reflect a seasonal variation whereby the highest rates occur in early spring and early fall, and rates are lowest in the summer.[31] Studies on asthma mortality have suggested that asthma mortality in children and young adults may peak in summer, whereas mortality among older adults peaks in winter. Potential explanations for this observed seasonality include plant allergens, acute respiratory infections, cold weather, and air pollution. For school-age children, the onset of school in September has been found to contribute to increased emergency department visits for asthma.[32]

Causes

Approximately 30% to 50% of the general population can be classified as atopic. Most asthmatics are atopic, and atopy is a significant risk factor for developing asthma.[33] Because atopy is strongly influenced by genetics, it follows that major aspects of asthma development are under genetic control. Indeed, those with a family history of asthma have long been known to be at increased risk for developing asthma.[34] However, asthma doesn't follow a simple Mendelian pattern, and a single chromosomal location has not been found to account for asthma. It is likely that there are many genes that can affect the development and severity of asthma, which contributes to the heterogeneity of this illness. Associations have been found between asthma and specific gene loci, such as the 17q21 locus.[35]

Although the relationship to atopy suggests a strong genetic component among the factors related to the etiology of asthma, there are many environmental risk factors as well. While causal relationships have not been proved, a wide range of specific exposures often precipitate symptoms in individuals with asthma. Common asthma triggers include dust mites, allergens from pets, cockroaches and rodents, cigarette smoking, secondhand smoke, molds, ambient air pollutants, cold conditions, and exercise.[23] A longitudinal study in children found that although IgE levels in umbilical cord blood were not predictive of subsequent development of asthma, IgE blood levels in blood samples taken at age one year were predictive.[36] This finding suggests that exposures within the first year of life may be substantial contributors to the risk of developing asthma in childhood.

There is also a relationship between asthma and obesity. Because obesity is associated with a generalized increase in inflammatory response, a causal role in asthma has been postulated.[37] Increased incidence of asthma and poorer asthma control have been observed at higher rates among people with elevated body mass index values.[38] Given the possibility that reduced physical activity among people with asthma could contribute to the likelihood of obesity, the relationship between asthma and obesity is likely complex in nature.

Ambient air pollutants have been shown to be important asthma triggers.[23] Associations between asthma and exposure to ozone and particulate matter have been commonly observed, but pollutants such as nitrogen dioxide and volatile organic compounds, along with community traffic density and proximity to heavily traveled roads, have also been found to be associated with adverse asthma-related health outcomes.[39] Incidence of asthma was also associated with traffic-related air pollution exposure from roadways near homes and schools.[40] Among school-age children active in sports, incidence of asthma was found to be higher in children living in communities with high ozone concentrations than among other children.[40]

Evidence-Based Interventions

Prevention

Because of the considerable uncertainty about how specific genetic and environmental factors contribute to the development of asthma at both the individual and population levels, there are few clear recommendations to prevent the development of asthma. Given the evidence regarding air pollutants as contributors to developing asthma, continuing to establish appropriate air pollutant restrictions for ozone and particulate matter may have benefit in reducing future asthma incidence and prevalence. Also, state and national public health alerts are issued when pollution concentrations exceed standards and could pose a threat to sensitive populations, including people with asthma.

Public health activity on asthma has focused primarily on means by which individuals with asthma can reduce or eliminate exacerbations that may pose a threat to their health or limit their quality of life. This has been done by promoting regular interaction with appropriate health care providers, providing and disseminating guidance about appropriate use of controller medications, educating patients about the nature of asthma as a chronic disease, and how to identify and avoid asthma triggers that may cause exacerbations. Because secondhand smoke is a known asthma trigger, efforts to discourage tobacco use in homes and other indoor environments or focusing smoking cessation efforts on people with asthma and their families is recommended. For potentially susceptible people, such as siblings and children of people with asthma, there may be benefit in extending environmental control measures applied to the individual with asthma (such as limiting exposure to pests and mold) to other members of the household. For example, dust mites can be effectively controlled by encasing mattresses and pillows in airtight covers, washing bedding every week, and removing wall-to-wall carpeting, especially in bedrooms. Because respiratory infections may have a considerable impact on asthma-related morbidity, it is recommended that people with asthma obtain pneumococcal, COVID-19, and annual influenza vaccinations.

Screening

Effective management can minimize the frequency and severity of asthma exacerbations; therefore, applying a proper diagnosis to individuals who have asthma is an important step in controlling the disease and reducing asthma-related adverse health outcomes. However, mild-to-moderate cases of asthma may be difficult to diagnose, especially among young children. In such cases, symptoms can often be confused with recurrent respiratory infections or bronchitis and may not be recognized as a chronic condition.

Because of asthma's impact on school attendance, as a major cause of hospitalization in children, and the preventable nature of asthma-related morbidity, population-based screening for asthma has received much attention as a potential intervention. However, many organizations, including the American Thoracic Society, have refrained from endorsing such screening efforts because of the lack of evidence that such approaches result in measurable improvements in health outcomes.[41] Population-based screening may be most effective in areas where there is likely to be a high prevalence of undiagnosed asthma and where access to high-quality care is likely to be available for newly diagnosed patients.

Treatment

The primary goal of asthma treatment is to control the condition and minimize exacerbations to avoid adverse asthma-related health outcomes. Most asthma medications can be described as controller medications or reliever (rescue) medications. The Global Initiative for Asthma promotes a stepwise approach for controller medications, depending on the severity of symptoms and lung function. Controller medications are generally taken daily on a long-term basis to control inflammation. Common types of controller medications include inhaled corticosteroids such as fluticasone, leukotriene modifiers such as montelukast, and long-acting $\beta 2$-agonists such as salmeterol. Reliever medications act quickly to address bronchoconstriction. These include rapid-acting β2-agonists and systemic corticosteroids. Frequent use of reliever medications (e.g., daily) may signify that a patient's asthma is not being well controlled and the treatment plan should be reevaluated. Prior to stepping up to higher doses of controller medication, it is important to evaluate if the current medications are being used correctly.[23] For more difficult-to-control asthma, targeted anti-inflammatory treatments can be used, such as monoclonal antibodies against specific molecules in the allergic inflammatory pathway.[42]

Moving Forward

The biggest impact for asthma moving forward would be to further delineate the genetic determinants of asthma and the interaction between these and environmental factors that lead to heterogeneity in this disease. Longitudinal cohorts of asthma patients are recommended to further understand the origins of asthma and the relationships between exposures and developmental changes over the life span. These could be integral to identifying high-risk individuals for whom interventions to prevent asthma might be recommended and to provide more specific therapeutic options. More research could help us better understand the usefulness of asthma phenotype classifications. Although effective medications for asthma control exist, there remain concerns about long-term side effects, such as growth restrictions in children, for which more data are required.

OCCUPATIONAL ASTHMA

Although the incidence of other occupational respiratory diseases is decreasing, occupational asthma continues to be problematic. Work-related asthma includes occupational asthma and asthma aggravated by work or the work environment, and is characterized by episodes of bronchoconstriction, airway inflammation, and airway hyperresponsiveness to agents or conditions present in the work environment.[43] Primary occupational asthma is distinguished from exacerbations of existing asthma by the presence of a workplace sensitizing agent, although symptoms usually do not appear until a few weeks to several years after the first exposure. The overall prevalence of occupational asthma varies from region to region, with estimates for the United States ranging between 10% and 23% of all adults with asthma.[44] Between 50% and 90% of individuals with occupational asthma will continue to have symptoms even after being removed from the source of the exposure.[45]

Establishing the presence of airflow obstruction is integral in making the diagnosis of occupational asthma.[46] It may be helpful to measure the peak expiratory flow rate several times daily for two to three weeks because correlating asthma to occupational exposure can be difficult. The fact that initial symptoms may occur only at home or after work can be misleading. Specific inhalation challenge with the suspected compound is not routinely performed because it is time consuming, is not widely available, and carries the risk of a potentially serious reaction.[46]

Descriptive Epidemiology

Several mechanisms have been identified that are associated with the development of work-related asthma: sensitization; reactive airways dysfunction syndrome (associated with a single, high exposure to irritant agents with onset of symptoms within hours); nonimmunologic airway irritation of preexisting asthma; and indoor environments with biologic contaminants.[44,46]

Agents are classified as high-molecular-weight compounds or low-molecular-weight compounds.[47] Atopy, or allergy, is an important risk factor for developing asthma from the high-molecular-weight compounds but not for the low-molecular-weight compounds.[48] High-molecular-weight compounds are proteins, polysaccharides, and peptides. Depending on the level of exposure, the prevalence of asthma from these compounds can be high. Asthma has been reported in 3% to 30% of animal handlers; 10% to 45% of workers exposed to biologic enzymes that are used, for example, in laundry detergents and other cleaning agents; 20% of bakers; and 70% of flight crews dispersing sterile irradiated screwworm flies.[45]

Examples of the low-molecular-weight compounds are isocyanates, wood dusts, metals, and drugs. Work-related asthma has been reported in 4% of workers exposed to the dust of western red cedar,[49] 5% to 10% of workers exposed to toluene diisocyanate, 29% to 40% of workers using epoxy resins, and 70% of workers exposed to platinum salts in processes such as metallurgy and photography.[50]

Causes

Criteria have been developed that characterize some chemicals as "asthmagens." Over 300 substances have been designated as asthma agents, the majority of which are sensitizing agents.[51] Materials having known or suspected allergic properties account for most cases of occupational asthma. The risk of developing occupational asthma is usually related to the magnitude of exposure for many agents, including western red cedar, toluene diisocyanate, baking products, and colophony fumes from soldering.[45]

The risk for persistent symptoms in workers diagnosed with occupational asthma was examined in 125 western red cedar workers.[49] All workers who remained at work continued to have symptoms. Among workers who left the work, those who were older, had a longer duration of exposure, and had a longer duration of symptoms were at higher risk for having persistent symptoms. Workers who develop toluene diisocyanate–related asthma and continue to be exposed to the compound have been found to have continued deterioration in pulmonary function.

Evidence-Based Interventions

The only way to prevent occupational asthma is to avoid work and work sites where exposure to certain levels of agents occurs. Thus, it is important for facility managers to know what agents have been associated with asthma and to inform their workers and then establish work practices that maintain exposures below known sensitization levels.[52] Material safety data sheets need to include information about components that may cause or exacerbate asthma. Workers need to be educated and trained about proper handling of materials and avoiding spills. Improved ventilation and the use of respirators can decrease the risk of disease. When sensitization occurs, often the only remedy for the affected worker is a transfer from the area of exposure. Deaths have been recorded when sensitized individuals have been reexposed at the workplace. Desensitization before exposure has not been shown to be effective.[53]

CYSTIC FIBROSIS

Significance

Cystic fibrosis (CF) is an inherited disease characterized by the production of abnormally thick and sticky mucus and decreased function of the cilia, resulting in respiratory infections and obstruction. It is a major source of severe chronic lung disease in children and young adults.[54] Although CF continues to result in premature death from its effects on the respiratory, gastrointestinal, and endocrine systems, major strides in screening and treatment have improved patient outcomes and survival for patients with CF.[55,56] (See Figure 18-5.) There are an estimated 40,000 patients in the United States with CF, and between 2015 and 2019 the average age of death of North American CF patients was 46.2 years.[57,58]

Pathophysiology

The primary genetic defect associated with CF is caused by a defect in a transmembrane conductance regulator (CFTR) gene that codes for proteins involved in the cellular transport of chloride. This genetic defect has been localized to chromosome 7, and more than 1,700 specific CFTR gene mutations have been identified.[59] Levels of the functional regulator protein are substantially reduced in patients with CF, affecting ion transport in sweat ducts, airways, pancreatic ducts, and elsewhere. The severity and level of organ involvement in CF is directly related to tissue levels of the protein. The primary manifestation of CF in the respiratory tract is abnormally thick and copious mucus in the airways that impairs microbial and mucociliary clearance. This often contributes to progressive cycles of respiratory infection and inflammation.[60] As more patients have survived into adulthood, extrapulmonary effects such as CF-induced diabetes and fibrotic and

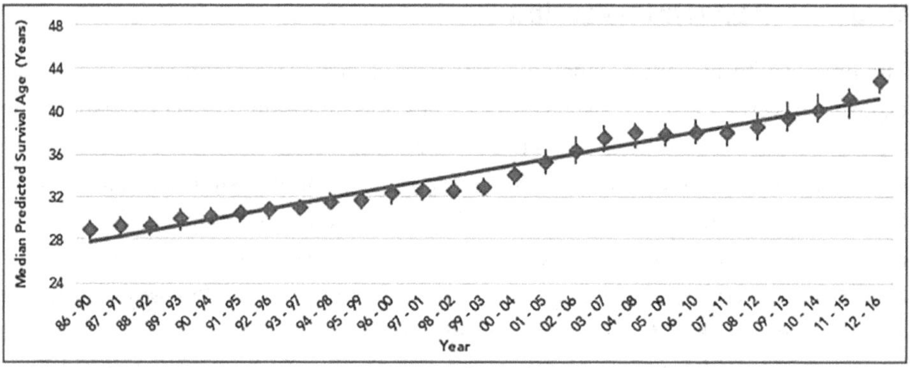

Source: Reprinted with permission of Cystic Fibrosis Foundation.[55]

Note: Data includes cystic fibrosis patients under care at Cystic Fibrosis Foundation–accredited care centers in the United States, who consented to have their data entered. Data are presented in five-year intervals.

Figure 18-5. Median Predicted Survival Age for Individuals With Cystic Fibrosis: United States, 1986–2016

cirrhotic liver disease are increasingly observed. Lung disease, however, remains the primary cause of morbidity and mortality from CF.

Descriptive Epidemiology

Cystic fibrosis is among the most common lethal genetic defects affecting Whites in the United States. Incidence varies greatly in the United States based on ethnicity, with incidence at 1 in 3,200 births for Whites, 1 in 15,000 births for African Americans, and 1 in 31,000 births for Asian Americans.[61] It is inherited in an autosomal recessive fashion, and estimates of the prevalence of the heterozygous form in individuals of Northern European descent ranges from 2% to 4%.[62,63] Individuals with the heterozygous form are not affected with CF.

A review of CF mortality records from 10 countries found that the median age of death was consistently highest in the United States. Although increases in life span were observed in all 10 countries over time, all 10 showed a shorter life span for women with CF than for men with CF.[64]

Causes

CF is a genetic illness. However, there are several classes of specific mutations within the target gene that can lead to the condition, and there are observed differences in disease severity associated with the different classes.[55] Among patients with CF, decrease in FEV1 and use of nutritional intervention have been established as markers for mortality risk.[65,66]

Evidence-Based Interventions

Prevention

Aside from genetic counseling and education for prospective parents, the prevention of CF is a difficult proposition.

Screening

Newborn screening for CF is now undertaken in all 50 states. The most common method used for screening is measurement of immunoreactive trypsinogen on dried blood spots, followed by direct gene analysis approach for confirmation. Among the benefits of early screening are the ability to begin nutritional interventions and secretion management early in the course of the disease.

Treatment

CFTR modulator therapy has shown promise for fundamentally changing the outcomes of cystic fibrosis; it has been shown to significantly improve FEV1 even in people with severe lung disease with cystic fibrosis.[67] CFTR modulators work by correcting the production and activity of malfunctioning protein made by the CFTR gene. Each modulator works only on specific mutations; currently, however, modulators are not available for all CFTR mutations. Standard therapy involves several other strategies. Airway clearance is the cornerstone of therapy, with medications to thin secretions and mechanical dislodgement of secretions with modalities such as chest physical therapy or percussive vests. Infections can be decreased using contact isolation and meticulous hand hygiene, monoclonal antibodies, and vaccines for influenza, pneumococcal disease, and COVID-19. Bronchodilators and inhaled corticosteroids are also typical therapies for cystic fibrosis.

Moving Forward

Future research and development are very promising and involve expanding CFTR modulator therapy and advancing gene therapy. Although CFTR modulator therapy is currently available for just a minority of CFTR mutations, expanding availability for more genetic mutations is a goal. Limiting the downstream consequences of lung and other organ damage by using modulators in younger patients is also an objective. Gene therapy approaches, incorporating copies of the normal CFTR gene in affected cells, remain promising. The goal is to place a copy of the gene for normal transmembrane conductance regulator protein in affected cells, resulting in production of the normal protein.[57]

INTERSTITIAL LUNG DISEASE

Interstitial lung disease refers to diseases that manifest in the interstitium, which includes the spaces between the pulmonary capillary cells and the pulmonary alveoli, the connective tissue surrounding blood vessels and bronchi, and the connective tissue of the pleura. Specific descriptors of this category of disease include pulmonary fibrosis, alveolitis, and pneumonitis.

Progressive dyspnea is the most common presenting concern. Pulmonary function testing may show abnormalities with a restrictive defect with decreased FVC, and these are helpful in following the course of the disease. The location and type of opacities on the chest radiograph can be helpful in diagnosing interstitial lung diseases. The diagnosis of interstitial lung disease can frequently be made by history and chest CT appearance; however, a lung biopsy is sometimes required if the diagnosis remains in doubt or if the disease process is severe or rapidly progressive.

SARCOIDOSIS

Sarcoidosis is an interstitial lung disease that is characterized by non-necrotizing granulomas and enlarged lymph nodes. Sarcoidosis can involve multiple organ systems, but the most common system affected is the lungs. Severity can range from asymptomatic to debilitation from severe fibrosis.

Descriptive Epidemiology

High-Risk Populations

Data from a private insurance database of 33.4 million insured adults, of whom 29,372 had sarcoidosis, revealed that the highest percentage of patients were in the age group of 55 to 64 years (31.2%) and 55% of cases occurred in patients 55 years of age or older. The rate of sarcoidosis among African Americans was more than twice as high as the rate among White Americans (17.8 vs 8.1/100,000). There was a higher prevalence of sarcoidosis among women than men in all ethnic groups.[68]

Geographic Distribution

The private insurance database mentioned earlier was used to evaluate for geographic differences in the rate of sarcoidosis in the United States. The country was split into the four US census regions: the Northeast (n = 11.1 million adults), South (n = 14.6 million adults), Midwest (n = 8.1 million adults), and West (n = 6.5 million adults). The West had a significantly lower incidence and prevalence of sarcoidosis than the other regions of the country.[68]

Causes

Interstitial lung disease can be caused by a wide variety of exposures, such as exposure to occupational dusts and fumes, medications, therapeutic radiation exposure, toxic gas inhalations, and infections such as COVID-19. However, the etiology of some interstitial lung diseases, such as idiopathic pulmonary fibrosis and sarcoidosis, is unknown.

Risk factors for developing many of the interstitial lung diseases remain poorly understood. An autopsy study on the risk factors for idiopathic pulmonary fibrosis found that laundry workers, barbers, beauticians, painters, production metalworkers, and production woodworkers were at greater risk for developing the disease.[69] Other studies on environmental factors and idiopathic pulmonary fibrosis have found increased odds ratios for exposure to wood dust, textile dust, metal dust, agricultural dust, and damp, moldy environments.[70–73] Smoking has been found to be a risk factor for idiopathic pulmonary fibrosis in several studies.[69,70,72] In a case-control study, a history of having ever smoked increased the risk for idiopathic pulmonary fibrosis by 60%.[70]

Occupational exposure to artificial food flavorings such as butter flavoring (diacetyl) applied to many different food products such as microwave popcorn has been associated with bronchiolitis obliterans.[74]

Evidence-Based Interventions

For interstitial lung diseases that develop from inhaling organic or inorganic dusts or fumes, limiting or avoiding the exposure will minimize or prevent the disease. Exposure to artificial butter flavoring, diacetyl, and other diketones has been observed from the commercial grinding and roasting of unflavored coffee beans.[75] These findings highlight the need for vigilance as the use of synthetic chemicals evolves to new settings, as well as the need to establish and maintain surveillance for illness associated with emerging industries and product use.

For many of the interstitial diseases, treatment is primarily supportive, treating the complications of respiratory and heart failure. Preventive care should include influenza and pneumococcal vaccines. Public health surveillance and clinician reporting of unusual diseases associated with occupational exposures is critical to early identification of emerging problems when intervention has the greatest potential for interrupting the emergence of disease.

OCCUPATIONAL LUNG DISEASES

This section covers five of the most common types of occupational lung diseases: (1) coal workers' pneumoconiosis, (2) silicosis, (3) asbestosis, (4) byssinosis, and (5) organic dust-related lung disease.

Significance

One of the most common occupational lung diseases, occupational chronic bronchitis (see COPD earlier in the chapter), and coughing are nonspecific but are often the first indications of work-related pulmonary pathology. Given a sufficient dose and duration of exposure, nearly all respirable agents can contribute to the development or aggravation of chronic lung diseases. It is not uncommon to have multiple occupational lung diseases present in the same workforce or even the same person. This is especially true for occupational bronchitis and occupational asthma.

Many chronic occupational lung diseases are defined by the agent associated with the specific disease and often named after the agent (e.g., silica inhalation causes silicosis, asbestos fiber inhalation causes asbestosis). Several distinct pathological processes have been associated with exposure to specific respirable dusts present in the occupational environment. Only a few of these diseases result from acute exposures. Most, especially pneumoconiosis, result from multiple years of exposure and are associated with an important hallmark of the disease process known as the disease latency period. This means that disease does not appear immediately, and typically at least 10, and commonly 20 or more, years pass between first exposure and the recognition of clinical disease. Some of these diseases may first appear and even progress many years after exposure has ended.

Occupational dusts are classified as either inorganic (e.g., coal dust, silica, asbestos) or organic (e.g., cotton dust, grain dust, mold spores). The respiratory conditions associated with most inorganic dusts are called pneumoconiosis and result from the direct effect of the dust on lung tissue. Chest X-ray is the primary diagnostic tool used to identify these diseases. Guidelines on how to classify chest radiographs for persons with pneumoconiosis have been published by the World Health Organization/International Labor Organization (ILO) since 1950. These guidelines describe and codify the radiographic abnormalities of the pneumoconiosis in a simple, reproducible manner by using two sets of standard comparison films. The guidelines were issued in 1971 and 1980, revised in 2000, and published in 2002.[3] In 2011 the ILO revised the guidelines to extend the classification to use with digital radiographic images.[4]

From 1968 to 2014 a total of 153,168 deaths from pneumoconiosis were recorded among US residents.[15] The US Occupational Safety and Health Administration (OSHA) has established national permissible exposure limits for all inorganic dusts associated with disease. Diseases resulting from exposure to most organic dusts are immunologically mediated. One exception to this latter classification is the condition related to cotton dust exposure; cotton dust is organic, but the condition is probably not immunologically mediated and is related to endotoxins present in the cotton dust.

Cigarette smoking increases the risk of lung disease in occupationally exposed workers. In most cases, the disease risks are additive—that is, the total disease risk is the sum of the risk from cigarette smoking and the risk from occupational exposure.

An exception to this is the multiplicative risk between asbestos exposure and cigarette smoking in the occurrence of lung cancer.

The following subsections briefly describe some important occupation-related chronic lung diseases.

Coal Workers' Pneumoconiosis

Coal workers' pneumoconiosis (CWP), first described in 1831 in a British coal miner, is known as black lung disease and is identified by a pattern of X-ray abnormalities and an exposure history. Through greater mechanization, coal production has increased while the workforce has declined; however, greater mechanization has led to dustier conditions. In 2013 there were approximately 123,000 coal-mining-sector employees in the United States.

Between 1968 and 2010, there occurred 73,849 US deaths with coal workers' pneumoconiosis noted on the death certificates. Deaths have significantly declined from a high of 2,870 in 1972 to 486 in 2010. For the decade from 1990 to 1999, more than three-fourths of all CWP decedents were residents of Pennsylvania, West Virginia, Virginia, and Kentucky. Pennsylvania alone accounted for about half of all CWP deaths in this period.[76] Although CWP has declined in the United States, the threat of CWP has significantly increased in developing countries seeking inexpensive sources of energy and using dust control measures and regulatory frameworks that are often rudimentary and ineffective.

Descriptive Epidemiology

The prevalence of CWP increases with increasing exposure to coal dust. In studies of CWP, years of mining are often used as a surrogate for dust exposure because information on dust exposure for individual miners is rarely complete.

Coal workers' pneumoconiosis is classified as simple CWP if rounded opacities less than one centimeter are seen on the chest radiograph (ILO opacities *p*, *q*, or *r*).[3] It is typical for the opacities to first appear in the upper lung fields of the chest X-ray and then to progress to involve all lung fields. The National Study of Coal Workers' Pneumoconiosis is maintained by the National Institute for Occupational Safety and Health (NIOSH). Data from that ongoing surveillance program shows that among US underground coal miners with 25 or more years of mining surveyed between 1973 and 1978, 34% had simple CWP. The prevalence of simple CWP declined to 4% during survey years 1996 to 1999.[77] It is uncommon in simple CWP for the radiographic abnormalities to progress after the individual has left the dusty environment.

Complicated CWP, often described as massive progressive fibrosis, is often preceded by recurrent infection, especially tuberculosis. Radiographically, it is defined as small opacities and the presence of large opacities (>1 cm) on the chest X-ray. Data from the national study suggest that the incidence of both simple and complicated CWP is declining, largely attributed to dust standards in mines being enforced, but may be increasing among younger individuals. In addition, although CWP prevalence in working coal miners declined substantially from 1970 to 1994, it increased from 1995 to 2006.[78]

Chronic exposure to coal dust can lead to the development of COPD, even in the absence of radiographic changes.[79] Coal miners with COPD have increased rates of dyspnea, cough, and phlegm production. The magnitude of the deficit in lung function attributable to chronic coal dust exposure is between 150 and 450 milliliters over an average lifetime of work in a coal mine, with a smaller percentage of individuals having deficits of greater than one liter.[80]

Causes

Coal workers' pneumoconiosis is related to the total dust burden in the lungs. The type of coal (known as coal rank, which is determined by the carbon content of the coal) is also important: the higher the rank, the greater the disease risk and dust biologic activity. Anthracite coal has the highest rank, followed by bituminous, subbituminous, and lignite. Coal workers' pneumoconiosis is caused by respirable coal mine dust (generally defined as dust particles <5μm in aerodynamic diameter). Usually, 10 or more years of exposure to coal dust must have elapsed before CWP can be diagnosed by a chest X-ray. Coal dust also may contain other harmful mineral dusts, such as silica dust, which increase the risk of other chronic lung diseases such as silicosis. The radiographic appearance of silicosis can be indistinguishable from CWP. The risk of CWP diagnosed by X-ray increases with the higher rank of coal, in part explaining the higher occurrence in miners from the eastern coal-producing regions of the United States compared with western areas. Miners who work underground, where dust control is problematic, are at higher risk than aboveground or surface miners.

Risk factors for the development of COPD in coal miners are the duration and extent of dust exposure, previous dust exposure, and the presence of other risk factors for obstructive lung disease, especially cigarette smoking. The average lifetime coal dust exposure among coal miners with symptoms of chronic lung disease was found to result in a loss in lung function equivalent to that associated with smoking 20 cigarettes per day over a lifetime.[80] Coal miners working in jobs with higher silica exposure, such as surface coal mine drillers, are at higher risk for the development of COPD.

Evidence-Based Interventions

Coal workers' pneumoconiosis can best be prevented by reducing coal dust exposure in mines and the workplace, engaging in comprehensive industrial hygiene monitoring to measure dust suppression, educating workers about disease risk and safe work practices, and, when excessive exposure circumstances are unavoidable, providing respiratory protection. Medical monitoring of coal miners is required, and periodic chest radiographs are intended to identify individuals who have CWP in its preliminary phases, thus enabling them to avoid further exposure and possibly preventing the disease's progression to more advanced stages. The use of the ILO pneumoconiosis grading system is critically important to allow quantification of changes over time and assessment of progression.

The Federal Coal Mine Health and Safety Act passed in 1969, and its amendments set limits on the amount of worksite respirable coal dust in the United States. For coal dust with less than 5% silica, the standard is 2 milligrams per cubic meter of air (mg/m^3). Although there is evidence that the current dust standards have contributed to the decrease in the occurrence of CWP, the Mine Safety and Health Administration monitoring data from the 1980s through 1999 show little change in the level of coal dust exposure exceedances. More than 8% of the 794,000 samples exceeded the permissible exposure limit. In 1995 NIOSH adopted a recommended exposure level of 1 mg/m^3, which was adopted because of concerns that the current standard did not protect against other lung conditions. Between 1995 and 2003 one-fourth of coal mine dust exposures recorded by the Mine Safety and Health Administration exceeded the recommended exposure level.[78]

Silicosis

Silicons constitute almost 28% of the earth's crust. It is the crystalline forms that are most toxic. Silica exists as five polymorphs, the most common being quartz, and these have many industrial applications. Occupational exposures occur worldwide, and although the disease is decreasing in developed countries, it is increasing in developing countries. In the United States, excessive exposures continue and are most frequently found in small operations that are seldom visited by regulatory agencies. Chronic inhalation of respirable particles of crystalline silica is the cause of silicosis. Like CWP, silicosis is characterized by a predominance of small, rounded X-ray abnormalities predominantly in the upper lung fields indicative of fibrosis. The histopathologic hallmark is the formation of silicotic nodules containing birefringent particles. Also, like CWP, silicosis can be divided into simple silicosis and complicated silicosis, or progressive massive fibrosis, based on the size of the opacities on the chest X-ray.

Unlike CWP, silicosis is characterized as acute, accelerated, or chronic. Fortunately, acute silicosis is uncommon today. It can occur, however, after high levels of exposure as in silica flour mills or in the now-outlawed use of silica for sandblasting. It is defined as acute silicosis if it appears in less than five years from first exposure. The acute form is often life-threatening and characterized by pulmonary edema, accumulation of proteinaceous fluid within alveoli, and interstitial inflammation. The most common form of the disease is chronic silicosis, which is defined as silicosis that appears 10 or more years after first exposure.

In its initial phases, the disease is not associated with declines in lung function, although cough and phlegm production are common. Chronic exposure to silica dust can also result in COPD, even without the X-ray manifestations of silicosis.[81] The disease may slowly progress over 20 to 40 years to the point of respiratory failure. Individuals with silicosis are at increased risk of developing tuberculosis.[82] Based on analyses of nine studies showing increased rates of lung cancer, silica is now categorized as a probable human carcinogen by the International Agency for Cancer Research.[83–85]

Descriptive Epidemiology

Hazardous exposure to respirable silica occurs in many different occupational settings, including surface and underground mining of ores containing silica, surface drilling, ceramics manufacturing, stone cutting, construction, silica flour mills, foundries, cement production, abrasive manufacturing and use, and sandblasting. In 2013, OSHA proposed a revised silica standard, at the time estimating that approximately 2.2 million workers were currently exposed to respirable crystalline silica, including 1.85 million workers in the construction industry and 320,000 workers in general industry and maritime workplaces.[86] As with CWP deaths, silicosis listed as a cause of death on a death certificate has declined from more than 1,000 annual deaths in the 1960s to a mean of 115 per year between 2010 and 2014.[15] Pennsylvania alone accounted for nearly 18% of all reported silicosis deaths from 1990 to 1999. Construction and mining industries accounted for more than a third of deaths from silicosis during that same period.

The prevalence of nonfatal silicosis in the United States is unknown. There are no national registries for the disease, and only a few states have surveillance requirements. By extrapolating from national mortality data, however, the Michigan state-based surveillance system and capture–recapture methodology estimated that from 1987 through 1996 there occurred 3,600 to 7,300 cases of silicosis annually.[87] The US Department of Labor estimated in 1980 that 59,000 of the workers who were then exposed to silica would eventually develop silicosis.[88]

Silicosis is most prevalent among workers involved in the dry drilling or grinding of rock with high silica content and other activities that generate large quantities of respirable particles. Largely reflecting the exposed workforce, silicosis is nine times more common in men than in women and more common among African American than White males. The most common industrial environments where silicosis occurs among men are mines, foundries, quarries, and silica flour mills.[78] Among women, silicosis occurs most commonly in the ceramics industry.

Causes

Silicosis is caused by acute or chronic inhalation of crystalline silica, which is present in quartz. A more toxic form of silica may be produced when quartz is heated or with freshly fractured quartz particles.[89] Foundry workers who are in occupations involving both heating and grinding quartz may be at greater risk of silicosis. A disturbing trend has been the continuing occurrence of silicosis deaths in young adults (aged 15–44 y) and reports of new occupations and tasks that place workers at risk for silicosis, such as fabricators and installers of engineered stone products containing quartz, and most recently, workers employed to extract natural gas by hydraulic fracturing who are exposed to the silica used in that process.[90]

Evidence-Based Interventions

The most effective method for preventing silicosis is primary prevention—eliminating exposure to respirable silica—and, in settings where silica dust occurs, verifying exposure reduction and maintenance through an industrial hygiene monitoring program. A secondary line of defense is worker education and training, use of protective equipment, and regulatory inspections and enforcement of existing worksite standards. The OSHA regulatory exposure limits for silica concentrations in the work environment were 0.1 mg/m^3 from 1989 to 1993. In 1993 this limit was modified (and effectively raised) based on a formula with a default limit of 5 mg/m^3 that is reduced as the silica content in a dust sample increases. NIOSH and the American Conference of Governmental Industrial Hygienists recommended an exposure limit of 0.05 mg/m^3. Under development by OSHA since 2013, a revised silica standard that became effective on June 23, 2016, reduces the permissible exposure limit for respirable crystalline silica to 50 micrograms per cubic meter of air, averaged over an eight-hour shift. It is estimated to prevent nearly 900 cases of silicosis each year and 600 deaths per year.[86] As with medical screening for conditions associated with other inorganic dusts, X-ray screening may identify individuals who have minimal disease, enabling these people to avoid additional exposure and possibly preventing progression to more advanced phases.

Asbestosis

There are four main types of commercially used asbestos fiber: chrysotile (serpentine mineral) and the amphibole minerals amosite, crocidolite, and anthophyllite. Another fibrous amphibole, tremolite, is a frequent contaminant of chrysotile ores as well as vermiculite. An estimated 27,500,000 workers were exposed to asbestos between 1940 and 1979.[91] Asbestos was widely used in construction materials, especially those used for insulation and acoustical products in many public, residential, and commercial buildings.

Most uses of asbestos have been eliminated, and many countries, but not the United States, have banned all use of asbestos.[92] Although its use in Europe, the United States, and many other countries has significantly decreased, the mining production of asbestos has been growing. Raw fiber continues to be used in less-developed countries.[93]

Current concerns in the United States focus on the potential for exposure to widely distributed, in-place asbestos-containing materials. The risk of adverse health effects from these sources of asbestos to workers or to building occupants depends on many factors, most specifically the status of the material—whether it is releasing asbestos fibers into the indoor environment, whether it is frequently disturbed, and how well contained fiber releases are from maintenance activities.

Adverse health effects from exposure to asbestos include pleural effusions, pleural thickening, plaques with and without calcification, malignant mesothelioma, lung cancer, and asbestosis. Of these, asbestosis is the most prevalent chronic lung condition. Approximately 107,000 asbestos-related deaths (from cancer or other diseases) occur worldwide each year.[94] For each year since 1998, asbestosis deaths outnumbered CWP deaths, displacing CWP as the most frequent type of pneumoconiosis death.

In its early stages, asbestosis is often clinically characterized by dry rales, or whistling or crackling noises, at the end of each inspiration. Often, clinical signs and pulmonary function abnormalities appear before chest X-ray abnormalities become apparent. Eventually, diffuse fibrosis can result in decreased lung capacity, decreased gas exchange, and severe shortness of breath. The X-ray abnormalities evident in people with asbestosis are predominantly small, irregular opacities in the lower lung fields (ILO *s*, *t*, and *u*). In addition, pleural thickening, or pleural plaques, often with calcification, can occur alone or in combination with asbestosis. Unlike CWP or silicosis, asbestosis deaths were increasing, from fewer than 100 in 1968 to more than 1,250 in 1999, but between 2000 and 2010 the number of US deaths leveled out at around 1,400 deaths per year[76] and decreased to a mean of 1,250 deaths per year between 2010 and 2014.[15]

Descriptive Epidemiology

In various surveys, between 6% and 40% of asbestos textile or insulation workers have detectable X-ray lung abnormalities. NHANES results indicate that 2.3% of US men and 0.2% of US women have pleural thickening upon chest X-ray.[95] In a study of 17,800 insulation workers in the United States, asbestosis was identified as the cause of death in 7% of the workers who died.[96,97]

Asbestos has thousands of uses, each of which present the possibility of exposure. Occupations and workers at risk span the life cycle of asbestos from removal from the ground to product manufacturing, to installation of products, to maintenance and removal, and finally to disposal. Although most uses of asbestos in newly manufactured products in the United States have been eliminated, today's exposure threats come from the long life of asbestos-containing products still present in building materials, which may pose a risk to workers during maintenance, repair, renovation, and demolition. A long latency period usually exists between exposure and the development of asbestosis, resulting in current cases seen today being a result of the legacy of exposures in the 1940s to 1970s.

Causes

Asbestosis is caused by exposure to airborne asbestos fibers. The magnitude of the risk of asbestosis depends on both the duration and the intensity of the exposure to asbestos dust. The more intense and prolonged the exposure, the greater the risk of developing the disease. Brief but very heavy exposure can also cause the disease.

Asbestos is unique among the pneumoconiosis-causing agents. Nonoccupational exposure to family members of workers bringing dust home on their clothes and those living in residences near mines and manufacturing facilities using asbestos have been associated with the occurrence of asbestos-associated disease.[98,99] Most recently, an environmental disaster was identified in Libby, Montana, where a large vermiculite mine and processing facility had been operating since the mid-1920s. The facility closed in 1990, and the community health impacts of the vermiculite asbestiform amphibole present in concentrations as high as 26% have been investigated. As a result of the research, 694 decedents were identified as having at least one asbestos-related cause of death and residing within the study area boundary. Workers, family members of workers, and community residents had significant excesses of asbestos-associated disease.[100]

Evidence-Based Interventions

Asbestosis can be prevented by eliminating exposure to asbestos. New asbestos-containing product manufacturing has been largely eliminated from the work environment in the United States and the EU countries, but the release of asbestos from existing materials must be controlled. Containment of asbestos in buildings may be initially less expensive than removal; however, containment is only a temporary solution, because product aging and deterioration will continue, and ongoing maintenance and repair can result in a further release of asbestos and eventual enforced removal under US Environmental Protection Agency regulations. National legislation requires accreditation of contractors who work with asbestos and training for asbestos abatement workers to ensure safety as well as to prevent "bystander" exposure. Safe work practices include identifying materials that contain asbestos; implementing rigorous operating procedures, such as wetting asbestos-containing materials; and wearing a self-contained breathing apparatus.

X-ray and pulmonary function screening may also help in protecting workers. Results from these examinations can encourage workers to avoid additional exposure, make them more aware of the need for strict work practices, and encourage them to participate in special health surveillance programs.

Byssinosis

Byssinosis is both an acute and a chronic airways disease caused by exposure to cotton dust. The acute phase of byssinosis is sometimes called Monday morning syndrome, in which chest tightness or shortness of breath occurs when workers return to cotton dust exposure following a weekend or days off. Symptoms usually resolve the second day. Progression of the disease is characterized by chronic cough and a decline in lung function. After more than 10 years of exposure, overall pulmonary function is often seen to decline. Byssinosis is similar in pathology to chronic bronchitis. A grading system has been developed for byssinosis.[101] In the United States, approximately 500,000 workers are potentially at risk for byssinosis,[102,103] although the disease is rarely fatal, claiming fewer than two lives per year between 2005 and 2014.[15]

Descriptive Epidemiology

It is estimated that more than 60 million people worldwide work in the textile or clothing industry and are at risk for developing byssinosis. The prevalence of byssinosis varies from a few percent to as high as 47% in some surveys.[104] In 1970 it was estimated that approximately 35,000 workers in the cotton textile mills had byssinosis.[102] Since regulation of cotton dust began in 1978, the degree of lung function impairment in cotton textile workers may have decreased.[102] There is no evidence of sex or race differences in risk of developing byssinosis.

Causes

Byssinosis results from exposure to the dust of cotton, flax, or hemp. Much has been learned about the causal agent of byssinosis, but the precise etiology is still being investigated. Evidence supports that it is not the cotton itself that is the causal agent but a bacterial endotoxin present in cotton dust.[105,106] Among cotton workers, the risk is highest among workers involved in the initial stages of processing: opening, picking, carding, stripping, and grinding raw cotton.

Evidence-Based Interventions

The best way to prevent byssinosis is to avoid exposure to cotton dust. Cotton dust concentrations in the workplace must be kept below OSHA's permissible exposure level. A technique known as cotton washing is effective but may not be feasible on a large scale. Employers must treat the acute phase of byssinosis as a sentinel health event, using it as an opportunity to reduce exposure among other workers with early symptoms.

Organic Dust–Related Lung Disease

A variety of chronic lung conditions can develop following short-term or long-term exposure to organic dusts (hypersensitivity pneumonitis) or toxic gases such as nitrogen oxides produced from the storage or decay of organic material (silo fillers disease).

Although agricultural workers are most frequently affected,[107] as with occupational asthma, there are more than 200 agents known to cause hypersensitivity pneumonitis, among them industrial chemicals such as metal-working fluids.[108]

In 2003 OSHA estimated that in 1996 there were 92,000 grain elevator and 68,000 grain mill employees working in approximately 5,200 grain elevator firms and 1,500 grain mill firms who were affected by the OSHA (2003) grain dust standard.[109] Grain dust is a mixture of different grains, bacteria and fungus, mites, inorganic material, and herbicides and pesticides. Grain-handlers' disease, caused by inhaling grain dust, is characterized by a drop in lung function over a work shift and by changes that persist over a harvest season.[110] Chronic grain dust exposure can result in chronic cough, phlegm, wheezing, and dyspnea, as well as a permanent decline in lung function. Pulmonary fibrosis may occur but is uncommon in workers with chronic grain dust exposure.[110]

Farmer's lung is caused by inhaling spores from moldy hay and is characterized by repeated attacks of fever, chills, malaise, coughing, and breathlessness.[111] The condition is a type of hypersensitivity pneumonitis or extrinsic allergic alveolitis that results from inhaling many different organic dusts. Most commonly, thermophilic *Actinomyces* or other fungi are present. Testing patient serum for specific precipitating antibodies can help identify which organisms or agents may be contributing to the disease. In a well-controlled research setting, inhalation chamber challenges have been used to identify offending agents. Such testing is not a routine practice. The chronic form occurs in fewer than 5% of patients who develop the acute form of the disease.[112] Lung function is abnormal in patients with the chronic form of the disease, with a decline in the FVC and a diffuse fibrosis evident on the chest X-ray.

Descriptive Epidemiology

Hypersensitivity pneumonitis is a rare disease with an increasing incidence, and little is known about the distribution of the disease outside the agricultural sector.[52,107] Some of the increase may be attributable to changes in agricultural practices and the movement to large-scale production of livestock in confined feeding operations.[113] Symptoms are often similar to asthma, COPD, and bronchitis; and initial acute attacks are often mistaken for pneumonia. No single clinical or laboratory test exists to establish the diagnosis. Chronic lung disease from inhaling grain dust is probably more common, but relatively little is known about its epidemiologic patterns.

Causes

Those at risk for the disease from inhaling biologically active organic dusts include farmers, grain handlers, woodworkers, bird breeders, mushroom workers, and animal handlers, including workers who clean pens and handle laboratory animals.[107] Environments where water-based machining fluids are used have also been associated with hypersensitivity pneumonitis, probably because of aerosolization of bacteria or fungi growing in the fluids.[108]

Evidence-Based Interventions

Agricultural dusts are regulated in the United States; NIOSH has proposed a limit of 4 mg/m^3 for grain dust. The concern over dust levels in grain-handling facilities has, in part, been because of the risk of explosions.[109] Improved design of grain elevators and livestock confinement spaces, proper ventilation, and education of farmworkers and rescue services can reduce the risk from dust and toxic gases.[112] Self-contained breathing devices should be worn by workers entering closed or poorly ventilated spaces or tanks containing liquid manure. Diseases caused by molds can be minimized by proper grain storage techniques. A critical factor in control of disease is worker knowledge of the circumstances in which exposures are likely to occur so that preventive precautions can be taken.

DISCUSSION QUESTIONS

1. Many modifiable factors contribute to the subsequent occurrence of chronic lung diseases in later life. Discuss four primary prevention actions that public health programs should promote that will reduce the likelihood of disabling lung diseases appearing in later life. What would be your top priority?
2. The causes of chronic occupational lung diseases have been known for over 200 years. Discuss the reasons why these diseases continue to frequently occur in US workers.
3. Disease and risk factor surveillance, along with epidemiologic analyses, are core public health functions. How would you defend the cost and importance of maintaining and expanding such activities in the current environment of expanding personal choice freedoms?
4. Among all the chronic diseases discussed in this book, where would you rank the public health importance of chronic lung disease, and what are the criteria you would use to perform such a ranking?
5. Discuss why it is important to integrate public health practices into mainstream individual clinical medicine services.

REFERENCES

1. National Center for Health Statistics. FastStats: leading causes of death. September 6, 2022. Available at: https://www.cdc.gov/nchs/fastats/leading-causes-of-death.htm. Accessed January 23, 2023.

2. Centers for Disease Control and Prevention, National Center for Health Statistics. National Vital Statistics System, Mortality 1999–2020 on CDC WONDER Online Database. Published 2021. Available at: http://wonder.cdc.gov/ucd-icd10.html. Accessed January 27, 2023.
3. International Labour Organization. *Guidelines for the Use of ILO International Classification of Radiographs of Pneumoconioses.* International Labour Organization; 2002.
4. International Labour Organization. *Guidelines for the Use of ILO International Classification of Radiographs of Pneumoconioses.* International Labour Organization; 2011.
5. Tamura T, Suganuma N, Hering KG, et al. Relationships (I) of international classification of high-resolution computed tomography for occupational and environmental respiratory diseases with the ILO international classification of radiographs of pneumoconioses for parenchymal abnormalities. *Ind Health.* 2015;53(3):260–270. doi:10.2486/indhealth.2014-0073
6. National Center for Health Statistics. Percentage of COPD, emphysema, or chronic bronchitis for adults aged 18 and over, United States, 2019–2021. Interactive Summary Health Statistics for Adults—2019–2021. Available at: https://wwwn.cdc.gov/NHISDataQueryTool/SHS_adult/index.html. Accessed January 23, 2023.
7. Tilert T, Dillon C, Paulose-Ram R, Hnizdo E, Doney B. Estimating the US prevalence of chronic obstructive pulmonary disease using pre- and post-bronchodilator spirometry: the National Health and Nutrition Examination Survey (NHANES) 2007–2010. *Respir Res.* 2013;14(1):103. doi:10.1186/1465-9921-14-103
8. National Center for Health Statistics. FastStats: chronic obstructive pulmonary disease (COPD) includes: chronic bronchitis and emphysema. September 6, 2022. Updated December 30, 2022. Available at: https://www.cdc.gov/nchs/fastats/copd.htm. Accessed January 23, 2023.
9. Ford ES, Murphy LB, Khavjou O, Giles WH, Holt JB, Croft JB. Total and state-specific medical and absenteeism costs of COPD among adults aged ≥ 18 years in the United States for 2010 and projections through 2020. *Chest.* 2015;147(1):31–45. doi:10.1378/chest.14-0972
10. Global Initiative for Chronic Obstructive Lung Disease. 2022 Gold Reports: global strategy for prevention, diagnosis and management of COPD. 2022. Available at: https://goldcopd.org/2022-gold-reports. Accessed January 23, 2023.
11. Rabe KF, Hurd S, Anzueto A, et al. Global strategy for the diagnosis, management, and prevention of chronic obstructive pulmonary disease: GOLD executive summary. *Am J Respir Crit Care Med.* 2007;176(6):532–555. doi:10.1164/rccm.200703-456SO
12. Perez TA, Castillo EG, Ancochea J, et al. Sex differences between women and men with COPD: a new analysis of the 3CIA study. *Respir Med.* 2020;171:106105. doi:10.1016/j.rmed.2020.106105
13. Ford ES, Croft JB, Mannino DM, Wheaton AG, Zhang X, Giles WH. COPD surveillance—United States, 1999–2011. *Chest.* 2013;144(1):284–305. doi:10.1378/chest.13-0809
14. Centers for Disease Control and Prevention. State-level estimates of COPD. Available at: https://www.cdc.gov/copd/data-and-statistics/state-estimates.html. Accessed March 27, 2023.
15. National Institute for Occupational Safety and Health. Work-related respiratory diseases (eWorld). 2022. Available at: https://wwwn.cdc.gov/eworld/Set/Work-Related_Respiratory_Diseases/88. Accessed January 23, 2023.
16. Johannessen A, Bakke PS, Hardie JA, Eagan TM. Association of exposure to environmental tobacco smoke in childhood with chronic obstructive pulmonary disease and respiratory symptoms in adults. *Respirology.* 2012;17(3):499–505. doi:10.1111/j.1440-1843.2012.02129.x

17. Blanc PD, Iribarren C, Trupin L, et al. Occupational exposures and the risk of COPD: dusty trades revisited. *Thorax.* 2009;64(1):6–12. doi:10.1136/thx.2008.099390
18. Hu G, Zhou Y, Tian J, et al. Risk of COPD from exposure to biomass smoke: a meta-analysis. *Chest.* 2010;138(1):20–31. doi:10.1378/chest.08-2114
19. Marsh S, Aldington S, Shirtcliffe P, Weatherall M, Beasley R. Smoking and COPD: what really are the risks? *Eur Respir J.* 2006;28(4):883–884. doi:10.1183/09031936.06.00074806
20. Eisner MD, Anthonisen N, Coultas D, et al. An official American Thoracic Society public policy statement: novel risk factors and the global burden of chronic obstructive pulmonary disease. *Am J Respir Crit Care Med.* 2010;182(5):693–718. doi:10.1164/rccm.200811-1757ST
21. Eisner MD, Balmes J, Katz PP, Trupin L, Yelin EH, Blanc PD. Lifetime environmental tobacco smoke exposure and the risk of chronic obstructive pulmonary disease. *Environ Health.* 2005;4(1):7. doi:10.1186/1476-069x-4-7
22. Shapiro S, Snider G, Rennard S. Chronic bronchitis and emphysema. In: Mason R, Murray J, Broaddus V, Nadel J, eds. *Murray and Nadel's Textbook of Respiratory Medicine.* WB Saunders Co; 2000.
23. Global Initiative for Asthma. 2022 GINA Main Report. Global Strategy for Asthma Management and Prevention. 2022. Available at: https://ginasthma.org/gina-reports. Accessed January 23, 2023.
24. Centers for Disease Control and Prevention. 2020 adult asthma data: prevalence tables and maps. Table L1: adult lifetime asthma prevalence and number by state or territory: BRFSS 2020. Updated March 11, 2022. Available at: https://www.cdc.gov/asthma/brfss/2020/tableL1.html. Accessed January 23, 2023.
25. Centers for Disease Control and Prevention. Asthma: AsthmaStats. August 6, 2022. Updated December 12, 2022. Available at: https://www.cdc.gov/asthma/asthma_stats/default.htm. Accessed January 23, 2023.
26. National Center for Health Statistics. FastStats: Asthma. September 6, 2022. Updated December 30, 2022. Available at: https://www.cdc.gov/nchs/fastats/asthma.htm. Accessed January 23, 2023.
27. Pearce N, Pekkanen J, Beasley R. How much asthma is really attributable to atopy? *Thorax.* 1999;54(3):268–272. doi:10.1136/thx.54.3.268
28. Barbee RA, Murphy S. The natural history of asthma. *J Allergy Clin Immunol.* 1998;102(4 pt 2): S65–S72. doi:10.1016/s0091-6749(98)70006-5
29. Sears M. Epidemiological trends in bronchial asthma. In: Kaliner M, Barnes P, Persson C, eds. *Asthma: Its Pathology and Treatment.* Marcel Dekker; 1991:1–49.
30. Qin X, Zahran HS, Malilay J. Asthma-related emergency department (ED) visits and post-ED visit hospital and critical care admissions, National Hospital Ambulatory Medical Care Survey, 2010-2015. *J Asthma.* 2021 May;58(5):565-572. doi: 10.1080/02770903.2020.1713149
31. Weiss KB. Seasonal trends in US asthma hospitalizations and mortality. *JAMA.* 1990;263(17):2323–2328.
32. Silverman RA, Ito K, Stevenson L, Hastings HM. The relationship of fall school opening and emergency department asthma visits in a large metropolitan area. *Arch Pediatr Adolesc Med.* 2005;159(9):818–823. doi:10.1001/archpedi.159.9.818

33. Arbes SJ, Gergen PJ, Vaughn B, Zeldin DC. Asthma cases attributable to atopy: results from the third National Health and Nutrition Examination Survey. *J Allergy Clin Immunol.* 2007;120(5):1139–1145. doi:10.1016/j.jaci.2007.07.056
34. Burke W, Fesinmeyer M, Reed K, Hampson L, Carlsten C. Family history as a predictor of asthma risk. *Am J Prev Med.* 2003;24(2):160–169. doi:10.1016/s0749-3797(02)00589-5
35. Moffatt MF, Gut IG, Demenais F, et al. A large-scale, consortium-based genomewide association study of asthma. *N Engl J Med.* 2010;363(13):1211–1221. doi:10.1056/NEJMoa0906312
36. Martinez FD, Wright AL, Taussig LM, Holberg CJ, Halonen M, Morgan WJ. Asthma and wheezing in the first six years of life. The Group Health Medical Associates. *N Engl J Med.* 1995;332(3):133–138. doi:10.1056/nejm199501193320301
37. Beuther DA, Weiss ST, Sutherland ER. Obesity and asthma. *Am J Respir Crit Care Med.* 2006;174(2):112–119. doi:10.1164/rccm.200602-231PP
38. Akinbami LJ, Fryar CD. Current asthma prevalence by weight status among adults: United States, 2001–2014. *Natl Cent Health Stat Data Brief.* 2016;(239):1–8.
39. Sarnat JA, Holguin F. Asthma and air quality. *Curr Opin Pulm Med.* 2007;13(1):63–66. doi:10.1097/MCP.0b013e3280117d25
40. McConnell R, Islam T, Shankardass K, et al. Childhood incident asthma and traffic-related air pollution at home and school. *Env Health Perspect.* 2010;118(7):1021–1026. doi:10.1289/ehp.0901232
41. Gerald LB, Sockrider MM, Grad R, et al. An official ATS workshop report: issues in screening for asthma in children. *Proc Am Thorac Soc.* 2007;4(2):133–141. doi:10.1513/pats.200604-103ST
42. King GG, Farrow CE, Chapman DG. Dismantling the pathophysiology of asthma using imaging. *Eur Respir Rev Off J Eur Respir Soc.* 2019;28(152):180111. doi:10.1183/16000617.0111-2018
43. Tarlo SM. Update on work-exacerbated asthma. *Int J Occup Med Env Health.* 2016;29(3):369–374. doi:10.13075/ijomeh.1896.00676
44. American Thoracic Society. Guidelines for assessing and managing asthma risk at work, school, and recreation. *Am J Respir Crit Care Med.* 2004;169(7):873–881. doi:10.1164/rccm.169.7.873
45. Blanc P. Occupational asthma in a national disability survey. *Chest.* 1987;92(4):613–617. doi:10.1378/chest.92.4.613
46. Tarlo SM, Balmes J, Balkissoon R, et al. Diagnosis and management of work-related asthma: American College of Chest Physicians consensus statement. *Chest.* 2008;134(3 suppl):1s–41s. doi:10.1378/chest.08-0201
47. Chan-Yeung M, Malo J. Natural history of occupational asthma. In: Bernstein I, Chan-Yeung M, Malo J, Bernstein D, eds. *Asthma in the Workplace.* 2nd ed. Marcel Dekker; 1999.
48. Beach J, Russell K, Blitz S, et al. A systematic review of the diagnosis of occupational asthma. *Chest.* 2007;131(2):569–578. doi:10.1378/chest.06-0492
49. Chan-Yeung M, Lam S, Koener S. Clinical features and natural history of occupational asthma due to western red cedar (*Thuja plicata*). *Am J Med.* 1982;72(3):411–415. doi:10.1016/0002-9343(82)90497-1
50. Mapp CE, Boschetto P, Maestrelli P, Fabbri LM. Occupational asthma. *Am J Respir Crit Care Med.* 2005;172(3):280–305. doi:10.1164/rccm.200311-1575SO

51. Rosenman KD, Beckett WS. Web based listing of agents associated with new onset work-related asthma. *Respir Med.* 2015;109(5):625–631. doi:10.1016/j.rmed.2015.03.004
52. Spagnolo P, Rossi G, Cavazza A, et al. Hypersensitivity pneumonitis: a comprehensive review. *J Investig Allergol Clin Immunol.* 2015;25(4):237–250.
53. Weeks J, Levy B, Wagner G, eds. *Preventing Occupational Disease and Injury.* American Public Health Association; 1991.
54. Boucher P, Knowles M, Yankaskas J. Cystic fibrosis. In: Mason R, Murray J, Broaddus V, Nadel J, eds. *Murray and Nadel's Textbook of Respiratory Medicine.* Vol 1. WB Saunders Co; 2000:1291–1324.
55. Cystic Fibrosis Foundation. Survival trending upward but what does this really mean? Available at: https://www.cff.org/community-posts/2017-11/survival-trending-upward-what-does-really-mean. Accessed March 27, 2023.
56. MacKenzie T, Gifford AH, Sabadosa KA, et al. Longevity of patients with cystic fibrosis in 2000 to 2010 and beyond: survival analysis of the Cystic Fibrosis Foundation patient registry. *Ann Intern Med.* 2014;161(4):233–241. doi:10.7326/m13-0636
57. Cabral B, Terlizzi V, Laselva O, Conte Filho C, Mota F. Anticipating new treatments for cystic fibrosis: a global survey of researchers. *J Clin Med.* 2022;11(5). doi:10.3390/jcm11051283
58. Cystic Fibrosis Foundation. About cystic fibrosis. Available at: https://www.cff.org/intro-cf/about-cystic-fibrosis. Accessed January 23, 2023.
59. Cystic Fibrosis Foundation. Types of CFTR mutations. Available at: https://www.cff.org/research-clinical-trials/types-cftr-mutations. Accessed January 23, 2023.
60. Flume PA, Van Devanter DR. State of progress in treating cystic fibrosis respiratory disease. *BMC Med.* 2012;10:88. doi:10.1186/1741-7015-10-88
61. Orenstein D, Rosenstein B, Stern R. Diagnosis of cystic fibrosis. In: Orenstein D, Roesnstein B, Stern R, eds. *Cystic Fibrosis Medical Care.* Lippincott, Williams and Wilkins; 2000:21–54.
62. Tsui LC, Buchwald M. Biochemical and molecular genetics of cystic fibrosis. *Adv Hum Genet.* 1991;20:153–266, 311–312. doi:10.1007/978-1-4684-5958-6_4
63. Schulz S, Jakubiczka S, Kropf S, Nickel I, Muschke P, Kleinstein J. Increased frequency of cystic fibrosis transmembrane conductance regulator gene mutations in infertile males. *Fertil Steril.* 2006;85(1):135–138. doi:10.1016/j.fertnstert.2005.07.1282
64. Fogarty A, Hubbard R, Britton J. International comparison of median age at death from cystic fibrosis. *Chest.* 2000;117(6):1656–1660. doi:10.1378/chest.117.6.1656
65. Kerem E, Reisman J, Corey M, Canny GJ, Levison H. Prediction of mortality in patients with cystic fibrosis. *N Engl J Med.* 1992;326(18):1187–1191. doi:10.1056/nejm199204303261804
66. Belkin RA, Henig NR, Singer LG, et al. Risk factors for death of patients with cystic fibrosis awaiting lung transplantation. *Am J Respir Crit Care Med.* 2006;173(6):659-666. doi:10.1164/rccm.200410-1369OC
67. Shteinberg M, Taylor-Cousar JL. Impact of CFTR modulator use on outcomes in people with severe cystic fibrosis lung disease. *Eur Respir Rev Off J Eur Respir Soc.* 2020;29(155):190112. doi:10.1183/16000617.0112-2019
68. Baughman RP, Field S, Costabel U, et al. Sarcoidosis in America. Analysis based on health care use. *Ann Am Thorac Soc.* 2016;13(8):1244–1252. doi:10.1513/AnnalsATS.201511-760OC

69. Scott J, Johnston I, Britton J. What causes cryptogenic fibrosing alveolitis? a case-control study of environmental exposure to dust. *BMJ*. 1990;301(6759):1015–1017. doi:10.1136/bmj.301.6759.1015
70. Hubbard R, Lewis S, Richards K, Johnston I, Britton J. Occupational exposure to metal or wood dust and aetiology of cryptogenic fibrosing alveolitis. *Lancet*. 1996;347(8997):284–289. doi:10.1016/s0140-6736(96)90465-1
71. Mapel DW, Samet JM, Coultas DB. Corticosteroids and the treatment of idiopathic pulmonary fibrosis. Past, present, and future. *Chest*. 1996;110(4):1058–1067. doi:10.1378/chest.110.4.1058
72. Baumgartner KB, Samet JM, Stidley CA, Colby TV, Waldron JA. Cigarette smoking: a risk factor for idiopathic pulmonary fibrosis. *Am J Respir Crit Care Med*. 1997;155(1):242–248. doi:10.1164/ajrccm.155.1.9001319
73. Taskar V, Coultas D. Exposures and idiopathic lung disease. *Semin Respir Crit Care Med*. 2008;29(6):670–679. doi:10.1055/s-0028-1101277
74. Centers for Disease Control and Prevention. Fixed obstructive lung disease among workers in the flavor-manufacturing industry—California, 2004–2007. *MMWR Morb Mortal Wkly Rep*. 2007;56(16):389–393.
75. Gaffney SH, Abelmann A, Pierce JS, et al. Naturally occurring diacetyl and 2,3-pentanedione concentrations associated with roasting and grinding unflavored coffee beans in a commercial setting. *Toxicol Rep*. 2015;2:1171–1181. doi:10.1016/j.toxrep.2015.08.003
76. Centers for Disease Control and Prevention. National Occupational Mortality Surveillance. 2016. Available at: https://www.cdc.gov/niosh/topics/noms/default.html. Accessed January 23, 2023.
77. National Institute for Occupational Safety and Health. *Worker Health Chartbook—2016*. National Institute for Occupational Safety and Health; 2004.
78. Laney AS, Weissman DN. Respiratory diseases caused by coal mine dust. *J Occup Environ Med*. 2014 Oct;56 Suppl 10(0 10):S18-22. doi: 10.1097/JOM.0000000000000260.
79. Oxman AD, Muir DC, Shannon HS, Stock SR, Hnizdo E, Lange HJ. Occupational dust exposure and chronic obstructive pulmonary disease. A systematic overview of the evidence. *Am Rev Respir Dis*. 1993;148(1):38–48. doi:10.1164/ajrccm/148.1.38
80. Lewis S, Bennett J, Richards K, Britton J. A cross sectional study of the independent effect of occupation on lung function in British coal miners. *Occup Env Med*. 1996;53(2):125–128. doi:10.1136/oem.53.2.125
81. Hnizdo E, Vallyathan V. Chronic obstructive pulmonary disease due to occupational exposure to silica dust: a review of epidemiological and pathological evidence. *Occup Env Med*. 2003;60(4):237–243. doi:10.1136/oem.60.4.237
82. Snider DE. The relationship between tuberculosis and silicosis. *Am Rev Respir Dis*. 1978;118(3):455–460. doi:10.1164/arrd.1978.118.3.455
83. Smith AH, Lopipero PA, Barroga VR. Meta-analysis of studies of lung cancer among silicotics. *Epidemiology*. 1995;6(6):617–624. doi:10.1097/00001648-199511000-00010
84. International Agency for Research on Cancer (IARC). *IARC Monographs on the Evaluation of Carcinogenic Risks to Humans*. Vol 68. *Silica, Some Silicates, Coal Dust and para-Aramid Fibrils*. World Health Organization. 1997. Available at: https://publications.iarc.fr/Book-And-Report-Series/Iarc-Monographs-On-The-Identification-Of-Carcinogenic-Hazards-To-Humans/

Silica-Some-Silicates-Coal-Dust-And-Em-Para-Em--Aramid-Fibrils-1997. Accessed January 23, 2023.

85. International Agency for Research on Cancer. *IARC Monographs on the Evaluation of Carcinogenic Risks to Humans*. Vol 100C. *Arsenic, Metals, Fibres, and Dusts*. World Health Organization. 2012. Available at: https://publications.iarc.fr/Book-And-Report-Series/Iarc-Monographs-On-The-Identification-Of-Carcinogenic-Hazards-To-Humans/Arsenic-Metals-Fibres-And-Dusts-2012. Accessed January 23, 2023.
86. Occupational Safety and Health Administration. Occupational exposure to respirable crystalline silica. Federal Register. 2016. Available at: https://www.federalregister.gov/documents/2016/03/25/2016-04800/occupational-exposure-to-respirable-crystalline-silica. Accessed January 23, 2023.
87. Rosenman KD, Reilly MJ, Henneberger PK. Estimating the total number of newly-recognized silicosis cases in the United States. *Am J Ind Med*. 2003;44(2):141–147. doi:10.1002/ajim.10243
88. Bates DV, Gotsch AR, Brooks S, Landrigan PJ, Hankinson JL, Merchant JA. Prevention of occupational lung disease. Task Force on Research and Education for the Prevention and Control of Respiratory Diseases. *Chest*. 1992;102(3 suppl):257S–276S. doi:10.1378/chest.102.3.257s
89. Vallyathan V, Castranova V, Pack D, et al. Freshly fractured quartz inhalation leads to enhanced lung injury and inflammation. Potential role of free radicals. *Am J Respir Crit Care Med*. 1995;152(3):1003–1009. doi:10.1164/ajrccm.152.3.7663775
90. Mazurek JM, Schleiff PL, Wood JM, Hendricks SA, Weston A. Notes from the field: update: silicosis mortality—United States, 1999–2013. *MMWR Morb Mortal Wkly Rep*. 2015;64(23):653–654.
91. American Thoracic Society. Diagnosis and initial management of nonmalignant diseases related to asbestos. *Am J Respir Crit Care Med*. 2004;170(6):691–715. doi:10.1164/rccm.200310-1436ST
92. Collegium Ramazzini. Asbestos is still with us: repeat call for a universal ban. *Am J Ind Med*. 2011;54(2):168–173. doi:10.1002/ajim.20892
93. LaDou J. The asbestos cancer epidemic. *Env Health Perspect*. 2004;112(3):285–290. doi:10.1289/ehp.6704
94. Collegium Ramazzini. The 18th Collegium Ramazzini statement: the global health dimensions of asbestos and asbestos-related diseases. *Scand J Work Environ Health*. 2016;42(1):86–90. doi:10.5271/sjweh.3541
95. Rogan WJ, Gladen BC, Ragan NB, Anderson HA. US prevalence of occupational pleural thickening. A look at chest x-rays from the first National Health and Nutrition Examination Survey. *Am J Epidemiol*. 1987;126(5):893–900. doi:10.1093/oxfordjournals.aje.a114726
96. Selikoff IJ, Hammond EC, Seidman H. Mortality experience of insulation workers in the United States and Canada, 1943–1976. *Annu N Y Acad Sci*. 1979;330:91–116. doi:10.1111/j.1749-6632.1979.tb18711.x
97. Markowitz SB, Levin SM, Miller A, Morabia A. Asbestos, asbestosis, smoking, and lung cancer. New findings from the North American insulator cohort. *Am J Respir Crit Care Med*. 2013;188(1):90–96. doi:10.1164/rccm.201302-0257OC
98. Anderson HA, Lilis R, Daum SM, Fischbein AS, Selikoff IJ. Household-contact asbestos neoplastic risk. *Annu N Y Acad Sci*. 1976;271:311–323. doi:10.1111/j.1749-6632.1976.tb23127.x

99. National Institute for Occupational Safety and Health. Report to Congress: Workers' Home Contamination Study conducted under the Workers' Family Protection Act. National Institute for Occupational Safety and Health; 1995.
100. Naik SL, Lewin M, Young R, Dearwent SM, Lee R. Mortality from asbestos-associated disease in Libby, Montana 1979–2011. *J Expo Sci Environ Epidemiol.* 2017;27(2):207–213. doi:10.1038/jes.2016.18
101. Bouhuys A, Schoenberg JB, Beck GJ, Schilling RS. Epidemiology of chronic lung disease in a cotton mill community. *Lung.* 1977;154(3):167–186. doi:10.1007/bf02713532
102. Glindmeyer HW, Lefante JJ, Jones RN, Rando RJ, Abdel Kader HM, Weill H. Exposure-related declines in the lung function of cotton textile workers. Relationship to current workplace standards. *Am Rev Respir Dis.* 1991;144(3 pt 1):675–683. doi:10.1164/ajrccm/144.3_Pt_1.675
103. Lai PS, Christiani DC. Long-term respiratory health effects in textile workers. *Curr Opin Pulm Med.* 2013;19(2):152–157. doi:10.1097/MCP.0b013e32835cee9a
104. Zuskin E, Ivankovic D, Schachter EN, Witek TJ. A ten-year follow-up study of cotton textile workers. *Am Rev Respir Dis.* 1991;143(2):301–305. doi:10.1164/ajrccm/143.2.301
105. Rylander R. Endotoxin in the environment—exposure and effects. *J Endotoxin Res.* 2002;8(4):241–252. doi:10.1179/096805102125000452
106. Shi J, Mehta AJ, Hang JQ, et al. Chronic lung function decline in cotton textile workers: roles of historical and recent exposures to endotoxin. *Environ Health Perspect.* 2010;118(11):1620–1624. doi:10.1289/ehp.0901178
107. Bang KM, Weissman DN, Pinheiro GA, Antao VC, Wood JM, Syamlal G. Twenty-three years of hypersensitivity pneumonitis mortality surveillance in the United States. *Am J Ind Med.* 2006;49(12):997–1004. doi:10.1002/ajim.20405
108. Kreiss K, Cox-Ganser J. Metalworking fluid-associated hypersensitivity pneumonitis: a workshop summary. *Am J Ind Med.* 1997;32(4):423–432. doi:10.1002/(sici)1097-0274(199710)32:4<423:aid-ajim16>3.0.co;2-5
109. Occupational Safety and Health Administration. Grain handling facilities standard. *Fed Regist.* 2003;68:12301–12303.
110. James AL, Cookson WO, Buters G, et al. Symptoms and longitudinal changes in lung function in young seasonal grain handlers. *Br J Ind Med.* 1986;43(9):587–591. doi:10.1136/oem.43.9.587
111. do Pico GA. Hazardous exposure and lung disease among farm workers. *Clin Chest Med.* 1992;13(2):311–328.
112. Speizer FE. Epidemiology of environmentally-induced chronic respiratory disease. *Chest.* 1981;80(1 suppl):21–22. doi:10.1378/chest.80.1_supplement.21s
113. Von Essen SG, Auvermann BW. Health effects from breathing air near CAFOs for feeder cattle or hogs. *J Agromedicine.* 2005;10(4):55–64. doi:10.1300/J096v10n04_08

19

Mental Disorders

Elizabeth Stein, MD, MS, Jerry Halverson, MD, and Ron Manderscheid, PhD

LEARNING OBJECTIVES

After completing this chapter, readers should be able to

1. Understand the different types of mental disorders and their collective burden on public health.
2. Identify the causes of mental health disorders, including modifiable risk factors.
3. Understand various individual treatments as well as community treatments for serious mental disorders.
4. Review the history of community approaches to serious mental disorders and how that affects the way populations with mental disorders are treated today.

INTRODUCTION

The care of persons with mental disorders is increasingly recognized as a central ingredient to overall health, and policymakers and health care leaders are making efforts to integrate it into other forms of health care. With this shift, the public health community recognizes mental disorders as one of the most serious chronic diseases, rivaling heart disease and cancer in years and quality of life lost and having linkages with most other chronic diseases. In 2020, of all adults in the United States, 21% suffered from a mental disorder in the last year (excluding substance use), and for 27% of these adults, the mental disorder qualified as a serious illness resulting in severe functional impairment that significantly interfered with major life activities.[1] More recently, the ongoing toll of the COVID-19 pandemic has emphasized the importance of recognizing and supporting access to treatment for mental disorders for all citizens.

Household surveys, National Syndromic Surveillance Program data, and anecdotal reports have sounded the alarm of increasing incidence of mental disorders in the United States during the COVID-19 pandemic. According to trends from the Centers for Disease Control and Prevention's (CDC) Household Pulse Survey, Cai et al.[2] found that the proportion of US adults with symptoms of anxiety disorder and/or depressive disorder quadrupled over the course of the pandemic, with the burden disproportionately borne by women and people of color. Among children and adolescents, emergency room visits for mental disorders have increased over 10% in January 2022 compared with January 2021 for admissions relating to anxiety, trauma, eating disorders, tics, and obsessive-compulsive disorders.[3] These increases were most profound among adolescent females. Following an earlier report from National Syndromic Surveillance Program data showing similar increases in mental health-related emergency room visits among children and adolescents in 2020, several pediatric associations and the US surgeon general declared a national emergency for these alarming trends in children's mental health.[4]

Despite research showing that treatment for such disorders can mitigate these life-shortening effects, people with mental disorders, relative to other chronic disease, are more likely to go without treatment. According to the National Alliance on Mental Illness, 46.2 % of adults with mental disorders as well as only 64.5% with serious mental disorders received treatment for their disorder in 2020. In US youth aged 6 to 17 years, only 50.6% with mental disorders received treatment.[5] In contrast, only about 15% of people with cardiovascular disease reported difficulty accessing routine health care.[6]

Given the significant morbidity and mortality associated with poor mental health, the public health community is seeking interventions to prevent mental disorders and to connect persons with these disorders to treatment. Yet several barriers pose challenges to this endeavor. Improving the population's relatively low mental health treatment access—a problem that stems from stigma, under-recognition by medical providers, superimposed on a poorly funded system with inadequate community mental health resources—requires a multisector approach by the government, health care system, criminal justice system, and community leaders.[7]

Efforts to increase access to treatment for mental disorders include federal legislation introduced by the Mental Health Parity and Addiction Equity Act of 2008 and the Patient Protection and Affordable Care Act of 2010 (ACA), which are leading to better access to health insurance and better integration of mental health treatment and primary care.[8] Despite these advances, much work remains to prevent, treat, and reduce the social burden of these debilitating chronic diseases. The COVID-19 pandemic has further decreased access to mental health treatment a result of the communal nature of the treatment and has led to enhanced use of telehealth alternatives to increase access.

SIGNIFICANCE

Mental disorders, including substance abuse, continue to be leading causes of death, disability, and human suffering in the United States and throughout the world.[9–11] The false dichotomy between physical and mental illness (sometimes called the "Cartesian dichotomy" because of René Descartes' philosophy of mind-body dualism) continues to bedevil both medicine and public health, and it is clear that the burden of mental

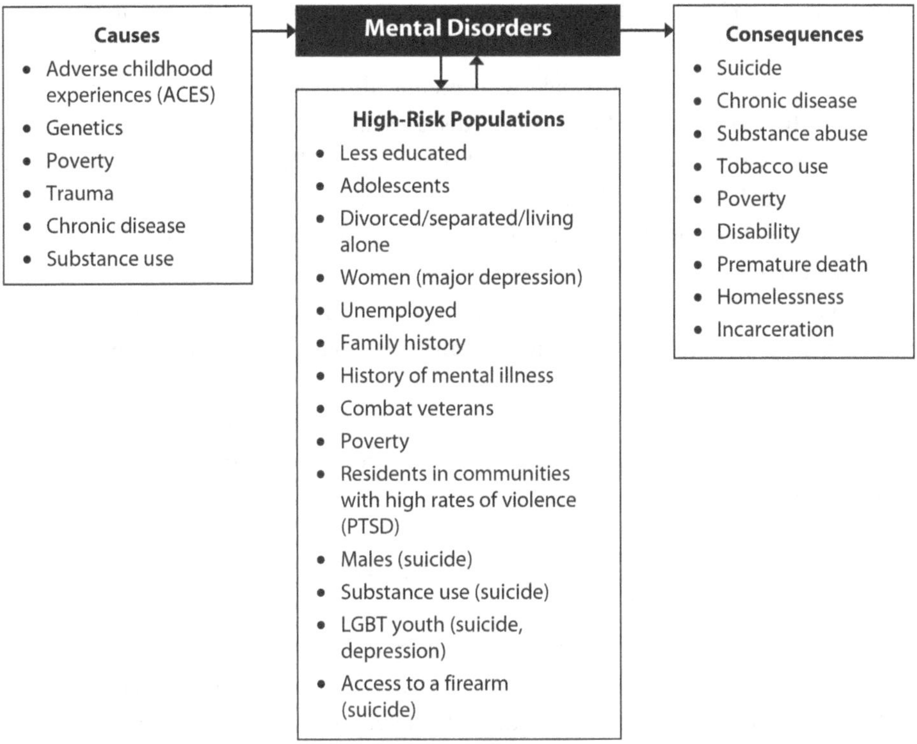

Figure 19-1. Mental Disorders: Causes, Consequences, and High-Risk Populations

disorders will continue to be underestimated unless there is some appreciation for the contribution that mental disorders make to the overall burden of illness in the United States and in the world.[12] Figure 19-1 summarizes the burden of mental disorders to individuals and to society.

Morbidity and Mortality

Mental disorder results in lost years of life because of its association with suicide and comorbid chronic or infectious diseases and in lost years of quality of life because of symptom burden. According to the 2019 Global Burden of Disease study, mental disorders are a leading cause of disability-adjusted life years lost because of morbidity and premature mortality. However, mental disorders are inextricably linked to other chronic diseases, so that when someone with depression dies of heart disease, the heart disease will be documented as the cause of death. Thus, this method of calculating mortality associated with mental disorders likely underestimates their true impact. Neuropsychiatric disorders are the leading cause of disability in the United States.[13] In addition, data from this study and the World Health Organization (WHO) show that mental disorders are the leading cause of global disability, accounting for 23% to 31% of the years of life with a disability worldwide.[14–16]

Although suicide among people with mental disorders garners the most public attention, in reality comorbid chronic diseases associated with mental disorders account for more person-years of life lost than suicide. The cause of this interaction with comorbid diseases is multifactorial, stemming from the effect of psychiatric illness itself on physiology and human behavior, poor access to care, and the effect of some psychiatric medications on human metabolism.[15,17]

In a growing body of literature, researchers point to an association between psychiatric conditions and alterations in immunity and metabolism as a cause of other chronic diseases. For instance, both stress and depression impair immune function, which could increase risk for both cancer and infectious diseases. States of stress and depression have been implicated in causing an inflammatory response; furthermore, inflammation itself may in turn induce the pathology of depression, initiating a feedback cycle that is hard to break.[18]

In addition to altering immunity, mental disorders are sometimes associated with behavior that increases risk for infectious diseases. For instance, Sartorius[19] has noted that people with schizophrenia are more likely to die from infectious diseases such as tuberculosis and HIV, in addition to chronic diseases such as heart disease and diabetes. Impaired judgment and decision-making, characteristic of psychosis found in schizophrenia and bipolar disorder, may result in risky behaviors such as unsafe sexual practices and injection drug use, putting these patients at greater risk for communicable diseases such as HIV and hepatitis C.[20,21] Depression and post-traumatic stress disorder (PTSD) also have associations with behaviors that increase comorbid disease risk and mortality, such as alcohol, tobacco, and substance use. In the 40-year Sterling County Study, participants who became depressed were more likely to start and less likely to quit smoking than those who had never been depressed. As noted by Murphy et al.,[22] "When depression and smoking coexist, the quality and quantity of life are doubly assaulted."

Yang et al.[23] showed that pre-pandemic psychiatric hospitalization was associated with elevated odds of any COVID-19 diagnosis (OR 1.44, 95% CI, 1.28–1.62), COVID-19 inpatient hospitalization (1.55, 1.34–1.78), and COVID-19-related death (2.03, 1.59–2.59). This association was greater for individuals with hospitalization for more than one psychiatric disorder.

In other cases, psychiatric medications increase the risk of developing chronic diseases. For instance, atypical antipsychotics significantly enhance the risk of diabetes and dyslipidemia through mechanisms causing weight gain and metabolic alterations.[24] Despite the negative impact of these side effects, it is important to consider evidence showing that relative to treated mental disorders, untreated mental disorders have significantly greater mortality and morbidity.[25]

Just as often as mental disorders increase risk for comorbid diseases, many chronic diseases perceived as physical affect mental physiology and increase the risk for mental disorders. Thus, the relationship between mental disorders and other chronic diseases can be bidirectional.[26] For example, depression occurs in 40% to 60% of patients who have experienced a heart attack, and one in four people with cancer suffers from depression.[17] These associations are particularly concerning, with emerging research showing that in patients with cancer, cardiovascular disease, or diabetes, comorbid psychiatric illness leads to increased morbidity and mortality.

The disabling effects of mental disorders are particularly striking in the large National Health Interview Survey of 2007. The researchers found that among people who reported having serious mental disorders in the general community-dwelling population, 35% had a history of homelessness or incarceration. Another disheartening finding of this study related to their treatment history, with fewer than two-thirds of these adults with serious mental disorders reporting that they had seen a mental health professional in the past year.[27]

New research showing that treating mental disorders can reduce or even eliminate the impact of these diseases on mortality and morbidity emphasizes the importance of connecting sufferers to treatment.[28] First, this study found that community-dwelling people with depression or anxiety died eight years earlier on average relative to people without these disorders. However, receipt of mental health services eliminated this disparity in age of death. Second, the study found that mediators between mental disorders and early death, such as education, income, smoking, exercise, body mass, and comorbid chronic disease, explained the increased mortality risk. Of these factors, comorbid diseases and behaviors such as smoking, exercise, and body mass were the strongest mediators of earlier death, and socioeconomic factors contributed more modestly. Last, by the authors' calculations, 3.5% of all mortality in the United States can be attributed to untreated depression and anxiety. Later in this chapter we further discuss the role of the recovery movement and the National Association of Mental Illness in bringing hope to people with mental disorders and helping them access effective treatment and support.

Finally, media attention has focused on the contribution of mental disorders to violence, such as mass shootings, with many pointing to untreated mental disorders as one of the drivers for these acts of violence.[29] These assertions further stigmatize people with mental disorders by fueling the public's pervasive belief that people with serious mental disorders are far more dangerous than the general population, an idea that was debunked as early as the 1990s.[30] For instance, a seminal study using data from the National Institute of Mental Health (NIMH) Epidemiologic Catchment Area Study of 1990 found that only a small fraction of violent crime (4%) is attributable to serious mental disorders such as schizophrenia and bipolar disorder.[31] The other 96% of violent acts stem from other causes such as substance use and antisocial personality disorder.

More recent research using data from the National Epidemiologic Survey on Alcohol and Related Conditions found a similar pattern, estimating that people with serious mental disorders and no comorbid substance use have a 12-month prevalence for violence of 2.9%, compared with 0.08% among people with no history of mental disorder or substance use.[32] Although the risk for violence is higher among people with serious mental disorders, the absolute risk of violence in this population is very low relative to the public perception that serious mental disorders account for a significant portion of our national violence problem.

Social Burden

Mental disorders have tremendous economic costs to individuals and to society as a whole. Some of these increased costs are easier to measure—such as health care and social service costs—than others. Other costs are less direct, stemming from the effect of mental disorders on families and caregivers, reduced productivity or employment, and morbidity and mortality as described previously.[33] For the individuals with mental disorders, longitudinal follow-up of the National Comorbidity Study showed that participants with mental disorders at baseline had lower odds of gainful employment and academic achievement 10 years later.[34,35] Another recent study of mental health and marital status found that people with mental disorders were less likely to get married. Among participants with mental disorders that did marry, researchers found a positive association between divorce and all 18 mental disorders.[36]

Untreated mental disorders in particular result in enormous social burden because of high volumes of people with mental disorders who are homeless or incarcerated. Before the closing of public psychiatric hospitals in the second half of the 20th century, people with serious mental disorders were institutionalized. The closing of these institutions shifted the burden to the community to care for people with serious mental disorders, but most communities lacked funding and resources to adequately meet their needs. Since this transition, the rate of people with mental disorders in prisons and jails has tripled in most estimates—with 20% of people in state prisons having a serious mental disorder up from 5% to 10% in the 1980s.[37] The prevalence of mental disorders is also high among people with unstable housing. For instance, in a study of Medicaid enrollees in Minnesota with unstable housing, half had a mental disorder.[38] Similarly, a 2012 survey by the National Alliance to End Homelessness[39] described characteristics of people who are chronically homeless and estimated that 30% to 50% have a serious mental disorder, most commonly schizophrenia or bipolar disorder.

PATHOPHYSIOLOGY

Mental disorders are commonplace, and more than 10 million adults in the United States have a serious mental disorder at any one time.[40,41] In the United States, mental disorders are defined by criteria outlined in the *Diagnostic and Statistical Manual of*

Mental Disorders (*DSM*),[42,43] published by the American Psychiatric Association (APA). The APA first released the *DSM* in 1952 and has published multiple updates since, most recently in 2013 with the release of the *DSM-5* and updated in 2022 with *DSM-5 TR*. The goal of the *DSM* is to provide standard criteria for the classification of mental disorders for use by clinicians and researchers. In addition to the *DSM-5*, behavioral health providers refer to the World Health Organization's *International Statistical Classification of Diseases and Related Health Problems*, Tenth Revision (*ICD-10*), to obtain codes for billing purposes.[44] The *ICD-10*, a manual that describes mental disorders in addition to other diseases, is used by clinicians in most non-US countries for both diagnostic and billing purposes. To assist US behavioral health providers, who rely on two different manuals for diagnosis and billing, the *DSM-5* lists corresponding *ICD-10* codes for each disorder. *ICD-11* has been implemented in 2022, but at the time of writing of this chapter, it has not been widely used in the United States. The categories for each manual are presented in Table 19-1.[45,46]

The biopsychosocial model, first described by George Engel in 1977, has helped shape our understanding of both the cause and the treatment of mental disorders. The model posits that mental disorders have biological (e.g., genetics), psychological (e.g., learned behavior and conditioning), and social (e.g., life stress, traumatic experiences, family and social support) components that contribute to the development of the illness, all of which need to be addressed during treatment.[45] For instance, research shows that genetics accounts for about 30% to 40% of the variance in major depressive disorder, with environmental factors causing the remaining 60% to 70%. These individual-specific environmental factors include more remote adverse events in childhood and recent stressors such as divorce and unemployment.[46] With the advent of the Human Genome Project, we have a greater appreciation for the biological and genetic underpinnings for most mental disorders. However, to truly prevent mental disorders, we must continue to recognize the role of environment and life experiences in the pathophysiology of these diseases.

Common serious mental disorders associated with high mortality, morbidity, and social burden include schizophrenia, mood disorders such as bipolar disorder and major depression, and anxiety or trauma-related disorders such as generalized anxiety disorder and PTSD. Thus, in this chapter we describe pathophysiology, epidemiology, prevention, and treatment in the context of each of these very different disorders along with suicide, one of the gravest potential consequences of these disorders. Substance use disorders are often included as mental health conditions; however, the magnitude of alcohol abuse as a public health problem is significant enough that this problem is discussed in Chapter 10 and thus is not included in this chapter. Likewise, although Alzheimer's disease and other dementias are included as mental disorders in the *ICD-10* and *DSM-5*, they are discussed in Chapter 20. Figure 19-1 summarizes populations at high risk for mental disorders.

Table 19-1. Comparison of *ICD-10* and *DSM-5* Categories

***ICD-10* Mental and Behavioral Disorders (F00–F99)[a]**

- F00–F09 Organic, including symptomatic, mental disorders
- F10–F19 Mental and behavioral disorders due to psychoactive substance use
- F20–F29 Schizophrenia, schizotypal, and delusional disorders
- F30–F39 Mood (affective) disorders
- F40–F49 Neurotic, stress-related, and somatoform disorders
- F50–F59 Behavioral syndromes associated with physiological disturbances and physical factors
- F60–F69 Disorders of adult personality and behavior
- F70–F79 Mental retardation
- F80–F89 Disorders of psychological development
- F90–F98 Behavioral and emotional disorders with onset usually occurring in childhood and adolescence
- F99 Unspecified mental disorder

***DSM-5* Categories**

- Neurodevelopmental Disorders:
  - Intellectual disabilities
  - Communication disorders
  - Autism spectrum disorder
  - Attention-deficit/hyperactivity disorder
  - Specific learning disorders
  - Motor disorders
  - Tic disorders
  - Other neurodevelopmental disorders
- Schizophrenia Spectrum and Other Psychotic Disorders
- Bipolar and related disorders
- Depressive disorders
- Anxiety disorders
- Obsessive-compulsive and related disorders
- Trauma- and stressor-related disorders
- Dissociative disorders
- Somatic symptom and related disorders
- Feeding and eating disorders
- Elimination disorders
- Sleep-wake disorders:
  - Insomnia disorder
  - Hypersomnolence disorder
  - Narcolepsy
  - Breathing-related sleep disorders
  - Parasomnias
- Sexual dysfunctions
- Gender dysphoria
- Disruptive, impulse-control, and conduct disorders
- Substance-related and addictive disorders (includes alcohol; see Ch. 10)
- Neurocognitive disorders (see categories Ch. 19)
- Personality disorders
- Paraphilic disorders
- Other mental disorders

(Continued)

Table 19-1. (Continued)

- Medication-induced movement disorders and other adverse effects of medications
- Other conditions that may be a focus of clinical attention:
  - Relational problems
  - Abuse and neglect
  - Educational and occupational problems
  - Housing and economic problems
  - Other problems related to the social environment
  - Problems related to crime or interaction with the legal system
  - Other health service encounters for counseling and medical advice
  - Problems related to other psychosocial, personal, and environmental circumstances
  - Other circumstances of personal history
  - Problems related to access to medical and other health care
  - Nonadherence to medical treatment

Source: Based on APA[42] and WHO.[44]

Note: DSM-5 = Diagnostic and Statistical Manual of Mental Disorders, Fifth Edition; *ICD-10 = International Classification of Diseases*, Tenth Revision.

[a]*ICD-10* codes corresponding to *DSM-5* disorders are specified in the original *DSM-5*.

Schizophrenia

Schizophrenia is a chronic and complex neuropsychiatric disorder that when untreated causes social and occupational dysfunction attributable to psychotic symptoms (e.g., auditory hallucinations, delusions, paranoia), disorganized speech and behavior, and negative symptoms (e.g., apathy, lack of motivation, social withdrawal). To meet *DSM-5* criteria for schizophrenia, symptoms must be present for at least six months.[42,43] The disorder most commonly develops in adolescence and young adulthood, usually developing in men between ages 18 and 24 years and in women between ages 25 and 35 years.[47]

The symptoms of schizophrenia likely stem from interrupted brain development in adolescence and early adulthood, which results in dysfunction in the transmission of several neurotransmitters, especially dopamine. This neural disturbance has both a genetic and environmental cause, as evidenced by studies showing 40% to 60% concordance among monozygotic twins.[48]

Because schizophrenia is a heterogeneous syndrome with many types, people with schizophrenia suffer diverse symptoms with varying degrees of severity. Although many people with schizophrenia struggle with disability, unemployment, or homelessness, many can treat their symptoms and go on to lead productive and full lives. For example, the late mathematician John Nash Jr., a Princeton professor memorialized in the movie *A Beautiful Mind*, spent several years in and out of psychiatric hospitals but was then able to manage his symptoms and make seminal contributions to the fields of economics, artificial intelligence, and political science.[49]

Mood Disorders: Depression and Bipolar Disorder

Within the category of mood disorders, major depressive disorder and bipolar disorder have the highest global burden in disability-adjusted life years.[16] For a diagnosis of major depressive disorder, people have a loss of interest in activities and depressed mood on most days for at least two weeks. Accompanying loss of interest and low mood are at least four other depressive symptoms, such as fatigue, poor concentration, hopelessness, guilt, irritability, restlessness, sluggishness, appetite change, feelings of worthlessness, insomnia, and suicidal thoughts. Likewise, in bipolar disorder, people suffer from episodes of major depression, but unlike major depressive disorder, people with bipolar disorder must have experienced an episode of mania or hypomania as well. Manic episodes may include symptoms of reduced need for sleep, elevated or irritable mood, rapid speech, delusions of grandeur, and even psychotic symptoms such as auditory hallucinations. A hypomanic episode is similar but with less severe symptoms and never includes symptoms of psychosis.[42,43]

Anxiety Disorders

Common anxiety disorders include generalized anxiety disorder, social anxiety disorder, and panic disorder. In generalized anxiety disorder, people suffer excess, exaggerated worry over everyday events to the extent that it affects their daily functioning. Social anxiety disorder is also marked by excess worry, but the worries are stimulated by fear of social interactions such as public speaking, meeting new people, or eating in front of people. In panic disorder, sufferers have panic attacks characterized by feelings of doom, racing heart, nausea, and shortness of breath, and they fear having future attacks to the degree that it affects their daily functioning.[42,43]

As they do with mental disorders, people with an anxiety disorder have a genetic tendency to develop the disorder; but environment contributes as well, with stress and learned behavior playing a role. Anxiety disorders can develop at any point in the life span but have different causes depending on the development stage. For children, school and social dynamics may be a source of anxiety, whereas older adults may develop anxiety in the context of dementia and stress from activities of daily living.[50] The disorder is characterized by disturbances in neurotransmitters and overactivation of stress responses by the sympathetic nervous system. People with anxiety disorders often suffer from comorbid depression.[42,43]

Post-Traumatic Stress Disorder

The most serious of the trauma-related disorders is PTSD, a mental disorder that occurs in people with symptoms of flashbacks reexperiencing of the event, hypervigilance, avoidance, insomnia, panic, and numbing after directly experiencing trauma in which they felt as if their life or the life of a loved one was in danger. The symptoms continue for longer than a month.[42,43]

In people who develop PTSD, traumatic exposures condition parts of the limbic system, including the amygdala, to activate even in the absence of threatening stimuli. The amygdala is a center for memory consolidation and feelings of fear and aggression, among other functions. When activated, the amygdala and its associated structures signal the activation of a neuroendocrine state that is characteristic of a flight-or-flight response. This includes an increase of adrenaline and the stress hormone cortisol—neurotransmitters and hormones that cause symptoms of PTSD. Chronic overactivation of these structures and the associated neuroendocrine response may lead to some of the negative health outcomes of PTSD such as increased risk for cognitive decline, diabetes, and heart disease. Like anxiety, comorbid depression commonly afflicts people with PTSD.[14,51]

Suicide

In the United States, firearms are the most commonly used methods for suicide in both men and women, followed by hanging for both sexes.[52] Although suicide overtly results from the behavior and environmental condition of the victim, many studies have elucidated underlying unique physiology in patients after they attempt or complete suicide. These studies find that patients who attempted suicide have decreased levels of the neurotransmitter serotonin in their cerebrospinal fluid and that these reductions correlated with degree of lethality, planning, and damage of the suicide attempt.[53,54]

DESCRIPTIVE EPIDEMIOLOGY

High-Risk Populations and Mental Disorders

Three major psychiatric epidemiological surveys have been conducted in the United States: the Epidemiologic Catchment Area Study,[55] the National Comorbidity Survey,[56] and the National Comorbidity Survey Replication.[57] These surveys were generally consistent in finding that 12-month mental disorders are highly prevalent, with 26% to 30% of the population meeting criteria for at least one *DSM-5* disorder. The more recent National Comorbidity Survey Replication found that non-Hispanic Blacks and Hispanics had a lower risk for mood and anxiety disorders relative to Whites; however, when these disorders were present, these populations tended to have more persistent symptoms.[58]

Schizophrenia

According to meta-analyses of international epidemiological surveys, the median lifetime prevalence of schizophrenia is about 4 in 1,000, with an incidence of about 1.5 per 1,000.[59,60]

Although some studies have measured higher incidence rates among men, who were 1.4 times more likely to be diagnosed, recent prevalence estimates by Saha et al.[60] found no gender differences in lifetime prevalence of the disorder.[61] The authors of one review proposed that higher suicide rates in men relative to women could explain the disparate findings in incidence and prevalence. The fact that the incidence data are based on clinical encounters rather than the epidemiological survey-based prevalence data may also explain this difference.[62]

The onset of schizophrenia typically occurs in the teen or early adult years, and onset before adolescence is rare. Women tend to have later onset, more prominent mood symptoms, and a better prognosis.[42,43] High-risk populations include people who are homeless and people in jails or prison. Other high-risk populations include migrants. According to a meta-analysis by Saha et al.,[60] migrant populations have a schizophrenia prevalence ratio of 1.8, relative to native-born populations. Other high-risk populations include the children of people with schizophrenia, who carry a sixfold higher risk of developing the disorder.[63]

Mood Disorders: Depression and Bipolar Disorder

Depression is sometimes referred to as the "common cold of mental illness," a phrase that highlights the prevalence of this disorder. In 2012 about 6.9% of community-dwelling, noninstitutionalized adults and 9.1% of youths aged 12 to 17 years had a major depressive episode in the past year. Recent estimates show that the lifetime prevalence for any *DSM-5* mood disorder is 17.5% for people aged older than 13 years—14.4% for major depressive disorder and 2.5% for bipolar disorder.[64]

Depression risk differs between groups: women have higher risk than men (2.7:1 in the Epidemiologic Catchment Area Study); adolescents have higher risk than adults and the elderly; people with less education have higher risk than people with more years of education; unemployed people have higher risk than employed; and separated or divorced people have nearly a threefold higher risk for depression relative to single or married persons.[65] In addition, poverty is known to be a risk factor for major depressive disorder, with higher rates of depression found in current and recent welfare recipients.[66] People with a parent with major depression have three times the risk of developing it themselves, with both genetics and learned behavior likely having a causative role.

Like schizophrenia and major depressive disorder, genetic studies demonstrate that bipolar disorder is highly heritable. Bipolar disorder tends to develop during young adulthood, is more prevalent in urban populations, and—unlike major depressive disorder—occurs about equally in men and women. Social class and ethnicity are not significant predictors of bipolar disorder. Individuals who cohabit, divorce, or never marry are more likely to have bipolar disorder than married individuals, and there is a dramatically higher prevalence rate for homeless people.[67]

Anxiety Disorders

According to data from the 2005 National Comorbidity Study, Kessler et al.[64] estimate that the lifetime prevalence for any anxiety disorder is 23.6%, excluding PTSD and obsessive-compulsive disorder (which are no longer categorized as anxiety disorders by the *DSM-5*). This lifetime prevalence of any anxiety disorder is accounted for by specific phobia (15.6%), social anxiety (10.7%), separation anxiety disorder (6.7%), generalized anxiety disorder (4.3%), panic disorder (3.8%), and agoraphobia (2.5%).

Anxiety is a common disorder affecting people across all phases of the life span, but certain groups are at higher risk for developing an anxiety disorder. One group with higher rates of anxiety, especially generalized anxiety disorder, are older adults with functional disabilities, cognitive impairment, or caregiver burden. Other high-risk populations include people who are childless, people with trauma exposure, and low-income groups.[50]

Post-Traumatic Stress Disorder

Rates of PTSD differ depending on population studied, but the estimate for national lifetime prevalence among the US community-dwelling population is 5.7%.[64] Although between 50% and 60% of people report having experienced a traumatic event in their lifetime, only about 7% go on to develop PTSD.[57] Studies find that people who experience an early life trauma, such as combat exposure or child abuse, are more likely to have subsequent traumatic exposures and that genetics may confer traits of either resilience or risk.[51,68] In addition to people with inherited risk, studies have identified several populations at high risk for PTSD because of environmental factors, including people in urban communities with high rates of violence, combat veterans, and first responders.

In studies of combat veterans, about 15% develop PTSD, and risk factors include being from disadvantaged backgrounds, having traumatic brain injury, and repeated exposure to trauma.[69–71] Other high-risk populations include people living in urban communities with high rates of violence. Studies of community-dwelling residents in Detroit find that Blacks are two times more likely to develop PTSD relative to Whites, a difference that was not significant after controlling for trauma exposure and central-city location. Most studies examining the apparent disparity of PTSD prevalence among Whites and Blacks attribute these differences to income, as evidenced by high rates of PTSD among White adults in low-income groups.[72,73]

Suicide

Suicide is the 10th leading cause of death in the United States, more common than homicide. Among people aged 15 to 24 years, it is the second leading cause of death, preceded by motor vehicle accidents.[74] According to CDC, the mortality rate for suicide is

13.9 per 100,000 for all US adults in 2019. The risk for suicide is higher for male relative to female individuals, people with access to a firearm relative to people without firearm access, and people of White race relative to people of other races.[75] Lesbian, gay, bisexual, and transgender youths also have higher risk of suicide, self-harm, and suicidal thoughts; however, protective factors such as social support from family and friends and school safety have been found to largely mediate this increased risk.[76,77] Other risk factors for suicide include being divorced or separated, having a history of previous suicide attempts, having a family history of suicide, experiencing a recent stressful life event, and substance use.[78,79]

Geographic Distribution

Considerable geographic variability exists in the degree of support people with mental disorders receive. Psychiatric hospitalization in New York City, for example, has been shown to vary according to socioeconomic status and proximity to general hospitals with psychiatric beds. Other predictors of psychiatric hospitalization included living in a high-poverty area, being African American, and living alone. One study found that the highest hospital admission rates were concentrated in those areas of the city in which social and economic disadvantages were greatest.[80] Another well-studied factor affecting the geographic distribution of mental disorders is poverty, with one study finding that the odds for depression were more than twice as high for people living in low-income neighborhoods relative to high-income neighborhoods.[81]

Time Trends

The 19th century witnessed dramatic growth in asylums in both Europe and the United States, and many psychiatrists argued forcefully at the time that serious mental disorders were increasing. However, the extant data are for prevalence rather than incidence, and the dramatic changes that occurred during the century can be attributed just as easily to the confluence of a number of social, political, and economic forces. Most authorities[82,83] believe that the incidence of serious mental disorders remained stable or declined slightly during the 20th century. In contrast, trends in the treatment of mental disorders in United States show marked change over the past century, as the treatment of serious mental disorders shifted from a model of public institutionalization to our current community health treatment model.

With the advent of antipsychotic medications that proved effective in treating many of the psychotic symptoms of serious mental disorders, social and political forces favored treating people with mental disorders in the community rather than housing them in public psychiatric institutions, a practice that was increasingly viewed as ostracizing and inhumane. This environment led to the Community Mental Health Centers and Mental Retardation Act of 1963, a pivotal event in mental health care in the United States.

This piece of legislation called for the closure of most public psychiatric institutions in favor of a community treatment model, allocating funding to states to open centers to treat community-dwelling residents with serious mental disorders. However, half of these centers never opened, and state mental health departments rarely receive adequate funding to care for these individuals. Experts in the field attribute this system overhaul to the increasing prevalence of people with serious mental disorders among incarcerated populations as well as to the increasing population of homeless individuals.[37,84,85]

More recently, the Mental Health Parity and Addiction Equity Act of 2008 and the ACA of 2010 have had an impact on the treatment of mental disorders in the United States.[86] The Mental Health Parity Act was intended to level the field between mental health and substance use insurance benefits and those of medical care. Specifically, this legislation was originally designed for private insurance plans of 50 or more enrollees that offered behavioral health insurance benefits. The concept of parity applied both to the actual insurance benefits and to how the benefits were managed. Two years later the ACA extended parity to all insurance offered through the state health insurance marketplaces and to insurance offered through the state Medicaid expansions. The US Department of Health and Human Services has estimated that the ACA extended parity to the health insurance of more than 62 million more Americans.[8]

Since the passage of the Mental Health Parity Act, advocates for mental health and policy experts have raised concerns that insurance companies are not being fully transparent about behavioral health and medical benefits, thus making it difficult for consumers to understand whether parity requirements are actually being followed. This concern has reached Congress, which has proposed draft legislation to enforce and monitor insurance parity.

Without question, the ACA represented the most significant change to behavioral health care in the half century since the passage of the Community Mental Health Centers and Mental Retardation Act of 1963. The ACA sought to extend health insurance coverage to an additional 40 million Americans while standardizing the categories of insurance benefits, including disease prevention and health promotion. It also eliminated all preexisting condition exclusion clauses in health insurance and permitted all young adults to remain on family policies until age 26.

To implement the new insurance coverage, state health insurance marketplaces were developed for all states. Because of federal-state controversy, about two-thirds of these marketplaces are operated by the US Department of Health and Human Services. In addition, the ACA provided for Medicaid expansions in all states to cover all persons up to 138% of the federal poverty level. To date, 31 states have undertaken a state Medicaid expansion.[87]

Other provisions of the ACA promoted the development of integrated behavioral health and primary care through medical and health homes, reform of financing systems away from encounter-based payments and toward case and capitation rates, and the implementation of consistent national performance measures. Many of the latter provisions of the ACA have not yet been fully realized.[88]

CAUSES

Modifiable Risk Factors

In the 2004 WHO Summary Report entitled "Prevention of Mental Disorders,"[89] authors describe social, economic, and environmental factors that either increase risk for mental disorders or serve as protective factors. Although genetic inheritance explains much of the variance in the development of mental disorders, external factors account for at least half. Unlike genetic factors, social contributors to mental disorders are modifiable and are therefore opportune targets for prevention. Figure 19-1 provides an outline of modifiable risk factors.

Some of these modifiable risk factors involve macro-level issues such as war, violence, poverty, and inequality—all of which increase the risk for mental disorders such as PTSD, alcohol use disorder, anxiety, and depression.[90,91] For example, one recent study found that US women living in states with high income inequality had an increased risk for developing depression.[92] Urban violence is associated with the development of PTSD symptoms, with a 2016 study finding that 70% of Black males in Baltimore suffered two or more symptoms of post-traumatic stress.[93]

Other modifiable risk factors stemming from the family and community context contribute to the development of mental disorders. Studies show that adverse childhood experiences—such as lack of secure attachment and family support, child abuse, parental mental disorders, or abuse by peer group—can increase the risk for depression and anxiety later in life.[94–97] In addition, early maternal factors such as postpartum depression and low birthweight have long been identified as risk factors for the later development of psychiatric disorder and behavioral problems.[98,99]

Individual factors that are associated with mental disorders are substance use and comorbid chronic diseases such as diabetes, heart disease, and cancer, as well as personal traits such as reduced resilience. A review studying the temporal associations between alcohol use disorder and mental disorders concluded that alcohol use disorders frequently precede major depression and anxiety disorders.[100] In patients who suffered a heart attack, one in five develops depression within three months of the event.[101] Last, studies of people commonly exposed to trauma (e.g., soldiers, people living in Israel, paramedics) find that those with stronger resilience traits are less likely to develop PTSD.[102–104]

Population-Attributable Risk

Few studies have been conducted to understand the modifiable risk factors for mental disorders, thus making estimates of population-attributable risk difficult. One area in which such research has been done involves risk factors for suicide. These studies estimate that for suicide, mental disorders have a population-attributable fraction of 47% to 74%.[105,106] Other studies counter that environmental factors such as firearm access and low socioeconomic status contribute equally or more to the population-attributable fraction for suicide deaths. For example, Australia and Switzerland had dramatic decreases in private firearm ownership in response to government policy changes, setting the stage for natural experiments on the population-attributable risk for suicide attributable to firearm ownership. Researchers found striking reductions in the suicide rate coinciding with the decrease in firearm ownership. In Switzerland researchers estimated that only 22% of the prevented firearm suicides resulted in people committing suicide by another method, and in Australia there was no evidence that people substituted other suicide methods.[107,108] In another Australian study, Page et al.[109] emphasized that poverty has an attributable risk fraction to suicide in young adults of 46% (males) and 58% (females), similar to the mental health population-attributable risk fraction of 48% (males) and 52% (females).

EVIDENCE-BASED INTERVENTIONS

Two approaches to eliminating the morbidity and mortality of mental disorders include (1) interventions to prevent the development of mental disorders and (2) interventions to treat existing mental disorders and promote recovery.

Prevention

Interventions to prevent mental disorders focus on decreasing or mitigating the effects of adverse childhood experiences, events shown to be associated with the later development of mental disorders. These early life interventions include enhancing social support, teaching parenting skills, improving early childhood education, and reducing—if not eliminating—school bullying. Poor social support, lack of good parenting, lack of quality early education, and child abuse all constitute risk factors for mental disorders. It is possible to enhance protective factors for children by promoting resilience, teaching social skills, and expanding a child's social network. The most successful primary prevention programs in mental health have a double focus: they work to reduce existing stressors and enhance the problem-solving competency of the children involved. As these children become more competent, they are better able to withstand or deal with those forces that would be likely to lead to deviancy, delinquency, or mental disorders.

A meta-analysis of 177 primary prevention mental health programs for children and adolescents supported the general efficacy of these programs, demonstrating that they reduced problems, enhanced academic performance, increased general levels of competencies, and had a positive influence across multiple measures of functioning.[110]

Interventions to Promote Recovery

In the 1990s, advocacy organizations such as National Alliance on Mental Illness began spearheading a recovery-oriented model for the treatment of mental disorders to promote the idea that people with mental disorders can live full lives with meaning and purpose. This concept emerged much earlier in the treatment of people with physical disability, likely because people with mental disorders face complex hurdles such as overcoming stigma and social problems associated with their disease, such as unemployment.[7]

For a mental health system to be recovery oriented, many criteria must be met beyond providing good clinical care. The recovery-oriented model acknowledges the complex psychosocial determinants of mental health, recognizing that people with persistent psychiatric symptoms can still recover but have nonclinical needs that must be met. These needs may include peer support from others with a mental disorder, social support through hobbies and activities, person-centered community supports such as childcare and transportation, and employment and educational opportunities. Moreover, recovery from mental illness requires a community with an integrated, multisector approach to mental health, where reemergence of symptoms does not result in arrest, loss of employment, or housing instability.[7]

Screening

In a summary report, the Center for Mental Health Services of the Substance Abuse and Mental Health Services Administration identified those programs in mental health and substance abuse prevention that hold the greatest promise in diminishing or preventing the development of a mental disorder or a substance use disorder.[111] The following programs are included:

- Universal screening of pregnant women for use of tobacco, alcohol, and illicit drugs.
- Home visitation for selected pregnant women, and some children up to 5 years.
- Supplemental educational services for vulnerable infants from disadvantaged families.
- Screening children and adolescents for behavioral disorders.
- Screening adolescents for tobacco or alcohol use, depression, and anxiety.
- Screening adults for depression, anxiety, and use of tobacco or alcohol.
- Psychoeducation to increase early ambulation of surgical patients and enhance adherence to prescribed regimens of care for patients with chronic diseases.

The report then identifies the following three practices with the most potential for reducing overall health care costs:

- Screening pregnant women for use of tobacco, alcohol, and illicit drugs.
- Screening for depression in persons with major chronic medical disease.
- Psycho-education for persons scheduled for major surgical procedures, persons with major chronic diseases, and selected other heavy users of health care services.

The effect sizes for these preventive services in randomized controlled trials ranged from 5% to 30%. Nitzkin and Smith[111] explain that the identified interventions often reduce mental illness burden rather than completely prevent mental illness and go on to assert, "the adverse consequences of the underlying disorders are such that the preventive services can be expected to pay for themselves in reduced health care costs and improved clinical and/or social outcomes."

More recently, the US Preventive Services Task Force recommended depression screening for all adults by primary care providers with the resources to treat or refer these patients, citing sufficient evidence that this practice results in moderate benefits. Studies find improved outcomes in clinical morbidity for patients who screened positive for depression and were subsequently treated with psychotherapy or antidepressant therapy.[112]

Treatment

As discussed, a major change that has occurred since the 1990s is an enhanced appreciation for the fact that many people with mental disorders do recover and go on to function effectively in society. Moreover, recent studies show that mortality caused by mental disorders can be reduced by appropriate treatment. Harrison et al.[113] analyzed projects by 69 investigators studying more than 1,000 individuals with schizophrenia from 14 countries around the world, with follow-up periods up to 25 years. The most important finding from this rigorous and well-designed investigation was that more than half the participants were rated as recovered at the end of the 15- to 25-year follow-up period.

Despite the high likelihood of recovery with appropriate treatment, many people with mental disorders do not get care relative to people with other chronic diseases. The *President's New Freedom Commission* report[114] identified three obstacles that prevent Americans from getting good mental health care: stigma, unfair treatment limitations imposed by private health insurance companies, and a fragmented mental health service delivery system. In addition to calling for major reform of the US health care system, this report underscored the importance of recovery and resilience and the fact that recovery is possible.

The treatments that have been shown in controlled studies to be effective for mental disorders and addictions vary across illness categories, and it is not possible to survey all treatments for all conditions within the confines of a chapter. However, the following general principles apply[115]:

- Medications effectively treat most mental disorders. For severe mental disorders, they are superior to psychosocial treatments alone.
- Combined treatments (medication plus psychosocial interventions) often produce the best results.

- Many psychotherapies are empirically supported, particularly cognitive-behavioral and interpersonal psychotherapies, and have equal efficacy vis-à-vis medication in mild-to-moderate cases of many conditions such as depression, anxiety, and PTSD.
- Other psychosocial treatments (e.g., family education, psychoeducation) and services (e.g., assertive community treatment [ACT] and supported employment for adults, multimodal treatment for children with conduct disorder) provide advantages for many conditions—particularly to promote rehabilitation and recovery in the most impaired individuals.

EXAMPLES OF EVIDENCE-BASED INTERVENTIONS

There are numerous examples of evidence-based interventions for both the prevention and treatment of mental disorders, varying according to type of mental disorder and target population. Here we focus on two areas: interventions for the prevention of depression and community psychiatry interventions for the treatment of serious mental disorders. For more examples of evidence-based interventions, refer to the Substance Abuse and Mental Health Services Administration's National Registry of Evidence Based Practices and Programs (http://nrepp.samhsa.gov) and WHO's summary report entitled "Prevention of Mental Disorders."[89]

Interventions for Preventing Depression

Interventions for mental disorders, including depression, take one of three major approaches depending on the target population: universal, selective, or indicated intervention. In universal interventions, the program applies to an entire population, such as incorporating social-emotional skills training into an elementary school curriculum. Selective interventions, in contrast, target individuals at high risk, such as through prenatal health and parenting education programs for low-income parents. Last, indicated interventions aim to reduce problem behavior and symptoms in children who are already displaying problems.

In a 2005 WHO summary report, the authors argue for community interventions that incorporate components of universal, selective, and indicated approaches to reduce the incidence of depression, citing literature reviews that find an overall 11% reduction in depressive symptoms post-intervention.[90] One promising approach is to improve parents' well-being and efficacy through therapy and education to improve the health of parents and transfer positive outcomes to the children of these individuals. A Cochrane review of indicated interventions for parents of young children with behavioral problems reported that behavioral and cognitive–behavioral group-based parenting interventions resulted in reduced child conduct problems and improved parental mental health and parenting skills.[116] These interventions aim to help parents learn coping skills and cognitive reframing techniques that they can pass on to their children, as well parenting skills such as to use positive reinforcement to increase desired behavior in their children. The reviewers of these intervention studies concluded that the modest costs of such programs are worth the potential benefits in long-term health, social change, and academic outcomes.[116]

Interventions for Serious Mental Disorders

The most powerful interventions for people living with serious mental disorders such as schizophrenia and bipolar disorder succeed by taking a biopsychosocial approach with multidisciplinary teams, aiming to improve the lives of individuals beyond their psychiatric symptoms. Two widely used models with a true biopsychosocial approach are the Clubhouse model and the Assertive Community Treatment (ACT) model.[117]

The Clubhouse model of psychosocial rehabilitation, forwarded by the International Center for Clubhouse Development in the 1970s, optimizes recovery in adults with mental disorders by engaging individuals as members of the Clubhouse. The Clubhouse includes day treatment facilities with access to education, psychiatric and general health care treatment, employment opportunities, social relationships, and housing. The members of the Clubhouse increase quality of life and gain a sense of purpose by participating in Clubhouse responsibilities such as clerical duties, reception, food service, and financial services. In this way, members become a critical part of the community and are granted access to outside jobs that often become permanent employment. The Clubhouse is staffed by multidisciplinary professionals with backgrounds in psychology, psychiatry, counseling, social work, and education. Membership is voluntary, and the amount that members contribute varies depending on member choice; moreover, members who choose to end participation are granted the lifetime right of reentry. Studies of the Clubhouse model find that members have improved outcomes in the areas of employment, quality of life, and perceived recovery from a mental disorder.[118,119] For more information, visit the website of the world's first clubhouse, Fountain House of New York City (http://www.fountainhouse.org).

Assertive Community Treatment

ACT is another stellar example of a cost-effective treatment for persons with severe mental disorders. Developed as a way to respond to the needs of the large numbers of mentally ill people released from state psychiatric hospitals in the 1970s as a result of deinstitutionalization, ACT is a team-based approach aimed at keeping clients connected with providers, reducing hospital admissions, and improving everyday functioning and quality of life. Assertive outreach, mobile treatment teams, and continuous treatment are essential components of ACT. Other important features include multidisciplinary staffing, integration of services, low client-to-staff ratios, home visits, a focus on ordinary problems in living, rapid access to needed services, and individualized treatment plans. This approach has been shown to be more effective than standard community care, hospital-based rehabilitation services, and typical case management. Multiple randomized clinical trials have documented that ACT, which targets the patients with the highest consumption of mental health services, reduces the costs associated with hospital care at the same time that it produces high levels of patient satisfaction.[120]

AREAS OF FUTURE RESEARCH

The needs of people with severe mental disorders clearly exceed the capacity of the current mental health community to treat these needs. The Annapolis Coalition on the Behavioral Health Workforce has noted:

> Across the nation there is a high degree of concern about the state of the behavioral health workforce and pessimism about its future. . . Most critically, there are significant concerns about the capability of the workforce to provide quality care. The majority of the workforce is uninformed about and unengaged in health promotion and prevention activities. . . There is overwhelming evidence that the behavioral health workforce is not equipped in skills or in numbers to respond adequately to the changing needs of the American population.[121]

As discussed, behavioral health integration within primary care is gaining recognition as an approach to this workforce dilemma. This collaborative care approach has been shown to be cost-effective in the treatment of depression, and it results in greater adherence to treatment goals and patient satisfaction.[122–124] Moreover, this approach to chronic disease management has been shown to be both efficient and effective, holding great promise in addressing the mental health needs of the nation.[125]

Other future areas of research include public health approaches to caring for people with serious mental disorders at risk for incarceration or housing instability and interventions to optimize reentry and recovery for persons with mental disorders leaving prison.[37] These developing areas of research include mental health courts and court-ordered outpatient treatment.

NIMH released a strategic plan, outlined in Table 19-2, for future research that recognizes the importance of addressing urgent mental health care needs at the same time as pursuing long-term basic science objectives.[126] NIMH also recognizes that advances in neuroscience and genomics should be considered within the context of environmental exposures and social factors known to influence mental health.[126]

Our understanding of mental disorders and their associations with increased morbidity and mortality continues to advance. Future research must focus on reducing the risk of early death for those with mental disorders by altering the mediators between

Table 19-2. National Institute of Mental Health Strategic Plan, 2015

Strategic Objective 1: Define the mechanisms of complex behaviors.
1.1 Describe the molecules, cells, and neural circuits associated with complex behaviors. 1.2 Identify the genomic and non-genomic factors associated with mental illnesses. 1.3 Map the connectomes for mental illnesses.
Strategic Objective 2: Chart mental illness trajectories to determine when, where, and how to intervene.
2.1 Characterize the developmental trajectories of brain maturation and dimensions of behavior to understand the roots of mental illnesses across diverse populations. 2.2 Identify clinically useful biomarkers and behavioral indicators that predict change across the trajectory of illness.
Strategic Objective 3: Strive for prevention and cures.
3.1 Develop new treatments based on discoveries in genomics, neuroscience, and behavioral science. 3.2 Develop ways to tailor existing and new interventions to optimize outcomes. 3.3 Test interventions for effectiveness in community practice settings.
Strategic Objective 4: Strengthen the public health impact of NIMH-supported research.
4.1 Improve the efficiency and effectiveness of existing mental health services through research. 4.2 Establish research-practice partnerships to improve dissemination, implementation, and continuous improvement of evidence-based mental health service. 4.3 Develop innovative service delivery models to improve dramatically the outcomes of mental health services received in diverse communities and populations. 4.4 Develop new capacity for research that evaluates the public health impact of mental health services innovations.

Source: Based on USDHHS, NIH, and NIMH.[126]
Note: NIMH = National Institute of Mental Health.

mental disorders and death, as well as through the provision of mental health services. Just as we have a national monitoring system for cancer, there is a need for a parallel system tracking early death relating to mental disorders or substance use conditions. Specific mental disorders and the contributing factors to early death from these disorders must be assessed so that we can track year-to-year progress in reducing the disparity in length of life.

REFERENCES

1. Substance Abuse and Mental Health Services Administration. *Results from the 2012 National Survey on Drug Use and Health: Mental Health Findings.* NSDUH series H-47, HHS publication (SMA) 13-4805. Rockville, MD: SAMHSA; 2013.
2. Cai C, Woolhandler S, Himmelstein DU, Gaffney A. Trends in anxiety and depression symptoms during the COVID-19 pandemic: results from the US Census Bureau's Household Pulse Survey. *J Gen Intern Med.* 2021;36(6):1841–1843. doi: 10.1007/s11606-021-06759-9.
3. Radhakrishnan L, Leeb RT, Bitsko RH, et al. Pediatric emergency department visits associated with mental health conditions before and during the COVID-19 pandemic—United States, January 2019–January 2022. *MMWR Morb Mortal Wkly Rep.* 2022;71:319–324.

4. Leeb RT, Bitsko RH, Radhakrishnan L, Martinez P, Njai R, Holland KM. Mental health–related emergency department visits among children aged <18 years during the COVID-19 pandemic—United States, January 1–October 17, 2020. *MMWR Morb Mortal Wkly Rep.* 2020;69:1675–1680.
5. National Alliance for Mental Illness. Mental Health by the numbers. Updated June 2022. Available at: https://www.nami.org/mhstats. Accessed January 27, 2023.
6. Dupre ME, Xu H, Granger BB, et al. Access to routine care and risks for 30-day readmission in patients with cardiovascular disease. *Am Heart J.* 2018;196:9–17.
7. Sheedy CK, Whitter M. *Guiding Principles and Elements of Recovery-Oriented Systems of Care: What Do We Know From the Research?* HHS Publication No. (SMA) 09-4439. Rockville, MD: Center for Substance Abuse Treatment, Substance Abuse and Mental Health Services Administration, 2009. Available at: https://www.naadac.org/assets/2416/sheedyckwhitterm2009_guiding_principles_and_elements.pdf. Accessed March 19, 2023.
8. Beronio K, Po R, Skopec L, Glied S. Affordable Care Act expands mental health and substance use disorder benefits and federal parity protections for 62 million Americans. February 19, 2013. Available at: https://aspe.hhs.gov/report/affordable-care-act-expands-mental-health-and-substance-use-disorder-benefits-and-federal-parity-protections-62-million-americans. Accessed January 27, 2023.
9. Mokdad AH, Marks JS, Stroup DF, Gerberding JL. Actual causes of death in the United States, 2000. *JAMA.* 2004;291(10):1238–1245.
10. Ustun TB. The global burden of mental disorders. *Am J Public Health.* 1999;89(9):1315–1318.
11. World Health Organization. Mental disorders. Updated June 8, 2022. Available at: https://www.who.int/news-room/fact-sheets/detail/mental-disorders. Accessed January 27, 2023.
12. Prince M, Patel V, Saxena S, et al. No health without mental health. *Lancet.* 2007;370(9590):859–877.
13. US Burden of Disease Collaborators. The state of US health, 1990–2010: burden of diseases, injuries, and risk factors. *JAMA.* 2013;310(6):591–606. doi:10.1001/jama.2013.13805
14. Kessler RC, Aguilar-Gaxiola S, Alonso J, et al. The global burden of mental disorders: an update from the WHO World Mental Health (WMH) surveys. *Epidemiol Psichiatr Soc.* 2009;18(1):23–33.
15. Vigo D, Thornicroft G, Atun R. Estimating the true global burden of mental illness. *Lancet Psychiatry.* 2016;3(2):171–178.
16. Whiteford HA, Ferrari AJ, Degenhardt L, Feigin V, Vos T. The global burden of mental, neurological and substance use disorders: an analysis from the Global Burden of Disease study 2010. *PLoS One.* 2015;10(2):e0116820.
17. American Psychiatric Association. *Coexisting Severe Mental Disorders and Physical Illness.* Washington, DC: American Psychiatric Association; 2003.
18. Leonard B. Stress, depression and the activation of the immune system. *World J Biol Psychiatry.* 2000;1(1):17–25.
19. Sartorius N. Physical illness in people with mental disorders. *World Psychiatry.* 2007:6(1):3–4.
20. Beyer JL, Taylor L, Gersing KR, Ranga K, Krishnan R. Prevalence of HIV infection in a general psychiatric outpatient population. *Psychosomatics.* 2007:48(1):31–37.

21. Swartz MS, Swanson JW, Hannon MJ, et al.; Five-Site Health and Risk Study Research Committee. Regular sources of medical care among persons with severe mental illness at risk of hepatitis C infection. *Psychiatr Serv.* 2003:54(6):854–859.
22. Murphy JM, Horton NJ, Monson RR, Laird NM, Sobol AM, Leighton AH. Cigarette smoking in relation to depression: historical trends from the Stirling County Study. *Am J Psychiatry.* 2003;160(9):1663–1669.
23. Yang H, Chen W, Hu Y, et al. Pre-pandemic psychiatric disorders and risk of COVID-19: a UK Biobank cohort analysis. *Lancet Healthy Longev.* 2020; 1: e69–e79
24. Newcomer JW, Haupt DW. *Schizophrenia, Metabolic Disturbance, and Cardiovascular Risk. Medical and Psychiatric Comorbidity Over the Course of Life.* Arlington, VA: American Psychiatric Publishing; 2006:331–349.
25. Baxter AJ, Harris MG, Khatib Y, Brugha TS, Bien H, Bhui K. Reducing excess mortality due to chronic disease in people with severe mental disorders: meta-review of health interventions. *Br J Psychiatry.* 2016;208(4):322–329.
26. Snoek FJ, Bremmer MA, Hermanns N. Constructs of depression and distress in diabetes: time for an appraisal. *Lancet Diabetes Endocrinol.* 2015;3(6):450–460.
27. Pratt LA. Characteristics of adults with serious mental illness in the United States household population in 2007. *Psychiatr Serv.* 2012;63(10):1042–1046.
28. Pratt LA, Druss BG, Manderscheid RW, Walker ER. Excess mortality due to depression and anxiety in the United States: results from a nationally representative survey. *Gen Hosp Psychiatry.* 2016;39:39–45.
29. Metzl JM, MacLeish KT. Mental illness, mass shootings, and the politics of American firearms. *Am J Public Health.* 2015;105(2):240–249.
30. Swanson JW, McGinty EE, Fazel S, Mays VM. Mental illness and reduction of gun violence and suicide: bringing epidemiologic research to policy. *Ann Epidemiol.* 2015;25(5):366–376.
31. Swanson JW. Mental disorder, substance abuse, and community violence: an epidemiological approach. In: Monahan J, Steadman H, eds. *Violence and Mental Disorder.* Chicago, IL: University of Chicago Press; 1994:101–136.
32. Van Dorn R, Volavka J, Johnson N. Mental disorder and violence: is there a relationship beyond substance use? *Soc Psychiatry Psychiatr Epidemiol.* 2012;47(3):487–503. doi:10.1007/s00127-011-0356-x
33. Sayers J. The world health report 2001—mental health: new understanding, new hope. *Bull World Health Organization.* 2001;79(11):1085.
34. Mojtabai R, Stuart EA, Hwang I, Eaton WW, Sampson N, Kessler RC. Long-term effects of mental disorders on educational attainment in the National Comorbidity Survey ten-year follow-up. *Soc Psychiatry Psychiatr Epidemiol.* 2015a;50(10):1577–1591.
35. Mojtabai R, Stuart EA, Hwang I, et al. Long-term effects of mental disorders on employment in the National Comorbidity Survey ten-year follow-up. *Soc Psychiatry Psychiatr Epidemiol.* 2015b;50(11):1657–1668.
36. Breslau J, Miller E, Jin R, et al. A multinational study of mental disorders, marriage, and divorce. *Acta Psychiatr Scand.* 2011;124(6):474–486.
37. Slate RN, Buffington-Vollum JK, Johnson WW. *The Criminalization of Mental Illness: Crisis and Opportunity for the Justice System.* 2nd ed. Durham, NC: Carolina Academic Press; 2013.

38. Diaz Vickery K, Guzman-Corrales L, Owen R, et al. Medicaid expansion and mental health: a Minnesota case study. *Fam Syst Health*. 2016;34(1):58–63.
39. National Alliance to End Homelessness. State of homelessness: 2022 edition. Available at: https://endhomelessness.org/homelessness-in-america/homelessness-statistics/state-of-homelessness. Accessed March 19, 2023.
40. Watanabe-Galloway S, Zhang W. Analysis of US trends in discharges from general hospitals for episodes of serious mental illness, 1995–2002. *Psychiatr Serv*. 2007:58(4):496–502.
41. National Advisory Mental Health Council. Health care reform for Americans with severe mental illnesses: report of the National Advisory Mental Health Council. *Am J Psychiatry*. 1993;150:1447–1465.
42. American Psychiatric Association. *Diagnostic and Statistical Manual of Mental Disorders*. 5th ed. Washington, DC: American Psychiatric Association; 2013.
43. American Psychiatric Association. *Diagnostic and Statistical Manual of Mental Disorders*. 5th ed. Text Revision. Washington, DC: American Psychiatric Association; 2022.
44. World Health Organization. *International Statistical Classification of Diseases and Related Health Problems*. 10th rev. Geneva, Switzerland: World Health Organization; 1992.
45. Engel GL. The need for a new medical model: a challenge for biomedicine. *Science*. 1977; 196(4286):129–136.
46. Hasler G. Pathophysiology of depression: do we have any solid evidence of interest to clinicians? *World Psychiatry*. 2010;9(3):155–161.
47. Castle DJ, Wessely S, Murray RM. Sex and schizophrenia: effects of diagnostic stringency, and associations with and premorbid variables. *Br J Psychiatry*. 1993;162:658–664.
48. Cardno AG, Gottesman II. Twin studies of schizophrenia: from bow-and-arrow concordances to Star Wars Mx and functional genomics. *Am J Med Genet*. 2000;97(1):12–17.
49. Funaki T. Nash: genius with schizophrenia or vice versa? *Pac Health Dialog*. 2009;15(2): 129–137.
50. Lenze EJ, Wetherell JL. A lifespan view of anxiety disorders. *Dialogues Clin Neurosci*. 2011;13(4):381–399.
51. Stein MB, Jang KL, Taylor S, Vernon PA, Livesley WJ. Genetic and environmental influences on trauma exposure and posttraumatic stress disorder symptoms: a twin study. *Am J Psychiatry*. 2002;159(10):1675–1681.
52. Centers for Disease Control and Prevention. Web-based Injury Statistics Query and Reporting System (WISQARS). 2022. Available at: https://www.cdc.gov/injury/wisqars. Accessed January 27, 2023.
53. Bach H, Arango V. Neuroanatomy of serotonergic abnormalities in suicide. In: Dwivedi Y, ed. *The Neurobiological Basis of Suicide*. Boca Raton, FL: CRC Press/Taylor and Francis; 2012.
54. Oquendo MA, Sullivan GM, Sudol K, et al. Toward a biosignature for suicide. *Am J Psychiatry*. 2014;171(12):1259–77. doi:10.1176/appi.ajp.2014.14020194
55. Robins LN, Regier DA, eds. *Psychiatric Disorders in America: The Epidemiologic Catchment Area Study*. New York, NY: The Free Press; 2001.
56. Kessler RC, McGonagle KA, Zhao S, et al. Lifetime and 12-month prevalence of *DSM-III-R* psychiatric disorders in the United States. Results from the National Comorbidity Survey. *Arch Gen Psychiatry*. 1994;51(1):8–19.

57. Kessler RC, Berglund P, Demler O, Jin R, Merikangas KR, Walters EE. Lifetime prevalence and age-of-onset distributions of DSM-IV disorders in the national comorbidity survey replication. *Arch Gen Psychiatry.* 2005;62(6):593–602.
58. Breslau J, Kendler KS, Su M, Gaxiola-Aguilar S, Kessler RC. Lifetime risk and persistence of psychiatric disorders across ethnic groups in the United States. *Psychol Med.* 2005;35(3): 317–327.
59. McGrath J, Saha S, Welham J, El Saadi O, MacCauley C, Chant D. A systematic review of the incidence of schizophrenia: the distribution of rates and the influence of sex, urbanicity, migrant status and methodology. *BMC Medicine.* 2004;2:13.
60. Saha S, Chant D, Welham J, McGrath J. A systematic review of the prevalence of schizophrenia. *PLoS Med.* 2005;2(5):e141.
61. Aleman A, Kahn RS, Selten J-P. Sex differences in the risk of schizophrenia: evidence from meta-analysis. *Arch Gen Psychiatry.* 2003;60(6):565–571.
62. Ochoa S, Usall J, Cobo J, Labad X, Kulkarni J. Gender differences in schizophrenia and first-episode psychosis: a comprehensive literature review. *Schizophr Res Treatment.* 2012;2012:e916198.
63. Owen MJ, Sawa A, Mortensen PB. Schizophrenia. *Lancet.* 2016;388(10039):86–97.
64. Kessler RC, Petukhova M, Sampson NA, Zaslavsky AM, Wittchen H-U. Twelve-month and lifetime prevalence and lifetime morbid risk of anxiety and mood disorders in the United States. *Int J Methods Psychiatr Res.* 2012;21(3):169–184.
65. Horwath E, Cohen RS, Weissman MM. Epidemiology of depressive and anxiety disorders. In: Tsuang MT, Tohen M, eds. *Textbook in Psychiatric Epidemiology.* 2nd ed. Hoboken, NJ: Wiley and Sons; 2002.
66. Siefert K, Bowman PJ, Heflin CM, Danziger S, Williams DR. Social and environmental predictors of maternal depression in current and recent welfare recipients. *Am J Orthopsychiatry.* 2000;70(4):510–522.
67. Tohen M, Angst J. Epidemiology of bipolar disorder. In: Tsuang M, Tohen M, eds. *Textbook in Psychiatric Epidemiology.* 2nd ed. New York, NY: Wiley and Sons; 2002.
68. Jang KL, Taylor S, Stein MB, Yamagata S. Trauma exposure and stress response: exploration of mechanisms of cause and effect. *Twin Res Hum Genet.* 2007;10(4):564–572.
69. Dannefer D. Cumulative advantage/disadvantage and the life course: cross-fertilizing age and social science theory. *J Gerontol B Psychol Sci Soc Sci.* 2003;58(6):S327–S337.
70. Howlett JR, Stein MB. Post-traumatic stress disorder: relationship to traumatic brain injury and approach to treatment. In: Laskowitz D, Grant G, eds. *Translational Research in Traumatic Brain Injury.* Boca Raton, FL: CRC Press/Taylor and Francis Group; 2016.
71. Sachs-Ericsson N, Joiner TE, Cougle JR, Stanley IH, Sheffler JL. Combat exposure in early adulthood interacts with recent stressors to predict PTSD in aging male veterans. *Gerontologist.* 2016;56(1):82–91.
72. Breslau N, Wilcox HC, Storr CL, Lucia VC, Anthony JC. Trauma exposure and posttraumatic stress disorder: a study of youths in urban America. *J Urban Health.* 2004;81(4): 530–544.
73. Parto JA, Evans MK, Zonderman AB. Symptoms of posttraumatic stress disorder among urban residents. *J Nerv Ment Dis.* 2011;199(7):436–439.

74. Drapeau CW, McIntosh JL. USA suicide 2013: official final data. Washington, DC: American Association of Suicidology; 2015.
75. Miller M, Azrael D, Barber C. Suicide mortality in the United States: the importance of attending to method in understanding population-level disparities in the burden of suicide. *Annu Rev Public Health.* 2012;33(1):393–408.
76. Eisenberg ME, Resnick MD. Suicidality among gay, lesbian and bisexual youth: the role of protective factors. *J Adolesc Health.* 2006;39(5):662–668.
77. Russell ST, Joyner K. Adolescent sexual orientation and suicide risk: evidence from a national study. *Am J Public Health.* 2001;91(8):1276–1281.
78. Mościcki EK. Epidemiology of suicide. *Int Psychogeriatr.* 1995;7(2):137–148.
79. Vijayakumar L, Kumar MS, Vijayakumar V. Substance use and suicide. *Curr Opin Psychiatry.* 2011;24(3):197–202.
80. Almog M, Curtis S, Copeland A, Congdon P. Geographical variation in acute psychiatric admissions within New York City 1990–2000: growing inequalities in service use? *Soc Sci Med.* 2004:59(2):361–376.
81. Galea S, Ahern J, Nandi A, Tracy M, Beard J, Vlahov D. Urban neighborhood poverty and the incidence of depression in a population-based cohort study. *Ann Epidemiol.* 2007;17(3):171–179.
82. Bresnahan M, Boydell J, Murray R, Susser E. Temporal variation in the incidence, course and outcome of schizophrenia. In: Murray RM, Jones PB, Susser E, van Os J, Cannon M, eds. *The Epidemiology of Schizophrenia.* Cambridge, UK: Cambridge University Press; 2003.
83. Warner R. Time trends in schizophrenia: changes in obstetric risk factors with industrialization. *Schizophr Bull.* 1995:21(3):483–500.
84. Pow JL, Baumeister AA, Hawkins MF, Cohen AS, Garand JC. Deinstitutionalization of American public hospitals for the mentally ill before and after the introduction of antipsychotic medications. *Harv Rev Psychiatry.* 2015;23(3):176–187.
85. Durham ML. The impact of deinstitutionalization on the current treatment of the mentally ill. *Int J Law Psychiatry.* 1989;12(2):117–131.
86. Sipe TA, Finnie RK, Knopf JA, et al.; Community Preventive Services Task Force. Effects of mental health benefits legislation: a community guide systematic review. *Am J Prev Med.* 2015;48(6):755–766.
87. Han B, Gfroerer J, Kuramoto SJ, Ali M, Woodward AM, Teich J. Medicaid expansion under the Affordable Care Act: potential changes in receipt of mental health treatment among low-income nonelderly adults with serious mental disorders. *Am J Public Health.* 2015;105(10): 1982–1989.
88. Caffrey MK. Integrated treatment for diabetes, depression gains notice, with help from ACA. *Am J Manag Care.* 2014;20(10 spec no):E1.
89. World Health Organization. *Prevention of Mental Disorders.* Geneva, Switzerland: World Health Organization; 2004.
90. Hosman C, Jane-Llopis E, Saxena S, eds. *Prevention of Mental Disorders: Effective Interventions and Policy Options.* Oxford, UK: Oxford University Press; 2005.
91. Yoshikawa H, Aber JL, Beardslee WR. The effects of poverty on the mental, emotional, and behavioral health of children and youth: implications for prevention. *Am Psychol.* 2012; 67(4):272–284.

92. Pabayo R, Kawachi I, Gilman SE. Income inequality among American states and the incidence of major depression. *J Epidemiol Commun Health*. 2014;68(2):110–115.
93. Smith JR, Patton DU. Posttraumatic stress symptoms in context: examining trauma responses to violent exposures and homicide death among Black males in urban neighborhoods. *Am J Orthopsychiatry*. 2016;86(2):212–223.
94. Beardslee WR, Brent DA, Weersing VR, et al. Prevention of depression in at-risk adolescents: longer-term effects. *JAMA Psychiatry*. 2013;70(11):1161–1170.
95. Khan A, McCormack HC, Bolger EA, et al. Childhood maltreatment, depression, and suicidal ideation: critical importance of parental and peer emotional abuse during developmental sensitive periods in males and females. *Front Psychiatry*. 2015;6:42.
96. Solantaus T, Salo S. Paternal postnatal depression: fathers emerge from the wings. *Lancet*. 2005;365(9478):2158–2159.
97. Weersing VR, Shamseddeen W, Garber J, et al. Prevention of depression in at-risk adolescents: predictors and moderators of acute effects. *J Am Acad Child Adolesc Psychiatry*. 2016;55(3):219–226.
98. Botellero VL, Skranes J, Bjuland KJ, et al. Mental health and cerebellar volume during adolescence in very-low-birth-weight infants: a longitudinal study. *Child Adolesc Psychiatry Mental Health*. 2016;10:6.
99. Kersten-Alvarez LE, Hosman CMH, Riksen-Walraven JM, van Doesum KTM, Smeekens S, Hoefnagels C. Early school outcomes for children of postpartum depressed mothers: comparison with a community sample. *Child Psychiatry Hum Dev*. 2012;43(2):201–218.
100. Falk DE, Yi H-Y, Hilton ME. Age of onset and temporal sequencing of lifetime DSM-IV alcohol use disorders relative to comorbid mood and anxiety disorders. *Drug Alcohol Depend*. 2008;94(1–3):234–245.
101. Larsen KK. Depression following myocardial infarction—an overseen complication with prognostic importance. *Dan Med J*. 2013;60(8):B4689.
102. Shoshani A, Slone M. The resilience function of character strengths in the face of war and protracted conflict. *Front Psychol*. 2015;6:2006.
103. Streb M, Häller P, Michael T. PTSD in paramedics: resilience and sense of coherence. *Behav Cogn Psychother*. 2014;42(4):452–463.
104. Szivak TK, Kraemer WJ. Physiological readiness and resilience: pillars of military preparedness. *J Strength Cond Res*. 2015;29(suppl 11):S34–S39.
105. Cavanagh JT, Carson AJ, Sharpe M, Lawrie SM. Psychological autopsy studies of suicide: a systematic review. *Psychol Med*. 2003;33(3):395–405.
106. Li Z, Page A, Martin G, Taylor R. Attributable risk of psychiatric and socio-economic factors for suicide from individual-level, population-based studies: a systematic review. *Soc Sci Med*. 2011;72(4):608–616.
107. Chapman S, Alpers P, Agho K, Jones M. Australia's 1996 gun law reforms: faster falls in firearm deaths, firearm suicides, and a decade without mass shootings. *Inj Prev*. 2006;12(6):365–372.
108. Reisch T, Steffen T, Habenstein A, Tschacher W. Change in suicide rates in Switzerland before and after firearm restriction resulting from the 2003 "Army XXI" reform. *Am J Psychiatry*. 2013;170(9):977–984.

109. Page A, Morrell S, Hobbs C, et al. Suicide in young adults: psychiatric and socio-economic factors from a case–control study. *BMC Psychiatry*. 2014;14:68.

110. Durlak J, Wells A. Evaluation of indicated preventive interventions (secondary prevention) mental health programs for children and adolescents. *Am J Community Psychol.* 1998; 26(5):775–802.

111. Nitzkin J, Smith SA. *Clinical Preventive Services in Substance Abuse and Mental Health Update: From Science to Services.* Rockville, MD: Center for Mental Health Services, Substance Abuse and Mental Health Services Administration; 2004.

112. Siu AL, US Preventive Services Task Force, Bibbins-Domingo K, et al. Screening for depression in adults: US Preventive Services Task Force recommendation statement. *JAMA*. 2016;315(4):380–387. doi: 10.1001/jama.2015.18392

113. Harrison G, Hopper K, Craig T, et al. Recovery from psychotic illness: a 15- and 25-year international follow-up study. *BR J Psychiatry.* 2001;178:506–517. doi:10.1192/bjp.178.6.506

114. Mental Health Commission. *President's New Freedom Commission on Mental Health.* 2001. Archived. Available at: https://govinfo.library.unt.edu/mentalhealthcommission/reports/FinalReport/toc.html. Accessed January 27, 2023.

115. Lehman AF, Goldman HH, Dixon LB, Print RC. *Evidence-Based Mental Health Treatments and Services: Examples to Inform Public Policy.* New York, NY: Milbank Memorial Fund; 2004.

116. Furlong M, McGilloway S, Bywater T, Hutchings J, Smith SM, Donnelly M. Cochrane review: behavioural and cognitive–behavioural group-based parenting programmes for early-onset conduct problems in children aged 3 to 12 years (review). *Evid Based Child Health.* 2013;8(2):318–692.

117. Brown LD. *Consumer-Run Mental Health: Framework for Recovery.* New York, NY: Springer Science & Business Media; 2011.

118. Macias C, Rodican CF, Hargreaves WA, Jones DR, Barreira PJ, Wang Q. Supported employment outcomes of a randomized controlled trial of ACT and Clubhouse models. *Psychiatr Serv.* 2006;57(10):1406–1415.

119. Mowbray CT, Woodward AT, Holter MC, MacFarlane P, Bybee D. Characteristics of users of consumer-run drop-in centers versus clubhouses. *J Behav Health Serv Res.* 2009;36(3): 361–371.

120. Burns T, Catty J, Dash M, Roberts C, Lockwood A, Marshall M. Use of intensive case management to reduce time in hospital in people with severe mental disorders: systematic review and meta-regression. *BMJ.* 2007;335(7615):336.

121. Annapolis Coalition. *An Action Plan for Behavioral Health Workforce Development: A Framework for Discussion.* SAMHSA/DHHS publication 280-02-0302. Rockville, MD: US Dept of Health and Human Services: 2007.

122. Hunkeler EM, Meresman JF, Hargreaves WA, et al. Efficacy of nurse telehealth care and peer support in augmenting treatment of depression in primary care. *Arch Fam Med.* 2000:9(8):700–708.

123. Katon W, Von Korff M, Lin E, et al. Collaborative management to achieve treatment guidelines: impact on depression in primary care. *JAMA.* 1995:273(13):1026–1031.

124. Katon W, Robinson P, Von Korff M, et al. A multifaceted intervention to improve treatment of depression in primary care. *Arch Gen Psychiatry.* 1996:53(10):924–932.

125. Manderscheid R, Kathol R. Fostering sustainable, integrated medical and behavioral health services in medical settings. *Ann Intern Med.* 2014;160(1):61–65. doi:10.7326/M13-1693

126. US Department of Health and Human Services, National Institutes of Health, National Institute of Mental Health. *NIMH Strategic Plan for Research.* 2015. NIH publication 02 2650. Available at: http://www.nimh.nih.gov/about/strategic-planning-reports/index.shtml. Accessed January 27, 2023.

20

Neurological Disorders

Sara Doyle, MD, MPH, Emily C. Davis, BS, and Edwin Trevathan, MD, MPH

LEARNING OBJECTIVES

After completing this chapter, readers should be able to

1. Convey the diversity and complexity of the different types of neurological disorders that impose a major public health burden.
2. Among neurological disorders outline the few opportunities for primary prevention, the greater opportunities for secondary prevention, and the importance of research to identify more modifiable risk factors for common neurological disorders.
3. Review available epidemiological data, often limited, on common neurological disorders.

INTRODUCTION

Neurological disorders, a large and heterogeneous group of disorders, are the leading cause of disability globally and thus play a major role in global public health.[1] Unfortunately, since 2014 mortality associated with neurological disorders has increased,[2] and in 2019 neurological disorders were responsible for 97.7 million disability-adjusted life years (DALYs).[3] Neurological disorders disproportionately affect subpopulations having ethnic, racial, and socioeconomic disparities,[4] and so reducing morbidity and mortality associated with neurological disorders will require a sustained focus on reducing neurological disorders–associated morbidity and mortality among the most vulnerable among us. Although there is limited research regarding the extent of these neurological disorders' disparities, we do know that mortality rates attributable to neurological disorders are disproportionately high among non-Hispanic Black populations and are likely associated with systemic (e.g., enslavement, segregation, discrimination) and structural factors in society that leave these populations with limited access to health resources, even in wealthy countries like the United States.[5]

Even common neurological disorders, such as Alzheimer's disease, Parkinson's disease, multiple sclerosis (MS), and the epilepsies, are associated with limited-to-no primary prevention opportunities, as few modifiable risk factors have been identified.

Traumatic brain injury (TBI) and spinal cord injury (SCI) offer significant opportunities for primary prevention. The morbidity and loss of productivity caused by low back pain and carpal tunnel syndrome (CTS) offer primary and secondary prevention opportunities.

More epidemiologic research using genetics, imaging, and biological markers for early recognition of Alzheimer's and related dementias, Parkinson's disease, MS, and epilepsy should be emphasized, and opportunities for prevention of injuries and health promotion among people with disabilities must be a public health priority (see Table 20-1). As we enter an era of "precision public health," it will become increasingly important to examine the interaction between these structural factors and genomic risk factors.[6]

Over the past few decades the incidence of some neurological disorders has increased among middle-aged adults.[7] Some of the potentially modifiable risk factors of these neurological disorders reach back to childhood, pregnancy, or even preconception. Public health professionals will need to work among younger populations for both primary and secondary prevention efforts to reduce the impact of neurological disorders in the general population. This chapter reviews some of the more common neurological disorders from a public health perspective.

EPILEPSY AND STATUS EPILEPTICUS

Epilepsy, which is the underlying condition predisposing an individual to repeated seizures, is a category of brain disorders operationally defined as (1) at least two unprovoked seizures occurring more than 24 hours apart, (2) one unprovoked (or reflex) seizure and a high probability of recurrent seizures, or (3) diagnosis of an epilepsy syndrome. Worldwide, epilepsy is the most common serious neurological disorder among children and young adults. As there are many types of epilepsy—each with different clinical manifestations, causes, comorbid conditions, and severity—the term *the epilepsies* is now being used to describe this heterogeneous group of brain disorders.[8]

Status epilepticus (SE), or prolonged seizures operationally defined as seizures lasting longer than five minutes, occurs as the first seizure in a least 25% of patients with epilepsy[9] and is the most common life-threatening neurological emergency among children. SE-associated mortality has been estimated at 10% to more than 25%, with a high risk of new neurological morbidity and disability among SE survivors. Access to effective, evidence-based SE diagnosis and management can reduce SE-associated mortality and morbidity.[10]

According to the 2019 Global Burden of Disease (GBD) study, the global age-standardized epilepsy burden, DALYs, totaled more than 18.3 million, with a higher prevalence for men than women. Epilepsy-associated mortality increased by 98.8% in the United States between 1999 and 2017, likely as a result of (1) the increased burden

Table 20-1. Neurological Diseases: Causes, Consequences, and High-Risk Groups

Disease	Causes	Consequences	High-Risk Groups
Epilepsy	• Genetic factors • Environmental exposures (often undefined) • Cerebral malformations • Trauma • Encephalitis or meningitis • Brain tumors or metastatic disease • Hypoxic injury • Strokes, vascular disease	• Increased risk of premature death • Increased risk of falls, burns, or drowning	• Family history • Central nervous system infections • Cerebral malaria survivors • Head injury • Children with developmental delay • Elderly with stroke
Parkinson's disease	• Genetic factors • Environmental triggers • Viral infection • Exposure to neurotoxins in the environment • Occupational exposures to heavy metals	• Motor impairment • Cognitive decline • Depression • Increased long-term care needs • Premature death	• Family history • Men • Whites • Certain occupations (e.g., teachers, health care workers, firefighters, farmers, welders)
Alzheimer's disease and other dementias	• Genetic factors • Long-term survival of chronic disease • Traumatic brain injury • Multi-infarct strokes • Diabetes, hypertension	• Premature death • Cognitive decline • Increased long-term care needs • Depression	• Family history • Elderly
Cerebral palsy	• Prematurity • Very low birthweight • High birthweight • Hypoxic–ischemic encephalopathy • Multiple births	• Feeding difficulties • Motor disability • Social isolation	• Premature births • Twins and multiple births • Family history • Neonatal hyperbilirubinemia
Autism spectrum disorders	• Genetic factors • Potential environmental exposures	• Social isolation • Anxiety • Impaired communication	• Family history • Males • Premature births • Advanced parental age
ALS	• Genetic factors • Exposures to lead, mercury, and other heavy metals	• Progressive weakness • Paralysis • Respiratory impairment • Premature death	• Family history • Men • Older adults
MS	• Genetic factors • Viral or other infectious diseases	• Intermittent motor, language, and/or cognitive impairment • Long-term care needs • Depression • Premature death	• Family history • Females • Young adults

(Continued)

Table 20-1. (Continued)

Disease	Causes	Consequences	High-Risk Groups
Guillain-Barré syndrome	• Genetic factors • Autoimmune response triggered by a recent viral or bacterial infection	• Temporary weakness and paralysis • Respiratory failure • Pneumonia • Deep vein thrombosis	• Family history • Whites • Living in northern latitudes
Tic disorders and Tourette syndrome	• Genetic factors • Potential environmental exposures	• Increased risk of school failure • Social isolation • Behavior problems	• Family history • Males
Traumatic brain injury and spinal cord injury	• Falls • Transportation-related injuries and automobile crashes • Sports or recreation injuries • Assaults • Alcohol and drug use	• Paralysis and death • Cognitive deficits[a] • Epilepsy[a] • Dementia[a] • Depression • Complications of immobility • Deep vein thrombosis	• Alcohol and drug abusers • Elderly • Children and adolescents • Men • Lower social/economic persons • Construction, farming, roofing, and logging occupations • Motorcyclists • Those who fail to wear seat belts
ADHD	• Genetic factors • Potential environmental exposures, injuries	• Poor self-esteem • Anxiety • Conduct disorder • Depression • Sleep problems • Substance abuse	• Males
Carpal tunnel syndrome	• Repetitive hand or wrist movements • Wrist trauma • Diabetes, hypothyroidism • Pregnancy	• Impaired hand use • Lost income and job loss	• Workers who engage in repetitive fine-motor movements (e.g., typists) • Food-processing workers, roofers, carpenters, and mill workers • Pregnant women
Low back pain	• Heavy lifting • Abdominal obesity • Cigarette smoking • Premature menopause • Genetic factors	• Disability • Lost income • Time away from work	• Occupations with heavy lifting (e.g., nursing, truck driving, warehouse, farming, lumber, construction work, mining) • Caregivers of disabled
Migraine and tension headaches	• Genetic factors • Depression • Stress • Environmental triggers (e.g., food)	• School absence • Lost income • Time away from work • Depression	• Family history of headache • Women • Low social and economic class

Note: ADHD = attention-deficit/hyperactivity disorder; ALS = amyotrophic lateral sclerosis; MS = multiple sclerosis.
[a]Complications of brain injury only.

of overall neurological disorders, with an associated all-neurological mortality; (2) an increase in epilepsy prevalence; and (3) increases in the prevalence of dementing disorders and malignant neoplasms as the cause of death among people with epilepsy.[11]

The epilepsy treatment gap, or the percentage of people with epilepsy who are untreated, remains very high in many parts of the world, and it is estimated to be 50% to 92% in low- and middle-income countries and as high as 10% in high-income countries, although few data on the epilepsy treatment gap are available in the United States.[12] People with epilepsy in the United States are significantly more likely to be insured under Medicaid, more likely to be disabled, and less likely to be employed compared with people without epilepsy.[13]

Significance

The severity of the epilepsies varies by epilepsy syndrome. For example, childhood epilepsy with centrotemporal spikes tends to undergo spontaneous remission in almost all children who have this disorder, but it may also be associated with learning disorders.[14] In contrast, Lennox-Gastaut syndrome is a profoundly severe epilepsy syndrome with multiple daily seizures that do not respond to treatment, with resulting intellectual disability and an increased risk of premature death.[15] Along with this increased risk of premature death, people with severe epilepsy syndromes have a high risk of disability and their epilepsy has a major negative impact on their quality of life. (Table 20-1).

More than 50% of people with epilepsy have comorbid conditions that interact with their epilepsy,[16] making treatment of their epilepsy more complex and increasing the risk of early disability and death. People with epilepsy are about eight times more likely to have comorbid conditions such as depression, anxiety, dementia, migraine, heart disease, arthritis, and obesity than the general population.[17] Furthermore, people with epilepsy may have impaired working memory, especially if seizures are not controlled with antiseizure drugs.[18]

Despite the availability of more than 25 approved antiseizure drugs in high-income countries, only about 66% of people with epilepsy achieve seizure-freedom. People with epilepsy in low- and middle-income countries are even less likely to achieve freedom from seizures, often because of interruptions in medication access.[16] Among some people with intractable focal epilepsy not controlled with medication, resection of the epileptogenic zone in the cerebral cortex may stop seizures or significantly reduce seizure frequency. Effectively managing the adverse effects of antiseizure drugs and treating comorbid depression increases a patient's quality of life.[19] Lack of seizure control limits the ability of individuals with epilepsy to maintain their independence, given their resulting inability to drive and/or work. Independence, driving, and cessation of seizures are consistently found to be the most important factors associated with quality of life among people with epilepsy.[20]

As noted, people with epilepsy have an increased risk of death, with high standardized mortality ratios, which are highest for childhood-onset symptomatic epilepsy syndromes, including Lennox-Gastaut syndrome and other severe epilepsy syndromes associated with other neurological conditions such as cerebral palsy or intellectual disability.[15] The reasons for excessive mortality among people with epilepsy are only partially understood. Seizures often result in falls, burns, or drowning, especially in low- and middle-income countries where adequate seizure control is hampered by limited access to basic antiseizure drugs.[21] Overall, in 2019 epilepsy was responsible for 18.3 million global years of healthy life lost to disability (YLDs).[22]

Sudden unexpected death in epilepsy (SUDEP) is second only to stroke among neurological disorders as the most common cause of the number of adult life years lost.[23] The incidence of SUDEP in children varies from 0.22 to 1.11 per 1,000 person-years and is estimated at 0.35 per 1,000 person-years in adults.[24] In the United States and Europe alone, sudden death among those with epilepsy accounts for approximately 7,000 deaths per year.[25] Sudden death is most common among young adults with intractable epilepsy (ongoing seizures despite optimal antiseizure medication) and has an incidence of about 2 to 10 per 1,000 person-years—many times higher than the risk of sudden death among age-matched people without epilepsy in the general population.[25,26] Maintaining seizure control, often with appropriate levels of antiseizure drugs, reduces the risk of sudden death.[21]

Pathophysiology

Excessive abnormal electrical discharges from cortical neurons and from specific structures adjacent to the cortex (e.g., the hippocampus) form the biological basis of seizures. The manifestations of seizures are as varied as the functions of the cortex; they defy simple rules for diagnosis, often resulting in both delays in diagnosis of potentially serious epilepsy and the erroneous diagnosis of epilepsy.[27]

Seizures that begin in a single region of the brain are classified as *focal seizures,* and seizures that start all over both hemispheres at the beginning of the seizure are classified as *generalized seizures.* People with generalized seizures tend to have altered consciousness at the onset of their seizures, whereas people with focal seizures often do not have altered consciousness until the electrical seizure has spread over the cortex.[28]

The degree of alteration of awareness caused by a seizure is usually a function of the size of the cortical surface involved in the seizure: the larger the amount of cortex involved in the seizure, the greater the degree of altered awareness. If a large portion of the cortex is involved in the seizure (especially if both hemispheres are actively seizing), then consciousness is almost always impaired. If the seizure starts in a single region of the brain, the manifestation of the seizure is a direct result of the disordered function of that brain region. Then, as the seizure spreads along the cortical surface, the seizure manifests additional cortical functions. Seizures that begin in a specific region of the brain tend to be *stereotypic*, with the clinical manifestation of each seizure onset being identical—a phenomenon that helps experienced clinicians make a diagnosis.[28-30]

The diagnosis of epilepsy is typically made by a clinician taking a detailed history, in high-income countries often in combination with an electroencephalogram.[28] Epilepsy screening and diagnosis in underserved communities may be enhanced by tools for epilepsy screening and diagnosis, especially in low- and middle-income countries.[31]

The mechanism involved in sudden death in epilepsy is unclear, but many such deaths occur during sleep when individuals are in a prone position after an apparent seizure. Central respiratory failure or dysfunction and/or cardiac arrhythmias during or after seizures appear to play a role.[26] Regardless, seizure-freedom on antiseizure medication significantly reduces the risk of sudden death.[32,33]

Descriptive Epidemiology

The prevalence of epilepsy has been estimated at about 6 to 9 per 1,000 in developed countries of Europe and Asia and in the United States. Using different methods, researchers have estimated the prevalence of epilepsy in both Rochester, Minnesota, and Atlanta, Georgia, at approximately 7 per 1,000; extrapolated to the total US population, an estimated two million Americans have active epilepsy.[34] Epilepsy rates are higher in low- and middle-income countries than in developed countries, with prevalence rates of 15 per 1,000 or even as high as 105 per 1,000.[35,36] The higher prevalence of epilepsy in these countries is largely unexplained and deserves further study.

Epilepsy incidence studies have been primarily conducted in high-income countries, like the United States, where the highest incidence of new-onset epilepsy is among the very young and the elderly. Between birth and age 65 years, the highest incidence occurs during the first year of life, with relatively high incidence during early childhood years. Beginning at age 65, the incidence of new-onset epilepsy rises sharply, as the aging population develops epilepsy as a secondary condition, one associated largely with strokes and vascular disease, dementias, and cancer.[37]

Epilepsy disproportionately affects the poor. In the United States, about half of adults with active epilepsy live in poverty.[38] Adults living in the United States between 2010 and 2013 with active epilepsy were more likely to be uninsured or insured by Medicaid, less likely to have private health insurance, less likely to be employed, more likely to be disabled, and more likely to report barriers to health care access and medication access than the general population.[13] These barriers mean that adults with epilepsy who are also poor are more likely not to get effective treatment for epilepsy and when compared with the general population will consequently experience higher disability and possibly mortality.[39]

Causes

Among infants and children who have an onset of epilepsy, genetic risk factors play an important role. Some forms of epilepsy—such as childhood absence epilepsy, benign Rolandic epilepsy, and juvenile myoclonic epilepsy—are primarily genetic disorders, with a minimal role for environmental triggers.[40] Other forms of epilepsy, such as focal epilepsy of mesial temporal lobe origin, are likely attributable to environmental–epigenetic interactions[41] or to a combination of environmental triggers (mostly yet to be discovered) with genetic predispositions.[42] Over the past few years much has been learned about susceptibility genes, including some preliminary identification of phenotypic and genotypic features,[43] but complex relationships between genes and the environment mean that much more study will be required over the next few decades.[44]

In general, anything that causes damage to the brain, alters the structure, or inflames the cerebral cortex can cause epilepsy: stroke, cerebral malformations, trauma, encephalitis, brain tumors or metastatic disease in the brain, and hypoxic injury to the cortex can all cause seizures and epilepsy. However, not all people who experience the same insult from a stroke or other injury to the cortex, or from encephalitis or a tumor, have seizures. Susceptibility genes appear to play a role in these situations as well.[45,46]

Epilepsy is a devastating feature of many different neurodevelopmental disorders when it is associated with developmental regression during the first 18 months of life.[47] The combination of developmental regression and new-onset epilepsy is often associated with a genetic susceptibility.[48]

Over the past several years some people have blamed vaccines for the development of epilepsy and developmental delays. The biologic plausibility of a vaccine-induced etiology is, however, weak to nonexistent. For example, in the 1980s the pertussis vaccine was claimed by some to have led to myoclonic epilepsy, encephalopathy, and developmental regression. It has since been proven that it is not this vaccine but instead the *SCN1A* gene mutation that causes severe myoclonic epilepsy of infancy (Dravet syndrome), regardless of vaccine history.[49,50] There is evidence that some vaccines, such as rubella, can reduce epilepsy incidence (Figure 20-1).[51]

Febrile seizures (especially febrile status epilepticus) are known to be associated with development of epilepsy, particularly focal epilepsy of temporal lobe origin. However, most children with febrile seizures and febrile status epilepticus do not develop epilepsy, and the relationship may be attributable to the underlying genes (or infections) causing the febrile seizures rather than the actual seizures themselves.[52,53]

Evidence-Based Interventions

Several vaccines are likely effective in preventing epilepsy caused by severe infections that damage the cerebral cortex, such as *Haemophilus influenzae* meningitis, meningococcal

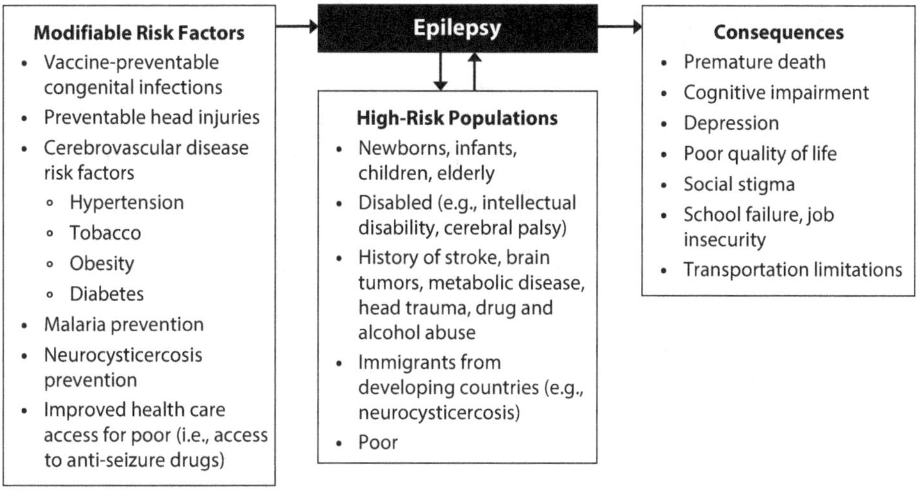

Note: For further information about high-risk populations for epilepsy, see England et al.[59]

Figure 20-1. Epilepsy: Causes, Consequences, and High-Risk Populations

meningitis, pertussis, and rubella vaccines.[51] Prevention of malaria in areas with endemic spread of *Plasmodium falciparum* may also prevent seizures and epilepsy.[54,55] Folic acid fortification of the grain supply and pre-conception supplementation has significantly reduced the incidence of neural tube defects and associated hydrocephalus (from Chiari II malformations) and is most effective where fortification is mandatory,[56] but we still do not know if other brain malformations that increase the risk of seizures have been reduced by folic acid fortification and supplementation. Prevention of congenital infections (i.e., cytomegalovirus, herpes, toxoplasmosis) prevents serious brain damage with associated epilepsy. Prevention of head injuries likely could, and perhaps already does, have an impact on the onset of epilepsy and associated neurological comorbidities, especially among adolescents. Among older adults, preventing cerebrovascular disease could have a major impact on the prevention of associated epilepsy.

Among people with drug-resistant focal onset epilepsy, surgical resection of the epileptogenic zone of cortex in rigorously selected people with epilepsy based upon standard evidence-based protocols can eliminate or reduce seizure frequency. Surgical resection also reduces the likelihood of death as well as the experience of depression and other comorbid conditions associated with epilepsy. One challenge is that referrals to epilepsy surgery centers are often delayed for many years.[57]

The ketogenic diet can reduce seizure frequency, especially in children who have severe generalized or multifocal epilepsy associated with encephalopathy.[58] Management of the ketogenic diet requires an experienced team of physicians and a dietician with ketogenic diet experience, typically available only at major referral centers in high-income countries.

Moving Forward

Reducing the consequences of epilepsy can, in part, be achieved through rapid diagnosis and appropriate early treatment for epilepsy, especially among children.[59] In the future it may be possible to identify genetically susceptible individuals and intervene early to prevent epilepsy. Intervening early among those with tuberous sclerosis complex, for which there is an animal model, provides an important insight into this opportunity as we learn more about epilepsy genomics.[60] Future epidemiological studies should emphasize the role of gene–environment interactions and seek to identify potentially modifiable risk factors for specific epilepsy syndromes.[61,62]

Prevention of the excessive morbidity and mortality associated with status epilepticus by following guidelines for prompt and systematic treatment of prolonged seizures in emergency departments and in communities should be a priority. Following newly published guidelines may prevent status epilepticus–associated morbidity and mortality.[63]

PARKINSON'S DISEASE

Parkinson's disease (PD), the second most common neurodegenerative disease after Alzheimer's disease, has characteristic motor and non-motor symptoms, with the non-motor symptoms often predating the better-known typical motor symptoms by decades. Studies of this prodromal phase have generated hypotheses regarding PD pathophysiology and may be a target for prevention or early intervention. There is currently no disease-modifying therapy for PD. Although PD is the most common cause of the group of motor symptoms or parkinsonism, other causes of parkinsonism include vascular- and drug-induced parkinsonism and other neurodegenerative diseases.[64] This section focuses only on Parkinson's disease.

Significance

Among these neurological disorders, which are the leading cause of disability worldwide, the prevalence of PD has increased the most since 1990. Both motor and non-motor symptoms of PD lead to significant morbidity and mortality. People with PD are at higher risk of serious injury and death associated with falls.[65] In 2016 alone PD accounted for over 350,000 years of life lost to disability or early death (DALYs) in the United States.[66]

Pathophysiology

The cause of the observed pathology in PD is not known, but the classic motor symptoms of PD (tremor, rigidity, slow movements, and postural instability) are driven by degeneration of dopaminergic neurons of the *substantia nigra pars compacta (SNPc)* in the midbrain. Motor symptoms are evident when about 60% to 80% of these neurons are lost.[64]

The reason for this specific degeneration is an area of active research, and hypotheses include oxidative stress and mitochondrial dysfunction.[67] The principle non-motor symptoms of PD are hyposmia, rapid eye movement sleep behavior disorder, constipation, orthostatic hypotension, and cognitive impairment. The pathophysiology of these symptoms is an active area of research, as it is likely that the process driving these symptoms causes PD. One leading hypothesis is the systematic deposition of abnormal α-synuclein protein aggregates—called Lewy bodies—in the central and peripheral nervous system cause cell dysfunction and cell death.[68]

Descriptive Epidemiology

PD is a clinical diagnosis, and this can complicate its study on the population level because of differential awareness of diagnosis, access to neurologic care, and diagnostic coding practices. There remains a need for high-quality epidemiology studies of PD, including cohort studies. A meta-analysis estimated that 6.1 million people lived with PD worldwide in 2016, and this figure is expected to double to 12 million by the year 2040, partially because of an aging population.[66] The incidence of PD is also increasing, especially in industrialized countries. The median age-adjusted incidence of PD is 14 per 100,000 per year. Among those aged 65 and over, the incidence is approximately 160 per 100,000 per year.[69] Several US studies report that age-adjusted incidence and prevalence are higher among men than among women, and higher among Whites than among African Americans, although access to diagnostic services may bias these data.[67]

Causes

Although the cause of PD and its specific pattern of neurodegeneration is not known, it is likely multifactorial. There is copious research into infectious, environmental, or toxic exposures and genetic causes.

Viral

A viral encephalitis epidemic in 1919 and the subsequent sequelae of parkinsonism provided neuropathological evidence of selective damage to the *substantia nigra*, although investigators have not found evidence of selective *substantia nigra* damage from other viral encephalitis cases or epidemics.[70]

Toxic/Environmental

In the 1980s there was a cluster of PD among intravenous drug users who injected MPTP (1-methyl-4-phenyl-1,2,3,6 tetrahydropyridine), a synthetic compound with heroin-like clinical effects.[64] A recent meta-analysis has reported some inconsistent evidence that rural living, drinking well water, and exposures to pesticides and paraquat are associated with an increased risk for PD. The relative risk for PD with each exposure ranges from 1.1 to 2.[69,71] Heavy metal exposure is also hypothesized as a risk factor, given that the prevalence of PD among male welders has been reported to be significantly higher than in controls from the general population.[72] Traumatic brain injury is associated with higher risk of PD close to the injury, but this risk decreases over time.[69]

Genetic

A genetic susceptibility for PD has been a major area of research in the last few decades, with studies estimating that 5% to 10% of PD cases have a genetic etiology. There are several known monogenic causes of PD; some are autosomal dominant and some recessive. Some genes confer increased risk of PD, perhaps from increased susceptibility to environmental factors.[64] Advancements in sequencing technology have led to genome-wide association studies for many neurologic diseases, including PD. Currently 90 genetic variants have been associated with increased risk of PD, but the significance of each of these variants is still unknown. There are no standard genetic testing panels for PD.[73]

Evidence-Based Interventions

There exists no treatment to prevent, cease, or reverse the degeneration of neurons in the *substantia nigra* among people with PD. All current treatments are individually targeted to improve motor and nonmotor symptoms. The mainstays of therapy for early PD are medications and exercise. The primary medications are dopamine replacement (i.e., levodopa) and medications that augment the dopamine/catecholamine pathways.[64] Unfortunately, over time these therapies become less effective, and among some people with PD, long-term therapy with dopamine agonists can be associated with emergence of dyskinesias or adverse psychiatric effects.[74] Since 2002, deep brain (basal ganglia) stimulation has been approved for patients with advanced motor symptoms of PD.[64]

Other movement disorders may present with parkinsonism but have different and distinct clinical trajectories. A specific diagnosis, even if treatment is unavailable, is independently therapeutic for patients and their families. Like other neurodegenerative diseases that present in later life, comorbid hypertension and vascular and metabolic disease can affect the brain and unmask or exacerbate the symptoms of the co-occurring PD. Adequate treatment of these conditions through medication or lifestyle interventions should not be neglected.[75]

Moving Forward

Further studies of the genetic–environmental interactions in PD may identify opportunities for prevention of PD in specific subpopulations of people at heightened risk and perhaps provide opportunities for disease-modifying therapy. Genetic screening of patients with Parkinson's disease and development of clear guidelines to interpret results and counsel patients may emerge as personalized medicine is implemented, at least in high-income countries.[73]

ALZHEIMER'S DISEASE AND RELATED DEMENTIAS

Dementia is a clinical diagnosis of progressive cognitive decline that leads to loss of independent function for an individual. Alzheimer's disease (AD) is the most common specific type of dementia, accounting for about 60% to 80% of dementia cases in adults. Other types of dementia include frontotemporal dementia, dementia with Lewy bodies, and vascular dementia.[76]

Significance

The global prevalence of dementia, which is already high, is expected to rise over the next few decades as the population ages. The costs and economic impact of dementia are very high. During 2020 in the United States, the combined medical and caregiving costs for persons with Alzheimer's dementia was over $500 billion.[77] Beyond this economic toll, caregivers for patients with dementia—often spouses or close family members—experience high rates of poor mental health.[78] Figure 20-2 lists the major Alzheimer's disease causes, consequences, and high-risk groups.

Pathophysiology

Dementia is a syndrome of progressive loss of multiple cognitive domains resulting from neuron loss or impaired neuron function, usually following a particular pattern depending on dementia type. While pathology of each of these types of dementia is known, the pathophysiologic mechanisms for each dementia type are largely unknown, but with

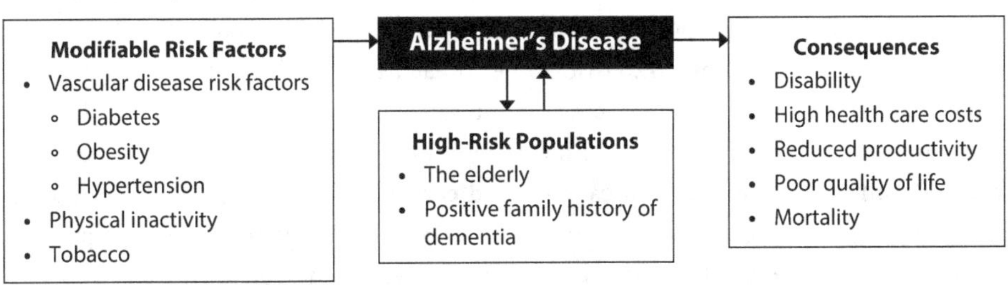

Note: For further information about high-risk populations for Alzheimer's disease, visit: http://www.alz.org.

Figure 20-2. Alzheimer's Disease: Causes, Consequences, and High-Risk Populations

several emerging hypotheses. Autopsy studies increasingly find overlapping pathologies though the patient carried only one clinical diagnosis.[78,79]

The pathological hallmark of AD is amyloid β plaques and *tau* neurofibrillary tangles. Cognitive symptoms correlate more strongly with degree of neurofibrillary pathology than with amyloid β pathology.[80] It is important to note that AD has a 15- to 30-year prodromal phase, which complicates prevention, early intervention, and treatment. Dominant hypotheses of triggers for this disease process are neuro-inflammation, vascular damage, aging, and dysfunction in the glymphatic system.[81] There is debate in the field about whether amyloid β aggregate formation itself drives the pathophysiology. Many individuals have AD pathology postmortem but without cognitive deficits during life,[78] raising the possibility of a major yet undiscovered mechanism and therefore additional modifiable risk factors.

In dementia with Lewy bodies, alpha synuclein protein aggregates are the dominant pathology. This is also seen in Parkinson's disease and other "alpha synucleinopathies." As in AD, inflammation is one hypothesized disease trigger, but research on this dementia type is less robust.[79] Dementia accompanies Parkinson's disease in about 25% to 30% of patients. Frontotemporal dementia (FTD) has multiple phenotypes and pathologic characteristics. The behavioral variant FTD has overlapping pathology with amyotrophic lateral sclerosis with TDP-43 aggregate deposition. FTD can also occur independently.[82]

Vascular cognitive impairment exhibits heterogeneity in clinical presentations and in pathology. As such, there are no unifying diagnostic criteria. Several cohort studies show co-occurrence of vascular pathology and primary neurodegenerative disease, such as AD. Vascular insult likely has a synergistic or threshold effect in terms of hastening onset of clinical dementia symptoms in these patients. Vascular insult alone can also lead to dementia symptoms.[75]

Descriptive Epidemiology

In 2019 alone, approximately 50 million people were living with dementia worldwide, and this number is projected to triple by 2050.[78] In the United States, approximately 6 million people are living with dementia. In high-income countries multiple studies have reported a declining incidence of dementia when comparing birth cohorts.[77,78]

The proportion of dementia attributable to each type of dementia varies between studies, likely because of different case definitions and whether postmortem pathology was considered. Typically, AD is the most common type (up to 80%), and other types each account for 5% to 8% of cases. As stated earlier, autopsy studies frequently show co-occurring pathologies. Vascular disease is a contributing pathology or the primary causal pathology in over 50% of dementia cases.[75] Therefore, targeting the risk factors for vascular disease offers potential for reducing the burden of dementia, including AD and other dementing illnesses, not just vascular dementia.

The incidence of AD increases from 2 per 1,000 persons in the 65 to 74 age group to 37 per 1,000 in the 85 and over age group. AD has a higher incidence in Black and Hispanic/Latino populations relative to Whites in the United States, and AD is twice as prevalent in women as in men.[80] Dementia with Lewy bodies and frontotemporal dementia are much less common.

Causes

While dementia has no single cause, there is a growing list of modifiable risk factors and associated genes.[78,81]

Modifiable Risk Factors

Experts now recognize 12 modifiable risk factors for dementia, and these factors begin to exert increase in risk during early and middle adulthood. These factors and their respective relative risks are low educational attainment (relative risk [RR] 1.6), hypertension (RR 1.6), hearing impairment (RR 1.9), smoking (RR 1.6), obesity (RR 1.6), depression (RR 1.9), physical inactivity (RR 1.4), diabetes (RR 1.5), low social contact (RR 1.6), excessive alcohol consumption (RR 1.2), traumatic brain injury (RR 1.8), and air pollution (RR 1.1). Given the high prevalence of each of these exposures, together they account for 40% of dementia cases worldwide.[78] Inadequate and poor-quality sleep during midlife is emerging as another highly prevalent and modifiable risk factor. Adults who consistently sleep six hours or less per night have a 30% to 40% greater risk of dementia compared with adults who get seven or more hours.[83] The issue of whether ingested aluminum might play a causal role in Alzheimer's disease remains unsettled, as some authors continue to argue that aluminum seems to play a role in amyloid aggregation and the potential pathogenic mechanisms of Alzheimer's disease (Figure 20-2).[84]

Genetics

Several well-known genetic variants are associated with an elevated risk of AD. The apolipoprotein E epsilon 4 allele is strongly associated with late-onset Alzheimer's disease, both for heterozygotes and homozygotes of this allele. Mutations in the amyloid β precursor protein (APP), presenilin 1 (PSEN1), and presenilin 2 (PSEN2) genes are associated with early onset AD. Using genome-wide association studies, researchers have identified other genetic variants associated with either increased or decreased risk of AD. With identification of rare mutations, a polygenic risk score for AD could be calculated, but a test like this is not yet available for clinical practice.[80,81] Several genetic mutations are associated with frontotemporal dementia, and there is overlap with other neurodegenerative diseases. For the behavioral variant of FTD, 15% to 20% of cases are monogenic, autosomal dominant inherited. Referral for genetic counseling is often helpful to family members of patients with FTD.[85]

Evidence-Based Interventions

There are no disease-modifying or -reversing therapies yet available for any type of dementia. Primary and secondary prevention efforts have modest impact, and yet some policies are not supportive of effective prevention strategies. Therapies slow or slightly mute the progressive symptoms of dementing illnesses.

Regular screening for hearing loss in high-risk occupations is imperative, as hearing aids reduce the risk of dementia for individuals with hearing loss. Medicare does not cover hearing aids—a policy gap that if closed could reduce or delay the onset of dementia.[78] Diagnosing and controlling hypertension in early and middle adulthood will reduce the burden of dementia, especially in countries like the United States, where over 40% of adults have hypertension. Screening for and treating common sleep disorders like obstructive sleep apnea and insomnia have the potential to prevent or delay the development of dementia.[83] Several studies have reported an association between reduced air pollution and slower cognitive decline or lower risk of dementia,[86] providing more incentives for policies to reduce air pollution.

Several pharmacologic therapies for symptoms related to dementia, including acetylcholinesterase inhibitors and N-methyl-D-aspartate receptor antagonists, have been introduced in high-income countries. Treatment of mood and behavioral symptoms may improve quality of life among people with all types of dementia. Socialization, exercise, and physical and occupational therapies are also helpful.[81] Advanced care planning is an essential component of dementia care,[78] and insurance coverage for this type of counseling has become mandatory in the United States following passage of the Affordable Care Act.

In 2021 the US Food and Drug Administration (FDA) provisionally approved aducanumab, a recombinant human IgG1 monoclonal antibody, for the treatment of patients with symptomatic Alzheimer's disease. This innovative medication promotes the clearance of amyloid β aggregates (plaques) from the brain and is hypothesized to stop or reverse progression of Alzheimer's dementia, but studies of aducanumab did not demonstrate consistent clinical benefit.[87] Unresolved safety concerns and questionable cost-effectiveness led a Centers for Medicare and Medicaid Services decision that Medicare would not cover aducanumab outside of a randomized controlled trial setting.

Moving Forward

Continued research into the modifiable risk factors for dementia, with attention to social and structural determinants of health, as well as the dissemination and implementation of research for interventions that address modifiable risk factors, should be prioritized. Continued investigation into the specific pathophysiology of dementia, along with other neurodegenerative diseases, is essential for the development of disease-modifying therapies. Effective policies that address cost and access of disease-modifying drugs must also be prioritized to meet this great challenge of dementia in the world's aging population.

CEREBRAL PALSY

Cerebral palsy (CP) describes a broad category of nonprogressive motor impairment syndromes attributable to abnormalities of brain structure or function with onset during early stages of brain development; impairments often change with developmental stage.[34,88] The CP syndromes each have different underlying neuroanatomical correlates and/or neuropathology.[89] Most people with cerebral palsy have *spasticity*, or significant resistance to passive movement, that becomes functionally worse as the velocity of movement increases. The spasticity alone can be limiting or disabling regardless of weakness, but typically individuals have both spasticity and muscle weakness.

In high-income countries 18% to 45% of children with cerebral palsy have *spastic diplegia*, with *diplegia* referring to weakness of all four limbs—the legs being more severely affected than the arms. People with spastic diplegia typically have some trunk weakness and struggle with balance, which when combined with spasticity place them at increased risk of falls and injuries. Infants with spastic diplegia often have normal or reduced muscle tone (resistance to passive movement) for the first few weeks or months of life and then develop obvious spasticity by the end of the first year.[90] Spastic diplegia is a clinical diagnosis but often is associated with brain magnetic resonance imaging (MRI) abnormalities in the "watershed" region between the distribution of the anterior cerebral artery and the middle cerebral artery, or periventricular leukomalacia.[91]

Spastic hemiplegic CP occurs in about a third of children with cerebral palsy and is characterized by more substantial hand and arm weakness than leg weakness contralateral to the side of the brain lesion. Spastic hemiplegic CP is often the result of an underlying intraventricular hemorrhage or the result of a stroke that occurred during intrauterine life or very early in the neonatal period.[92] Strokes early in life among children with sickle cell disease can present with deficits of hemiparesis, especially common in communities of African ancestry.[93]

Spastic quadriplegic CP accounts for about 10% to 30% of cases of cerebral palsy in high-income countries and is associated with severe impairment of both the arms and the legs, where the legs are typically more severely affected. *Double hemiplegia* refers to less common cases of quadriplegia in which the arms are bilaterally more severely affected than their legs. Brain malformations and hypoxic-ischemic encephalopathy are important causes of spastic quadriplegia cerebral palsy.[94]

CP is often associated with intellectual disability. The frequency of associated intellectual disability and the severity of the intellectual disability is typically less with the types of cerebral palsy that involve smaller areas of cortical abnormality (e.g., spastic diplegia) and almost uniformly present and severe among those whose cerebral palsy reflects widespread cortical dysfunction or damage (e.g., spastic quadriplegia). Coexisting morbidities, including feeding problems, visual impairment, and epilepsy, often exacerbate the level of disability, complicate the medical management, and impair the community participation of people with CP.[88,94]

There are racial and socioeconomic disparities associated with cerebral palsy, with Black children about 29% more likely to have CP and Asian children 20% less likely to have CP compared with other populations. However, when controlled for birth weight, there is no reported difference.[95] The risk of spastic CP is 50% higher for Black versus White children—a comparison that remains after adjusting for socioeconomic status. For socioeconomic status, low versus high socioeconomic status was associated with a 67% increased risk of CP.[96]

Significance

CP is associated with significant morbidity, including with epilepsy and status epilepticus, feeding and swallowing difficulty with associated aspiration pneumonias, and severe orthopedic problems often requiring multiple surgeries.[92] In many countries, having a child with cerebral palsy has a negative impact on the entire family's economic well-being because of the increased care needs and is associated with high rates of divorce and other family stressors. Long-term disability, particularly with limited mobility, can have a substantial impact on family dynamic. However, the Danish system for family support has successfully kept parents working and living together with their affected child.[97]

Descriptive Epidemiology

The prevalence of CP among school-aged children has ranged from about 2 to 4 per 1,000, with the majority of studies reporting a prevalence of about 2 to 3 per 1,000. Boys are more likely to have CP than girls, with a sex ratio of 1.1:1 to 1.5:1.[92] Cerebral palsy incidence is measured approximately 2.08 per 1,000 live births, but within the group of children born with a body weight below 1,500 grams, the frequency of CP is 70 times higher when compared with children with a body weight over 2,500 grams at birth.[98]

The relationship between race and the risk of CP is complex. Studies in metropolitan Atlanta have demonstrated that Black children had lower prevalence rates of cerebral palsy than did White children if their birthweight was less than 2,500 grams, but higher rates if their birthweight was 2,500 grams or more. Noting this, it is most likely that the increased risk of CP in Black children is attributable to their higher risk of a low birthweight.[95]

Causes

Prematurity is the most common risk factor for CP. A bimodal distribution of birthweight among children with CP has been reported—one peak at about 1,000 grams, and a second peak at about 3,000 grams. About one-fourth of children with CP were born weighing less than 1,500 grams, compared with about 1% of the general population; about half of children with CP were born weighing less than 2,500 grams, compared with about 5% of the general population. Children from multiple births have a high risk of CP, primarily because of the increased risk of prematurity in multiple births. Death of a co-twin in utero is also a significant risk factor for CP. Children with CP also have higher rates of birth defects than do children in the general population.[92,99]

Acute chorioamnionitis and funisitis are significant risk factors for CP.[100–102] Zika virus infection during pregnancy often results in brain damage associated with microcephaly, CP, and intellectual disability.[103] Among infants with clinical findings that are consistent with congenital Zika, 54% had epilepsy and 100% had motor abnormalities.[104] At two-year follow-up, there was significant impairment in children with congenital Zika and CP.[105]

Evidence-Based Interventions

The primary prevention for CP largely depends on efforts to prevent prematurity,[94] but a few other opportunities for prevention exist. Magnesium sulfate given before preterm birth has been shown to offer neuroprotection to the fetus and seems to be a factor in reducing the rates of prematurity-associated CP.[106,107] A Cochrane Collaboration analysis suggested that treating 63 at-risk women would prevent one baby from having CP (95% confidence interval [CI], 43–87).[108] A report suggested that, among very premature infants (>26 weeks gestational age), antenatal administration of magnesium sulfate may increase the risk of necrotizing enterocolitis and death,[109] but other studies have shown no relationship between antenatal magnesium sulfate and necrotizing enterocolitis.[110]

About 5% of CP is preventable after neonatal encephalopathy with neonatal hypothermia treatment.[111] Placental inflammatory villitis is associated with poor neurological outcomes among infants who had hypoxic–ischemic encephalopathy and who underwent hypothermia therapy.[112]

People with CP benefit from improved nutrition and may benefit from physical therapy. People with CP often have malnutrition associated with swallowing and chewing dysfunction. Individuals with CP often require more feeding time in general, which has been estimated at more than three hours a day. Interventions such as gastrostomy tubes are effective in improving nutrition among these children with CP.[1] CP and epilepsy frequently coexist; effective treatment of epilepsy frequently improves quality of life and reduces the risk of premature death among children with CP and epilepsy.

Moving Forward

Antenatal magnesium sulfate, while currently recommended in guidelines by major obstetric societies, is an important ongoing area of research. The prevention, early diagnosis, and treatment of chorioamnionitis and funisitis will also remain an important area of investigation. In addition, the development of a Zika virus vaccine is a global health priority.

AUTISM SPECTRUM DISORDERS

Autism spectrum disorders (ASD) are a group of disorders of the developing brain that tend to have the following characteristics: social impairments manifested by difficulty interacting and communicating, repetitive and stereotypic behaviors, and a limited repertoire of interests or activities. These manifestations of ASD may be recognized during the first two years of life. ASD is an umbrella-like diagnostic category that subsumes a heterogeneous group of developing brain disorders, or neurodevelopmental disorders, that includes the clinical syndromes previously classified as autistic disorder, Asperger's syndrome, and Pervasive Developmental Disorder–Not Otherwise Specified (PDD-NOS). People with autistic disorder have abnormalities of language, severe impairment of reciprocal social behavior, and severely restricted behaviors and interests. Some people with an ASD, who were previously classified as having Asperger's syndrome, have a relative preservation of cognitive, language, and communication skills, but with abnormalities of reciprocal social behavior.[34] The ASD phenotype and concomitant extent of disability vary, but approximately 30% of individuals with ASD are nonverbal and between one-third and two-thirds also have an intellectual disability.[114]

The connection between ASD prevalence and socioeconomic status remains unclear, though initial studies showed an increased prevalence of ASD in wealthy populations,[115] likely a result of referral bias and enhanced access to diagnostic services and to other structural advantages of the wealthy.[116] ASD has likely been underdiagnosed in low-income populations. A diagnostic delay of ASD in low-income families of about one year compared with higher-income families has been reported.[96]

Since 2018, there has been an increase in diagnoses of ASD among non-Hispanic Black populations, surpassing the number of individuals diagnosed in White populations.[117] Although statistically significant racial differences in incidence have not yet been established, it is important to analyze further how race/ethnicity affects ASD, as with other neurological disorders.

Significance

Whereas ASD has a significant economic impact in high-income countries, the economic costs of ASD are not well characterized in low- and middle-income countries. In 2015, care for individuals with autism spectrum disorders cost approximately $268 billion, more than the cost of stroke and hypertension combined,[118] and yet this may be an underestimate of the true cost of ASD to society. The United Nations estimated in 2015 that about 80% of individuals with ASD are underemployed or unemployed, with as many as 50% to 75% being unemployed. ASD also affects the economic activity of families. In Australia loss of productivity for parents of children with ASD was estimated to make up 89% of the total family cost of ASD. Substantial impacts have also been highlighted in the United States and the United Kingdom.[119]

Through young adulthood, the mortality risk among people with ASDs is twofold higher than that of the general population, with the highest ASD-associated mortality risk among those with epilepsy or intellectual disability comorbidities.[120] Suicide has been shown to be a large contributor to premature death in individuals with ASD.[121] ASD is responsible for 4.31 million global DALYs in 2019.[122] Attention-deficit/hyperactivity disorder (ADHD), anxiety, depression, and epilepsy are common comorbid conditions among people with ASD and contribute to the DALYs.[123] The connection between ASD and depression is particularly important. Recent studies show a lifetime depression diagnosis of up to 40.2% in populations with ASD—four times higher than the rate of depression within the general population.[124] ASD-associated comorbid conditions also include learning disabilities, migraine, sleep disorders, and gastrointestinal disorders,[125] which further contribute to health care costs.

Pathophysiology

Research has conclusively demonstrated that ASDs are the manifestation of widespread dysfunction of neural networks involving the interrelationships of language and the social and emotional functions of the cerebral cortex.[34,126]

Descriptive Epidemiology

The prevalence of ASDs in the United States has been estimated at 1 in 59, or about 1.7% of the population,[127] with the prevalence estimated at about 1.5% of individuals in developed countries worldwide.[119] All population-based studies have documented a significantly higher prevalence among boys than among girls, with reported ratios ranging from 2:1 to 5:1, with a more recent estimate of 3:1.[128] It seems as if females are less likely to be diagnosed even if they meet the diagnostic criteria. It is also possible that ASD manifests differently in females because of differences in the female brain.[129]

There is debate as to whether the prevalence of ASD has increased over the past 20 years, given changes in case definitions and societal beliefs regarding the origins of behavioral abnormalities, as well as growth in special education programs for children with ASDs from earlier times when such programs were more limited or simply nonexistent.[34,126] In the most comprehensive ASD prevalence studies from the United States, which reported the highest ASD prevalence rates, both health and educational records were abstracted.[114] Some authors have suggested that some of the increased prevalence is attributable to diagnostic substitution related to educational services.[130] Regardless, it is now clear that the ASD prevalence among adults, at least in the United Kingdom, is similar to the prevalence among children reported from the United States.[131]

Causes

Infants and young children who are later diagnosed with ASD may appear normal for the first few months of life, but almost all with ASD are predestined to have ASD from before birth, as determined by their genetic predisposition. ASD is highly heritable, though the mechanism is still mostly unknown because of the complexity of the interactions.[34,123,126] Twin studies have demonstrated evidence of the strong genetic component for autism, with estimated heritability ranging from 40% to 90%.[132] More than 100 genes have been identified to be associated with ASD.[133,134] Likewise, known genetic disorders such as fragile X syndrome, tuberous sclerosis, untreated phenylketonuria, Down syndrome, and neurofibromatosis all have high rates of coexisting autism.[135]

Some parents who witness their children developmentally regress during the first two years of life, when vaccines are administered, have blamed vaccines for their child's ASD. Multiple studies from many countries have now reported no causal relationship between autism and vaccines. Yet, concerns remain for some parents who find it difficult to believe that they witnessed a temporal relationship that was genetically driven and not caused by exposure to vaccines.[136–138] Andrew Wakefield's now discredited 1998 study that hypothesized a relationship between the measles, mumps, and rubella (MMR) vaccine and autism was retracted by *The Lancet*.[139] Wakefield was sanctioned for "dishonestly and irresponsibly" conducting his research, in which study participants were referred to Wakefield by plaintiffs' lawyers, the published data were falsified, and Wakefield falsely claimed that the studies were approved by a university ethics committee.[140–142] These false claims still have severe consequences, most recently in the conversation about COVID-19 vaccination.[143]

Gene–environment interactions are important areas of ASD research.[135,144] Some risk factors for ASD have been identified as advanced parental age, birth trauma (particularly hypoxia),[145] maternal obesity, and diabetes mellitus. Other environmental factors can contribute, though no clear causal relationship has been established.[123] A variety of risk factors currently being investigated include various hormonal factors, immune mechanisms, and potential environmental toxins.[34,146]

Evidence-Based Interventions

There are no proven ways to prevent or cure autism spectrum disorders. However, identifying children with signs and symptoms of language delays or regression and social impairment early and enrolling them in early intervention programs before the age of 3 is associated with improved developmental outcomes in some children. Therefore, community programs aimed at early diagnosis and intervention are currently emphasized.[147,148] There is now evidence that parent-mediated interventions among high-risk infants could reduce the risk of autism[149]; more research is needed to reproduce and further define these potentially effective parenting interventions.

Moving Forward

In addition to more genetic and gene–environment interaction research, further implementation on potential interventions such as parent-mediated interventions of high-risk infants is especially important. Research on the role of potentially modifiable risk factors such as maternal diabetes and parental age is likewise important.

AMYOTROPHIC LATERAL SCLEROSIS AND MOTOR NEURON DISEASE

Amyotrophic lateral sclerosis (ALS), also known as Lou Gehrig's disease, is the most common motor neuron disease worldwide, with onset in adulthood of relentlessly progressive muscle weakness leading to death from respiratory failure and related complications, typically within three to five years of symptom onset.[150] A degenerative disease, ALS is caused by the selective death of the upper and lower motor neurons in the spinal cord, brain stem, and brain. About two-thirds of cases start with limb weakness, and about one-third start with dysarthria or dysphagia. Non-motor symptoms include impaired executive function, behavioral abnormalities, and frontotemporal dementia occurring in 15% to 20% of ALS patients.[82] Progressive bulbar palsy, primary lateral sclerosis, and progressive muscle atrophy are phenotypic variants of degenerative motor neuron disease. These variants, which are rare and have different clinical courses, are not discussed here but are mentioned for completeness and so that the public health practitioner is aware of them and can ensure patients are referred to specialist care. For infants, children, and adolescents, spinal muscular atrophy (SMA) is the most common motor neuron disease and is inherited in an autosomal-recessive manner.[151]

Significance

ALS is rare, with global incidence of about 1 to 3 per 100,000 person-years. The mean age of onset of ALS is 55 years. Thus, ALS attacks adults during the peak of their working lives, and the consequent economic and psychosocial burden for affected families and local communities is significant.[82,150]

Pathophysiology

Discovery of various genes causing ALS has spurred hypotheses for the pathophysiologic mechanisms driving ALS. Various abnormal protein aggregates are seen in the damaged neurons as well as proliferation of glial cells and inflammatory cells. The most common protein aggregate is the TAR DNA-binding protein 43 (TDP-43); however, different protein aggregates are seen in specific ALS genetic subtypes. The mechanism by which these misfolded proteins ultimately cause cell death is likely multifactorial. The three dominant hypotheses are disrupted protein folding, dysfunctional RNA trafficking, and impaired cytoskeletal dynamics leading to energy failure. It remains unclear why these disrupted processes selectively affect motor neurons in ALS.[82]

Descriptive Epidemiology

ALS is rare, and population-based studies rely on patient registries maintained by countries or regions, like the European ALS Epidemiology Consortium. A recent meta-analysis of epidemiologic studies estimates the global incidence of ALS to be 2.2 per 100,000 person-years and prevalence to be 4 to 6 per 100,000 persons. These studies are limited by variable case definitions and differential access to neurologic care. Overall, ALS appears to be more common in Europe and North America versus Asia and Latin America[82,152] though notably, in the mid-20th century, epidemics of ALS were reported in Guam, New Guinea, and the Kii Peninsula in the Western Pacific. These case clusters were thought to be the result of a toxin from a nut in the cycad tree. The incidence rates of ALS in these regions have now returned to less than 1 in 100,000.[153] In the United States the overall incidence and prevalence is 1.86 and 5.2 per 100,000, respectively. ALS has a higher prevalence in men (6.4) versus women (4.0), in White (5.4) populations versus Black (2.3), and in the Midwest (5.5) versus other regions of the United States.[154] Spinal muscular atrophy has a birth prevalence of approximately 8 to10 cases per 100,000 live births.[151] A genetic screening test for spinal muscular atrophy is available and now part of standard newborn screening in many US states.

Causes

The exact cause of ALS is unknown, and the current working hypothesis is that the disease is an interplay between complex genetic and environmental factors.[82] Classically, ALS is parsed into "familial" and "sporadic" disease, though this may be an oversimplification resulting from incomplete penetrance and genetic pleiotropy. Currently, about 10% of ALS cases have a positive family history of the disease.[155]

Genetic

Since 1990, the number of ALS genes identified has increased rapidly, and now at least 30 genes are associated with an increased risk of ALS. In familial ALS, mutations in the following four genes are most frequent: C9orf72, TARDBP, SOD1 and FUS.[82,155] These mutations are also seen in sporadic ALS. Genome-wide association studies observe rare variants more frequently in sporadic ALS.[155]

Toxic/Environmental

Even with an expanding list of susceptibility genes, these do not yet account for all ALS cases. Experts postulate an environmental or toxic factor at play in the pathogenesis. Unfortunately, as ALS is a rare disease with a poor prognosis, studies to identify an exposure are subject to bias and remain inconclusive.[82] As with other neurodegenerative diseases, it is also possible that the disease process could start decades prior to symptoms, and this also limits identification. Some studies have reported increased risk of ALS with exposure to heavy metals (e.g., lead, mercury, manganese) and pesticides, but negative reports have also been published. Some studies observe higher-risk occupations include military service, welding, and jobs with high exposure to electromagnetic radiation. Finally, head trauma may be a risk factor, as studies of chronic traumatic encephalopathy find overlapping pathologic features with ALS.[82]

Evidence-Based Interventions

No treatments are available to reverse or stop the neurodegenerative process of ALS. There are, however, two FDA-approved medications for ALS: riluzole and edaravone. These medications prolong survival by about two or three months. Pulmonary hygiene and mechanical ventilation (both invasive and noninvasive) confer about a seven-month survival benefit by preventing hypoxia and pneumonia.[156] Maintaining adequate nutrition and preventing aspiration with gastric feeding is also important. Early involvement of palliative care to facilitate goals of care conversations, advance directive planning, and symptom management is important for quality of life and to maintain patient autonomy.[150]

In 2016 FDA approved nusinersen (Spinraza) for the treatment of spinal muscular atrophy. This is an antisense oligonucleotide that led to improvement in motor, electrophysiologic tests and survival in 40% to 50% of children receiving the infusions.[151] State-based newborn screening programs that include spinal muscular atrophy provide a mechanism for its early diagnosis and treatment.

Moving Forward

As with other progressive neurodegenerative diseases, understanding the biology and pathophysiology of ALS is critical to identify opportunities for prevention and improve therapeutic targets. Internal environmental risk factors (i.e., the gut microbiome) and their association with ALS is an area of active research. Drugs that use antisense oligonucleotide technology (similar to nusinersen) and viruses to achieve wide distribution in the central nervous system are in preclinical trials.[82] Although SMA is rare, the cumulative effect of growing numbers of infants and children identified with SMA via newborn screening and taking expensive drugs like nusinersen long term will have an impact on health care budgets. Policies that reduce the costs of these medications will become more essential over time.

MULTIPLE SCLEROSIS AND OTHER INFLAMMATORY DISEASES OF THE CENTRAL NERVOUS SYSTEM

Multiple sclerosis (MS) is the best-known inflammatory disorder of the central nervous system (CNS). In the last 15 years, other CNS inflammatory diseases with distinct pathology and epidemiology have been identified. In this section, we discuss MS, neuromyelitis optica spectrum disorders (NMOSDs), and acute disseminated encephalomyelitis (ADEM) and briefly mention "MS mimics" for completeness and to raise awareness for public health surveillance.

Public Health Significance

In 2010, estimated DALYs totaled 1.1 million for MS.[1] Most recent population studies estimate that over 700,000 people live with MS in the United States alone.[157] Population studies of NMOSD and other inflammatory disorders are emerging. We predict increased recognition of the morbidity conferred by these disorders in the coming years.

Pathophysiology

In both MS and NMOSD, acute inflammation in the CNS causes damage to the myelin that coats the nerve axon and leads to dysfunction of the neuron. Symptoms depend on where in the CNS the demyelination occurs. There are characteristic susceptible anatomic locations for MS, NMOSD, and other CNS inflammatory diseases.[158] Most individuals with MS and NMOSD have relapsing–remitting courses where symptoms improve to some degree after each exacerbation. However, radiographic studies show permanent scarring from these events, and pathologic studies show ongoing, evolving inflammation even in the absence of clinical symptoms.[159]

MS is an immune-mediated disease thought to be a reaction to an antigen in the CNS, which is classically an immune-privileged site because of the blood–brain barrier. The exact trigger of the auto-reaction to myelin is unknown and is an area of active investigation. Innate immune cells—macrophages and CD8+ T cells—are present in early stages, but the inflammatory response evolves over time. There is no specific blood or cerebral spinal fluid marker to diagnose MS. Diagnosis is made by clinical history, radiographic findings, and if needed, lumbar puncture.[158,159]

Unlike in cases of MS, there is a putative antibody causing most cases of NMOSD. Antibodies against aquaporin-4 channel (AQP-4), which is a receptor on the astrocyte foot processes, cause "seropositive" NMOSD. These antibodies can be associated with systemic autoimmune disease, like systemic lupus erythematosus, or can be paraneoplastic, though this is rare. About 25% of "seronegative" NMOSD is caused by antibodies against myelin oligodendrocyte glycoprotein (MOG). This is called MOG antibody disease and appears to have a slightly different epidemiology.[160] NMOSD is a relapsing disease, its attacks usually more severe than in MS and the recoveries less complete.

Usually ADEM has a monophasic course followed by complete recovery, but some patients can go on to develop MS or NMOSD. ADEM is typically seen in children and usually follows an infection or vaccination. Specific antibodies for the monophasic syndrome have not been identified.[160]

Descriptive Epidemiology

Overall, these diseases are rare. Large epidemiologic studies have been conducted for MS and, to a lesser extent, NMOSD. Important for the public health practitioner is that MS and NMOSD have characteristic geographic distributions.

Multiple Sclerosis

The prevalence of multiple sclerosis varies by geographic region, following a gradient from low to high prevalence with increasing distance from the equator. With more population migration, there is some evidence that this gradient is disappearing within the United States. A 2017 population-based epidemiologic study in the United States estimated that the 2010 prevalence of MS was about 309 per 100,000.[157] MS is more common in women than men at nearly a 3:1 ratio.[69,157] In addition, MS is generally more common in White populations than Black, but this difference is attenuating. The age group with the highest incidence of MS is 25 to 35 years, but with improving treatments, the highest age-specific prevalence is 55 to 64 years.[69,157]

Neuromyelitis Optica Spectrum Disorders

Overall, the global prevalence of NMOSD is about 4 to 5 per 100,000, and it is more common in Black populations and in women. The prevalence of NMOSD in Blacks is 10 per 100,000 persons, and is 5 to 10 times higher in women when compared with men.[160] NMOSD can occur any time during the life span. Contrary to multiple sclerosis, NMOSDs are more common in countries close to the equator.

Other Neuroinflammatory Disorders

As other neuroinflammatory disorders are rare diseases and case definitions can vary as pathophysiology research progresses, epidemiologic studies are limited. A recent study of pediatric demyelinating disease using Korean health insurance data found that demyelinating diseases, particularly ADEM, are more commonly diagnosed in the summer, consistent with the infectious trigger hypothesis.[161]

Causes

Multiple Sclerosis

As for ALS, the cause of MS is unknown. It is currently thought to be a complex interaction between genetic susceptibility and environmental exposures. A large cohort study recently published provided strong evidence that infection with Epstein-Barr virus (EBV) is a leading cause of multiple sclerosis.[162] MS is nonetheless rare after Epstein-Barr infection, so other environmental and genetic risk factors likely play a role. Other modifiable risk factors consistently identified by epidemiologic studies are vitamin D deficiency, high body weight in early life, and cigarette smoking, but the strength of association of these factors is not nearly as strong as that of Epstein-Barr infection.[163] Genome-wide association studies have identified over 100 gene variants associated with increased risk of MS, and most of these genes are linked to immune regulatory function.[164]

Focus on vitamin D as a protective factor for MS arose from the geographic prevalence gradient of MS (i.e., higher prevalence at higher latitudes) and a lower incidence of MS in coastal Norwegian villages whose residents have a high consumption of fatty fish rich in vitamin D compared with agricultural villages at the same latitude. Although still an active area of investigation, vitamin D does seem to have a protective effect. Compared with individuals in the lowest quintile of serum vitamin D levels, individuals in the highest quintile had a 62% lower risk of developing MS.[163]

High body weight (>95th percentile) in childhood and early adulthood (body mass index >30 kg/m^2) is associated with 1.5 to 2.5 higher risk of developing MS. Hypothesized mechanisms are lower vitamin D levels or the immunomodulatory effects of adipose tissue.[163]

Current smokers have a 1.5 greater risk of developing MS compared with nonsmokers; however, the mechanism is unknown. Hypotheses include vascular, immune system, or direct neurotoxic effects of cigarette smoke. The population-attributable risk of cigarette smoking on multiple sclerosis is 6% to 7%.[163]

Neuromyelitis Optica Spectrum Disorders

As stated earlier, a specific antibody is associated with most cases of NMOSD. Increasing evidence shows that this antibody is generated peripherally and then crosses the blood–brain barrier into the CNS. There are emerging studies for genetic and modifiable environmental risk factors. Case-control studies dominate the latter. As this is a rare disease that can cause significant disability, these studies are subject to significant bias and thus no risk factors have yet been conclusively identified.[165]

Evidence-Based Interventions

There is no screening for MS, NMOSD, or other neuroinflammatory disorders. Research regarding modifiable risk factors is most robust for MS. Public health efforts to improve nutrition, physical activity, and smoking prevention and cessation are likely to have a modest effect on decreasing MS incidence or disease severity.[163]

MS and NMOSD have no cure. Most cases of ADEM are monophasic, though this clinical syndrome is unlikely to be a unique etiologic entity.[160] For central nervous system inflammatory diseases, there is treatment for acute exacerbations, usually involving high-dose steroids, and there is chronic maintenance therapy, which involves immunosuppressive or immunomodulatory therapies.[165] For MS, the last decade has brought medical therapies for relapsing–remitting disease that have led to longer remissions and that while expensive, are considered cost-effective because of reduced disability and increased productivity.[166] For NMOSD, there are no disease-specific treatment guidelines. Acute treatment and chronic immunosuppression are extrapolated from treatments for MS and from retrospective observational studies.[165] For ADEM, acute treatment usually includes high-dose steroids or plasma exchange.[160] Guidelines regularly updated by the American Academy of Neurology are an important resource for clinicians (https://www.aan.com). The built environment and accessibility for people with motor disabilities is especially important for individuals who are disabled because of CNS inflammatory disorders.

Moving Forward

Continued population-based surveillance data and epidemiological research of modifiable risk factors, including gene–environment interaction studies with particular attention to the infectious triggers, are needed.

GUILLAIN-BARRÉ SYNDROME

Guillain-Barré syndrome (GBS) is an acute post-infectious demyelinating disease of the peripheral nervous system affecting motor and sensory motor neurons throughout the body. The onset is characterized by weakness that progresses over many hours to many days. Typically, onset of weakness is accompanied by vague uncomfortable sensory complaints, with progression from the legs and arms to the trunk and chest muscles. In some with GBS, weakness progresses to involve muscles essential for respiration, and patients require mechanical ventilation; early diagnosis and treatment may prevent progression and requirement for mechanical ventilation. GBS, the leading cause of acute paralysis in humans,[167] is an immune-mediated disease, which usually occurs 2 to 4 weeks after an infection.[168]

The rate of demyelination and associated clinical deterioration is often faster in children than among adults, with children recovering faster as well. Most people with GBS have complete or near-complete recovery of their weakness; however, short-term mortality and morbidity remain significant. Standard case definitions for GBS have improved both clinical research efforts and epidemic investigations.[169]

There is a paucity of research examining a possible relationship between GBS and race, and the estimate of the overall incidence are difficult because of the low incidence. COVID-19 infection has been linked to an increase in cases of GBS, with 15 cases per 100,000 cases of COVID-19.[170] High rates of GBS have been reported with other infections that occur in outbreaks or epidemics such as *Campylobacter*, Epstein-Barr, and Zika.

Significance

GBS has a highly variable course, with some patients requiring only short hospital stays, whereas others have prolonged periods of hospitalization followed by lengthy periods of rehabilitation. Although most people with GBS eventually fully recover neurological function, mortality rates of more than 5% have been reported, often from complications of respiratory failure or autonomic dysfunction with associated cardiac arrythmias.[171] Up to 20% of patients with GBS cannot walk within one year of symptom onset.[172] COVID-19 appears to be connected strongly with demyelinating GBS,[173] though mortality rates remain similar to those within populations without COVID infections.[170]

Pathophysiology

GBS results from an autoimmune response directed against the myelin sheath of peripheral nerves, typically triggered by a recent viral or bacterial infection, or less commonly, a noninfectious agent.[169,174,175] Antibodies created to fight the infection can cross-react with epitopes on peripheral nerves and roots and lead to demyelination.[176] Demyelination affects motor and sensory nerve function, and some patients have both bulbar involvement and autonomic dysfunction, which is associated with high rates of cardiac arrhythmias.[177,178]

Descriptive Epidemiology

The reported incidence of GBS has varied considerably, with annual incidence rates in the United States ranging from less than 0.5 to more than 2 per 100,000.[179,180] There are few estimates of GBS in low- and middle-income countries, which face additional barriers to identification and treatment, such as poor hygiene and increased exposure to infection.[181] This is an important research gap to fill.

Unlike other autoimmune disorders, GBS incidence increases by approximately 20% for every 10-year increase in age. It is also slightly higher in incidence in men than in women.[179] Some studies have also reported higher rates for Whites than for African Americans, though the relationship between race/ethnicity and incidence is not well understood.[169] Overall, GBS was responsible for 44,400 global YLDs in 2019.[182]

Causes

Infections that trigger peripheral nerve myelin–directed autoimmune responses have long been the focus of research and are thought to be the primary risk factors for GBS. Gastrointestinal and upper respiratory infections a few weeks before onset of weakness are typical and are more common among GBS cases than among controls. *Campylobacter*,[183] Epstein-Barr virus, and cytomegalovirus have received the most attention from past investigators,[184] and more recently 42 cases of Guillain-Barré syndrome occurred during a Zika virus outbreak.[185]

Concern regarding the increased risk of GBS following the swine flu vaccine in 1976 and 1977 received considerable attention. Studies of swine flu vaccine administered after 1977 have not shown any association with GBS, suggesting that there was a unique immunologic reaction to the vaccine used in 1976 and 1977 that has not occurred since that time.[186,187] There was some concern that the SARS-CoV-2 vaccination could cause a similar increase in GBS,[188,189] but COVID-19 infection is more frequently associated with GBS than is the vaccine.

Evidence-Based Interventions

The best primary prevention opportunities are the prevention of infectious triggers of GBS and the control of epidemics of agents known to be frequently associated with GBS clusters, such as *Campylobacter* and Zika. Rapid diagnosis and supportive care, including respiratory care and mechanical ventilation if needed, remain the mainstay of treatment. If the demyelinating disorder is treated early in the course of the disease, plasmapheresis or intravenous gamma globulin can shorten the course and may reduce the odds of requiring mechanical ventilation.[169] It is important that public health officials remain vigilant and respond rapidly to potential epidemics of GBS.[179]

Moving Forward

Supporting the development and maintenance of surveillance systems to detect GBS outbreaks in a timely fashion is a key public health priority. Rapid diagnosis and appropriate treatment reduce the respiratory failure and mortality associated with GBS. Therefore, guidelines at the community level to assist in rapid diagnosis and research in rapid diagnostic methods are important. Continued research on the relationship between COVID-19 and other emerging infections is a priority.

TIC DISORDERS AND TOURETTE SYNDROME

Tics are stereotypic, purposeless, and sudden movements that may be transiently suppressed. In some people tics resemble purposeful movement and yet are involuntary. Tics have been generally classified as simple and chronic. Simple tic disorders are those in which a single motor tic manifestation occurs in an individual—such as eye blinks, jaw-jutting movements, or throat clearing—without evolution of multiple different motor tic manifestations and without vocal tics. Chronic multifocal tic disorders manifest in multiple different simple and complex motor tics, often accompanied by vocal tics that are most commonly noises such as snorts or consonant sounds, as well as bursts of involuntary expletive speech (coprolalia). Simple tics often undergo spontaneous remission, especially among children, within a year of onset. Chronic multifocal tics, when in association with vocal tics, that last for greater than a year are typically lifelong in duration and are classified as Tourette syndrome (TS).[190]

Tics and TS are both associated with a reduction in quality of life. They are both comorbid with obsessive-compulsive disorder (OCD) and ADHD, with up to 60% of individuals having one or the other in addition to tics.[191] There is also serious social stigma associated with tics that can cause individuals to be depressed. Added to this is that medication used for management of tics and TS can cause depression.[192]

It was previously thought that tics and TS were limited to childhood and adolescence, but now it is clear that both can extend into adulthood. Although the maximum severity occurs around 10 to 12 years of age, approximately 10% to 20% of individuals have symptoms that extend into adulthood and some worsen with age.[193] Adult onset of tics is rare, but it occurs particularly in individuals with underlying neurodevelopmental or neuropsychiatric disorders (e.g., Down syndrome, Huntington's disease, neuroacanthocytosis), head trauma, basal ganglia stroke, HIV infection, neuroleptic and antiepileptic drug side effects, or cocaine abuse.[194] Obsessive-compulsive disorder particularly has been shown to appear up to several years following tics.[195] Some evidence also suggests that low socioeconomic status is a risk factor for tics and TS.[196]

Significance

Although most people with tics are not disabled and often are not aware that their movements are abnormal, some people with TS are significantly impaired. TS is not associated with intelligence impairment nor does it negatively affect life expectancy, but it nonetheless has an impact on quality of life.[185] This is particularly the case when tics and TS are associated with other comorbid conditions.

As mentioned briefly earlier, TS is commonly associated with OCD, as well as anxiety mood disorders and ADHD.[190,197–200] These psychiatric comorbidities often persist until adulthood, even following TS remission.[190] The impact of this is that individuals with TS, particularly when tics continue into adulthood, are at a substantially higher risk for suicide.[201]

A major challenge for both clinical and epidemiological investigations is the lack of laboratory or radiographic diagnostic tests for tic disorders or TS. Furthermore, distinguishing TS from simple tic disorders is difficult using just medical record review and self-reported data. As recently as a decade ago, a phenomenon of mass hysteria was associated with tics and symptoms of TS. As documented at a high school in Le Roy, New York, between 2011 and 2012, there was a psychiatric connection between the development of tics and local incidence. Students in Le Roy experienced an "outbreak" of tics within their female population particularly, causing great stress to families and extensive media coverage in the region. It has been hypothesized that the more people got tics, the more people thought that they too would—increasing the incidence.[202] The mechanism here isn't yet clear. More recently documented has been an increase in incidence of tics as a result of watching TS videos on TikTok.[203]

Pathophysiology

The tics and other movement abnormalities in TS are considered to be a manifestation of disinhibition within the cortico-striato-thalamo circuits of the brain. The exact cause of the abnormality manifested by tics is not known but is hypothesized to relate to an abnormality of the gamma-aminobutyric acid (GABA) system.[204] There is also a genetic component.[195] Some evidence also shows changes in dopaminergic modulation.[193]

Descriptive Epidemiology

Tic disorders are very common among children, but the published estimates range considerably according to the research method used. The prevalence of TS has been reported to be between 3 and 9 per 1,000 individuals.[195] Overall, the best estimates for the prevalence of TS, including relatively mild cases, are approximately 0.3% to 1% of the population.[205] Boys have a higher prevalence of TS than girls, with male-to-female ratios reported to be as high as 4.7:1. These estimates might not be entirely accurate if symptoms are subtle and manageable, as individuals might not think there is a problem.[206] TS seems to occur worldwide.[200]

Causes

TS has a strong familial predisposition, although parents are often diagnosed as a result of manifestations in their children, underscoring the likely underascertainment from medical record reviews.[198] Evidence of linkage to the centromeric region of chromosome 5 in a single large family with TS has been reported.[207] Within the last decade a few candidate susceptibility genes have also been reported.[208]

The association of simple tics with Group A beta-hemolytic streptococci has been reported, but this association has been questioned as a causal factor for chronic tic disorders,[209] and it has not been found to be a causal factor in exacerbations of tic and obsessive-compulsive symptoms.[210]

Evidence-Based Interventions

There are no proven methods for preventing tic disorders or TS. Management of the comorbid behavioral and learning conditions, such as ADHD, is important, and public health professionals should be aware of the mental health needs of people with TS.[190] Evidence shows that behavioral treatments can be effective, so early identification is important to maintain quality of life.[211]

Moving Forward

Future epidemiological studies of TS will need to address the potential factors (genetic and environmental) that might have an impact on the severity of these tic disorders, with an emphasis on factors that may exacerbate tics in susceptible individuals. Further research on the comorbid conditions and experiences of people with tics and TS, to improve quality of life and reduce suicide rates, is needed.

TRAUMATIC BRAIN INJURY

Traumatic brain injury (TBI) remains a clinical diagnosis; there are yet no laboratory biomarkers for clinical practice to objectively assess the severity of injury. TBIs are classified as mild (concussion), moderate, and severe.[212] Variable case definitions and applications of this classification system often make comparisons between studies complicated. Long-term effects of TBI, including multiple concussions, have emerged as an important issue for public health professionals, offering opportunities for primary prevention.

Significance

TBI is a leading cause of long-term disability and death in the United States and worldwide. The estimated total cost of TBI in the United States alone in 2000 was over $60 billion.[213] While falls leading to TBI are most common in older adults, TBI is a significant pediatric concern, especially when considering nonaccidental trauma. In the United States, the DALY burden of abusive head trauma in children aged 0 to 4 years far exceeds the DALY burden for all severe burns.[196]

Cognitive impairment as a long-term consequence of TBI, including mild TBI or concussion, has been firmly established. TBI is also an established risk factor for dementia with a dose–response association and higher risk with repeated mild concussions (see Dementia section earlier in this chapter). Chronic traumatic encephalopathy (CTE) is a neurodegenerative disease, with clinical manifestations and diagnosed postmortem, associated with repetitive concussions. Gaps remain in the understanding of the neurodegenerative process and in defining a specific predictive syndrome for CTE during life. Currently, researchers define traumatic encephalopathy syndrome (TES) as the cognitive-behavioral syndrome associated with CTE pathology. In 2014, diagnostic criteria were published for TES. These criteria were sensitive but not specific. By these criteria, a diagnosis of TES had a nocebo effect and actually worsened symptoms for patients and did not accurately predict CTE pathology. In 2019 the NINDS reconvened an expert panel to revise these criteria to be used for research purposes only.[212]

Descriptive Epidemiology

In 2016, the global incidence of TBI was estimated at 370 per 100,000 person-years. Overall, the incidence of TBI has increased over the last two decades, though this trend varies by sociodemographic index. The US incidence of TBI, which is likely underestimated, was 330 per 100,000 person-years, a rate largely unchanged from 1990 to 2016.

TBI is more frequent in older age groups; the incidence of nonfatal TBI in persons older than 75 years of age is over five times greater than for persons aged 55 to 64. Stratifying by gender, men have a consistently higher incidence of both mild and moderate-to-severe TBI compared with women, though this difference attenuates in older age groups. There were over 61,000 TBI-related deaths in the United States in 2017.[214,215]

Causes

Causes of TBI and TBI-related death vary by gender and age group. In the United States, the three leading causes of nonfatal TBIs requiring hospitalization are unintentional falls (51%), motor vehicle crashes (24%), and other unintentional injury (7.7%). For men, the three leading causes of TBI-related death are suicide (45%), unintentional falls (25%), and motor vehicle crashes (19%). For women, the leading causes are unintentional falls (49%), motor vehicle crashes (21%), and suicide (19%).[214] Alcohol and drug use are interactive risk factors for motor vehicle crashes, falls, transportation-related injuries and automobile crashes, sports or recreation injuries, and assaults.

Evidence-Based Interventions

Prevention of falls, suicide prevention—particularly among men—and motor vehicle safety are essential to prevent traumatic brain injury. Currently, the US Preventive Services Task Force has a grade B recommendation for exercise interventions for fall prevention in community-dwelling adults aged 65 and older who are at increased risk for falls and do not have osteoporosis. Other multifactorial exercise interventions have a grade C recommendation for select populations. While vitamin D supplementation is often recommended for older adults, it is no longer recommended for primary fall prevention. The National Institute of Aging also recommends exercise training as well as regular medical care to check hearing and vision and manage medications, particularly anticoagulant use (Figure 20-3).[214,216]

Among people with chronic effects of TBI, including CTE, interventions to prevent suicide and promote mental health are a public health priority. US suicide rates are increasing, reflected in the TBI surveillance data, especially among men. Among people who have survived the acute effects of TBI, the rates of suicide are six times higher in men than in women.[214] The Substance Abuse and Mental Health Services Administration maintains resources of best practices to assess and protect individuals with suicidal ideation or attempts.

In the last few decades, the reduction in motor vehicle injuries and deaths has been a major public health success, attributable to increased use of seat belts, airbags, child safety seats, motorcycle helmets, stricter laws regarding driving while intoxicated, and graduated licensing of young drivers. Consistent helmet use for cyclists and motorcyclists remains imperative.[214]

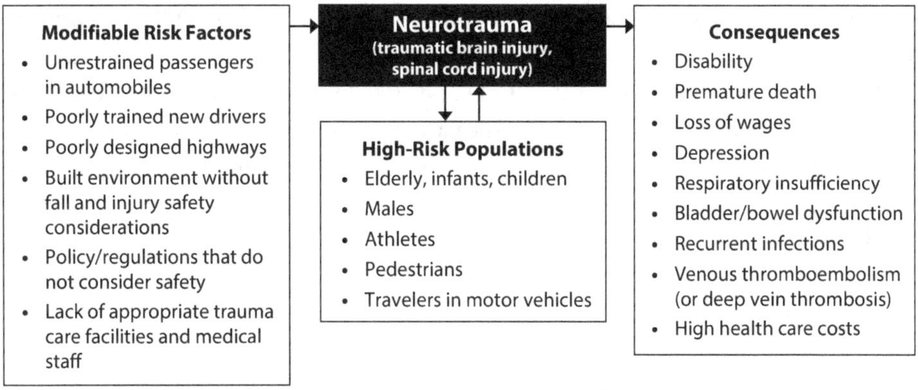

Note: For further information about high-risk populations for neurotrauma, visit http://www.biausa.org and http://www.pva.org.

Figure 20-3. Neurotrauma: Causes, Consequences, and High-Risk Populations

Moving Forward

A biomarker to diagnose and quantify the degree of TMI antemortem has been an active area of study for years. Recently, researchers demonstrated the specificity of a point-of-care test using small, noncoding RNA in the saliva of rugby athletes.[217] Prognosticating outcomes after TBI with attention to health disparities, particularly mild TBI, is also an active area of research and relevant for patient counseling and resource connection. Dedicated attention to health disparities in TBI outcomes is also necessary.[218] TES and CTE remain important areas of research.[212]

SPINAL CORD INJURY

Significance

About 17,730 Americans sustain a spinal cord injury (SCI) each year. The average lifetime health care cost for a typical 25-year-old with SCI varies by the severity and level of injury. For incomplete motor impairment, the estimated lifetime direct cost is $2 to $3 million; for complete motor impairment, the direct cost is more than $5 million. The indirect costs of SCI are much higher.[219]

Descriptive Epidemiology

The estimated annual incidence of SCI in the United States is 54 per million. Worldwide, the incidence varies from 12 to 60 per million per year. SCI incidence has a bimodal age distribution, with the first peak between ages 15 and 29 years, and a second peak at

65 years of age and older. SCI is more common in men (78% of cases) than in women, and more common in non-Hispanic White populations (60%) than Black populations (23%).[220] Prevalence is estimated at 11 to 112 per 100,000 persons. Mortality from SCI is high but has declined considerably over the past several decades. This decline is attributable to improved emergency medical services (especially emergency neurosurgical care), development of specialty centers for care, improved professional training, and lower death rates from infections and other secondary conditions.[219–221]

Causes

The three most common causes of SCI throughout the world are motor vehicle crashes, falls, and violence.[221] In the United States, 40% of injuries are from motor vehicle crashes, 32% from falls, 14% from violence, and 8% from sports.[219] As with TBI, alcohol and drug use increase the risk of SCI.[220] SCI can also occur as a result of infections, inflammatory disease, and vascular occlusions that interrupt blood flow to the spinal cord.

Evidence-Based Interventions

As with TBI, improving the built environment, promoting policies that improve safety, and injury prevention education for the community can all contribute to primary prevention of SCI. SCI outcomes immediately after the injury are better with a well-coordinated emergency medical system to access skilled medical and surgical trauma care. Emergency trauma center systems that cross state lines and national borders have decreased time to care while reducing mortality and morbidity (Figure 20-3).[222]

Opportunities for secondary prevention among people with SCIs include depression, dysautonomia, bowel/bladder dysfunction, pressure ulcers, airway management problems, secondary pulmonary conditions and pneumonia, spasticity, deep vein thrombosis, osteoporosis, and scoliosis. The University of Alabama Spinal Cord Injury Model System maintains an excellent website with resource and practice information on each of these domains (see Resources).

ATTENTION-DEFICIT/HYPERACTIVITY DISORDER

Attention-deficit/hyperactivity disorder (ADHD) is a syndrome defined by the following diagnostic criteria: onset during preschool years, inattention, impulsivity, and overactivity.[223] Over 70% of individuals with ADHD also struggle with comorbid conditions, including anxiety, conduct disorder, learning disorders, OCD, epilepsy, tic disorders, depression, bipolar disorder, and sleep disorders.[224] Individuals with ADHD are also more likely to have problems with substance abuse and to smoke cigarettes.[225,226] Males are more likely than females to be diagnosed with ADHD.[227]

Significance

ADHD is strongly associated with various behavior problems, including oppositional defiant behavior disorder and conduct disorders. Children with both ADHD and conduct disorder have higher risk for neurocognitive impairment.[228] ADHD tends to persist into adulthood and may predict serious antisocial behavior, involvement with police, and substance misuse in adolescence.[226,229]

Adolescents and young adults with ADHD have high rates of suicidal ideation and suicide attempts compared with the general population.[230] Treatment of ADHD with medication seems to reduce the risk of concurrent and subsequent depression.[231]

Pathophysiology

No single area of the brain that is damaged or dysfunctional alone results in ADHD. Rather, ADHD is the result of abnormal functioning of neural networks and connections. Neural connections between the prefrontal cortex and the striatum of the brain (the caudate nuclei and the putamen) are areas of dysfunction among people with ADHD. The frontal and prefrontal areas of the brain, as well as the more posterior regions of the brain, exhibit abnormal functioning relative to attention. Systems involving visual attention and orientation seem to be especially dysfunctional.[226] When performing cognitive tasks, people with ADHD tend to activate broader regions of the cortex as compared with people who have less difficulty focusing—probably explaining distractibility among those with ADHD.[232]

Descriptive Epidemiology

ADHD occurs in about 3% to 4% of all school-age children (95% CI). More recent numbers for 2015 to 2016 show an increase to about 10% of children within the United States being diagnosed with ADHD,[233] but global trends from 2019 show an overall prevalence of less than 2%.[234] It is difficult to determine whether this increase in diagnosis results from increased prevalence or from increased community awareness of ADHD symptoms and medication management options.

Although reported prevalence rates of ADHD among US school-age children are higher than they were 30 years ago, ADHD signs and symptoms in children were reported early in the 20th century.[235] ADHD prevalence rates now are not significantly different from those reported in the late 20th century.[226] Prevalence rates for ADHD vary by use of diagnostic criteria in different areas of the United States, with significant differences in treatment patterns from one part of the country to another. Once considered to be a disorder of childhood, ADHD is now known to occur in up to 4% of adults[226]; about half of those with ADHD diagnosed in childhood have ADHD symptoms persisting into adulthood.[236]

Causes

Attention-deficit/hyperactivity disorder is a familial disorder, and the genetics of ADHD have been explored with both twin studies and traditional family genetic studies. About 76% of ADHD is said to be attributable to inherited genetic susceptibility, similar to what has been reported in autism and in schizophrenia.[237] Most cases of ADHD are multifactorial and involve single nucleotide polymorphisms or the interaction of many different genes. However, genetic syndromes such as fragile X syndrome, tuberous sclerosis complex, 22q11 microdeletion, and Williams syndrome are associated with very high rates of ADHD.[238] Recently a synaptosomal-associated protein (SNAP-25), a presynaptic plasma membrane protein expressed specifically in neuronal cells, has been found to have several polymorphisms associated with ADHD in family and case-control studies.[239]

Evidence-Based Interventions

Primary prevention opportunities for ADHD are not established. However, given the high frequency of comorbid conditions among adolescents and adults diagnosed with ADHD as children, identification of children with ADHD also identifies those who are at higher risk of cigarette smoking, substance abuse, depression, and other mental illnesses; therefore, to reach this population public health professionals should increase their efforts to seek opportunities for focused health promotion. Consensus guidelines for diagnosis, evaluation, and treatment of ADHD have optimized outcomes. Early diagnosis and treatment can prevent school failure and improve long-term academic and social outcomes.[226]

Moving Forward

A better understanding of how the presence of these comorbid conditions can alter the diagnosis management of ADHD is important. Ongoing studies of media and technology use in childhood may reveal a possible relationship with emergence of ADHD symptoms.

CARPAL TUNNEL SYNDROME

Carpal tunnel syndrome (CTS), the most common compression neuropathy, is caused by entrapment of the median nerve at the wrist as it passes under the transverse carpal ligament, resulting in sensory changes and, in more severe cases, weakness of the muscles of the hand. The diagnosis is made from typical history and examination findings consistent with dysfunction of the median nerve distal to the wrist. Diagnosis of CTS is aided by abnormal median nerve conduction studies.[240] Of note, median nerve compression can also be found incidentally in nerve conduction studies performed for unrelated symptoms, but here only clinical CTS is reviewed.

Significance

CTS is the most expensive upper-extremity musculoskeletal disorder in the United States, with estimated annual costs exceeding $2 billion, primarily from surgical releases. The median number of work days missed is 27 for occupation-related CTS.[241]

Descriptive Epidemiology

Reporting and diagnosis of CTS in high-income countries has increased over the past few decades, possibly with the introduction of improved diagnostic techniques. In Rochester, Minnesota, the adjusted annual rates increased from 258 per 100,000 in 1981 through 1985 to 424 in 2000 through 2005. One study from Sweden reported a prevalence of about 3.8% in the general population of adults.[242] A prospective study of workers who performed hand-intensive activities found a 7.8% prevalence of CTS.[241] Variable case definitions limit comparability of large population-based studies.

Causes

Wrist trauma is strongly associated with development of CTS. Other risk factors include diabetes, obesity, hypothyroidism, pregnancy, rheumatoid arthritis, osteoarthritis in the wrist, and repetitive hand or wrist movements, which are often work-related.[243] Although CTS is common, the population-attributable fraction of these risk factors has not been reported.

Evidence-Based Interventions

Prevention of CTS by enhancing worker safety programs and training in ergonomics hazard prevention in the workplace deserves significant attention based on the prevalence and cost of CTS. Preventing and managing other risk factors like diabetes is also essential.[240] Most mild-to-moderate cases (defined both clinically and on electrophysiologic studies) can be managed nonsurgically. Hand orthoses are usually first line, though large studies do not consistently support their benefit. Corticosteroid injections may provide short-term relief, but clinical benefit is not clear. For severe cases—severe symptoms with hand muscle weakness and/or denervation—carpal tunnel release surgery may be helpful.[240,243]

Moving Forward

Studies of workplace interventions focusing on primary prevention of CTS, followed by enhanced policies aimed toward primary prevention, should be a priority.[244]

LOW BACK PAIN

The leading cause of disability globally, low back pain (LBP) is experienced by most adults at some time during their lives. LBP is an important public health concern in all countries because of the individual morbidity, rising health care costs, inequitable occupational exposures, and overall economic impact.[245]

Significance and Descriptive Epidemiology

The prevalence of low back pain is increasing, with worldwide estimated point prevalence is 15% to 30%. Symptom length can vary, and the median one-year prevalence of LBP is approximately 37%, while the lifetime prevalence is 60% to 80%.[245,246] LBP accounted for 60.1 million years lived with disability worldwide in 2015.[245] Nested analyses within cohort studies have reported that obesity and smoking are associated with increased risk of back pain with odds ratios of 1.5 and 1.3, respectively. There may be a genetic susceptibility, as studies report heritable mutations in genes involved in pain perception and signaling.[247]

Causes

Occupational exposure accounts for 30% to 40% of LBP.[248] The occupations associated with the highest risk of LBP are agricultural and forestry workers (RR 3). Service workers and manual production laborers likewise have increased risk of LBP (RR 1.5).[246] Mechanical factors such as sitting, having awkward postures, and bending and lifting have been identified as leading causes. However, several systematic reviews conclude that it is unlikely that these activities independently cause LBP.[247] LBP is a symptom with many causes, though the exact cause for a patient is usually unknown. Given that imaging studies (MRI, CT, and X-ray) have low specificity, guidelines for managing LBP consistently recommend against routine use of imaging.

Evidence-Based Interventions

Generalized primary prevention efforts have not proven effective in the general population, especially as the cause of LBP is unknown in most patients. Treatment guidelines for patients with LBP emphasize exercise, education, and psychological interventions as first-line treatment. Pharmacotherapy with nonsteroidal anti-inflammatory drugs is second line, and opioid use should be sparing. For chronic LBP, steroid joint injections and surgery are second-line treatments in select patients.[249] There is no evidence that workplace interventions (e.g., general education, lift training or assistive devices, ergonomic furniture) prevent LBP.[247,249]

There are certain acute symptoms, often termed red flag symptoms, for which the patient should urgently be referred for more extensive medical evaluation and imaging. These symptoms are thoracic back pain, weakness of the legs, loss of sensation in a "saddle distribution," loss of bowel or bladder continence, fever, and systemic symptoms (including history of cancer). While a minority of patients with these symptoms ultimately have a serious disorder, early intervention can prevent long-term morbidity.[245]

To reduce the cost of LBP, clinical decision-making tools have been effective in reducing the number of imaging studies ordered by clinicians. Public education about management and prevention of LBP has been effective in changing beliefs about pain in some countries.[249]

Moving Forward

Preventing and effectively managing the burden of LBP will require a public health approach with explicit plans for implementing and evaluating policies to reduce risk factors for LBP at the community level and in the workforce. There are some clinical system research efforts to develop an integrated, multidisciplinary treatment pathway approach for patients with LBP. Integrating occupational health practices and government disability policy in a graduated return-to-work intervention is another area of innovation.[249]

MIGRAINE AND TENSION-TYPE HEADACHE

About one-third of men and approximately one-half of women experience episodic tension-type headache. For the most affected, headaches have minimal impact on their lives; but for the small percentage of people who have evolution of chronic daily headache, the degree of impairment and even disability is often significant. An estimated 20% of women and about 5% to 10% of men experience migraine.[250] The estimates from 2019 show that migraines and tension-type headaches were responsible for 46.6 million global YLDs.[251]

Migraine prevalence in the United States is highest among Native American populations, second among Whites, and third in Black and Hispanic populations.[252] There are additional reports of race-based disparities in diagnoses and treatment of migraines and headaches within African American populations.[253]

Significance

Migraine is among the more prevalent disabling neurological disorders. Children with migraine headaches average twice as many days absent from school as children without migraines.[254] Worldwide, migraine is one of the leading causes of disability, especially among children and young adults, and yet migraine is considered a low health care priority in most countries.[255] Migraine often coexists with cardiovascular disease, psychiatric disorders, and sleep disorders, which all negatively affect quality of life.[256]

Descriptive Epidemiology

The International Headache Society diagnostic criteria for migraine have become the gold standard used by clinicians.[257] The mean global prevalence of tension-type headaches has been estimated at 42%,[258] although the practical application of headache classification schemes in the general population is difficult, as the clinical manifestations of migraine and other types of headache often overlap. Migraines affect approximately 12% of the US population, though global estimates are higher.[256] Migraine typically presents in childhood or adolescence; new onset of migraine after 40 years is very rare. Migraine prevalence is two to four times higher among women than men and is twice as high among low-income populations. Women often experience exacerbation of migraines around menopause.[259]

Causes

Risk factors for migraine headaches include a positive family history, depression, epilepsy, female sex, and low socioeconomic status.[260] Given the high frequency of maternal migraine history among people with migraine, a mitochondrial DNA pattern of inheritance has long been hypothesized. Reports have verified that two common mitochondrial DNA polymorphisms are highly associated with migraine headache and likely account for a very high proportion of familial cases of migraine.[261] Depression and stress have long been known to be important risk factors for other types of headaches.[262]

Among people with headaches, especially migraine, specific triggers that precipitate headaches are well defined and require that clinicians and patients become familiar with the triggers unique to each person affected. The most common triggers include onset of menses, dietary changes or specific foods (e.g., cheeses, chocolate, nuts), extreme fatigue, or variation in sleep patterns. Patient surveys have been developed to identify potential triggers in order to develop prevention strategies.[263] Excessive use of painkillers, including narcotics for headache, can cause rather than cure or prevent headaches.[264]

Evidence-Based Interventions

The best opportunities for improving quality of life and preventing headaches among people with migraines include sustained medical care, enhanced by a medical home, and education regarding avoiding migraine triggers. Although chronic stress is a major contributor to episodic tension-type headaches, prevention of chronic stress is difficult and typically involves major upstream interventions to address the social determinants of health. Reducing intake of caffeine, tobacco, and alcohol may reduce migraine frequency in susceptible individuals. It is also important to improve sleep, diet, and hydration.[265]

People with frequent migraine headaches often benefit from daily prophylactic treatment; medications such as propranolol, tricyclic drugs, and cyproheptadine have all been helpful. Drugs that can abort migraine attacks if given shortly after headache onset, such as ergotamine tartrate and sumatriptan, can be helpful but require careful expert medical management to minimize adverse events.[266,267] People with disabling episodic tension-type headache, especially those with chronic daily headache, benefit from stress management and psychophysiological techniques such as biofeedback.[268] In addition, treatment for coexisting depression is sometimes important for people with chronic daily headaches.[269]

Moving Forward

Efficient methods of educating the public regarding good sleep hygiene, avoidance of triggers, and the importance of the medical home may reduce the morbidity related to migraine in the community.

DISCUSSION QUESTIONS

1. The neurologic diseases described in this chapter vary considerably regarding their potential for prevention. What are the implications of these differences for public health practice?
2. Some of these neurologic diseases, like low back pain, lead to considerable pain, suffering, and disability. Describe methods that are used in public health to compare and contrast these diseases with other diseases.
3. For each neurologic disease discussed in this chapter, describe the differing roles for primary, secondary, and tertiary prevention.
4. Describe the role of the social determinants of health (e.g., income, education, race/ethnicity, place of residence) in the prevention and control of each of these neurologic diseases.

REFERENCES

1. Whiteford HA, Ferrari AJ, Degenhardt L, Feigin V, Vos T. The global burden of mental, neurological and substance use disorders: an analysis from the Global Burden of Disease Study 2010. *PLoS One*. 2015;10(2):e0116820. doi:10.1371/journal.pone.0116820
2. Pakpoor J, Goldacre M. Neuroepidemiology: the increasing burden of mortality from neurological diseases. *Nat Rev Neurol* 2017;13(9):518–519. doi:10.1038/nrneurol.2017.112
3. Global Burden of Disease Collaborators. Global burden of diseases: neurological disorders. *Lancet*. 2020. Available at: https://www.thelancet.com/gbd/summaries. Accessed January 27, 2023.
4. Williams DR, Lawrence JA, Davis BA. Racism and health: evidence and needed research. *Annu Rev Public Health*. 2019;40:105–125. doi:10.1146/annurev-publhealth-040218-043750
5. Woolf SH, Chapman D, Hyung Lee J, et al. The price of inequities: avertable deaths from neurological diseases in the past decade. *Neurology* 2023;2023;101(7 suppl 1):S9–S16. doi:10.1212/WNL.0000000000207561
6. Khoury MJ, Iademarco MF, Riley WT. Precision public health for the era of precision medicine. *Am J Prev Med*. 2016;50(3):398–401. doi:10.1016/j.amepre.2015.08.031
7. Pritchard C, Rosenorn-Lanng E, Silk A, Hansen L. Controlled population-based comparative study of USA and international adult [55–74] neurological deaths 1989–2014. *Acta Neurol Scand*. 2017;136(6):698–707. doi:10.1111/ane.12789
8. Fisher RS, Acevedo C, Arzimanoglou A, et al. ILAE official report: a practical clinical definition of epilepsy. *Epilepsia*. 2014;55(4):475–482. doi:10.1111/epi.12550
9. Pujar SS, Martinos MM, Cortina-Borja M, et al. Long-term prognosis after childhood convulsive status epilepticus: a prospective cohort study. *Lancet Child Adolesc Health*. 2018;2(2):103–111. doi:10.1016/S2352-4642(17)30174-8
10. Lv RJ, Wang Q, Cui T, Zhu F, Shao XQ. Status epilepticus-related etiology, incidence and mortality: a meta-analysis. *Epilepsy Res*. 2017;136:12–17. doi:10.1016/j.eplepsyres.2017.07.006
11. DeGiorgio CM, Curtis A, Carapetian A, Hovsepian D, Krishnadasan A, Markovic D. Why are epilepsy mortality rates rising in the United States? A population-based multiple cause-of-death study. *BMJ Open*. 2020;10(8):e035767. doi:10.1136/bmjopen-2019-035767
12. Kwon CS, Wagner RG, Carpio A, Jette N, Newton CR, Thurman DJ. The worldwide epilepsy treatment gap: a systematic review and recommendations for revised definitions—a report from the ILAE Epidemiology Commission. *Epilepsia*. 2022;63(3):551–564. doi:10.1111/epi.17112
13. Thurman DJ, Kobau R, Luo YH, Helmers SL, Zack MM. Health-care access among adults with epilepsy: the US National Health Interview Survey, 2010 and 2013. *Epilepsy Behav*. 2016;55:184–188. doi:10.1016/j.yebeh.2015.10.028
14. Panayiotopoulos CP, Michael M, Sanders S, Valeta T, Koutroumanidis M. Benign childhood focal epilepsies: assessment of established and newly recognized syndromes. *Brain*. 2008;131(pt 9):2264–2286. doi:10.1093/brain/awn162
15. Autry AR, Trevathan E, Van Naarden Braun K, Yeargin-Allsopp M. Increased risk of death among children with Lennox-Gastaut syndrome and infantile spasms. *J Child Neurol*. 2010;25(4):441–447. doi:10.1177/0883073809348355
16. Thijs RD, Surges R, O'Brien TJ, Sander JW. Epilepsy in adults. *Lancet*. 2019;393(10172):689–701. doi:10.1016/S0140-6736(18)32596-0

17. Keezer MR, Sisodiya SM, Sander JW. Comorbidities of epilepsy: current concepts and future perspectives. *Lancet Neurol.* 2016;15(1):106–115. doi:10.1016/S1474-4422(15)00225-2
18. Poole BJ, Phillips NL, Stewart E, Harris IM, Lah S. Working memory in pediatric epilepsy: a systematic review and meta-analysis. *Neuropsychol Rev.* 2021;31(4):569–609. doi:10.1007/s11065-021-09491-7
19. Luoni C, Bisulli F, Canevini MP, et al. Determinants of health-related quality of life in pharmacoresistant epilepsy: results from a large multicenter study of consecutively enrolled patients using validated quantitative assessments. *Epilepsia.* 2011;52(12):2181–2191. doi:10.1111/j.1528-1167.2011.03325.x
20. Noe K. Balancing safety and independence for people with epilepsy under threat of SUDEP. *Epilepsy Curr.* 2020;20(5):276–277. doi:10.1177/1535759720944938
21. Surges R, Sander JW. Sudden unexpected death in epilepsy: mechanisms, prevalence, and prevention. *Curr Opin Neurol.* 2012;25(2):201–207. doi:10.1097/WCO.0b013e3283506714
22. Global Burden of Disease Collaborators. Global burden of diseases: epilepsy. *Lancet.* 2020. Available at: https://www.thelancet.com/gbd/summaries. Accessed January 23, 2023.
23. Nevalainen O, Simola M, Ansakorpi H, et al. Epilepsy, excess deaths and years of life lost from external causes. *Eur J Epidemiol.* 2016;31(5):445–453. doi:10.1007/s10654-015-0095-5
24. Abdel-Mannan O, Taylor H, Donner EJ, Sutcliffe AG. A systematic review of sudden unexpected death in epilepsy (SUDEP) in childhood. *Epilepsy Behav.* 2019;90:99–106. doi:10.1016/j.yebeh.2018.11.006
25. Thurman DJ, Hesdorffer DC, French JA. Sudden unexpected death in epilepsy: assessing the public health burden. *Epilepsia.* 2014;55(10):1479–1485. doi:10.1111/epi.12666
26. Lhatoo S, Noebels J, Whittemore V; NINDS Center for SUDEP Research. Sudden unexpected death in epilepsy: identifying risk and preventing mortality. *Epilepsia.* 2015;56(11):170016. doi:10.1111/epi.13134
27. Jetté N, Wiebe S. Initial evaluation of the patient with suspected epilepsy. *Neurol Clin.* 2016;34(2):339–350, vii. doi:10.1016/j.ncl.2015.11.008
28. Guerrini R. Epilepsy in children. *Lancet.* 2006;367(9509):499–524. doi:10.1016/S0140-6736(06)68182-8
29. Duncan JS, Sander JW, Sisodiya SM, Walker MC. Adult epilepsy. *Lancet.* 2006;367(9516):1087–1100. doi:10.1016/S0140-6736(06)68477-8
30. Berg AT, Berkovic SF, Brodie MJ, et al. Revised terminology and concepts for organization of seizures and epilepsies: report of the ILAE Commission on Classification and Terminology, 2005–2009. *Epilepsia.* 2010;51(4):676–685. doi:10.1111/j.1528-1167.2010.02522.x
31. Aliyu MH, Abdullahi AT, Iliyasu Z, et al. Bridging the childhood epilepsy treatment gap in northern Nigeria (BRIDGE): rationale and design of pre-clinical trial studies. *Contemp Clin Trials Commun.* 2019;15:100362. doi:10.1016/j.conctc.2019.100362
32. Hughes JR. A review of sudden unexpected death in epilepsy: prediction of patients at risk. *Epilepsy Behav.* 2009;14(2):280–287. doi:10.1016/j.yebeh.2008.12.004
33. Tomson T, Nashef L, Ryvlin P. Sudden unexpected death in epilepsy: current knowledge and future directions. *Lancet Neurol.* 2008;7(11):1021–1031. doi:10.1016/S1474-4422(08)70202-3

34. Yeargin-Allsopp M, Boyle C, van Naarden-Braun K, Trevathan E. The epidemiology of developmental disabilities. In: Accardo P, ed. *Capute and Accardo's Neurodevelopmental Disabilities in Infancy and Childhood*. Baltimore, MD: Paul H. Brookes Publishing; 2008:61–104.
35. Birbeck GL, Kalichi EM. Epilepsy prevalence in rural Zambia: a door-to-door survey. *Trop Med Int Health*. 2004;9(1):92–95.
36. Prischich F, De Rinaldis M, Bruno F, et al. High prevalence of epilepsy in a village in the Littoral Province of Cameroon. *Epilepsy Res*. 2008;82(2–3):200–210. doi:10.1016/j.eplepsyres.2008.09.004
37. Hauser WA, Annegers JF, Rocca WA. Descriptive epidemiology of epilepsy: contributions of population-based studies from Rochester, Minnesota. *Mayo Clin Proc*. 1996;71(6):576–586. doi:10.4065/71.6.576
38. US Centers for Disease Control and Prevention Epilepsy Program. About one-half of adults with active epilepsy and seizures have annual family incomes under $25,000: the 2010 and 2013 US National Health Interview Surveys. *Epilepsy Behav*. 2016;58:33–34.
39. Wicker E, Cole JW. Sudden unexpected death in epilepsy (SUDEP): a review of risk factors and possible interventions in children. *J Pediatr Pharmacol Ther*. 2021;26(6):556–564. doi:10.5863/1551-6776-26.6.556
40. Lagae L. What's new in: "genetics in childhood epilepsy." *Eur J Pediatr*. 2008;167(7):715–722. doi:10.1007/s00431-008-0690-5
41. Kobow K, Blümcke I. Epigenetic mechanisms in epilepsy. *Prog Brain Res*. 2014;213:279–316. doi:10.1016/B978-0-444-63326-2.00014-4
42. Aronica E, Gorter JA. Gene expression profile in temporal lobe epilepsy. *Neuroscientist*. 2007;13(2):100–108. doi:10.1177/1073858406295832
43. Lewis-Smith D, Ganesan S, Galer PD, et al. Phenotypic homogeneity in childhood epilepsies evolves in gene-specific patterns across 3251 patient-years of clinical data. *Eur J Hum Genet*. 2021;29(11):1690–1700. doi:10.1038/s41431-021-00908-8
44. Petrovski S, Kwan P. Unraveling the genetics of common epilepsies: approaches, platforms, and caveats. *Epilepsy Behav*. 2013;26(3):229–233. doi:10.1016/j.yebeh.2012.09.007
45. Yang H, Song Z, Yang GP, et al. The ALDH2 rs671 polymorphism affects post-stroke epilepsy susceptibility and plasma 4-HNE levels. *PLoS One*. 2014;9(10):e109634. doi:10.1371/journal.pone.0109634
46. Diamond ML, Ritter AC, Failla MD, et al. IL-1β associations with posttraumatic epilepsy development: a genetics and biomarker cohort study. *Epilepsia*. 2015;56(7):991–1001. doi:10.1111/epi.13100
47. Trevathan E. Seizures and epilepsy among children with language regression and autistic spectrum disorders. *J Child Neurol*. 2004;19(suppl 1):S49–S57. doi:10.1177/088307380401900106
48. McTague A, Howell KB, Cross JH, Kurian MA, Scheffer IE. The genetic landscape of the epileptic encephalopathies of infancy and childhood. *Lancet Neurol*. 2016;15(3):304–316. doi:10.1016/S1474-4422(15)00250-1
49. Berkovic SF, Harkin L, McMahon JM, et al. De-novo mutations of the sodium channel gene SCN1A in alleged vaccine encephalopathy: a retrospective study. *Lancet Neurol*. 2006;5(6):488–492. doi:10.1016/S1474-4422(06)70446-X

50. Verbeek NE, van der Maas NA, Sonsma AC, et al. Effect of vaccinations on seizure risk and disease course in Dravet syndrome. *Neurology*. 2015;85(7):596–603. doi:10.1212/WNL.0000000000001855
51. Vezzani A, Fujinami RS, White HS, et al. Infections, inflammation and epilepsy. *Acta Neuropathol*. 2016;131(2):211–234. doi:10.1007/s00401-015-1481-5
52. Scheffer IE, Harkin LA, Grinton BE, et al. Temporal lobe epilepsy and GEFS+ phenotypes associated with SCN1B mutations. *Brain*. 2007;130(pt 1):100–109. doi:10.1093/brain/awl272
53. Camfield P, Camfield C. Febrile seizures and genetic epilepsy with febrile seizures plus (GEFS+). *Epileptic Disord*. 2015;17(2):124–33. doi:10.1684/epd.2015.0737
54. Boivin MJ, Kakooza AM, Warf BC, Davidson LL, Grigorenko EL. Reducing neurodevelopmental disorders and disability through research and interventions. *Nature*. 2015;527(7578):S155–S160. doi:10.1038/nature16029
55. Kariuki SM, Kakooza-Mwesige A, Wagner RG, et al. Prevalence and factors associated with convulsive status epilepticus in Africans with epilepsy. *Neurology*. 2015;84(18):1838–1845. doi:10.1212/WNL.0000000000001542
56. Atta CA, Fiest KM, Frolkis AD, et al. Global birth prevalence of spina bifida by folic acid fortification status: a systematic review and meta-analysis. *Am J Public Health*. 2016;106(1):e24–e34. doi:10.2105/AJPH.2015.302902
57. Engel J. The current place of epilepsy surgery. *Curr Opin Neurol*. 2018;31(2):192–197. doi:10.1097/WCO.0000000000000528
58. Ghosh S, Sinha JK, Khan T, et al. Pharmacological and therapeutic approaches in the treatment of epilepsy. *Biomedicines*. 2021;9(5):470. doi:10.3390/biomedicines9050470
59. England MJ, Liverman CT, Schultz AM, Strawbridge LM. Epilepsy across the spectrum: promoting health and understanding. A summary of the Institute of Medicine report. *Epilepsy Behav*. 2012;25(2):266–276. doi:10.1016/j.yebeh.2012.06.016
60. Jeong A, Wong M. Tuberous sclerosis complex as a model disease for developing new therapeutics for epilepsy. *Expert Rev Neurother*. 2016;16(4):437–447. doi:10.1586/14737175.2016.1151788
61. Larsen J, Johannesen KM, Ek J, et al. The role of SLC2A1 mutations in myoclonic astatic epilepsy and absence epilepsy, and the estimated frequency of GLUT1 deficiency syndrome. *Epilepsia*. 2015;56(12):e203–e208. doi:10.1111/epi.13222
62. Lal D, Reinthaler EM, Dejanovic B, et al. Evaluation of presumably disease causing SCN1A variants in a cohort of common epilepsy syndromes. *PLoS One*. 2016;11(3):e0150426. doi:10.1371/journal.pone.0150426
63. Glauser T, Shinnar S, Gloss D, et al. Evidence-based guideline: treatment of convulsive status epilepticus in children and adults: report of the Guideline Committee of the American Epilepsy Society. *Epilepsy Curr*. 2016;16(1):48–61. doi:10.5698/1535-7597-16.1.48
64. Zesiewicz TA. Parkinson disease. *Continuum (Minneap Minn)*. 2019;25(4):896–918. doi:10.1212/CON.0000000000000764
65. Almeida LR, Valença GT, Negreiros NN, Pinto EB, Oliveira-Filho J. Recurrent falls in people with Parkinson's disease without cognitive impairment: focusing on modifiable risk factors. *Parkinsons Dis*. 2014;2014:432924. doi:10.1155/2014/432924

66. GBD Parkinson's Disease Collaborators. Global, regional, and national burden of Parkinson's disease, 1990–2016: a systematic analysis for the Global Burden of Disease Study 2016. *Lancet Neurol.* 2018;17(11):939–953. doi:10.1016/S1474-4422(18)30295-3
67. Elbaz A, Carcaillon L, Kab S, Moisan F. Epidemiology of Parkinson's disease. *Rev Neurol (Paris).* 2016;172(1):14–26. doi:10.1016/j.neurol.2015.09.012
68. Adler CH, Beach TG. Neuropathological basis of nonmotor manifestations of Parkinson's disease. *Mov Disord.* 2016;31(8):1114–1119. doi:10.1002/mds.26605
69. Ascherio A, Schwarzschild MA. The epidemiology of Parkinson's disease: risk factors and prevention. *Lancet Neurol.* 2016;15(12):1257–1272. doi:10.1016/S1474-4422(16)30230-7
70. Tanner CM, Goldman SM. Epidemiology of Parkinson's disease. *Neurol Clin.* 1996;14(2):317–335. doi:10.1016/S0733-8619(05)70259-0
71. Breckenridge CB, Berry C, Chang ET, Sielken RL Jr., Mandel JS. Association between Parkinson's disease and cigarette smoking, rural living, well-water consumption, farming and pesticide use: systematic review and meta-analysis. *PLoS One.* 2016;11(4):e0151841. doi:10.1371/journal.pone.0151841
72. Sriram K, Lin GX, Jefferson AM, et al. Modifying welding process parameters can reduce the neurotoxic potential of manganese-containing welding fumes. *Toxicology.* 2015;328:168–178. doi:10.1016/j.tox.2014.12.015
73. Cook L, Schulze J, Verbrugge J, et al. The commercial genetic testing landscape for Parkinson's disease. *Parkinsonism Relat Disord.* 2021;92:107–111. doi:10.1016/j.parkreldis.2021.10.001
74. LeWitt PA, Fahn S. Levodopa therapy for Parkinson disease: a look backward and forward. *Neurology.* 2016;86(14 suppl 1):S3–S12. doi:10.1212/WNL.0000000000002509
75. Graff-Radford J. Vascular cognitive impairment. *Continuum (Minneap Minn).* 2019;25(1):147–164. doi:10.1212/CON.0000000000000684
76. McKhann GM, Knopman DS, Chertkow H, et al. The diagnosis of dementia due to Alzheimer's disease: recommendations from the National Institute on Aging-Alzheimer's Association workgroups on diagnostic guidelines for Alzheimer's disease. *Alzheimers Dement.* 2011;7(3):263–269. doi:10.1016/j.jalz.2011.03.005
77. Aranda MP, Kremer IN, Hinton L, et al. Impact of dementia: health disparities, population trends, care interventions, and economic costs. *J Am Geriatr Soc.* 2021;69(7):1774–1783. doi:10.1111/jgs.17345
78. Livingston G, Huntley J, Sommerlad A, et al. Dementia prevention, intervention, and care: 2020 report of the Lancet Commission. *Lancet.* 2020;396(10248):413–446. doi:10.1016/S0140-6736(20)30367-6
79. Amin J, Erskine D, Donaghy PC, et al. Inflammation in dementia with Lewy bodies. *Neurobiol Dis.* 2022;168:105698. doi:10.1016/j.nbd.2022.105698
80. Rabinovici GD. Late-onset Alzheimer disease. *Continuum (Minneap Minn).* 2019;25(1):14–33. doi:10.1212/CON.0000000000000700
81. Scheltens P, De Strooper B, Kivipelto M, et al. Alzheimer's disease. *Lancet.* 2021;397(10284):1577–1590. doi:10.1016/S0140-6736(20)32205-4
82. Brown RH Jr., Al-Chalabi A. Amyotrophic lateral sclerosis. *N Engl J Med.* 2017;377(16):1602. doi:10.1056/NEJMc1710379

83. Sabia S, Fayosse A, Dumurgier J, et al. Association of sleep duration in middle and old age with incidence of dementia. *Nat Commun.* 2021;12(1):2289. doi:10.1038/s41467-021-22354-2
84. Pogue AI, Lukiw WJ. Aluminum, the genetic apparatus of the human CNS and Alzheimer's disease (AD). *Morphologie.* 2016;100(329):56–64. doi:10.1016/j.morpho.2016.01.001
85. Seeley WW. Behavioral variant frontotemporal dementia. *Continuum (Minneap Minn).* 2019;25(1):76–100. doi:10.1212/CON.0000000000000698
86. Slomski A. Air quality and brain health. *JAMA.* 2022;327(15):1430-1431. doi:10.1001/jama.2022.3691
87. Day GS, Scarmeas N, Dubinsky R, et al. Aducanumab use in symptomatic Alzheimer disease evidence in focus: a report of the AAN Guidelines Subcommittee. *Neurology.* 2022;98(15):619–631. doi:10.1212/WNL.0000000000200176
88. van Lieshout P, Candundo H, Martino R, Shin S, Barakat-Haddad C. Onset factors in cerebral palsy: a systematic review. *Neurotoxicology.* 2017;61:47–53. doi:10.1016/j.neuro.2016.03.021
89. Folkerth RD. The neuropathology of acquired pre- and perinatal brain injuries. *Semin Diagn Pathol.* 2007;24(1):48–57. doi:10.1053/j.semdp.2007.02.006
90. Stanley F, Blair E, Alberman E. *Cerebral Palsies: Epidemiology and Causal Pathways.* London, UK: MacKeith Press; 2000.
91. Robinson MN, Peake LJ, Ditchfield MR, Reid SM, Lanigan A, Reddihough DS. Magnetic resonance imaging findings in a population-based cohort of children with cerebral palsy. *Dev Med Child Neurol.* 2009;51(1):39–45. doi:10.1111/j.1469-8749.2008.03127.x
92. Yeargin-Allsopp M, Van Naarden Braun K, Doernberg NS, Benedict RE, Kirby RS, Durkin MS. Prevalence of cerebral palsy in 8-year-old children in three areas of the United States in 2002: a multisite collaboration. *Pediatrics.* 2008;121(3):547–554. doi:10.1542/peds.2007-1270
93. Kirkham FJ, DeBaun MR. Stroke in children with sickle cell disease. *Curr Treat Options Neurol.* 2004;6(5):357–375. doi:10.1007/s11940-996-0028-4
94. Pakula AT, Van Naarden Braun K, Yeargin-Allsopp M. Cerebral palsy: classification and epidemiology. *Phys Med Rehabil Clin N Am.* 2009;20(3):425–452. doi:10.1016/j.pmr.2009.06.001
95. Wu YW, Xing G, Fuentes-Afflick E, Danielson B, Smith LH, Gilbert WM. Racial, ethnic, and socioeconomic disparities in the prevalence of cerebral palsy. *Pediatrics.* 2011;127(3):e674–e681. doi:10.1542/peds.2010-1656
96. Durkin MS, Yeargin-Allsopp M. Socioeconomic status and pediatric neurologic disorders: current evidence. *Semin Pediatr Neurol.* 2018;27:16–25. doi:10.1016/j.spen.2018.03.003
97. Michelsen SI, Flachs EM, Madsen M, Uldall P. Parental social consequences of having a child with cerebral palsy in Denmark. *Dev Med Child Neurol.* 2015;57(8):768–775. doi:10.1111/dmcn.12719
98. Sadowska M, Sarecka-Hujar B, Kopyta I. Cerebral palsy: current opinions on definition, epidemiology, risk factors, classification and treatment options. *Neuropsychiatr Dis Treat.* 2020;16:1505–1518. doi:10.2147/NDT.S235165
99. Allen MC. Neurodevelopmental outcomes of preterm infants. *Curr Opin Neurol.* 2008;21(2):123–128. doi:10.1097/WCO.0b013e3282f88bb4

100. Shalak LF, Laptook AR, Jafri HS, Ramilo O, Perlman JM. Clinical chorioamnionitis, elevated cytokines, and brain injury in term infants. *Pediatrics*. 2002;110(4):673–80. doi:10.1542/peds.110.4.673
101. Kim CJ, Romero R, Chaemsaithong P, Chaiyasit N, Yoon BH, Kim YM. Acute chorioamnionitis and funisitis: definition, pathologic features, and clinical significance. *Am J Obstet Gynecol*. 2015;213(4 suppl):S29–S52. doi:10.1016/j.ajog.2015.08.040
102. Park HW, Choi YS, Kim KS, Kim SN. Chorioamnionitis and patent ductus arteriosus: a systematic review and meta-analysis. *PLoS One*. 2015;10(9):e0138114. doi:10.1371/journal.pone.0138114
103. Rasmussen SA, Jamieson DJ, Honein MA, Petersen LR. Zika virus and birth defects—reviewing the evidence for causality. *N Engl J Med*. 2016;374(20):1981–1987. doi:10.1056/NEJMsr1604338
104. Pessoa A, van der Linden V, Yeargin-Allsopp M, et al. Motor abnormalities and epilepsy in infants and children with evidence of congenital Zika virus infection. *Pediatrics*. 2018;141(suppl 2):S167–S179. doi:10.1542/peds.2017-2038F
105. Carvalho AL, Ventura P, Taguchi T, Brandi I, Brites C, Lucena R. Cerebral palsy in children with congenital Zika syndrome: a 2-year neurodevelopmental follow-up. *J Child Neurol*. 2020;35(3):202–207. doi:10.1177/0883073819885724
106. Hirtz DG, Weiner SJ, Bulas D, et al. Antenatal magnesium and cerebral palsy in preterm infants. *J Pediatr*. 2015;167(4):834–839.e3. doi:10.1016/j.jpeds.2015.06.067
107. Teela KC, De Silva DA, Chapman K, et al. Magnesium sulphate for fetal neuroprotection: benefits and challenges of a systematic knowledge translation project in Canada. *BMC Pregnancy Childbirth*. 2015;15:347. doi:10.1186/s12884-015-0785-8
108. Doyle LW, Crowther CA, Middleton P, Marret S, Rouse D. Magnesium sulphate for women at risk of preterm birth for neuroprotection of the fetus. *Cochrane Database Syst Rev*. 2009(1):CD004661. doi:10.1002/14651858.CD004661.pub3
109. Kamyar M, Clark EA, Yoder BA, Varner MW, Manuck TA. Antenatal magnesium sulfate, necrotizing enterocolitis, and death among neonates <28 weeks gestation. *AJP Rep*. 2016;6(1):e148–e154. doi:10.1055/s-0036-1581059
110. Hong JY, Hong JY, Choi YS, et al. Antenatal magnesium sulfate treatment and risk of necrotizing enterocolitis in preterm infants born at less than 32 weeks of gestation. *Sci Rep*. 2020;10(1):12826. doi:10.1038/s41598-020-69785-3
111. Garfinkle J, Wintermark P, Shevell MI, Platt RW, Oskoui M; Registry CCP. Cerebral palsy after neonatal encephalopathy: how much is preventable? *J Pediatr*. 2015;167(1):58–63.e1. doi:10.1016/j.jpeds.2015.02.035
112. Mir IN, Johnson-Welch SF, Nelson DB, Brown LS, Rosenfeld CR, Chalak LF. Placental pathology is associated with severity of neonatal encephalopathy and adverse developmental outcomes following hypothermia. *Am J Obstet Gynecol*. 2015;213(6):849.e1–e7. doi:10.1016/j.ajog.2015.09.072
113. Gulati S, Sondhi V. Cerebral palsy: an overview. *Indian J Pediatr*. 2018;85(11):1006–1016. doi:10.1007/s12098-017-2475-1
114. Christensen DL, Braun KVN, Baio J, et al. Prevalence and characteristics of autism spectrum disorder among children aged 8 years—autism and developmental disabilities monitoring

network, 11 sites, United States, 2012. *MMWR Surveill Summ.* 2018;65(13):1–23. doi:10.15585/mmwr.ss6513a1

115. Treffert DA. Epidemiology of infantile autism. *Arch Gen Psychiatry.* 1970;22(5):431–438. doi:10.1001/archpsyc.1970.01740290047006
116. Wing L. Childhood autism and social class: a question of selection? *Br J Psychiatry.* 1980;137:410–417. doi:10.1192/bjp.137.5.410
117. Yuan J, Li M, Lu ZK. Racial/ethnic disparities in the prevalence and trends of autism spectrum disorder in US children and adolescents. *JAMA Netw Open.* 2021;4(3):e210771. doi:10.1001/jamanetworkopen.2021.0771
118. Leigh PJ, Grosse SD, Cassady D, Melnikow J, Hertz-Picciotto I. Spending by California's Department of Developmental Services for persons with autism across demographic and expenditure categories. *PLoS One.* 2016;11(3):e0151970. doi:10.1371/journal.pone.0151970
119. Rogge N, Janssen J. The economic costs of autism spectrum disorder: a literature review. *J Autism Dev Disord.* 2019;49(7):2873–2900. doi:10.1007/s10803-019-04014-z
120. Schendel DE, Overgaard M, Christensen J, et al. Association of psychiatric and neurologic comorbidity with mortality among persons with autism spectrum disorder in a Danish population. *JAMA Pediatr.* 2016;170(3):243–250. doi:10.1001/jamapediatrics.2015.3935
121. Hirvikoski T, Mittendorfer-Rutz E, Boman M, Larsson H, Lichtenstein P, Bölte S. Premature mortality in autism spectrum disorder. *Br J Psychiatry.* 2016;208(3):232–238. doi:10.1192/bjp.bp.114.160192
122. Global Burden of Disease Collaborators. Global burden of diseases: autism spectrum disorders. *Lancet.* 2020. Available at: https://www.thelancet.com/gbd/summaries. Accessed January 27, 2023.
123. Lord C, Brugha TS, Charman T, et al. Autism spectrum disorder. *Nat Rev Dis Primers.* 2020;6(1):5. doi:10.1038/s41572-019-0138-4
124. Hudson CC, Hall L, Harkness KL. Prevalence of depressive disorders in individuals with autism spectrum disorder: a meta-analysis. *J Abnorm Child Psychol.* 2019;47(1):165–175. doi:10.1007/s10802-018-0402-1
125. Al-Beltagi M. Autism medical comorbidities. *World J Clin Pediatr.* 2021;10(3):15–28. doi:10.5409/wjcp.v10.i3.15
126. Trevathan E, Shinnar S. Epidemiology of autism spectrum disorders. In: Tuchman R, Rapin I, eds. *Autism: A Neurological Disorder of Early Brain Development.* London, UK: MacKeith Press; 2006: 20–36.
127. Hyman SL, Levy SE, Myers SM; Council on Children with Disabilities, Section on Developmental and Behavioral Pediatrics. Identification, evaluation, and management of children with autism spectrum disorder. *Pediatrics.* 2020;145(1):e20193447. doi:10.1542/peds.2019-3447
128. Loomes R, Hull L, Mandy WPL. What is the male-to-female ratio in autism spectrum disorder? A systematic review and meta-analysis. *J Am Acad Child Adolesc Psychiatry.* 2017;56(6):466–474. doi:10.1016/j.jaac.2017.03.013
129. van Eijk L, Zietsch BP. Testing the extreme male brain hypothesis: is autism spectrum disorder associated with a more male-typical brain? *Autism Res.* 2021;14(8):1597–1608. doi:10.1002/aur.2537

130. Shattuck PT. The contribution of diagnostic substitution to the growing administrative prevalence of autism in US special education. *Pediatrics*. 2006;117(4):1028–1037. doi:10.1542/peds.2005-1516
131. Brugha TS, McManus S, Bankart J, et al. Epidemiology of autism spectrum disorders in adults in the community in England. *Arch Gen Psychiatry*. 2011;68(5):459–465. doi:10.1001/archgenpsychiatry.2011.38
132. Gaugler T, Klei L, Sanders SJ, et al. Most genetic risk for autism resides with common variation. *Nat Genet*. 2014;46(8):881–885. doi:10.1038/ng.3039
133. Sanders SJ, He X, Willsey AJ, et al. Insights into autism spectrum disorder genomic architecture and biology from 71 risk loci. *Neuron*. 2015;87(6):1215–1233. doi:10.1016/j.neuron.2015.09.016
134. Satterstrom FK, Kosmicki JA, Wang J, et al. Large-scale exome sequencing study implicates both developmental and functional changes in the neurobiology of autism. *Cell*. 2020;180(3):568–584.e23. doi:10.1016/j.cell.2019.12.036
135. Miles JH. Autism spectrum disorders—a genetics review. *Genet Med*. 2011;13(4):278–294. doi:10.1097/GIM.0b013e3181ff67ba
136. Gerber JS, Offit PA. Vaccines and autism: a tale of shifting hypotheses. *Clin Infect Dis*. 2009;48(4):456–461. doi:10.1086/596476
137. Gadad BS, Li W, Yazdani U, et al. Administration of thimerosal-containing vaccines to infant rhesus macaques does not result in autism-like behavior or neuropathology. *Proc Natl Acad Sci (USA)*. 2015;112(40):12498–12503. doi:10.1073/pnas.1500968112
138. Jain A, Marshall J, Buikema A, Bancroft T, Kelly JP, Newschaffer CJ. Autism occurrence by MMR vaccine status among US children with older siblings with and without autism. *JAMA*. 2015;313(15):1534–1540. doi:10.1001/jama.2015.3077
139. Lancet editors. Retraction—ileal-lymphoid-nodular hyperplasia, non-specific colitis, and pervasive developmental disorder in children. *Lancet*. 2010;375(9713):445. doi:10.1016/S0140-6736(10)60175-4
140. General Medical Council. *Fitness to Practise Panel Hearing—Dr. Andrew Jeremy Wakefield*. GMC reference 2733564. London, UK: General Medical Council; 2009:1–95.
141. Offit P. *Autism's False Prophets: Bad Science, Risky Medicine, and the Search for a Cure*. New York, NY: Columbia University Press; 2008.
142. Godlee F, Smith J, Marcovitch H. Wakefield's article linking MMR vaccine and autism was fraudulent. *BMJ*. 2011;342:c7452. doi:10.1136/bmj.c7452
143. Motta M, Stecula D. Quantifying the effect of Wakefield et al. (1998) on skepticism about MMR vaccine safety in the US. *PLoS One*. 2021;16(8):e0256395. doi:10.1371/journal.pone.0256395
144. de la Torre-Ubieta L, Won H, Stein JL, Geschwind DH. Advancing the understanding of autism disease mechanisms through genetics. *Nat Med*. 2016;22(4):345–361. doi:10.1038/nm.4071
145. Modabbernia A, Velthorst E, Reichenberg A. Environmental risk factors for autism: an evidence-based review of systematic reviews and meta-analyses. *Mol Autism*. 2017;8:13. doi:10.1186/s13229-017-0121-4
146. Sandin S, Schendel D, Magnusson P, et al. Autism risk associated with parental age and with increasing difference in age between the parents. *Mol Psychiatry*. 2016;21(5):693–700. doi:10.1038/mp.2015.70

147. Estes A, Munson J, Rogers SJ, Greenson J, Winter J, Dawson G. Long-term outcomes of early intervention in 6-year-old children with autism spectrum disorder. *J Am Acad Child Adolesc Psychiatry.* 2015;54(7):580–587. doi:10.1016/j.jaac.2015.04.005
148. Centers for Disease Control and Prevention. Learn the signs. Act early. Available at: http://www.cdc.gov/ncbddd/actearly/index.html. Accessed January 27, 2023.
149. Green J, Charman T, Pickles A, et al. Parent-mediated intervention versus no intervention for infants at high risk of autism: a parallel, single-blind, randomised trial. *Lancet Psychiatry.* 2015;2(2):133–140. doi:10.1016/S2215-0366(14)00091-1
150. Riva N, Agosta F, Lunetta C, Filippi M, Quattrini A. Recent advances in amyotrophic lateral sclerosis. *J Neurol.* 2016;263(6):1241–1254. doi:10.1007/s00415-016-8091-6
151. Wurster CD, Ludolph AC. Nusinersen for spinal muscular atrophy. *Ther Adv Neurol Disord.* 2018;11:1756285618754459. doi:10.1177/1756285618754459
152. Brown CA, Lally C, Kupelian V, Flanders WD. Estimated prevalence and incidence of amyotrophic lateral sclerosis and SOD1 and C9orf72 genetic variants. *Neuroepidemiology.* 2021;55(5):342–353. doi:10.1159/000516752
153. Chio A, Logroscino G, Traynor BJ, et al. Global epidemiology of amyotrophic lateral sclerosis: a systematic review of the published literature. *Neuroepidemiology.* 2013;41(2):118–130. doi:10.1159/000351153
154. Mehta P, Kaye W, Raymond J, et al. Prevalence of amyotrophic lateral sclerosis—United States, 2015. *MMWR Morb Mortal Wkly Rep.* 2018;67(46):1285–1289. doi:10.15585/mmwr.mm6746a1
155. Hardiman O, Al-Chalabi A, Chio A, et al. Amyotrophic lateral sclerosis. *Nat Rev Dis Primers.* 2017;3:17071. doi:10.1038/nrdp.2017.71
156. Khamankar N, Coan G, Weaver B, Mitchell CS. Associative increases in amyotrophic lateral sclerosis survival duration with non-invasive ventilation initiation and usage protocols. *Front Neurol.* 2018;9:578. doi:10.3389/fneur.2018.00578
157. Wallin MT, Culpepper WJ, Campbell JD, et al. The prevalence of MS in the United States: a population-based estimate using health claims data. *Neurology.* 2019;92(10):e1029–e1040. doi:10.1212/WNL.0000000000007035
158. Thompson AJ, Banwell BL, Barkhof F, et al. Diagnosis of multiple sclerosis: 2017 revisions of the McDonald criteria. *Lancet Neurol.* 2018;17(2):162–173. doi:10.1016/S1474-4422(17)30470-2
159. Dendrou CA, Fugger L, Friese MA. Immunopathology of multiple sclerosis. *Nat Rev Immunol.* 2015;15(9):545–558. doi:10.1038/nri3871
160. Flanagan EP, Cabre P, Weinshenker BG, et al. Epidemiology of aquaporin-4 autoimmunity and neuromyelitis optica spectrum. *Ann Neurol.* 2016;79(5):775–783. doi:10.1002/ana.24617
161. Yoon HH, Park JY, Kim SY, et al. Epidemiology of demyelinating diseases in Korean pediatric patients. *J Child Neurol.* 2021;36(2):141–147. doi:10.1177/0883073820959543
162. Bjornevik K, Cortese M, Healy BC, et al. Longitudinal analysis reveals high prevalence of Epstein-Barr virus associated with multiple sclerosis. *Science.* 2022;375(6578):296–301. doi:10.1126/science.abj8222
163. Ascherio A, Munger KL. Epidemiology of multiple sclerosis: from risk factors to prevention—an update. *Semin Neurol.* 2016;36(2):103–114. doi:10.1055/s-0036-1579693

164. Sawcer S, Franklin RJ, Ban M. Multiple sclerosis genetics. *Lancet Neurol.* 2014;13(7): 700–709. doi:10.1016/S1474-4422(14)70041-9
165. Carnero Contentti E, Correale J. Neuromyelitis optica spectrum disorders: from pathophysiology to therapeutic strategies. *J Neuroinflammation.* 2021;18(1):208. doi:10.1186/s12974-021-02249-1
166. Chevalier J, Chamoux C, Hammes F, Chicoye A. Cost-effectiveness of treatments for relapsing remitting multiple sclerosis: a French societal perspective. *PLoS One.* 2016;11(3): e0150703. doi:10.1371/journal.pone.0150703
167. Malek E, Salameh J. Guillain-Barre syndrome. *Semin Neurol.* 2019;39(5):589–595. doi:10.1055/s-0039-1693005
168. Dimachkie MM, Barohn RJ. Guillain-Barré syndrome and variants. *Neurol Clin.* 2013;31(2): 491–510. doi:10.1016/j.ncl.2013.01.005
169. Willison HJ, Jacobs BC, van Doorn PA. Guillain-Barré syndrome. *Lancet.* 2016;388(10045): 717–727. doi:10.1016/S0140-6736(16)00339-1
170. Palaiodimou L, Stefanou MI, Katsanos AH, et al. Prevalence, clinical characteristics and outcomes of Guillain-Barré syndrome spectrum associated with COVID-19: a systematic review and meta-analysis. *Eur J Neurol.* 2021;28(10):3517–3529. doi:10.1111/ene.14860
171. Kalita J, Ranjan A, Misra UK. Outcome of Guillain-Barre syndrome patients with respiratory paralysis. *QJM.* 2016;109(5):319–323. doi:10.1093/qjmed/hcv190
172. Shahrizaila N, Lehmann HC, Kuwabara S. Guillain-Barré syndrome. *Lancet.* 2021; 397(10280):1214–1228. doi:10.1016/S0140-6736(21)00517-1
173. Filosto M, Cotti Piccinelli S, Gazzina S, et al. Guillain-Barré syndrome and COVID-19: an observational multicentre study from two Italian hotspot regions. *J Neurol Neurosurg Psychiatry.* 2021;92(7):751–756. doi:10.1136/jnnp-2020-324837
174. Burns TM. Guillain-Barré syndrome. *Semin Neurol.* 2008;28(2):152–167. doi:10.1055/s-2008-1062261
175. Pritchard J. What's new in Guillain-Barré syndrome? *Postgrad Med J.* 2008;84(996):532–538. doi:10.1136/jnnp.2006.097709
176. Wouk J, Rechenchoski DZ, Rodrigues BCD, Ribelato EV, Faccin-Galhardi LC. Viral infections and their relationship to neurological disorders. *Arch Virol.* 2021;166(3):733–753. doi:10.1007/s00705-021-04959-6
177. Dimario FJ, Edwards C. Autonomic dysfunction in childhood Guillain-Barré syndrome. *J Child Neurol.* 2012;27(5):581–586. doi:10.1177/0883073811420872
178. van den Berg B, Walgaard C, Drenthen J, Fokke C, Jacobs BC, van Doorn PA. Guillain-Barré syndrome: pathogenesis, diagnosis, treatment and prognosis. *Nat Rev Neurol.* 2014;10(8): 469–482. doi:10.1038/nrneurol.2014.121
179. Sejvar JJ, Baughman AL, Wise M, Morgan OW. Population incidence of Guillain-Barré syndrome: a systematic review and meta-analysis. *Neuroepidemiology.* 2011;36(2):123–133. doi:10.1159/000324710
180. Webb AJ, Brain SA, Wood R, Rinaldi S, Turner MR. Seasonal variation in Guillain-Barré syndrome: a systematic review, meta-analysis and Oxfordshire cohort study. *J Neurol Neurosurg Psychiatry.* 2015;86(11):1196–1201. doi:10.1136/jnnp-2014-309056

181. Papri N, Islam Z, Leonhard SE, Mohammad QD, Endtz HP, Jacobs BC. Guillain-Barré syndrome in low-income and middle-income countries: challenges and prospects. *Nat Rev Neurol.* 2021;17(5):285–296. doi:10.1038/s41582-021-00467-y
182. Global Burden of Disease Collaborators. Global burden of diseases: Guillain-Barré syndrome. *Lancet.* 2020. Available at: https://www.thelancet.com/gbd/summaries. Accessed January 23, 2023.
183. Parker CT, Huynh S, Heikema AP, Cooper KK, Miller WG. Complete genome sequences of Campylobacter jejuni strains RM3196 (233.94) and RM3197 (308.95) isolated from patients with Guillain-Barré syndrome. *Genome Announc.* 2015;3(6). doi:10.1128/genomeA.01312-15
184. Taheraghdam A, Pourkhanjar P, Talebi M, et al. Correlations between cytomegalovirus, Epstein-Barr virus, anti-ganglioside antibodies, electrodiagnostic findings and functional status in Guillain-Barré syndrome. *Iran J Neurol.* 2014;13(1):7–12.
185. Watrin L, Ghawche F, Larre P, Neau JP, Mathis S, Fournier E. Guillain-Barré syndrome (42 cases) occurring during a Zika virus outbreak in French Polynesia. *Medicine (Baltimore).* 2016;95(14):e3257. doi:10.1097/MD.0000000000003257
186. Kuwabara S. Guillain-Barré syndrome: epidemiology, pathophysiology and management. *Drugs.* 2004;64(6):597–610. doi:10.2165/00003495-200464060-00003
187. McGrogan A, Madle GC, Seaman HE, de Vries CS. The epidemiology of Guillain-Barré syndrome worldwide. A systematic literature review. *Neuroepidemiology.* 2009;32(2): 150–163. doi:10.1159/000184748
188. Allen CM, Ramsamy S, Tarr AW, et al. Guillain-Barré syndrome variant occurring after SARS-CoV-2 vaccination. *Ann Neurol.* 2021;90(2):315–318. doi:10.1002/ana.26144
189. Chun JY, Park S, Jung J, et al. Guillain-Barré syndrome after vaccination against COVID-19. *Lancet Neurol.* 2022;21(2):117–119. doi:10.1016/S1474-4422(21)00416-6
190. Gunduz A, Okun MS. A review and update on Tourette syndrome: where is the field headed? *Curr Neurol Neurosci Rep.* 2016;16(4):37. doi:10.1007/s11910-016-0633-x
191. Cavanna AE, Rickards H. The psychopathological spectrum of Gilles de la Tourette syndrome. *Neurosci Biobehav Rev.* 2013;37(6):1008–1015. doi:10.1016/j.neubiorev.2012.10.011
192. Cavanna AE, Seri S. Tourette's syndrome. *BMJ.* 2013;347:f4964. doi:10.1136/bmj.f4964
193. Robertson MM, Eapen V, Singer HS, et al. Gilles de la Tourette syndrome. *Nat Rev Dis Primers.* 2017;3:16097. doi:10.1038/nrdp.2016.97
194. Ueda K, Black KJ. A comprehensive review of tic disorders in children. *J Clin Med.* 2021;10(11). doi:10.3390/jcm10112479
195. Novotny M, Valis M, Klimova B. Tourette syndrome: a mini-review. *Front Neurol.* 2018;9:139. doi:10.3389/fneur.2018.00139
196. Miller LL, Scharf JM, Mathews CA, Ben-Shlomo Y. Tourette syndrome and chronic tic disorder are associated with lower socio-economic status: findings from the Avon Longitudinal Study of Parents and Children cohort. *Dev Med Child Neurol.* 2014;56(2):157–163. doi:10.1111/dmcn.12318
197. Kossoff EH, Singer HS. Tourette syndrome: clinical characteristics and current management strategies. *Paediatr Drugs.* 2001;3(5):355–363. doi:10.2165/00128072-200103050-00004

198. Faridi K, Suchowersky O. Gilles de la Tourette's syndrome. *Can J Neurol Sci*. 2003;30(suppl 1): S64–S71. doi:10.1017/s0317167100003267

199. Lombroso PJ, Scahill L. Tourette syndrome and obsessive-compulsive disorder. *Brain Dev*. 2008;30(4):231–237. doi:10.1016/j.braindev.2007.09.001

200. Hirschtritt ME, Lee PC, Pauls DL, et al. Lifetime prevalence, age of risk, and genetic relationships of comorbid psychiatric disorders in Tourette syndrome. *JAMA Psychiatry*. 2015;72(4):325–333. doi:10.1001/jamapsychiatry.2014.2650

201. Fernández de la Cruz L, Rydell M, Runeson B, et al. Suicide in Tourette's and chronic tic disorders. *Biol Psychiatry*. 2017;82(2):111–118. doi:10.1016/j.biopsych.2016.08.023

202. Goldstein DM, Hall K. Mass hysteria in Le Roy, New York: how brain experts materialized truth and outscienced environmental inquiry. *Am Ethnologist*. 2015;42(4):640-657.

203. Jargon J. Teen girls are developing tics. Doctors say TikTok could be a factor. *Wall Street Journal*. Updated October 19, 2021. Available at: https://www.wsj.com/articles/teen-girls-are-developing-tics-doctors-say-tiktok-could-be-a-factor-11634389201. Accessed January 23, 2023.

204. Thenganatt MA, Jankovic J. Recent advances in understanding and managing Tourette syndrome. *F1000Res*. 2016;5:F100. doi:10.12688/f1000research.7424.1

205. Quezada J, Coffman KA. Current approaches and new developments in the pharmacological management of Tourette syndrome. *CNS Drugs*. 2018;32(1):33–45. doi:10.1007/s40263-017-0486-0

206. Ueda K, Black KJ. Recent progress on Tourette syndrome. *Fac Rev*. 2021;10:70. doi:10.12703/r/10-70

207. Laurin N, Wigg KG, Feng Y, Sandor P, Barr CL. Chromosome 5 and Gilles de la Tourette syndrome: linkage in a large pedigree and association study of six candidates in the region. *Am J Med Genet B Neuropsychiatr Genet*. 2009;150B(1):95–103. doi:10.1002/ajmg.b.30779

208. Bertelsen B, Stefansson H, Riff Jensen L, et al. Association of AADAC deletion and Gilles de la Tourette syndrome in a large European cohort. *Biol Psychiatry*. 2016;79(5):383–391. doi:10.1016/j.biopsych.2015.08.027

209. Harris K, Singer HS. Tic disorders: neural circuits, neurochemistry, and neuroimmunology. *J Child Neurol*. 2006;21(8):678–689. doi:10.1177/08830738060210080901

210. Leckman JF, King RA, Gilbert DL, et al. Streptococcal upper respiratory tract infections and exacerbations of tic and obsessive-compulsive symptoms: a prospective longitudinal study. *J Am Acad Child Adolesc Psychiatry*. 2011;50(2):108–118.e3. doi:10.1016/j.jaac.2010.10.011

211. Whittington C, Pennant M, Kendall T, et al. Practitioner review: treatments for Tourette syndrome in children and young people—a systematic review. *J Child Psychol Psychiatry*. 2016;57(9):988–1004. doi:10.1111/jcpp.12556

212. Katz DI, Bernick C, Dodick DW, et al. National Institute of Neurological Disorders and Stroke consensus diagnostic criteria for traumatic encephalopathy syndrome. *Neurology*. 2021;96(18):848–863. doi:10.1212/WNL.0000000000011850

213. Faul M, Coronado V. Epidemiology of traumatic brain injury. *Handb Clin Neurol*. 2015;127:3–13. doi:10.1016/B978-0-444-52892-6.00001-5

214. Peterson AB, Thomas KE. Incidence of nonfatal traumatic brain injury-related hospitalizations—United States, 2018. *MMWR Morb Mortal Wkly Rep*. 2021;70(48): 1664–1668. doi:10.15585/mmwr.mm7048a3

215. GBD 2016 Traumatic Brain Injury and Spinal Cord Injury Collaborators. Global, regional, and national burden of traumatic brain injury and spinal cord injury, 1990–2016: a systematic analysis for the Global Burden of Disease Study 2016. *Lancet Neurol.* 2019;18(1):56–87. doi:10.1016/S1474-4422(18)30415-0

216. Grossman DC, Curry SJ, Owens DK, et al. Interventions to prevent falls in community-dwelling older adults: US Preventive Services Task Force recommendation statement. *JAMA.* 2018;319(16):1696–1704. doi:10.1001/jama.2018.3097

217. Di Pietro V, O'Halloran P, Watson CN, et al. Unique diagnostic signatures of concussion in the saliva of male athletes: the Study of Concussion in Rugby Union through MicroRNAs (SCRUM). *Br J Sports Med.* 2021;55(24):1395–1404. doi:10.1136/bjsports-2020-103274

218. Schneider ALC, Huie JR, Boscardin WJ, et al. Cognitive outcome 1 year after mild traumatic brain injury: results from the TRACK-TBI Study. *Neurology.* 2022;98(12):e1248–e1261. doi:10.1212/WNL.0000000000200041

219. National Spinal Cord Injury Statistical Center. *National Spinal Cord Injury Statistical Center, Facts and Figures at a Glance.* Birmingham, AL: University of Alabama at Birmingham; 2019.

220. van den Berg ME, Castellote JM, Mahillo-Fernandez I, de Pedro-Cuesta J. Incidence of spinal cord injury worldwide: a systematic review. *Neuroepidemiology.* 2010;34(3):184–192. doi:10.1159/000279335

221. Furlan JC, Sakakibara BM, Miller WC, Krassioukov AV. Global incidence and prevalence of traumatic spinal cord injury. *Can J Neurol Sci.* 2013;40(4):456–464. doi:10.1017/s0317167100014530

222. Rubiano AM, Carney N, Chesnut R, Puyana JC. Global neurotrauma research challenges and opportunities. *Nature.* 2015;527(7578):S193–S197. doi:10.1038/nature16035

223. American Psychiatric Association. *Diagnostic and Statistical Manual of Mental Disorders.* 5th ed. Washington, DC: American Psychiatric Association; 2013.

224. Pehlivanidis A, Papanikolaou K, Mantas V, et al. Lifetime co-occurring psychiatric disorders in newly diagnosed adults with attention deficit hyperactivity disorder (ADHD) or/and autism spectrum disorder (ASD). *BMC Psychiatry.* 2020;20(1):423. doi:10.1186/s12888-020-02828-1

225. McClernon FJ, Kollins SH. ADHD and smoking: from genes to brain to behavior. *Ann N Y Acad Sci.* 2008;1141:131–147. doi:10.1196/annals.1441.016

226. Thapar A, Cooper M. Attention deficit hyperactivity disorder. *Lancet.* 2016;387(10024):1240–1250. doi:10.1016/S0140-6736(15)00238-X

227. Bax AC, Bard DE, Cuffe SP, McKeown RE, Wolraich ML. The association between race/ethnicity and socioeconomic factors and the diagnosis and treatment of children with attention-deficit hyperactivity disorder. *J Dev Behav Pediatr.* 2019;40(2):81–91. doi:10.1097/DBP.0000000000000626

228. Jensen CM, Steinhausen HC. Comorbid mental disorders in children and adolescents with attention-deficit/hyperactivity disorder in a large nationwide study. *Atten Defic Hyperact Disord.* 2015;7(1):27–38. doi:10.1007/s12402-014-0142-1

229. Langley K, Fowler T, Ford T, et al. Adolescent clinical outcomes for young people with attention-deficit hyperactivity disorder. *Br J Psychiatry.* 2010;196(3):235–240. doi:10.1192/bjp.bp.109.066274

230. Chou WJ, Liu TL, Hu HF, Yen CF. Suicidality and its relationships with individual, family, peer, and psychopathology factors among adolescents with attention-deficit/hyperactivity disorder. *Res Dev Disabil.* 2016;53–54:86–94. doi:10.1016/j.ridd.2016.02.001

231. Chang Z, D'Onofrio BM, Quinn PD, Lichtenstein P, Larsson H. Medication for attention-deficit/hyperactivity disorder and risk for depression: a nationwide longitudinal cohort study. *Biol Psychiatry.* 2016;80(12):916–922. doi:10.1016/j.biopsych.2016.02.018

232. Brennan AR, Arnsten AF. Neuronal mechanisms underlying attention deficit hyperactivity disorder: the influence of arousal on prefrontal cortical function. *Ann N Y Acad Sci.* 2008;1129:236–245. doi:10.1196/annals.1417.007

233. Xu G, Strathearn L, Liu B, Yang B, Bao W. Twenty-year trends in diagnosed attention-deficit/hyperactivity disorder among US children and adolescents, 1997–2016. *JAMA Netw Open.* 2018;1(4):e181471. doi:10.1001/jamanetworkopen.2018.1471

234. Global Burden of Disease Collaborators. GBD cause and risk summaries: attention-deficit/hyperactivity disorder. Global Burden of Disease. *Lancet.* 2019. Available at: https://www.thelancet.com/gbd/summaries. Accessed January 27, 2023.

235. Still GF. *The Goulstonian Lectures on Some Abnormal Psychical Conditions in Children.* London, UK: Lancet; 1902.

236. Caye A, Spadini AV, Karam RG, et al. Predictors of persistence of ADHD into adulthood: a systematic review of the literature and meta-analysis. *Eur Child Adolesc Psychiatry.* 2016;25(11):1151–1159. doi:10.1007/s00787-016-0831-8

237. Thapar A, Cooper M, Eyre O, Langley K. What have we learnt about the causes of ADHD? *J Child Psychol Psychiatry.* 2013;54(1):3–16. doi:10.1111/j.1469-7610.2012.02611.x

238. Bastain TM, Lewczyk CM, Sharp WS, et al. Cytogenetic abnormalities in attention-deficit/hyperactivity disorder. *J Am Acad Child Adolesc Psychiatry.* 2002;41(7):806–810. doi:10.1097/00004583-200207000-00012

239. Liu YS, Dai X, Wu W, et al. The association of SNAP25 gene polymorphisms in attention deficit/hyperactivity disorder: a systematic review and meta-analysis. *Mol Neurobiol.* 2017;54(3):2189–2200. doi:10.1007/s12035-016-9810-9

240. LeBlanc KE, Cestia W. Carpal tunnel syndrome. *Am Fam Physician.* 2011;83(8):952–958.

241. Dale AM, Harris-Adamson C, Rempel D, et al. Prevalence and incidence of carpal tunnel syndrome in US working populations: pooled analysis of six prospective studies. *Scand J Work Environ Health.* 2013;39(5):495–505. doi:10.5271/sjweh.3351

242. Atroshi I, Gummesson C, Johnsson R, Ornstein E, Ranstam J, Rosén I. Prevalence of carpal tunnel syndrome in a general population. *JAMA.* 1999;282(2):153–158. doi:10.1001/jama.282.2.153

243. Karjalanen T, Raatikainen S, Jaatinen K, Lusa V. Update on efficacy of conservative treatments for carpal tunnel syndrome. *J Clin Med.* 2022;11(4). doi:10.3390/jcm11040950

244. Trillos-Chacon MC, Castillo MJ, Tolosa-Guzman I, Sanchez Medina AF, Ballesteros SM. Strategies for the prevention of carpal tunnel syndrome in the workplace: a systematic review. *Appl Ergon.* 2021;93:103353. doi:10.1016/j.apergo.2020.103353

245. Hartvigsen J, Hancock MJ, Kongsted A, et al. What low back pain is and why we need to pay attention. *Lancet.* 2018;391(10137):2356–2367. doi:10.1016/S0140-6736(18)30480-X

246. Driscoll T, Jacklyn G, Orchard J, et al. The global burden of occupationally related low back pain: estimates from the Global Burden of Disease 2010 study. *Ann Rheum Dis.* 2014;73(6):975–981. doi:10.1136/annrheumdis-2013-204631

247. Balagué F, Mannion AF, Pellisé F, Cedraschi C. Non-specific low back pain. *Lancet.* 2012;379(9814):482–491. doi:10.1016/S0140-6736(11)60610-7

248. Punnett L, Prüss-Utün A, Nelson DI, et al. Estimating the global burden of low back pain attributable to combined occupational exposures. *Am J Ind Med.* 2005;48(6):459–469. doi:10.1002/ajim.20232

249. Foster NE, Anema JR, Cherkin D, et al. Prevention and treatment of low back pain: evidence, challenges, and promising directions. *Lancet.* 2018;391(10137):2368–2383. doi:10.1016/S0140-6736(18)30489-6

250. Barnes NP. Migraine headache in children. *BMJ Clin Evid.* 2015;2015:0318.

251. Global Burden of Disease Collaborators. GBD cause and risk summaries: headache disorders. *Lancet.* October 2020. Available at: https://www.thelancet.com/pb-assets/Lancet/gbd/summaries/diseases/headache-disorders.pdf. Accessed January 27, 2023.

252. Loder S, Sheikh HU, Loder E. The prevalence, burden, and treatment of severe, frequent, and migraine headaches in US minority populations: statistics from National Survey studies. *Headache.* 2015;55(2):214–228. doi:10.1111/head.12506

253. Charleston L. Headache disparities in African-Americans in the United States: a narrative review. *J Natl Med Assoc.* 2021;113(2):223–229. doi:10.1016/j.jnma.2020.09.148

254. Mack KJ. New daily persistent headache in children and adults. *Curr Pain Headache Rep.* 2009;13(1):47–51. doi:10.1007/s11916-009-0010-4

255. World Health Organization. *Atlas of Headache Disorders and Resources in the World 2011.* Geneva, Switzerland: World Health Organization, 2011.

256. Burch RC, Buse DC, Lipton RB. Migraine: epidemiology, burden, and comorbidity. *Neurol Clin.* 2019;37(4):631–649. doi:10.1016/j.ncl.2019.06.001

257. Headache Classification Committee of the International Headache Society. *The International Classification of Headache Disorders, 3rd edition. Cephalalgia.* 2018;38(1):1–211. doi:10.1177/0333102417738202

258. Ferrante T, Manzoni GC, Russo M, et al. Prevalence of tension-type headache in adult general population: the PACE study and review of the literature. *Neurol Sci.* 2013;34 (suppl 1):S137–S138. doi:10.1007/s10072-013-1370-4

259. Merikangas KR. Contributions of epidemiology to our understanding of migraine. *Headache.* 2013;53(2):230–246. doi:10.1111/head.12038

260. Bigal ME, Lipton RB, Winner P, et al. Migraine in adolescents: association with socioeconomic status and family history. *Neurology.* 2007;69(1):16–25. doi:10.1212/01.wnl.0000265212.90735.64

261. Zaki EA, Freilinger T, Klopstock T, et al. Two common mitochondrial DNA polymorphisms are highly associated with migraine headache and cyclic vomiting syndrome. *Cephalalgia.* 2009;29(7):719–728. doi:10.1111/j.1468-2982.2008.01793.x

262. Jensen R, Stovner LJ. Epidemiology and comorbidity of headache. *Lancet Neurol.* 2008;7(4):354–361. doi:10.1016/S1474-4422(08)70062-0

263. Kelman L. The triggers or precipitants of the acute migraine attack. *Cephalalgia.* 2007;27(5):394–402. doi:10.1111/j.1468-2982.2007.01303.x

264. Hawkes N. Too frequent use of painkillers can cause rather than cure headaches. *BMJ.* 2012;345:e6281. doi:10.1136/bmj.e6281

265. Raucci U, Boni A, Evangelisti M, et al. Lifestyle modifications to help prevent headache at a developmental age. *Front Neurol.* 2020;11:618375. doi:10.3389/fneur.2020.618375

266. Diener HC, Charles A, Goadsby PJ, Holle D. New therapeutic approaches for the prevention and treatment of migraine. *Lancet Neurol.* 2015;14(10):1010–1022. doi:10.1016/S1474-4422(15)00198-2

267. Richer L, Billinghurst L, Linsdell MA, et al. Drugs for the acute treatment of migraine in children and adolescents. *Cochrane Database Syst Rev.* 2016;4:CD005220. doi:10.1002/14651858.CD005220.pub2

268. Smitherman TA, Wells RE, Ford SG. Emerging behavioral treatments for migraine. *Curr Pain Headache Rep.* 2015;19(4):13. doi:10.1007/s11916-015-0486-z

269. Zebenholzer K, Lechner A, Broessner G, et al. Impact of depression and anxiety on burden and management of episodic and chronic headaches—a cross-sectional multicentre study in eight Austrian headache centres. *J Headache Pain.* 2016;17:15. doi:10.1186/s10194-016-0603-3

21

Arthritis and Other Musculoskeletal Diseases

Jon Arnason, MD, Ann Chodara, MD, Shivani Garg, MD, MS,
Karen Hansen, MD, MS, Julie Hildebrand, MD, Tiffany Lin, MD,
and Christie M. Bartels, MD, MS

LEARNING OBJECTIVES

After completing this chapter, readers should be able to

1. Describe the population prevalence and consequences of arthritis, including osteoarthritis as the most common condition.
2. Compare and contrast risk factors for osteoporosis and gout.
3. Characterize sociodemographics, risk factors, and outcomes of key inflammatory arthritis conditions, including rheumatoid arthritis, spondyloarthritis, and lupus.
4. Name primary or secondary intervention strategies to reduce arthritis incidence, prevalence, or arthritis-related disability.

INTRODUCTION

Arthritis and osteoporosis are the most frequent causes of disability among adults in the United States, and the number of adults experiencing activity-limiting arthritis is estimated to increase 50% by 2040.[1–3] Arthritis prevalence has increased for two decades—affecting more than 50% of adults aged 65 years or older.[3] More than 100 diseases make up the spectrum of arthritis and musculoskeletal disorders, with a variety of upstream causes and downstream consequences (Figure 21-1). Many have unknown causes with little proven primary or secondary prevention. However, osteoarthritis (OA) accounts for significant US disability and economic cost and is amenable to primary and secondary prevention, including weight loss and exercise.

About 58.5 million US adults—one in five—reported doctor-diagnosed arthritis,[1,3] and 12 million adults older than 50 years have osteoporosis.[4] More than 25 million adults have arthritis-attributable activity limitations.[1] Three million have self-reported gout (up from an estimated 2.1 million in 1995), and five million have fibromyalgia.[5] The number of US adults with arthritis is expected to rise to 78.4 million (26% of the population) by 2040.[2]

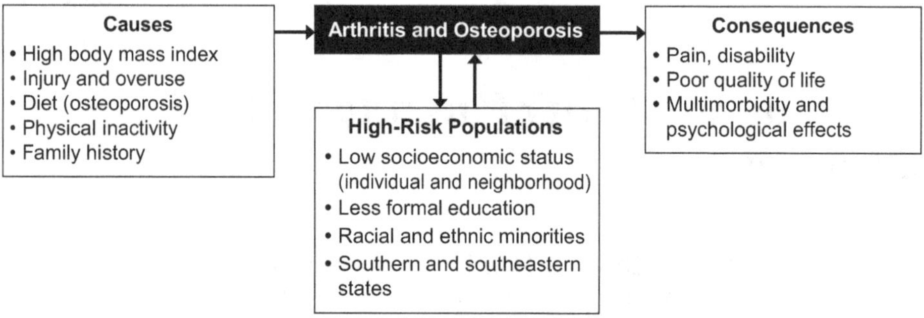

Figure 21-1. Arthritis: Causes, Consequences, and High-Risk Populations

The age- and sex-stratified prevalence of arthritis was estimated from the National Health Interview Survey, which asked, "Have you ever been told by a doctor or other health professional that you have some form of arthritis, rheumatoid arthritis, gout, lupus, or fibromyalgia?"[6] Arthritis prevalence is slightly higher in women than in men and rises with age. By age 65, nearly 50% of adults have doctor-diagnosed arthritis versus 7% of those aged 18 to 44 years (Figure 21-2).[7]

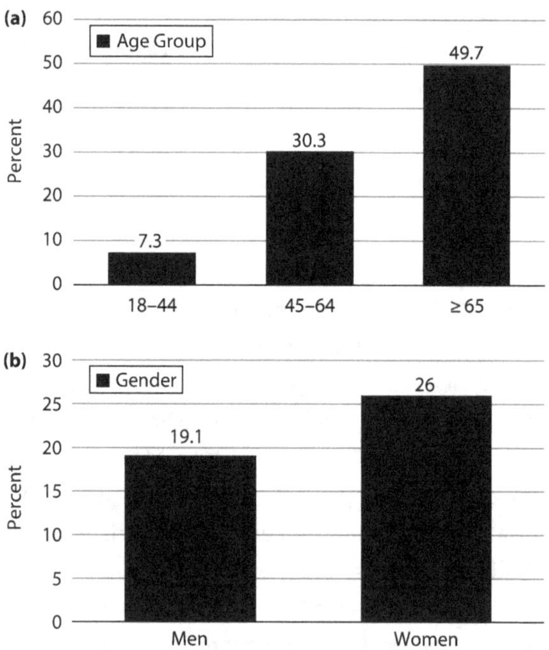

Note: Answered yes to the question, "Have you ever been told by a doctor or other health professional that you have some form of arthritis, rheumatoid arthritis, gout, lupus, or fibromyalgia?"

Figure 21-2. Prevalence of Doctor-Diagnosed Arthritis (a) by Age and (b) by Gender: National Health Interview Survey, United States, 2010–2012

High costs are associated with rising prevalence and incidence of arthritis. US arthritis-related direct and indirect annual costs are over $300 billion,[3] and biologic medications for immune-mediated arthritis equaled approximately 30% of all US prescription expenditures. Total costs for all arthritis conditions were $304 billion, including $164 million in lost wages.[1] The Centers for Disease Control and Prevention (CDC) has taken steps to address the high costs related to arthritis through programs and support at state and national levels.[1] CDC helps fund state health departments to increase physical activity and educational programs with community organizations. Nationally, CDC also partners to increase access to physical activity programs and self-management materials. Specific national organizations include the YMCA (http://www.ymca.net) through its Enhance Fitness program and other initiatives. The National Recreation and Park Association, in concert with CDC and the Arthritis Foundation, promotes programs across 32 states designed to encourage increased activity for all those with arthritis, such as Active Living Every Day, Arthritis Foundation Aquatic Exercise, and Walk With Ease.

This chapter reviews the epidemiology of OA, rheumatoid arthritis (RA), gout, fibromyalgia, osteoporosis, axial spondyloarthritis, and systemic lupus erythematosus (SLE), and describes opportunities for their prevention and control. Although osteoporosis is not a form of arthritis, it is included because of its significant musculoskeletal-related public health burden.

OSTEOARTHRITIS

Osteoarthritis (also known as OA or degenerative joint disease) is a progressive disease characterized by focal loss of articular cartilage with formation of osteophytes, bone remodeling, and loss of function. Osteoarthritis is the most common type of arthritis and the most frequent cause of disability in the United States.[4]

Osteoarthritis is characterized by pain, crepitus, stiffness after immobility, and limitation of movement. It often affects weight-bearing knees and hips, as well as hands, feet, and the spine. The prevalence of OA varies by definition of the disease[8]: radiographic, symptomatic, or self-report.[9] Approximately one-third of people older than 45 years have radiographic evidence of knee OA, and about half of those have symptoms.[10,11] Radiographic imaging findings of OA are not well correlated to symptoms (Figure 21-3). The American College of Rheumatology (ACR) has established definitions and guidelines for hand, hip, and knee OA.[12,13]

Pathophysiology

The pathogenesis of OA is incompletely understood,[14] but it is likely multifactorial, given systemic and local biomechanical factors. Cartilage destruction is a hallmark, specifically the degradation of type II collagen. OA was previously thought to be a noninflammatory

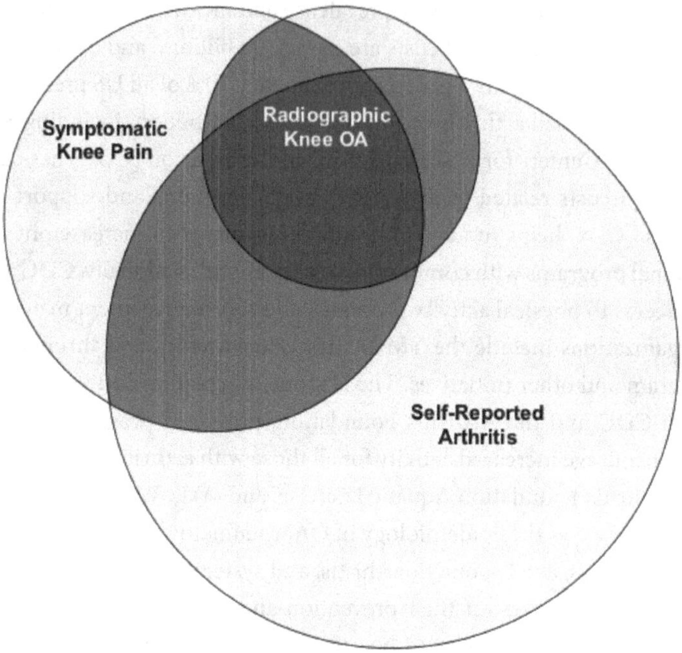

Figure 21-3. Schematic Showing Discordance Between Self-Reported Arthritis, Symptomatic Knee Pain, and Radiographic Knee Osteoarthritis (OA)

arthropathy; however, recent studies have shown activation of some innate immune response in OA joints, with pro-inflammatory cytokines and growth factors and remodeling, including stimulation of matrix metalloproteinases that degrade cartilage.[15] These are potential targets for disease modification in OA, which to date has been limited.

Many propose that specific obesity-related mechanisms lead to OA.[16] These include relative loss of muscle mass and strength, mechanical stress, and systemic inflammation. It is known that obesity causes abnormal joint loading, resulting in adverse changes to the composition, structure, and properties of articular cartilage. Low-grade systemic inflammation is also now considered a hallmark of obesity, resulting in elevations of interleukin (IL)-1ß, IL-6, tumor necrosis factor-alpha (TNF-α), and acute phase reactants C-reactive protein, which might contribute to OA. An overall schematic of upstream and downstream causes and consequences is shown in Figure 21-4.

Public Health Impact

Data from the 2017 Global Burden of Disease study estimate the incidence of hip and knee OA at 195 cases per 100,000. Incidence increases with age, and OA is more common in women. Incidence varies by region and high- and low-income areas, and it is lower in

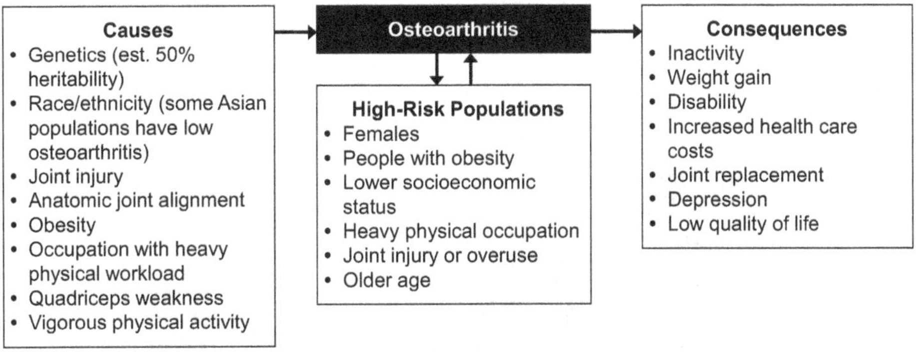

Figure 21-4. Osteoarthritis: Causes, Consequences, and High-Risk Populations

Black than White Americans. One study estimated a one-in-four lifetime risk of developing hip osteoarthritis.[17] Lifetime risk of knee OA is 40% in men and 47% in women.[18]

OA affects an estimated 32.5 million Americans,[4] with 300 million people affected by hip and knee OA globally and rising. OA prevalence increases with age, though reported rates differ between radiographic and symptomatic OA at the hand, hip, and knee.

Through 2014, $65.5 billion per year of medical costs was attributable to OA. In that period, adults with OA earned $4,000 less than counterparts without OA; estimated lost US work earnings totaled $71.3 billion.[2] The burden of disability from knee OA is considered as great as heart disease and is increasing.

Geographic distribution of doctor-diagnosed arthritis is shown in Figure 21-5.[19] Note the southern state predominance.

Time Trends

Over time OA has been increasing. It affected 21 million Americans in 1990, and it now impacts over 32.5 million US adults.[20]

Modifiable Risk Factors

Modifiable risk factors for incident OA include joint injury or overuse, occupations requiring repetitive knee bending and squatting, and overweight/obesity (Table 21-1). In people who are obese or overweight, weight loss is an important factor affecting the mechanical and inflammatory pathways. Every five-point increase in body mass index (BMI) is associated with a 35% increased risk of developing knee OA; this association is stronger for women than men.[21] Studies estimate that 24.6% of all incident knee pain relates to high BMI.[22] The Nurses' Health Study noted those with highest BMI at age 18 had a fivefold increase in hip replacement related to hip OA.[23]

Physical activity is another important modifiable lifestyle risk factor. In adults with knee OA, a dose-response relationship exists between greater levels of physical activity

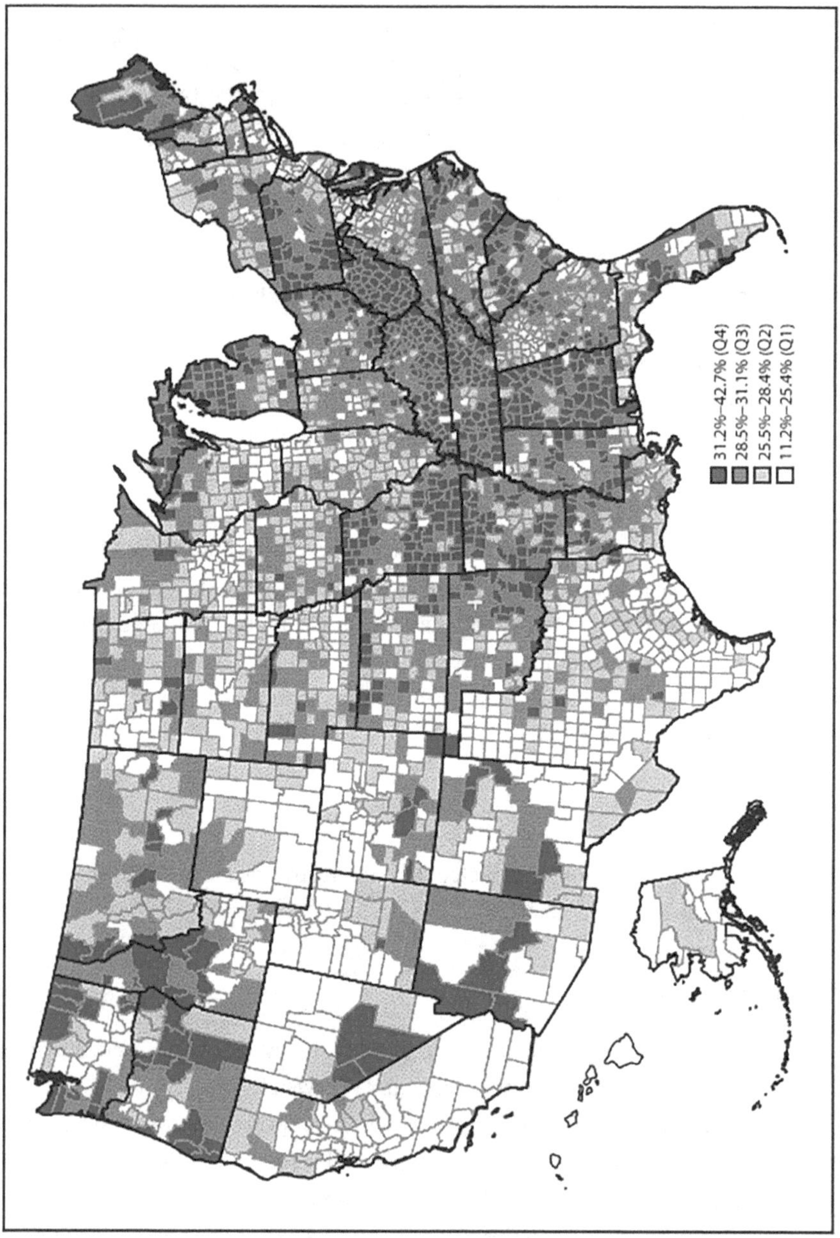

Source: Reprinted from Barbour et al.[19]

Figure 21-5. Variation in Physician-Diagnosed Arthritis Rates by County

Table 21-1. Modifiable Risk Factors for Osteoarthritis in the United States

Magnitude	Risk Factor[a]
Strong (relative risk 4)	Joint trauma
Moderate (relative risk 2–4)	Repetitive occupational usage
	Obesity
Weak (relative risk 2)	Muscle weakness
	Nutritional deficiencies

[a]Risk factors differ in their magnitude based on the osteoarthritis site.

and reduced disability and improved quality of life.[24] Interventions targeting activity may achieve treatment goals of preventing or decreasing damage, reducing pain, and improving function.

The Population Attributable Risk (PAR) of knee OA with elevated BMI and occupational exposure to squatting/kneeling is 4% versus 7% from lifting/carrying loads.[25]

Evidence-Based Interventions

Prevention

Although OA has no cure, managing risk factors is important in slowing progression. Randomized controlled trials have focused on lifestyle changes targeting exercise and diet for primary and secondary prevention of OA. A recent meta-analysis noted that diet and exercise provide moderate pain relief more than diet alone and that these interventions moderately improve physical function.[26]

Considering modifiable risk factors, national public health recommendations include reducing obesity to no more than 15% among adults, increasing the proportion of physically active adults, and reducing injuries, especially work-related injuries.[27]

CDC, in collaboration with the Arthritis Foundation and other partners, released a National Public Health Agenda for Osteoarthritis in 2010 and 2020 to guide governments, organizations, insurers, and others to improve care of osteoarthritis. CDC-recommended evidence-based community programs include the Active Living Everyday, Walk With Ease, Fit & Strong!, Arthritis and Chronic Disease Self-Management, and Arthritis Foundation Aquatics programs.[28]

Screening

Screening and early detection of OA are not feasible at present. Symptomatic patients may require radiographs for diagnosis.

Treatment

The American College of Rheumatology and Arthritis Foundation released clinical practice guidelines for management of hand, hip, and knee osteoarthritis in 2019.[29] These summarize evidence and recommendations for pharmacologic and physical, psychosocial, and mind-body approaches. Strong recommendations are made regarding the role of exercise, orthosis and bracing, self-management programs, weight loss, tai chi, and assistive device use, as well as consideration for oral and topical nonsteroidal anti-inflammatory drugs (NSAIDs) and intra-articular steroids. Other oral and topical pharmacologic treatments are available. Intra-articular hyaluronic acid has conditionally not been recommended because of a lack of evidence.

Physical activity is a non-pharmaceutical treatment for OA. Recommended activities include low-impact weight-bearing exercises such as walking or resistance training, water aerobics, or stationary bicycling. There is currently no evidence to link physical activity with prevention of OA. Research shows light or moderate physical activity does not increase risk of OA. The most effective use of physical activity in the treatment of OA may be to employ it as a rehabilitation tool and as a means to reduce other comorbidities.

A multidisciplinary approach is important for optimal osteoarthritis management. If conservative management is unsuccessful, surgical interventions are available, including bariatric surgery for weight loss and joint replacement for individuals with moderate-to-severe pain and limitations in activities that reduce quality of life. Thigh muscle strength predicted the risk of knee replacement in women, supporting the role of physical therapy and quadriceps strengthening.[30]

Moving Forward

Many nonemergent procedures were delayed during the COVID-19 pandemic, and consequently patients experienced disrupted access to care and lifestyle changes, including decreased physical activity, that affect arthritis. One prospective study noted significant worsening in pain and physical function and decrease in activity in patients who had delayed hip or knee replacement as a result of the lockdown.[31]

Overall, research in OA presently aims to control pain and increase function, though assessing success is challenging because of variation in outcomes reporting. In addition to studying the influence of exercise and diet, researchers continue to investigate the use of intra-articular platelet-rich plasma, mechanical treatments, and procedural options for pain control. Clinical trials have investigated substances that arrest OA progression or reduce pain. There is a need to develop chondroprotective strategies to prevent the occurrence and progression of OA and to develop population-based approaches to address risk factors such as obesity.

RHEUMATOID ARTHRITIS

Rheumatoid arthritis (RA) is a chronic inflammatory autoimmune disease that most notably affects the joints by attacking the joint lining. If untreated, joint inflammation causes painful swelling that can lead to bone erosion and joint deformity. RA can also damage other tissues, including the skin, eyes, lungs, heart, and blood vessels. The disease course can have periods of flares and remission, and the severity of disease varies by individual.

Pathophysiology

RA is a debilitating chronic inflammatory immune disorder with an unknown etiology affecting three women for every man.[32] Autoimmune-mediated joint inflammation causes pain, stiffness, and swelling, which may lead to joint damage, loss of function, and decreased quality of life. The pathophysiology of RA consists of pathways leading to the swelling and breakdown of joints, commonly in the hands and feet. Genetic and environmental interactions in a susceptible host trigger immune dysfunction in the form of "autoimmunity." These autoimmune pathways, which mistakenly target the body's own tissues, trigger an influx of lymphocytes (i.e., T cells and B cells) stimulating the production of cytokines, including TNF-α, IL-1, and IL-6. These inflammatory mediators are overproduced and overexpressed, leading to unremitting inflammation, with subsequent damage to and destruction and disfigurement of the joint.[33] The complex interplay of the immune system results in a variety of white blood cells, synovial fibroblasts, and dendritic cells being involved in the inflammatory and destructive process.

Significance

RA is common, affecting 0.5% to 1% of adults in the United States. The disease can have a significant negative impact on ability to work and perform activities of daily living. Historically, RA decreased an individual's life expectancy by ten years[34]; however, recent studies show improving survival rates, attributed to advances in treatment of rheumatoid arthritis and associated comorbid conditions.[35,36] See Figure 21-6, which illustrates causes, consequences, and at-risk populations.

In 2020 a meta-analysis determined the annual combined direct and indirect costs of rheumatoid arthritis per patient to range between $2,408 to $83,845 in US dollars, with increased medication cost for biologic therapies the largest contributor to cost.[37] Of note, cost of hospitalizations trended lower.[38] The authors estimated intangible costs of quality-of-life deterioration at $10.3 billion and premature mortality at $9.6 billion.[39] The indirect cost of RA from loss of work and productivity has been estimated as nearly three times greater than the cost of treating the disease.[40]

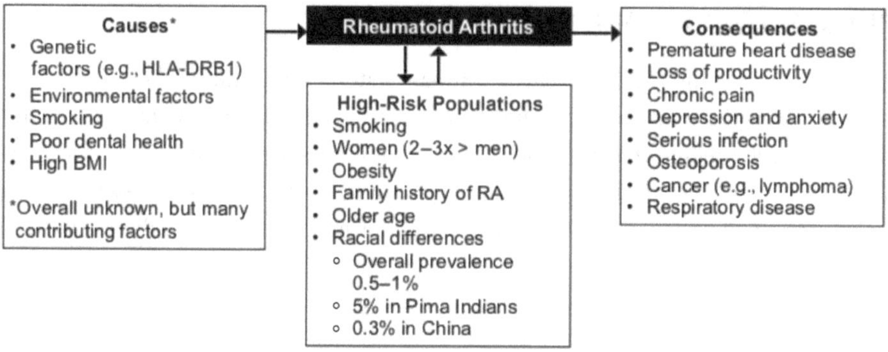

Note: BMI = body mass index; HLA-DRB1 = shared epitope; RA = rheumatoid arthritis.

Figure 21-6. Rheumatoid Arthritis: Causes, Consequences, and High-Risk Populations

Public Health Impact

RA is a chronic inflammatory disease, marked by episodes of disease flares and long-term inflammation. Sustained remission generally requires long-term immunosuppressive medications. As a result, patients with RA may be more likely to experience chronic pain, loss of productivity, and depression and anxiety, particularly in patients at lower socioeconomic levels.[41] High RA disease activity is also associated with an increased risk of infection, osteoporosis, interstitial lung disease, cardiovascular disease, and certain malignancies.[42,43] Patients with RA have a higher mortality rate than the general population, with cardiovascular disease the most frequent cause of death.[44] Patients with RA are at high risk for many comorbid conditions, due to a combination of chronic inflammation, immune system dysfunction, and immunosuppression, as well as higher rates of smoking, obesity, and other factors. Historically, mortality has been up to 50% higher in RA compared with the general population, but more recent studies suggest improvements, likely reflecting the impact of advances in diagnosis and improvements in treatment.[35,36]

Descriptive Epidemiology

RA is the most common form of inflammatory arthritis worldwide with a prevalence typically ranging from 0.5% to 1.0%, and US prevalence of 1.1%.[45] Pima Indians (5.3%) and Chippewa Indians (6.8%) carry a higher risk.[46] RA disproportionately affects women, who have a two- to threefold risk compared with men; women older than 65 years of age have the highest prevalence of RA.[47] Typical onset for both men and women occurs between the ages of 30 and 50 years.[47] Those identified as overweight or obese have a 35% increased risk of developing RA at 18 years of age and a nearly 50% increased risk as an adult. Women with a history of ten cumulative years of obesity have a 37% increased risk of developing RA at a younger age.[48] Significant disparities exist in risk for rheumatoid arthritis, with higher risk in non-Hispanics and Blacks and people with lower socioeconomic status, and lower risk with higher education levels.[40]

Geographic Distribution

The geographic distribution of RA is highly variable. Prevalence of RA is greater in more industrialized countries, such as in Northern Europe and North America. This geographic variability most likely points to genetic differences and environmental exposures.[32] The varying prevalence may be partially attributable to urbanization.[49] RA is difficult to control, with only 75% to 80% of patients in the industrialized world (and a much lower percentage of patients in underdeveloped countries) attaining the treatment goal of low disease activity or remission.[50]

Time Trends

An overall decrease in RA incidence has been observed over the past four decades.[51] In the disease course of RA over the past decade, trends have shown a decrease in RA activity from a high to a moderate level, presumably attributable to clinicians implementing more modern and aggressive treatment methods.[52,53] Over the past twenty years the long-term prognosis for RA patients has improved, which is also attributed to earlier diagnosis and improved treatment approaches.[54]

Causes

Although the precise etiology of RA remains largely unknown, current research points to many contributors, including genetic susceptibilities and environmental exposures as key factors related to the development and severity of RA.[55] Genetic factors, including a genetic risk marker called the shared epitope (HLA–DRB1), may contribute as much as 50% to 60% to the development of RA in the general population.[32,56] A family history of RA increases an individual's risk three- to ninefold.[57] The remaining contributions are believed to come from modifiable, environmental risk factors.

Modifiable Risk Factors

Modifiable risk factors, such as smoking, increase risk for developing RA or promote progression of RA and are amenable to change. Those who smoke are twice as likely to develop RA as nonsmokers and are much more likely with both smoking and the shared epitope.[55,57] The combination of smoking and being overweight also increases an RA-prone individual's arthritis risk 60%, highlighting more gene–environment interactions.[55] Poor oral health, possibly related to the presence of specific bacteria and epigenetic citrullination, may have a role in the development of RA.[58] Many other factors remain under investigation.

Evidence-Based Interventions

Prevention

Early screening and aggressive treatment hold promise to reduce long-term disease burden.[59,60] There is a period during development of RA without clinical RA but with elevated disease-related biomarkers and autoantibodies.[61] This has been termed preclinical RA. Identifying individuals at risk for RA allows preclinical interventions and possibly better outcomes.[57] Furthermore, reducing the number of ever-smokers may reduce rates of RA incidence and prevalence. High BMI may predict worse RA response, and intervention focusing on diet may possibly have a long-term effect in the development and pathway of RA.[32]

Screening

No clear-cut, cost-effective, presymptomatic screening tool is recommended for RA detection; however, early identification at the onset of RA symptoms leads to more effective treatment and positive outcomes.[57] Some investigators are testing identifying a high-risk group with a high probability of developing clinical RA to treat them to prevent onset of the disease (NIH Clinical Trial NCT02603146, completion est. 2023).[62] Once clinical symptoms are present, usual RA screening tests include bilateral hand and foot X-rays, rheumatoid factor and cyclic citrullinated peptide antibody testing, and inflammatory markers.

Treatment

Our ability to treat RA has changed dramatically over the past twenty years, first with the advent of new oral disease-modifying antirheumatic drugs (DMARDs). More recently the development of biologic agents and targeted synthetic DMARD agents has further advanced treatment options for RA. The ACR guidelines recommend starting treatment early, with the ideal approach involving a treat-to-target approach with the goal of achieving low disease activity.[58]

Pharmacotherapy at the onset of symptoms with analgesics and NSAIDs improves function, reduces pain, and lessens stiffness. In both early and established RA, a common treatment approach is the use of traditional DMARDs (i.e., methotrexate, sulfasalazine, and leflunomide).[32] This reduces the disease activity of RA, allowing many individuals with RA to achieve remission and minimize joint damage and deformity.[60] Second-line biologic agents (like tumor necrosis factor inhibitors and other cytokine inhibitors) and targeted synthetic DMARD agents such as JAK inhibitors block immune system signals involved in the inflammatory process, reducing damage to the joints. These agents have substantially reduced joint destruction, deformity, functional limitation, and disability in a way that was unimaginable 20 years ago. Often, prednisone or intramuscular steroids can help until the other therapy (such as a DMARD) becomes effective, though long-term use is discouraged. Biologic and targeted synthetic DMARD agents have improved control of RA; however, many of these agents are associated with increased risk for infection and other side effects. The 2021 ACR guideline for the treatment of RA provides detailed recommendations for the management of rheumatoid arthritis.[58]

As a nondrug therapy, physical activity can reduce the impact of RA on symptoms.[32,63] Physical therapy with the goal of aerobic fitness and muscle strengthening has been shown to be safe and effective in RA patients, without evidence of joint or bone damage related to the prescribed exercise regimen.[64]

Moving Forward

Research clarifying RA pathophysiology will provide a better understanding of which pharmacologic agents to use to tailor patient-specific treatment plans. In patients with rheumatoid arthritis, glucocorticoid therapy has been associated with worse outcomes from COVID-19 infection. Adverse outcomes from COVID-19 infection were not seen in association with other pharmacologic agents used for treatment of RA, though many restricted activity to avoid risk resulting from immunosuppression.[65] Identifying more biomarkers for prognosis and flare could guide treatment decisions. Health disparities should also be addressed, from diagnosing to delivering optimal care to patients of lower socioeconomic status and in less affluent countries. Further studies need to address the risks and cost-effectiveness of treatments, including the appropriate use of biologic and targeted synthetic DMARD treatment for advanced and moderate RA patients.

Improved pharmacologic and nonpharmacologic therapies, along with continued research on RA etiology, will help the mission for remission in RA disease. Innovation and improved understanding may ultimately provide a long-term cure. Similarly, advances in the field may make it possible to intervene and prevent development of rheumatoid arthritis.

CRYSTAL ARTHROPATHIES

Crystal deposits are a common cause of inflammatory arthritis. Gout, for example, is attributable to uric acid crystals, and calcium pyrophosphate and basic calcium phosphate deposits can also cause inflammation. Although clinical manifestations vary, the crystals induce inflammation in a similar manner by being taken up by macrophages, where they activate the NPLR3 inflammasome, a part of the innate immune system.[66] A definitive diagnosis of gout and calcium pyrophosphate deposition (CPPD) usually requires an examination of aspirated material with a polarized microscope. Radiographs are not sensitive or specific, but ultrasound and dual-energy

CT have a higher specificity.[67] If those diagnostics are not available, algorithms can help make a provisional diagnosis.

Gout

Gout has been known since antiquity and has historically been associated with affluence, given dietary and metabolic risks. Acute gout most often involves the first metatarsophalangeal joint and causes severe pain and swelling, but polyarticular inflammation and a more chronic tophaceous gout, with uric acid aggregates called tophi, are also common.[68]

Significance

Gout is possibly the most common inflammatory arthritis worldwide. It can lead to irreversible joint damage if untreated.

Pathophysiology

Uric acid is the final product of purine metabolism in primates, who unlike other mammals lack uricase, which converts uric acid to more soluble metabolites. Among primates, only humans get gout, probably related to diet. Hyperuricemia, serum uric acid concentration of greater than 6.5 mg/dL, can be caused either by increased urate production or decreased renal excretion and may lead to the crystallization of monosodium urate, which can trigger acute gout or form tophi.

Descriptive Epidemiology

Gout is common worldwide, with an incidence in 2017 of 0.097% and prevalence of 0.54%.[69] National Health and Nutrition Examination Survey data estimate the US prevalence of gout between 2015 and 2016 as 3.9% among adults; 5.2% in men and 2.7% in women,[70] and 4.8% in Black patients and 4.0% in White.[71]

The Framingham Heart Study reported a US gout incidence of 1.4 per 1,000 person-years in women and 4.0 per 1,000 person-years in men.[72] The incidence of gout is increased in the United States, Scandinavian countries, and South Korea. The incidence of gout increases with age and is higher in men than in women, who have lower incidence until after menopause.[73]

High-Risk Populations

Not every person with hyperuricemia develops gout, but elevated serum uric acid levels are associated with increased risk of incident and recurrent gout.[74] Risk factors for hyperuricemia include decreased renal clearance of uric acid (which is genetically determined), inborn metabolic errors, male gender, alcohol consumption, diet excessive in meat, seafood, and fructose-sweetened beverages, lead exposure, and certain medications, especially some diuretics.[73] There is a linear trend of increasing prevalence of gout with increasing BMI.[75] Hyperuricemia can also be regarded as a manifestation of the metabolic syndrome, along with obesity, hyperlipidemia, and hypertension. Accordingly, there is an association with cardiovascular disorders, erectile dysfunction, atrial fibrillation, obstructive sleep apnea, and venous thromboembolism.

Genome-wide and targeted sequencing has identified numerous genes associated with urate levels and risk of gout, including genes encoding proteins of the NLRP3 inflammasome and transmembrane urate transporters in the kidneys, gut, and liver.[76]

Geographic Distribution

The prevalence of gout in the United States and Europe is 3% to 4% of adults but possibly lower in Scandinavian populations; it varies among Asian countries with 1.13% in China, but it is increasing there and in South Korea. The highest prevalence, greater than 10%, has been reported in some Oceanic ethnic groups.[73]

Modifiable Risk Factors

Modifiable risk factors include obesity, diet of purine-rich food such as meat, high-fructose beverages, excessive alcohol intake, and lead exposure.

Evidence-Based Interventions

Prevention

Primary prevention includes lifestyle modifications such as weight reduction and diet modification. Various diets have been studied for their impact on uric acid and the incidence of gout.[77] This includes Mediterranean, DASH, low purine, and weight loss diets as well as specific food items such as coffee and cherries. Foods may influence uric acid but have a small effect on the incidence of gout. A weight loss diet is recommended for those who are obese, and everyone with hyperuricemia and gout should limit their intake of meat, fructose-sweetened beverages, and alcohol. A study of over 50,000 male health professionals estimated that more than half of incident gout cases were prevented by the combination of DASH-style diet, no alcohol intake, and no diuretic use.[78] Limiting lead exposure is also important for those in high-risk occupations.

Treatment

Treatment guidelines for gout are updated regularly.[79] Acute gout can be treated with colchicine or NSAIDs, but for those who are unable to take or tolerate those medications, steroids can be used, either oral, intramuscular, or intraarticular.

While asymptomatic hyperuricemia may not need treatment, uric acid lowering with allopurinol, a xanthine oxidase inhibitor, is recommended for those with tophaceous gout, joint damage, or frequent acute gout attacks. The dose should be adjusted over time to bring the serum uric acid below 6 mg/dL. Patients of Southeast Asian and African descent should be screened for the HLA–B*5801 allele prior to starting allopurinol, as it confers higher risk of cutaneous reactions. Febuxostat can be used for those who cannot tolerate allopurinol, but it may be associated with increased risk of cardiovascular events. Severe tophaceous gout that does not respond to other means may be treated with pegloticase, a recombinant uricase.

Recurrent attacks of gout can continue while uric acid is being lowered below the target of 6 mg/dL or amid tophi. The risk of acute attacks is reduced if colchicine or NSAIDs are taken along with the uric acid lowering medication until reaching targets.

Calcium Pyrophosphate Deposition

In calcium pyrophosphate deposition (CPPD), which was first described in the 1960s, calcium pyrophosphate crystals form within cartilage. It is often asymptomatic but can also cause chronic arthritis with acute flares resembling gout, sometimes called pseudogout. It most often involves knees and wrists but can affect any joint, including the spine.

In CPPD there are abnormalities of cartilage pyrophosphate metabolism. Mutations of the Ankh gene, which encodes protein of a transmembrane phosphate transporter, and the TNFRSF11B gene, which plays a role in bone cell regulation, have been associated with CPPD.[80]

CPPD prevalence increases with age and is often found incidentally on radiographs as chondrocalcinosis. It is associated with osteoarthritis, low BMI, low cortical bone density, metabolic conditions such as hyperparathyroidism, hemochromatosis, and hypophosphatasia in addition to abnormalities in renal handling of phosphate and magnesium.[81] Classification criteria have been proposed to facilitate further epidemiologic research.[82]

Acute CPPD is treated similarly to gout, but in chronic disease, hydroxychloroquine, colchicine, and agents typically used for rheumatoid arthritis are tried, with variable success.[83]

Basic Calcium Phosphate Deposition

Basic calcium phosphate deposition, which includes calcium hydroxyapatite, can cause inflammation.[84] The epidemiology of this condition is less well known than gout, but common manifestations include soft tissue inflammation with chronic or acute calcific tendinitis or periarthritis and rare destructive arthritis such as Milwaukee shoulder. Currently, like CPPD, there are no recommendations for prevention, and treatment is limited to NSAIDs and steroids.

FIBROMYALGIA

Fibromyalgia is a common syndrome of chronic, widespread pain, fatigue, sleep disturbances, and often cognitive and somatic symptoms.[85,86] The pain is diffuse and sometimes involves the entire body. The fatigue of fibromyalgia is both physical and mental, affecting concentration and thinking, termed fibro-fog.

The diagnosis of fibromyalgia is clinical, aided by diagnostic criteria. The revised 2010 ACR criteria from 2016, and the more recent collaborative American Pain Society criteria differ in some ways, but both consider fibromyalgia a disorder of generalized pain along with somatic and cognitive symptoms. Soft tissue tenderness is common in fibromyalgia but is no longer required for diagnosis.[87,88]

Fibromyalgia often coexists with other painful conditions, including arthritis and autoimmune diseases. It can also be regarded as one of several central sensitivity syndromes, along with chronic fatigue syndrome, interstitial cystitis, irritable bowel syndrome, temporomandibular joint dysfunction, myalgic encephalopathy, and autonomic dysfunction, among others.[89]

Significance

Fibromyalgia may mimic other conditions and often goes undiagnosed. Patients make frequent health care visits and undergo numerous diagnostic tests. Since fibromyalgia often accompanies other painful conditions and mental health problems such as depression, it is important to distinguish from a coexisting illness and treat accordingly. Fibromyalgia is a common cause of work disability, and thus maintaining physical function is important.[90]

Pathophysiology

The cause of fibromyalgia is unknown. but there is evidence for alterations in central nervous system pain and sensory processing.[91] Patients with fibromyalgia sense stimuli such as heat, cold, and pressure at the same level as those without the condition but are more likely to report the sensation as painful. In addition, such patients have hyperalgesia and allodynia, suggesting altered sensory processing, centrally or in peripheral nociceptors. Stress and psychologic trauma increase the risk of fibromyalgia, and chronic inflammation may also contribute. Sleep disturbance may play a central role in the pathophysiology.[92]

Descriptive Epidemiology

The prevalence of fibromyalgia according to the modified 2010 ACR criteria was 5.4% with a ratio of females to males of 2.3:1.[93] The prevalence may be higher in some subgroups, such as in patients with other painful conditions, depression, and anxiety or other rheumatic conditions.

High-Risk Populations

Fibromyalgia is more common in women than in men, and is found among those who suffer from other painful conditions, as well as infections, psychological conditions such as anxiety or depression, and distress following catastrophic events.[85]

Causes

No fibromyalgia-specific genes have been identified, but several candidate genes have been proposed, many of which are expressed in the central nervous system and have a role in pain perception and neuronal differentiation. Epigenetic factors may also be relevant, as fibromyalgia may have a hypomethylated DNA pattern in genes implicated in stress response, autonomic system response, and subcortical neuronal abnormalities.[94]

Modifiable Risk Factors

Women who sleep poorly are more likely to develop fibromyalgia than those who sleep well. Regular physical activity is also protective.[95] Prompt treatment of painful conditions may also reduce the risk of progression to fibromyalgia. Fibromyalgia is more common in obese people.

Evidence-Based Interventions

Prevention

Treating other painful conditions, disrupted sleep, depression, anxiety, and obesity may reduce the risk of progression to fibromyalgia, but since there is currently insufficient understanding of the pathogenesis of fibromyalgia, no specific means of prevention are universally agreed upon.

Treatment

Fibromyalgia is a complicated disease with physical, psychological, and social components. No single treatment leads to full resolution of all symptoms; thus, a combination of treatments is needed. Evidence- and expert opinion-based guidelines recommend patient education, psychological therapies for mood disorders and to improve coping ability, pharmacotherapy, and a multimodal rehabilitation program.[96] If there is a concurrent painful condition, such as arthritis, it should be treated, and efforts should be made to improve sleep quality, increase physical activity, and promote good diet and healthy lifestyle. Those who are unable to exercise on their own benefit from the supervision of experienced trainers.

Although many medications have been tried for fibromyalgia, only a few have been found to be helpful. Those include medications classified as antidepressants or antiepileptic medications. Pain medications do not help, and opiates should be avoided. Local therapies and complementary and alternative medicine such as special diets, acupuncture, manual therapies, transcranial electromagnetic treatment, cannabinoids, and Naltrexone (an opiate antagonist) have been used with varying success.[86]

AXIAL SPONDYLOARTHRITIS

The axial spondyloarthritides are a family of autoinflammatory conditions that involve the spine and sacroiliac joints. They include ankylosing spondylitis, psoriatic arthritis, inflammatory bowel disease–associated arthritis, and reactive arthritis. These conditions cause inflammation in the axial skeleton, including the spine and sacroiliac joints, which results in fatigue, pain, and stiffness. These conditions may also result in peripheral arthritis, enthesitis (inflammation of insertion sites where tendon or ligament meets bone), and non-joint extra-articular features such as uveitis (inflammation of the middle layer of the eye), psoriasis, and inflammatory bowel disease.[97]

Figure 21-7 shows the Assessment of Spondyloarthritis International Society's 2009 Axial Spondyloarthritis Classification Criteria, which is a useful framework when considering a diagnosis of axial spondyloarthritis.[96] Subtypes of spondyloarthritis are shown in Figure 21-8.

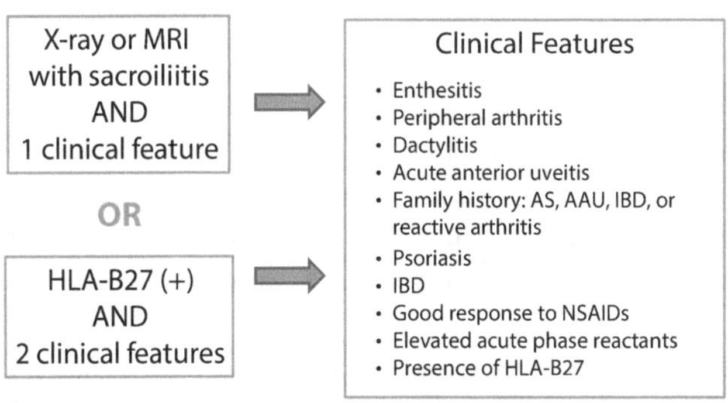

Source: Based on Rudwaleit et al.[98]

Note: AAU = acute anterior uveitis; AS = axial spondyloarthritis; IBD = inflammatory bowel disease; MRI = magnetic resonance imaging; NSAID = nonsteroidal anti-inflammatory drug.

[a]Presence of inflammatory back pain for ≥3 months with age of onset <45 years.

Figure 21-7. 2009 ASAS Axial Spondyloarthritis Classification Criteria

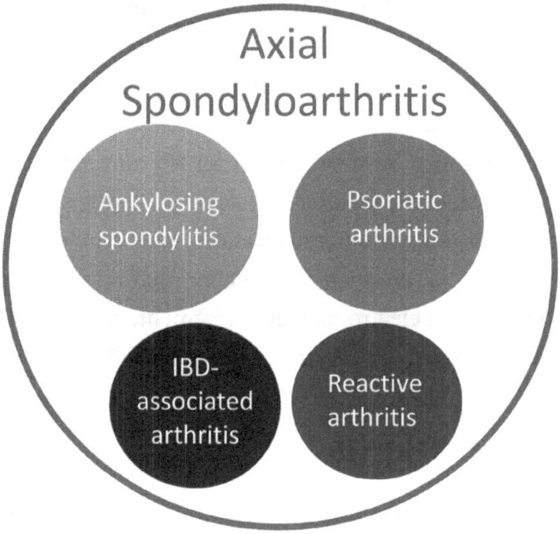

Note: IBD = inflammatory bowel disease. IBD can include conditions such as Crohn's disease or ulcerative colitis.

Figure 21-8. Types of Spondyloarthritis

Significance

The prevalence of axial spondyloarthritis is 0.9% to 1.4% in the United States,[99] with no statistically significant sex differences. Untreated, these diseases can result in structural and functional impairments and a decreased quality of life. Heart conduction disturbances, osteoporosis and vertebral fractures, and aortic insufficiency may occur as complications of the disease. Because of the inflammatory nature of this condition, patients are also at greater risk for cardiovascular disease.

Pathophysiology

The most common symptom of axial spondyloarthritis is an insidious onset of low back pain. Patients may gradually develop ankylosis (abnormal stiffening and immobility of a joint from fusion of the bones) at the entheses, which is the location where ligaments, tendons, and capsules are attached to the bone. Processes involving affected entheses are inflammation, bone erosion, and syndesmophyte (spur) formation. In contrast to RA and lupus, dysregulation of the innate immune system is believed to play a large role in the pathogenesis of this condition. Tumor necrosis factor, interleukin-17, and interleukin-22 are important mediators of inflammation.[100] Interleukin-22 also appears to play a role in bone proliferation.[100] In patients with reactive arthritis, cross-reactivity against enteric and genitourinary organisms is believed to drive the inflammatory process, though triggers are unclear in many spondyloarthritis cases.

Descriptive Epidemiology

High-Risk Populations

Axial spondyloarthritis is a polygenic disease. The strongest risk factor is HLA-B27. While the frequency of HLA-B27 varies by specific disease, it is most commonly seen in 90% of ankylosing spondylitis cases, although only 5% to 6% of individuals with HLA-B27 develop ankylosing spondylitis. Twin studies suggest ankylosing spondylitis has over 90% heritability. Genome-wide association studies have identified many other genes that contribute in smaller magnitudes to the risk of developing axial spondyloarthritis.[97]

Geographic Distribution

Very little information on geographic distribution of spondyloarthritis exists, as most data are specific to ankylosing spondylitis. A systematic literature review on ankylosing spondylitis found a prevalence per 10,000 of 31.9 in North America, 23.8 in Europe, 16.7 in Asia, 10.2 in Latin America, and 7.4 in Africa.[101] Incidence of ankylosing spondylitis reflects the prevalence of HLA-B27 seropositivity. HLA-B27 is highly prevalent in the circumpolar Arctic and the sub-Arctic regions of Eurasia, North America, and some parts of Melanesia. It is very high in some North American Indian populations.[102] HLA-B27 is rare among the genetically unmixed native populations of South America, Australia, and certain parts of equatorial and southern Africa.[103]

Evidence-Based Interventions

Prevention

There is no known primary prevention for axial spondyloarthritis. Secondary prevention includes NSAIDs and immunosuppressive therapies to control inflammation; physical activity; and management of traditional cardiovascular risk factors, including hypertension, hyperlipidemia, diabetes mellitus, and tobacco use, to reduce the risk of myocardial infarction and stroke.

Screening

The presence of four of five inflammatory back pain symptoms (details in Figure 21-9), with morning stiffness and improvement with activity, is 77% sensitive for axial spondyloarthritis.[104] A musculoskeletal examination may reveal spinal and sacroiliac joint tenderness with abnormal occiput to wall and modified Schober's tests.

Inflammatory markers are elevated in only 50% of patients, and HLA-B27 may be positive. X-rays, particularly of the sacroiliac joints and spine, can detect structural changes such as joint erosion and bone sclerosis at a late stage of disease. However, structural X-ray

1. Age of onset: <40 y
2. Insidious onset
3. Improvement with exercise
4. No improvement with rest
5. Pain at night

4/5 criteria indicates IBP
(77% sensitivity, 91.7% specificity)

Additional features:
Morning stiffness >30 min, alternating buttock pain, response to NSAIDs

Note: NSAIDs = non steroidal anti-inflammatory drugs.
Source: Based on Sieper et al.[104]

Figure 21-9. Inflammatory Back Pain (IBP) Features

changes may not be evident early. Magnetic resonance imaging is useful in this setting to visualize synovitis within the sacroiliac joint, and subchondral bone edema.

Treatment

There is no cure for axial spondyloarthritis. Treatment is aimed at relieving pain, stiffness, and fatigue and reducing and preventing structural damage. Active physical therapy is recommended for all patients to maintain function and mobility. NSAIDs are first-line pharmacotherapy. DMARDs, then biologics, may be considered in patients with predominantly peripheral arthritis that has not responded to NSAIDs.[105] Evidence-based guidelines recommend: physical therapy, NSAIDs, DMARDs, local glucocorticoid injections in certain situations, TNF inhibitors, IL-17 inhibitors, and JAK inhibitors as outlined in the 2019 update of the American College of Rheumatology/Spondylitis Association of America/Spondyloarthritis Research and Treatment Network Recommendations for the Treatment of Ankylosing Spondylitis and Nonradiographic Axial Spondyloarthritis.[105]

Moving Forward

Magnetic resonance imaging protocols need to be further refined to increase their diagnostic sensitivity and specificity. In addition, it remains unclear whether inclusion of magnetic resonance imaging of the spine may increase sensitivity for diagnosis. Likewise, selection of treatments can be difficult. Finally, nonradiographic axial spondyloarthritis requires further study to determine if individuals with this condition have a distinctly different profile with regard to prognosis and disease progression that would inform clinical management.

OSTEOPOROSIS

Significance

Osteoporosis is the most common human bone disease. For epidemiologic studies, the World Health Organization defines osteoporosis as a femoral neck or total hip bone mineral density value measured 2.5 standard deviations at or below the mean for normal young White women. National Health and Nutrition Examination Survey data estimated that 12 million people aged 50 years or older in the United States (5.1% in men; 16.5% in women) had osteoporosis.[4] The US Preventive Services Task Force (USPSTF) estimates that 71% of women will sustain osteoporotic fractures in their lifetime.[106] The costs of osteoporosis care in the United States are projected to exceed $25 billion by 2025.[107]

Pathophysiology

Osteoporosis is often defined as a systemic skeletal disorder characterized by microarchitectural deterioration of bone tissue, increased bone fragility, and susceptibility to fracture. Bone density is measured in grams of mineral per area or volume, and bone quality refers to architecture, turnover, damage accumulation (e.g., micro-fractures), and mineralization.

The pathogenesis of osteoporosis is complex and involves the interplay between genetics, hormones, nutrition, lifestyle, and environmental factors. Bone mineral density in adulthood is largely determined by the amount of bone accrued by early to middle adult life, but also taken into account is the rate of decline in bone mass during middle to late adult life. The usual clinical manifestation of osteoporosis is low-trauma fractures of the spine, hip, wrist, or other skeletal regions. In older adults virtually all low-trauma fractures (except digits, face, and skull) are related to osteoporosis.[108] Many epidemiologic studies have used fracture as a measure of osteoporosis, given the lack of access to technology to measure bone mineral density. However, the availability of dual-energy X-ray absorptiometry (DXA) for measurement of bone mineral density has allowed for the study of factors related to low bone mineral density.

Descriptive Epidemiology

High-Risk Populations

Osteoporosis is often considered a disease of postmenopausal women. Peak bone mass, usually achieved in the third decade, is lower in women than in men. Bone mass

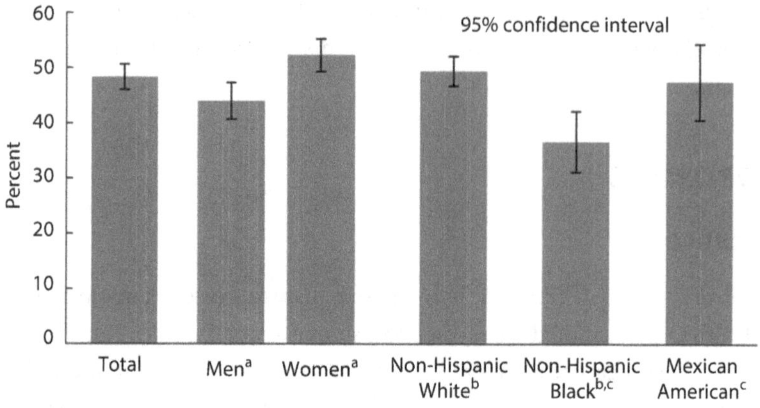

Source: Reprinted from Looker and Frenk.[110]

Note: Age-adjusted by the direct method to the year 2000 US Census Bureau estimates using age groups 65–79 and 80 and over. World Health Organization diagnostic criteria were used to define osteoporosis as a bone mineral density (BMD) value at the femur neck or lumbar spine that falls more than 2.5 standard deviation units below the mean BMD for young non-Hispanic White females. BMD at the femur neck and lumbar spine was measured using dual-energy X-ray absorptiometry (DXA).

[a]Significant difference between men and women, (p <0.05).

[b]Significant difference between non-Hispanic White and non-Hispanic Black, (p <0.05).

[c]Significant difference between non-Hispanic White and Mexican American, (p <0.05).

[d]Significant difference between non-Hispanic Black and Mexican American, (p <0.05).

Figure 21-10. Age-Adjusted Percentage of Adults 65 Years and Over With Low Bone Mass at the Femur Neck or Lumbar Spine, by Sex, Race, and Hispanic Origin: United States, 2005–2010

begins to decline in the fourth decade of life, by 0.5% to 1.0% per year. Accelerated loss occurs during the menopausal transition. Not surprisingly, women have a higher prevalence of osteoporosis than men (Figure 21-10).[109,110] Consequently, age-specific incidence rates for hip fracture are higher among women than men through the ninth decade.

In the West, Hispanic and White populations have lower bone mineral density, a higher prevalence of osteoporosis and fracture, and a greater rate of decline in bone mineral density than Black populations.[109] Risk of fragility fracture by sex, age, and race/ethnicity shows highest risk in women, persons older than 80 years, and Non-Hispanic Whites, respectively.[111]

Twin and family studies suggest that genetic factors may explain as much as 85% of the variation in age-specific bone mineral density in the population.[112] Genetics play the largest role in peak bone mass and also play a role in the rate of bone loss with aging. In genome-wide association studies, hundreds of associations with osteoporosis were identified including genes that regulate osteoclasts (RANKL, OPG, and RANK). Other genes affect calcium metabolism and the estrogen receptor gene.[113] A combination of genomic, transcriptomic, proteomic, and metabolomic research approaches will be needed to unravel the hundreds of genome-wide association studies ostensibly linked to osteoporosis.[114]

Clinical factors associated with a high risk for osteoporosis and subsequent fractures include older age, low body weight, weight loss, physical inactivity, a low-trauma fracture at or after age 50, current smoking, excessive alcohol consumption, and recent systemic glucocorticoids.[115]

Modifiable Risk Factors

A number of lifestyle factors, diseases, and medications are associated with osteoporosis and consequent fractures (Table 21-2).[115] Although most of these are associated with osteoporosis as defined by low bone mineral density, some are associated only with osteoporotic fractures because of their relationship with falls (e.g., reduced visual acuity, Parkinson's disease, excessive alcohol consumption). Risk factors for osteoporosis may reduce peak bone mass and strength during growth and development (e.g., anorexia), increase bone resorption (e.g., menopause), or decrease bone formation (e.g., glucocorticoids). Recent studies have identified the molecular mechanisms involved in regulation of osteoclast and osteoblast development and function; these are the cells that are responsible for bone resorption and formation, respectively.[116]

The Fracture Risk Assessment Tool (FRAX) is an online calculator that incorporates risk factors that can, in combination with bone mineral density, predict a person's ten-year absolute risk for osteoporotic fracture.[117,118] The risk factors within FRAX were derived from a series of meta-analyses of data obtained from population-based longitudinal cohort studies with fracture outcomes. FRAX risk factors include age, sex, race, height, weight, low-trauma fracture after age 50, parental history of hip fracture, smoking, use of glucocorticoids, excessive alcohol intake, and presence of RA as a prototype chronic systemic inflammatory disease.

Table 21-2. Modifiable Risk Factors for Osteoporosis and Osteoporotic Fractures

Magnitude	Risk Factor
Strong (relative risk >4)	Immobility Low body weight and weight loss Current or recent use of glucocorticoids
Moderate (relative risk 2–4)	Current smoking Excessive alcohol intake Low calcium intake or low sunlight exposure
Weak (relative risk <2)	Current use of antidepressants Current use of proton-pump inhibitors

Evidence-Based Interventions

Prevention

Osteoporosis prevention focuses on reaching peak bone mass during growth and development and slowing the rate of bone loss with aging. Measures aimed at promoting peak bone mass during childhood and adolescence include consuming adequate calories, calcium, and vitamin D; performing regular weight-bearing activities; and avoiding smoking. Overly strenuous athletics such as the "female athlete triad" of amenorrhea, low body weight, and low bone mineral density should be avoided.[119] To slow bone loss, clinicians should discuss hormone therapy in menopause. Proportional contributions of several factors are shown in Table 21-3.

Clinicians should also address risk factors for falling, particularly in older adults at high risk of fracture. Simple measures that reduce falls include wearing shoes indoors, providing adequate lighting, installing handrails, and removing throw rugs and extension cords. In addition, strength and balance exercises are recommended to reduce falls.[120] Finally, correcting vision impaired by cataracts or other causes is an important intervention to reduce falls.

Screening

The diagnosis of osteoporosis can be made by DXA scan or by clinical judgment (e.g., an older adult with a low-trauma compression or hip fracture). USPSTF recommends osteoporosis screening for all women aged 65 years and older without previous fractures or secondary causes of osteoporosis. The task force also recommends screening women younger than 65 years with additional risk factors. It does not recommend screening for men without prior fractures or secondary causes of osteoporosis.[121] In a recent review, the USPSTF found evidence that screening for osteoporosis reduced the risk of hip fracture and that osteoporosis medications reduce the risk of vertebral and nonvertebral fractures.[122]

Treatment

Several medications are approved by the US Food and Drug Administration (FDA) for the prevention or treatment of osteoporosis; these drugs work by decreasing bone

Table 21-3. Attributable Risks for Hip Fractures

Factor	Best Estimate, %	Range, %
Nonuse of hormone replacement	19	6-31
Thin body build	18	10.5-26
Cigarette smoking	10	4-16

resorption (antiresorptive agents), by increasing bone formation (anabolic agents), or by applying both mechanisms. All FDA-approved osteoporosis drugs must have reduced the risk of spine fractures in randomized placebo-controlled clinical trials. Most drugs must also have reduced the risk of non-spine fractures, including hip fractures, in such trials. Because a detailed discussion of these individual treatments is beyond the scope of this chapter, readers are referred to a series of recently published reviews of osteoporosis therapies.[122,123]

In the United States, an FDA-approved osteoporosis medication is recommended for older adults with low-trauma hip or compression fractures, a T-score of −2.5 or lower, a 20% or greater ten-year probability of major osteoporotic fracture, or a 3% or greater ten-year probability of hip fracture.[123] Initiation of an osteoporosis drug is recommended if an adult aged 40 years or older is taking at least 5 mg of prednisone daily for three months and has a FRAX score of 10% or higher.[124]

Examples of Evidence-Based Interventions

Population-based public health interventions for improving bone health in the United States include programs to increase physical activity, reduce falls, and reduce tobacco use, among other approaches. Key among these is the CDC compendium of falls prevention resources and implementation guides.[125]

Moving Forward

Focus group participants have identified several areas for future research.[126] Patients identified the need to increase public awareness of osteoporosis; reduce diagnostic delays; and improve communication about the causes of osteoporosis, the role of diet and exercise, and the efficacy and side effects of osteoporosis medications. To that end, the COVID-19 pandemic has further reduced rates of bone density testing, estimation of fracture risk using FRAX, and onset of osteoporosis therapies, as documented in a recent systematic review.[127] The widening treatment gap highlights the need for new, pragmatic approaches to diagnose and treat osteoporosis.

Future efforts are needed to improve fracture risk prediction tools and address racial and ethnic disparities in the diagnosis and treatment of osteoporosis. The International Osteoporosis Foundation has identified a number of key areas to improve health care delivery. These include increased screening for osteoporosis; development of coordinated, multidisciplinary care for secondary fracture prevention, including fracture liaison services; supporting the wide use of evidence-based guidelines to treat osteoporosis; establishing public health policies designed to maximize peak bone mass; and increasing public knowledge of healthy diets that include adequate calcium intake.

SYSTEMIC LUPUS ERYTHEMATOSUS

Systemic lupus erythematosus, commonly called lupus, is a chronic autoimmune disorder that can affect almost every organ of the body. In lupus the immune system, which normally functions to protect against viruses or bacteria, becomes overactive, forming antibodies that attack the self, called autoantibodies. These autoantibodies can deposit in tissues and organs, including the skin, joints, kidneys, brain, heart, lungs, and blood.

Lupus predominantly affects women of childbearing age. It is more common in Black, Hispanic, Asian, Native American, and Alaskan Native women than White women.[128] Lupus prevalence ranges from 40 to 400 per 100,000 population, with the highest prevalence in Black women.[129] Symptoms of lupus can mimic other diseases, and no single laboratory test can definitively diagnose systemic lupus. Diagnosis requires a positive antinuclear antibodies (ANA) result, as well as laboratory and clinical criteria. Antimalarials, steroids, and other cytotoxic therapies are used to suppress the immune system to treat lupus. Lupus can be life-threatening or cause irreversible organ damage. Thus, early detection and treatment is key.

Etiopathogenesis and Pathophysiology

Lupus is a multifactorial disease whose exact etiology remains unknown. Genetic, immunologic, thyroid, and environmental factors play a role. Familial rates and high concordance in identical twins suggest a genetic contribution in lupus, although there is no obvious pattern of inheritance. Twin concordance is 25% to 50%. Nearly 100 genes or genomic loci have been identified as associated with lupus, most affecting function of the immune system.[130] In addition, female sex and hormones are risk factors. Women are nine to ten times more at risk of developing lupus, and the risk of lupus is 14 times more in Klinefelter syndrome (a.k.a. 47, XXY). This suggests an association with genes on the X chromosome, although over ninety genetic loci may contribute, and a singular genetic cause has not been identified. Next, estrogens increase the production of B-cell activation factor and modulate other pro-inflammatory cells. Causal association between oral contraceptives and lupus flares has not been established, but hormonal oral contraceptives are often avoided in severe lupus.[131] Environmental triggers of lupus can include medications, ultraviolet rays and sun exposure, smoking, and viral infections, among others.[132]

The pathogenesis of lupus is complex and evolving. A break in the self-tolerance in genetically susceptible individuals leads to activation of autoimmunity when exposed to environmental triggers. Cell damage caused by infectious and environmental triggers exposes "spilled" self-antigens, leading to activation of T and B cells. T cells activate autoreactive B cells that lead to autoantibody production, a hallmark of lupus. These autoantibodies are pathogenic and cause organ damage by immune complex deposition, complement activation, and altered cell function leading to cell death (apoptosis).

Activated B cells can also serve as antigen-presenting cells creating a loop, leading to more autoimmunity without intervention.[133]

Descriptive Epidemiology

Geographic Distribution and Disparities

In 2018 an estimated 204,295 individuals (95% CI, 160,902–261,725) in the United States. fulfilled the ACR classification criteria for definite lupus.[128] The pooled prevalence of lupus from five CDC-funded lupus registries was 72.8 per 100,000 people.[128] Prevalence was nine times higher among women than men (128.7 vs. 14.7/100,000). Female prevalence was the highest among Black women (230.9/100,000), followed by Hispanic (120.7/100,000), White (84.7/100,000), and Asian/Pacific Islander (84.4/100,000) women. Among men, the pooled prevalence of lupus was the highest in Black men (26.7/100,000), followed by Hispanic (18.0/100,000), Asian/Pacific Islander (11.2/100,000), and White (8.9/100,000) men. The American Indian/Alaska Native population had the highest race-specific lupus estimates, both among women (270.6/100,000) and men (53.8/100,000). Race- and sex-specific prevalence rates for each registry are shown in Table 21-4.[128]

National incidence data are difficult to obtain because it is relatively difficult to locate and adjudicate cases. However, lupus incidence estimates from the five CDC-funded lupus registries were 5.1 per 100,000 person-years overall (95% CI, 4.6–5.6), higher in women than in men (8.7 vs. 1.2/100,000 person-years), and highest among Black women (15.9/100,000 person-years). The American Indian/Alaska Native population had the second highest race-specific lupus estimates for women (10.4/100,000) and men (3.8/100,000). Incidence in Hispanic women with lupus was 6.7 per 100,000. On the basis

Table 21-4. Prevalence of Systemic Lupus Erythematosus by Race/Ethnicity and Sex in Five State-Specific Registries

Prevalence	Michigan	Georgia	Alaska	California	New York City
Sex					
Female	9.3	145.8	271	149.7	138.3
Male	1.5	17.5	54	22.9	19.4
Race/ethnicity					
White	47.5	39.9	NA	NA	NA
Black	111.6	128	NA	NA	NA
Asian	NA	NA	NA	94.7	56.2
Hispanic	NA	NA	NA	90.5	82.2
American Indian	NA	NA	178	NA	NA

Source: Based on Izmirly et al.[128]

Note: NA = not applicable; SLE = systemic lupus erythematosus. SLE is per 100,000.

Table 21-5. Incidence of Systemic Lupus Erythematosus by Race/Ethnicity and Sex in Five State-Specific Registries

Incidence	Michigan	Georgia	Alaska	California	New York City
Sex					
Female	9.3	10.6	8.4	NA	NA
Male	1.5	1.9	2.7	NA	NA
Race/ethnicity					
White	7.9	9.4	NA	NA	NA
Black	3.7	3.2	NA	NA	NA
Asian	NA	NA	NA	4.2	3.8
Female				8.9	6.6
Male				0.3	0.5
Hispanic	NA	NA	NA	4.1	4.0
Female				7.2	6.5
Male				0.6	1.3
American Indian	NA	NA	7.4	0.6	NA

Source: Based on Izmirly et al.[134]
Note: NA = not applicable; SLE = systemic lupus erythematosus. SLE is per 100,000.

of these data, it is estimated that 14,263 persons (95% CI, 11,563–17,735) were newly diagnosed with lupus in the United States in 2018.[128] Race- and sex-specific incidence rates by registry are shown in Table 21-5.[134]

Time Trends

There are no recent US studies to determine if prevalence and incidence of lupus are changing. In the United Kingdom, the incidence of lupus has been declining, with a 1.8% decrease in new lupus cases (1999–2012) after a peak in 2000. Still, prevalence of lupus in the United Kingdom showed a 3.1% increase annually from 1999 to 2012.[135]

US lupus mortality improved with ten-year survival for lupus patients: adjusted standardized mortality ratio in 1968 versus 2013 was 4.5 (95% CI, 4.2–4.8) versus 3.4 (95% CI, 3.2–3.6) per million persons. However, the lupus-specific reduction in mortality (24.4%) was smaller than mortality reduction in non-lupus causes (43.9%) during the same 46-year period.[136]

Public Health Impact

Health disparities exist with lupus and are associated with early morbidity and mortality. Women younger than 40 years with lupus are at 52 times higher risk of cardiovascular disease compared with age-matched healthy peers.[137] Moreover, the incidence of end-stage kidney disease (or kidney failure) is 18 to 20 times higher in lupus compared with non-lupus patients (4.1 vs. 0.3/1,000 person-years).[138] Lupus ranks fifth as a leading cause of mortality in young Black or Hispanic women aged 25 to 40 years.[139] The main causes of death include active SLE disease, organ failure, infection, cancers, or cardiovascular disease.[140] In a large international SLE cohort (1958–2001), observed all-cause deaths in lupus were 2.4 times higher than the expected (standardized mortality ratio 2.4; CI, 2.3–2.5). Standardized mortality was even higher for those who were female, of Black race, younger age, or who had SLE for less than one year.[140]

Annual per-patient medical direct costs have been estimated to be $34,146 for SLE and $73,306 for patients with lupus nephritis.[141] Infection and lupus flares were the top two causes for SLE hospitalization.[142] Average length of hospital stay was 8.5 days, with mean direct costs of $20,934 per admission. Compared with many other chronic health conditions, lupus and lupus nephritis were the most costly.[143] Indirect SLE costs, including work absence, have been estimated at $1,287–$20,603 per year. Higher indirect costs were associated with being female, of advancing age, and neuropsychiatric, with renal organ damage from SLE.

Black patients are disproportionately affected by SLE, and have increased prevalence, severity, damage, renal involvement, and mortality and also have worse quality of life.[144,145] Black patients had a threefold higher risk of developing lupus nephritis than did other populations. Furthermore, the burden of cardiovascular disease was found to be 19 times higher in Black people with lupus.[146] Recent studies have shown that Black people with SLE have three to four times higher risk of mortality compared with White people (standardized mortality ratio in Black women = 3.38).[147] In addition, death occurred much younger (51 vs. 64 years). Mortality was four times higher in Hispanic and Asian women with SLE.[148]

Modifiable Risk Factors

Postmenopausal hormone replacement therapy can cause mild-to-moderate flares in patients with SLE, but not severe flares.[149] Nonetheless, the risk versus benefit of hormone replacement should be discussed with patients. Several medications, including procainamide, hydralazine, and TNF-inhibitors, can cause a reversible drug-induced lupus. Also, sulfa-drugs can cause flares in patients with SLE and thus are to be avoided.[150] Ultraviolet rays and sun exposure increase cell death (apoptosis) and can trigger SLE. It is therefore recommended that patients use sunscreen and limit exposure. Because infections can lead to flares, vaccination against influenza and SARS-CoV-2 is highly encouraged. Likewise, given their immune problems, patients with SLE are advised of the importance of pneumococcal and meningococcal vaccination. Smoking can trigger lupus flares, particularly skin manifestations and cardiovascular disease in lupus.

In addition, smoking may reduce the efficacy of lupus medications. Thus, SLE patients are encouraged to quit smoking.[132]

Evidence-Based Interventions

Screening and Diagnosis

As a multisystem disease, SLE manifests clinical features that vary considerably, from manifesting as a mild disease with mucocutaneous involvement and joint pain to being a severe life-threatening disease with multiorgan involvement. ANA are the hallmark required for most diagnoses and the initial test to screen for SLE. ANA and immunofluorescence testing are the gold standard. ANA testing with a titer of 1:80 or greater is 98% sensitive; negative ANA makes lupus unlikely. However, specificity is low (57%–88%) and can be seen in several other autoimmune disorders, as well as in a proportion of the healthy; thus ANA does not confirm diagnosis.[151,152] A positive ANA in a setting of clinical manifestations of lupus should prompt referral and specific autoantibody testing, (ds-DNA antibodies, Smith antibodies, anti-phospholipid antibodies, complements). These autoantibodies can help support diagnosis, predicting disease course, and clinical features.[153,154]

ACR first developed the SLE classification criteria in 1971, then revised it in 1997.[153] The criteria were further revised by the Systemic Lupus International Collaborating Clinics (SLICC) group in 2012 to increase sensitivity.[154] In 2019 the European League Against Rheumatism (EULAR) and ACR developed classification criteria for SLE via an international Delphi forum.[155] The criteria include positive ANA at least once as a required entry criterion, followed by additive weighted criteria grouped in seven clinical and three immunological domains (Figure 21-11). Patients with ten or more points or a lupus nephritis (LN) biopsy are classified as SLE. The new criteria had a sensitivity of 96.1% and specificity of 93.4% (vs. 82.8% and 93.4% for ACR 1997 and 96.7% and 83.7% for SLICC 2012).[155,156] These criteria are for research, yet they can assist in diagnosis of SLE.

Treatment

The treatment of lupus depends on severity of disease. In mild-to-moderate lupus anti-malarial agents and low doses of corticosteroids are commonly used. In severe disease high-dose corticosteroids and immunosuppressive agents are used to control disease. Treatment in SLE aims at remission, low disease activity, and flare prevention. Hydroxychloroquine is recommended in all patients with lupus (dose ≤5 mg/kg). It reduces the risk of disease flare, organ damage, and cardiovascular disease and improves pregnancy outcomes and survival.[157–159] Hydroxychloroquine is safe even to use during pregnancy and breastfeeding. An annual eye exam is recommended to monitor for macular toxicity, although the risk of toxicity is less than 2% at ten years.[160]

Entry criterion

Antinuclear antibodies (ANA) at a titer of ≥1:80 on HEp-2 cells or an equivalent positive test (ever)

↓

If absent, do not classify as SLE

If present, apply additive criteria

↓

Additive criteria

Do not count a criterion if there is a more likely explanation than SLE.

Occurrence of a criterion on at least one occasion is sufficient.

SLE classification requires at least one clinical criterion and ≥10 points.

Criteria need not occur simultaneously.

Within each domain, only the highest weighted criterion is counted toward the total score§.

Clinical domains and criteria	Weight
Constitutional	
Fever	2
Hematologic	
Leukopenia	3
Thrombocytopenia	4
Autoimmune hemolysis	4
Neuropsychiatric	
Delirium	2
Psychosis	3
Seizure	5
Mucocutaneous	
Non-scarring alopecia	2
Oral ulcers	2
Subacute cutaneous OR discoid lupus	4
Acute cutaneous lupus	6
Serosal	
Pleural or pericardial effusion	5
Acute pericarditis	6
Musculoskeletal	
Joint involvement	6
Renal	
Proteinuria >0.5g/24h	4
Renal biopsy Class II or V lupus nephritis	8
Renal biopsy Class III or IV lupus nephritis	10

Immunology domains and criteria	Weight
Antiphospholipid antibodies	
Anti-cardiolipin antibodies OR	
Anti-β2GP1 antibodies OR	
Lupus anticoagulant	2
Complement proteins	
Low C3 OR low C4	3
Low C3 AND low C4	4
SLE-specific antibodies	
Anti-dsDNA antibody* OR	
Anti-Smith antibody	6

Total score:

↓

Classify as Systemic Lupus Erythematosus with a score of 10 or more if entry criterion fulfilled.

Source: Aringer et al.[155] Reprinted with permission of John Wiley & Sons.

Figure 21-11. The 2019 European League Against Rheumatism and American College of Rheumatology Lupus Classification Criteria

Unfortunately, nonadherence to hydroxychloroquine is up to 80% with disparities noted.[161] Depending on clinical presentation and severity, other immunomodulatory agents (methotrexate, azathioprine, mycophenolate, or voclosporin) and biological agents (belimumab, rituximab, anifrolumab) could be started. Steroid-sparing immunomodulatory agents can improve disease control and outcomes. In persistently active or flaring extrarenal disease, biological therapies, such as belimumab, may be added. Newer agents, such as anifrolumab and voclosporin, can be used in nephritis or severe disease refractory to first-line oral immunomodulatory or biological therapies.[162,163]

Patients with SLE should also be assessed for their antiphospholipid antibody status (blood-clotting antibodies), and counseled regarding infectious and cardiovascular diseases risk. Preventive strategies include regular blood pressure monitoring, counseling for smoking cessation, administering vaccinations, and providing aspirin or statin for high-risk patients and should be tailored by risk profiles.[164]

Moving Forward

Future studies examining biomarkers or predictors that determine the susceptibility to develop SLE could guide early detection and treatment. In addition, research is needed on biomarkers and predictors of severe disease and poor outcomes, such as cardiovascular disease, kidney failure, and mortality. Causes of heterogeneity in SLE and responses to therapy could identify subsets of SLE at risk of poor outcomes or to help personalize therapy. Moreover, along with new drug discovery, strategies to optimize therapies and evidence-based strategies to reduce disparities in lupus will improve health and survival of all lupus patients.[155]

DISCUSSION QUESTIONS

1. Discuss the magnitude of arthritis burden and relationship between aging, obesity, and arthritis. Recognizing osteoarthritis as the most common arthritis, name potential primary and secondary intervention strategies.
2. Describe gene environment interactions in rheumatoid arthritis and how smoking and obesity might affect rheumatoid arthritis incidence and severity.
3. Osteoporosis is greatest in which sociodemographic populations? What can be done for primary and secondary osteoporosis and fragility fracture prevention?
4. Systemic lupus erythematosus is a multisystem disease that disproportionately affects young women. Describe two health disparities in SLE.

ACKNOWLEDGMENTS

The authors of this chapter thank Monica Messina and Mindy Jones for their administrative support.

REFERENCES

1. Centers for Disease Control and Prevention. Arthritis related statistics. Updated October 12, 2021. Available at: https://www.cdc.gov/arthritis/data_statistics/arthritis-related-stats.htm. Accessed January 30, 2023.
2. Hootman JM, Helmick CG, Barbour KE, Theis KA, Boring MA. Updated projected prevalence of self-reported doctor-diagnosed arthritis and arthritis-attributable activity limitation among US adults, 2015–2040. *Arthritis Rheumatol.* 2016;68(7):1582–1587. doi:10.1002/art.39692
3. Theis KA, Murphy LB, Guglielmo D, et al. Prevalence of arthritis and arthritis-attributable activity limitation—United States, 2016–2018. *MMWR Morb Mortal Wkly Rep.* 2021; 70(40):1401–1407. doi:10.15585/mmwr.mm7040a2
4. United States Bone and Joint Initiative. *The Burden of Musculoskeletal Diseases in the United States (BMUS).* 4th ed. Rosemont, IL: US Bone and Joint Initiative; 2020. Available at: https://www.boneandjointburden.org/fourth-edition. Accessed January 30, 2023.
5. Lawrence RC, Felson DT, Helmick CG, et al. Estimates of the prevalence of arthritis and other rheumatic conditions in the United States. Part II. *Arthritis Rheum.* 2008;58(1):26–35. doi:10.1002/art.23176
6. Barbour KE, Helmick CG, Boring M, Brady TJ. Vital signs: prevalence of doctor-diagnosed arthritis and arthritis-attributable activity limitation—United States, 2013–2015. *MMWR Morb Mortal Wkly Rep.* 2017;66(9):246–253. doi:10.15585/mmwr.mm6609e1
7. Centers for Disease Control and Prevention, US Department of Health and Human Services. Summary health statistics for US Adults: National Health Interview Survey, 2010. January 2012. Available at: https://www.cdc.gov/nchs/data/series/sr_10/sr10_252.pdf.
8. Felson DT, Zhang Y. An update on the epidemiology of knee and hip osteoarthritis with a view to prevention. *Arthritis Rheum.* 1998;41(8):1343–1355. doi:10.1002/1529-0131(199808)41:8<1343::aid-art3>3.0.co;2-9
9. Hannan MT Anderson JJ, Zhang Y, Levy D, Felson DT. Bone mineral density and knee osteoarthritis in elderly men and women. The Framingham Study. *Arthritis Rheum.* 1993;36(12): 1671–1680. doi:10.1002/art.1780361205
10. Felson DT, Naimark A, Anderson J, Kazis L, Castelli W, Meenan RF. The prevalence of knee osteoarthritis in the elderly. The Framingham Osteoarthritis Study. *Arthritis Rheum.* 1987;30(8):914–918. doi:10.1002/art.1780300811
11. Jordan JM, Helmick CG, Renner JB, et al. Prevalence of knee symptoms and radiographic and symptomatic knee osteoarthritis in African Americans and Caucasians: the Johnston County Osteoarthritis Project. *J Rheumatol.* 2007;34(1):172–180.
12. Altman R, Alarcón G, Appelrouth D, et al. The American College of Rheumatology criteria for the classification and reporting of osteoarthritis of the hand. *Arthritis Rheum.* 1990;33(11):1601–1610. doi:10.1002/art.1780331101
13. Kolasinski SL, Neogi T, Hochberg MC, et al. 2019 American College of Rheumatology/ Arthritis Foundation guideline for the management of osteoarthritis of the hand, hip, and knee. *Arthritis Care Res (Hoboken).* 2020;72(2):149–162. doi:10.1002/acr.24131
14. Bijlsma JW, Knahr K. Strategies for the prevention and management of osteoarthritis of the hip and knee. *Best Pract Res Clin Rheumatol.* 2007;21(1):59–76. doi:10.1016/j.berh.2006.08.013

15. van den Bosch MHJ, van Lent P, van der Kraan PM. Identifying effector molecules, cells, and cytokines of innate immunity in OA. *Osteoarthritis Cartilage.* 2020;28(5):532–543. doi:10.1016/j.joca.2020.01.016
16. Vincent KR, Conrad BP, Fregly BJ, Vincent HK. The pathophysiology of osteoarthritis: a mechanical perspective on the knee joint. *PM&R.* 2012;4(5s):s3–s9. doi:10.1016/j.pmrj.2012.01.020
17. Murphy LB, Helmick CG, Schwartz TA, et al. One in four people may develop symptomatic hip osteoarthritis in his or her lifetime. *Osteoarthritis Cartilage.* 2010;18(11):1372–1379. doi:10.1016/j.joca.2010.08.005
18. Murphy L, Schwartz TA, Helmick CG, et al. Lifetime risk of symptomatic knee osteoarthritis. *Arthritis Rheum.* 2008;59(9):1207–1213. doi:10.1002/art.24021
19. Barbour KE, Moss S, Croft JB, et al. Geographic variations in arthritis prevalence, health-related characteristics, and management—United States, 2015. *MMWR Surveillance Summaries.* 2018;67(4);1–28. Available at: https://www.cdc.gov/mmwr/volumes/67/ss/ss6704a1.htm. Accessed January 31, 2023.
20. Centers for Disease Control and Prevention. Osteoarthritis (OA). Updated July 27, 2020. Available at: https://www.cdc.gov/arthritis/basics/osteoarthritis.htm. Accessed January 30, 2023.
21. Jiang L, Tian W, Wang Y, et al. Body mass index and susceptibility to knee osteoarthritis: a systematic review and meta-analysis. *Joint Bone Spine.* 2012;79(3):291–297. doi:10.1016/j.jbspin.2011.05.015
22. Silverwood V, Blagojevic-Bucknall M, Jinks C, Jordan JL, Protheroe J, Jordan KP. Current evidence on risk factors for knee osteoarthritis in older adults: a systematic review and meta-analysis. *Osteoarthritis Cartilage.* 2015;23(4):507–515. doi:10.1016/j.joca.2014.11.019
23. Karlson EW, Mandl LA, Aweh GN, Sangha O, Liang MH, Grodstein F. Total hip replacement due to osteoarthritis: the importance of age, obesity, and other modifiable risk factors. *Am J Med.* 2003;114(2):93–98. doi:10.1016/s0002-9343(02)01447-x
24. Fransen M, McConnell S, Harmer AR, Van der Esch M, Simic M, Bennell KL. Exercise for osteoarthritis of the knee. *Cochrane Database Syst Rev.* 2015;1(1):CD004376. doi:10.1002/14651858.CD004376.pub3
25. Vrezas I, Elsner G, Bolm-Audorff U, Abolmaali N, Seidler A. Case-control study of knee osteoarthritis and lifestyle factors considering their interaction with physical workload. *Int Arch Occup Environ Health.* 2010;83(3):291–300. doi:10.1007/s00420-009-0486-6
26. Hall M, Castelein B, Wittoek R, Calders P, Van Ginckel A. Diet-induced weight loss alone or combined with exercise in overweight or obese people with knee osteoarthritis: a systematic review and meta-analysis. *Semin Arthritis Rheum.* 2019;48(5):765–777. doi:10.1016/j.semarthrit.2018.06.005
27. Chang HJ, Finn DJ, Dunlop DD, Tamez D, Chang RW. Arthritis and other musculoskeletal diseases. In: Remington PL, Brownson RC, Wegner MV, eds. *Chronic Disease Epidemiology and Control.* 4th ed. American Public Health Association; 2016:chap. 20.
28. Centers for Disease Control and Prevention. Physical activity programs. Updated April 16, 2021. Available at: https://www.cdc.gov/arthritis/interventions/physical-activity.html. Accessed January 30, 2023.

29. Kolasinski SL, Neogi T, Hochberg MC, et al. 2019 American College of Rheumatology/Arthritis Foundation guideline for the management of osteoarthritis of the hand, hip, and knee. *Arthritis Rheumatol.* 2020;72(2):220–233. doi:10.1002/art.41142
30. Culvenor AG, Wirth W, Ruhdorfer A, Eckstein F. Thigh muscle strength predicts knee replacement risk independent of radiographic disease and pain in women: data from the Osteoarthritis Initiative. *Arthritis Rheumatol.* 2016;68(5):1145–1155. doi:10.1002/art.39540
31. Endstrasser F, Braito M, Linser M, Spicher A, Wagner M, Brunner A. The negative impact of the COVID-19 lockdown on pain and physical function in patients with end-stage hip or knee osteoarthritis. *Knee Surg Sports Traumatol Arthrosc.* 2020;28(8):2435–2443. doi:10.1007/s00167-020-06104-3
32. Scott DL, Wolfe F, Huizinga TW. Rheumatoid arthritis. *Lancet.* 2010;376(9746):1094–1108. doi:10.1016/s0140-6736(10)60826-4
33. Aletaha D, Smolen JS. Diagnosis and management of rheumatoid arthritis: a review. *JAMA.* 2018;320(13):1360–1372. doi:10.1001/jama.2018.13103
34. Chehata JC, Hassell AB, Clarke SA, et al. Mortality in rheumatoid arthritis: relationship to single and composite measures of disease activity. *Rheumatology (Oxford).* 2001;40(4):447–452. doi:10.1093/rheumatology/40.4.447
35. Sparks JA, Chang SC, Liao KP, et al. Rheumatoid arthritis and mortality among women during 36 years of prospective follow-up: results from the Nurses' Health Study. *Arthritis Care Res (Hoboken).* 2016;68(6):753–762. doi:10.1002/acr.22752
36. Zhang Y, Lu N, Peloquin C, et al. Improved survival in rheumatoid arthritis: a general population-based cohort study. *Ann Rheum Dis.* 72017;76(2):408–413. doi:10.1136/annrheumdis-2015-209058
37. Hresko A, Lin TC, Solomon DH. Medical care costs associated with rheumatoid arthritis in the US: a systematic literature review and meta-analysis. *Arthritis Care Res (Hoboken).* 2018;70(10):1431–1438. doi:10.1002/acr.23512
38. Hsieh PH, Wu O, Geue C, McIntosh E, McInnes IB, Siebert S. Economic burden of rheumatoid arthritis: a systematic review of literature in biologic era. *Ann Rheum Dis.* 2020;79(6):771–777. doi:10.1136/annrheumdis-2019-216243
39. Birnbaum H, Pike C, Kaufman R, Marynchenko M, Kidolezi Y, Cifaldi M. Societal cost of rheumatoid arthritis patients in the US. *Curr Med Res Opin.* 2010;26(1):77–90. doi:10.1185/03007990903422307
40. Xu Y, Wu Q. Prevalence trend and disparities in rheumatoid arthritis among US adults, 2005–2018. *J Clin Med.* 2021;10(15):3289. doi:10.3390/jcm10153289
41. Matcham F, Scott IC, Rayner L, et al. The impact of rheumatoid arthritis on quality-of-life assessed using the SF-36: a systematic review and meta-analysis. *Semin Arthritis Rheum.* 2014;44(2):123–130. doi:10.1016/j.semarthrit.2014.05.001
42. Jin S, Hsieh E, Peng L, et al. Incidence of fractures among patients with rheumatoid arthritis: a systematic review and meta-analysis. *Osteoporos Int.* 2018;29(6):1263–1275. doi:10.1007/s00198-018-4473-1
43. De Cock D, Hyrich K. Malignancy and rheumatoid arthritis: epidemiology, risk factors and management. *Best Pract Res Clin Rheumatol.* 2018;32(6):869–886. doi:10.1016/j.berh.2019.03.011

44. England BR, Baker JF, Sayles H, et al. Body mass index, weight loss, and cause-specific mortality in rheumatoid arthritis. *Arthritis Care Res (Hoboken).* 2018;70(1):11–18. doi:10.1002/acr.23258
45. Fina-Aviles F, Medina-Peralta M, Mendez-Boo L, et al. The descriptive epidemiology of rheumatoid arthritis in Catalonia: a retrospective study using routinely collected data. *Clin Rheumatol.* 2016;35(3):751–757. doi:10.1007/s10067-014-2801-1
46. Silman AJ, Pearson JE. Epidemiology and genetics of rheumatoid arthritis. *Arthritis Res.* 2002;4(suppl 3):S265–S272. doi:10.1186/ar578
47. Rindfleisch JA, Muller D. Diagnosis and management of rheumatoid arthritis. *Am Fam Physician.* 2005;72(6):1037–1047.
48. Lu B, Hiraki LT, Sparks JA, et al. Being overweight or obese and risk of developing rheumatoid arthritis among women: a prospective cohort study. *Ann Rheum Dis.* 2014;73(11):1914–1922. doi:10.1136/annrheumdis-2014-205459
49. Kalla AA, Tikly M. Rheumatoid arthritis in the developing world. *Best Pract Res Clin Rheumatol.* 2003;17(5):863–875. doi:10.1016/s1521-6942(03)00047-0
50. Putrik P, Ramiro S, Kvien TK, Sokka T, Uhlig T, Boonen A. Variations in criteria regulating treatment with reimbursed biologic DMARDs across European countries. Are differences related to country's wealth? *Ann Rheum Dis.* 2014;73(11):2010–2021. doi:10.1136/annrheumdis-2013-203819
51. Doran MF, Crowson CS, Pond GR, O'Fallon WM, Gabriel SE. Frequency of infection in patients with rheumatoid arthritis compared with controls: a population-based study. *Arthritis Rheum.* 2002;46(9):2287–2293. doi:10.1002/art.10524
52. Aga AB, Lie E, Uhlig T, et al. Time trends in disease activity, response and remission rates in rheumatoid arthritis during the past decade: results from the NOR-DMARD Study 2000–2010. *Ann Rheum Dis.* 2015;74(2):381–388. doi:10.1136/annrheumdis-2013-204020
53. Welsing PM, Fransen J, Van Riel PL. Is the disease course of rheumatoid arthritis becoming milder? Time trends since 1985 in an inception cohort of early rheumatoid arthritis. *Arthritis Rheum.* 2005;52(9):2616–2624. doi:10.1002/art.21259
54. Markusse IM, Akdemir G, Dirven L, et al. Long-term outcomes of patients with recent-onset rheumatoid arthritis after 10 years of tight controlled treatment: a randomized trial. *Ann Intern Med.* 2016;164(8):523–531. doi:10.7326/M15-0919
55. de Hair MJ, Landewé RB, van de Sande MG, et al. Smoking and overweight determine the likelihood of developing rheumatoid arthritis. *Ann Rheum Dis.* 2013;72(10):1654–1658. doi:10.1136/annrheumdis-2012-202254
56. MacGregor AJ, Snieder H, Rigby AS, et al. Characterizing the quantitative genetic contribution to rheumatoid arthritis using data from twins. *Arthritis Rheum.* 2000;43(1):30–37. doi:10.1002/1529-0131(200001)43:1<30::aid-anr5>3.0.co;2-b
57. Karlson EW, van Schaardenburg D, van der Helm-van Mil AH. Strategies to predict rheumatoid arthritis development in at-risk populations. *Rheumatology.* 2014;55(1):6–15. doi:10.1093/rheumatology/keu287
58. Fraenkel L, Bathon JM, England BR, et al. 2021 American College of Rheumatology guideline for the treatment of rheumatoid arthritis. *Arthritis Rheumatol.* 2021;73(7):1108–1123. doi:10.1002/art.41752

59. Gibofsky A. Comparative effectiveness of current treatments for rheumatoid arthritis. *Am J Manag Care*. 2012;18(13 suppl):S303–S314.
60. Demoruelle MK, Deane KD. Treatment strategies in early rheumatoid arthritis and prevention of rheumatoid arthritis. *Curr Rheumatol Rep*. 2012;14(5):472–480. doi:10.1007/s11926-012-0275-1
61. Deane KD, O'Donnell CI, Hueber W, et al. The number of elevated cytokines and chemokines in preclinical seropositive rheumatoid arthritis predicts time to diagnosis in an age-dependent manner. *Arthritis Rheum*. 2010;62(11):3161–3172. doi:10.1002/art.27638
62. Arkema EV, Goldstein BL, Robinson W, et al. Anti-citrullinated peptide autoantibodies, human leukocyte antigen shared epitope and risk of future rheumatoid arthritis: a nested case-control study. *Arthritis Res Ther*. 2013;15(5):R159. doi:10.1186/ar4342
63. Lee J, Dunlop D, Ehrlich-Jones L, et al. Public health impact of risk factors for physical inactivity in adults with rheumatoid arthritis. *Arthritis Care Res (Hoboken)*. 2012;64(4):488–493. doi:10.1002/acr.21582
64. Hakkinen A, Sokka T, Kautiainen H, Kotaniemi A, Hannonen P. Sustained maintenance of exercise induced muscle strength gains and normal bone mineral density in patients with early rheumatoid arthritis: a 5 year follow up. *Ann Rheum Dis*. 2004;63(8):910–916. doi:10.1136/ard.2003.013003
65. D'Silva KM, Wallace ZS. COVID-19 and rheumatoid arthritis. *Curr Opin Rheumatol*. 2021;33(3):255–261. doi:10.1097/bor.0000000000000786
66. Mulay SR, Anders HJ. Crystallopathies. *N Engl J Med*. 2016;374(25):2465–2476. doi:10.1056/nejmra1601611
67. Dalbeth N, Gosling AL, Gaffo A, Abhishek A. Gout. *Lancet*. 2021;397(10287):1843–1855. doi:10.1016/s0140-6736(21)00569-9
68. Neogi T. Gout. *N Engl J Med*. 2011;364(5):443–452. doi:10.1056/nejmcp1001124
69. Mattiuzzi C, Lippi G. Recent updates on worldwide gout epidemiology. *Clin Rheumatol*. 2020;39(4):1061–1063. doi:10.1007/s10067-019-04868-9
70. Chen-Xu M, Yokose C, Rai SK, Pillinger MH, Choi HK. Contemporary prevalence of gout and hyperuricemia in the United States and decadal trends: the National Health and Nutrition Examination Survey, 2007–2016. *Arthritis Rheumatol*. 2019;71(6):991–999. doi:10.1002/art.40807
71. Zhu Y, Pandya BJ, Choi HK. Prevalence of gout and hyperuricemia in the US general population: the National Health and Nutrition Examination Survey 2007–2008. *Arthritis Rheum*. 2011;63(10):3136–3141. doi:10.1002/art.30520
72. Bhole V, de Vera M, Rahman MM, Krishnan E, Choi H. Epidemiology of gout in women: fifty-two-year followup of a prospective cohort. *Arthritis Rheum*. 2010;62(4):1069–1076. doi:10.1002/art.27338
73. Dehlin M, Jacobsson L, Roddy E. Global epidemiology of gout: prevalence, incidence, treatment patterns and risk factors. *Nat Rev Rheumatol*. 2020;16(7):380–390. doi:10.1038/s41584-020-0441-1
74. Shiozawa A, Szabo SM, Bolzani A, Cheung A, Choi HK. Serum uric acid and the risk of incident and recurrent gout: a systematic review. *J Rheumatol*. 2017;44(3):388–396. doi:10.3899/jrheum.160452

75. Singh JA. Veterans Affairs databases are accurate for gout-related health care utilization: a validation study. *Arthritis Res Ther*. 2013;15(6):r224. doi:10.1186/ar4425
76. Major TJ, Dalbeth N, Stahl EA, Merriman TR. An update on the genetics of hyperuricaemia and gout. *Nat Rev Rheumatol*. 2018;14(6):341–353. doi:10.1038/s41584-018-0004-X
77. Danve A, Sehra St, Neogi T. Role of diet in hyperuricemia and gout. *Best Pract Res Clin Rheumatol*. 2021;35(4):101723. doi:10.1016/j.berh.2021.101723
78. McCormick N, Rai SK, Lu N, Yokose C, Curhan GC, Choi HK. Estimation of primary prevention of gout in men through modification of obesity and other key lifestyle factors. *JAMA Netw Open*. 2020;3(11):e2027421. doi:10.1001/jamanetworkopen.2020.27421
79. Fitzgerald JD, Dalbeth N, Mikuls T, et al. 2020 American College of Rheumatology guideline for the management of gout. *Arthritis Care Res (Hoboken)*. 2020;72(6):744–760. doi:10.1002/acr.24180
80. Williams CJ, Rosenthal AJ. Pathogenesis of calcium pyrophosphate deposition disease. *Best Pract Res Clin Rheumatol*. 2021;35(4):101718. doi:10.1016/j.berh.2021.101718
81. Abhishek A. Calcium pyrophosphate deposition disease: a review of epidemiologic findings. *Curr Opin Rheumatol*. 2016;28(2):133–139. doi:10.1097/bor.0000000000000246
82. Tedeschi SK, Pascart T, Latourte A, et al. Identifying potential classification criteria for calcium pyrophosphate deposition disease (CPPD): item generation and item reduction. *Arthritis Care Res (Hoboken)*. 2022;74(10):1649–1658 doi:10.1002/acr.24619
83. Parperis K, Papachristodoulou E, Kakoullis L, Rosenthal AK. Management of calcium pyrophosphate crystal deposition disease: a systematic review. *Semin Arthritis Rheum*. 2021;51(1): 84–94. doi:10.1016/J.Semarthrit.2020.10.005
84. Rosenthal AK. Basic calcium phosphate crystal-associated musculoskeletal syndromes: an update. *Curr Opin Rheumatol*. 2018;30(2):168–172. doi:10.1097/bor.0000000000000477
85. Bair MJ, Krebs EE. Fibromyalgia. *Ann Intern Med*. 2020;172(5):ITC33–ITC48. doi:10.7326/aitc202003030
86. Sarzi-Puttini P, Giorgi V, Marotto D, Atzeni F. Fibromyalgia: an update on clinical characteristics, aetiopathogenesis and treatment. *Nat Rev Rheumatol*. 2020;16(11):645–660. doi:10.1038/s41584-020-00506-w
87. Wolfe F, Clauw DJ, Fitzcharles MA, et al. 2016 revisions to the 2010/2011 fibromyalgia diagnostic criteria. *Semin Arthritis Rheum*. 2016;46(3):319–329. doi:10.1016/j.semarthrit.2016.08.012
88. Arnold LM, Bennett RM, Crofford LJ, et al. AAPT diagnostic criteria for fibromyalgia. *J Pain*. 2019;20(6):611–628. doi:10.1016/j.jpain.2018.10.008
89. Fitzcharles MA, Perrot S, Häuser W. Comorbid fibromyalgia: a qualitative review of prevalence and importance. *Eur J Pain*. 2018;22(9):1565–1576. doi:10.1002/ejp.1252
90. Wolfe F, Walitt BT, Katz RS, Häuser W. Social Security work disability and its predictors in patients with fibromyalgia. *Arthritis Care Res (Hoboken)*. 2014;66(9):1354–1363. doi:10.1002/acr.22305
91. Sluka KA, Clauw DJ. Neurobiology of fibromyalgia and chronic widespread pain. *Neuroscience*. 2016;338:114–129. doi:10.1016/j.neuroscience.2016.06.006
92. Choy EH. The role of sleep in pain and fibromyalgia. *Nat Rev Rheumatol*. 2015;11(9): 513–520. doi:10.1038/nrrheum.2015.56

93. Jones GT, Atzeni F, Beasley M, Flüß E, Sarzi-Puttini P, Macfarlane GJ. The prevalence of fibromyalgia in the general population: a comparison of the American College of Rheumatology 1990, 2010, and modified 2010 classification criteria. *Arthritis Rheumatol.* 2015;67(2): 568–575. doi:10.1002/art.38905
94. D'Agnelli S, Arendt-Nielsen L, Gerra MC, et al. Fibromyalgia: genetics and epigenetics insights may provide the basis for the development of diagnostic biomarkers. *Mol Pain.* 2019;15:1744806918819944. doi:10.1177/1744806918819944
95. Skarpsno ES, Nilsen TIL, Sand T, Hagen K, Mork PJ. The joint effect of insomnia symptoms and lifestyle factors on risk of self-reported fibromyalgia in women: longitudinal data from the Hunt Study. *BMJ Open.* 2019;9(8):e028684. doi:10.1136/bmjopen-2018-028684
96. Macfarlane GJ, Kronisch C, Dean LE, et al. EULAR revised recommendations for the management of fibromyalgia. *Ann Rheum Dis.* 2017;76(2):318–328. doi:10.1136/annrheumdis-2016-209724
97. Sieper J, Poddubnyy D. Axial spondyloarthritis. *Lancet.* 2017;390(10089):73–84. doi:10.1016/s0140-6736(16)31591-4
98. Rudwaleit M, Landewé R, van der Heijde D, et al. The development of Assessment of Spondyloarthritis International Society classification criteria for axial spondyloarthritis (part I): classification of paper patients by expert opinion including uncertainty appraisal. *Ann Rheum Dis.* 2009;68(6):770–776. doi:10.1136/ard.2009.108217
99. Reveille JD, Witter JP, Weisman MH. Prevalence of axial spondylarthritis in the United States: estimates from a cross-sectional survey. *Arthritis Care Res (Hoboken).* 2012;64(6): 905–910. doi:10.1002/acr.21621
100. Smith JA, Colbert RA. Review: the interleukin-23/interleukin-17 axis in spondyloarthritis pathogenesis: Th17 and beyond. *Arthritis Rheumatol.* 2014;66(2):231-241. doi:10.1002/art.38291
101. Dean LE, Jones GT, MacDonald AG, Downham C, Sturrock RD, Macfarlane GJ. Global prevalence of ankylosing spondylitis. *Rheumatology (Oxford).* 2014;53(4):650–657. doi:10.1093/rheumatology/ket387
102. Gofton JP, Chalmers A, Price GE, Reeve CE. Hl-a 27 and ankylosing spondylitis in B.C. Indians. *J Rheumatol.* 1984;11(5):572–573.
103. Lawrence RC, Everett DF, Benevolenskaya LI, et al. Spondyloarthropathies in circumpolar populations: I. Design and methods of United States and Russian studies. *Arctic Med Res.* 1996;55(4):187–194.
104. Sieper J, van der Heijde D, Landewe R, et al. New criteria for inflammatory back pain in patients with chronic back pain: a real patient exercise by experts from the Assessment of Spondyloarthritis International Society (ASAS). *Ann Rheum Dis.* 2009;68(6):784–788. doi:10.1136/ard.2008.101501
105. Ward MM, Deodhar A, Gensler LS, et al. 2019 update of the American College of Rheumatology/Spondylitis Association of America/Spondyloarthritis Research and Treatment Network recommendations for the treatment of ankylosing spondylitis and nonradiographic axial spondyloarthritis. *Arthritis Rheumatol.* 2019;71(10):1599–1613. doi:10.1002/art.41042
106. Curry SJ, Krist AH, Owens DK, et al. Screening for osteoporosis to prevent fractures: US Preventive Services Task Force recommendation statement. *JAMA.* 2018;319(24): 2521–2531. doi:10.1001/jama.2018.7498

107. Burge R, Dawson-Hughes B, Solomon DH, Wong JB, King A, Tosteson A. Incidence and economic burden of osteoporosis-related fractures in the United States, 2005–2025. *J Bone Miner Res.* 2007;22(3):465–475. doi:10.1359/jbmr.061113
108. Stone KL, Seeley DG, Lui LY, et al. BMD at multiple sites and risk of fracture of multiple types: long-term results from the study of osteoporotic fractures. *J Bone Mineral Res.* 2003;18(11):1947–1954. doi:10.1359/jbmr.2003.18.11.1947
109. Wright NC, Looker AC, Saag KG, et al. The recent prevalence of osteoporosis and low bone mass in the United States based on bone mineral density at the femoral neck or lumbar spine. *J Bone Mineral Res.* 2014;29(11):2520–2526. doi:10.1002/jbmr.2269
110. Looker AC, Frenk SM. Percentage of adults aged 65 and over with osteoporosis or low bone mass at the femur neck or lumbar spine: United States, 2005–2010. National Center for Health Statistics, Centers for Disease Control and Prevention. 2015. Available at: http://www.cdc.gov/nchs/data/hestat/osteoporsis/osteoporosis2005_2010.htm. Accessed September 14, 2016.
111. United States Bone and Joint Initiative. Fragility fractures. Available at: https://boneandjointburden.org/fourth-edition/iva2/fragility-fractures. Accessed January 30, 2023.
112. Spector TD, Williams FMK. The UK Adult Twin Registry (TwinsUK). *Twin Res Human Genetics.* 2006;9(6):899–906. doi:10.1375/twin.9.6.899
113. Kumar J, Swanberg M, McGuigan F, Callreus M, Gerdhem P, Akesson K. LRP4 association to bone properties and fracture and interaction with genes in the WNT- and BMP signaling pathways. *Bone.* 2011;49(3):343–348. doi:10.1016/j.bone.2011.05.018
114. Al-Barghouthi BM, Farber CR. Dissecting the genetics of osteoporosis using systems approaches. *Trends Genet.* 2019;35(1):55–67. doi:10.1016/j.tig.2018.10.004
115. Espallargues M, Sampietro-Colom L, Estrada MD, et al. Identifying bone-mass-related risk factors for fracture to guide bone densitometry measurements: a systematic review of the literature. *Osteoporos Int.* 2001;12(10):811–822. doi:10.1007/s001980170031
116. Boyce BF, Yao Z, Zhang Q, et al. New roles for osteoclasts in bone. *Ann N Y Acad Sci.* 2007;1116:245–254. doi:10.1196/annals.1402.084
117. Centre for Metabolic Bone Diseases, University of Sheffield. FRAX Fracture Risk Assessment Tool. 2008. Available at: https://frax.shef.ac.uk/FRAX. Accessed January 30, 2023.
118. De Laet C, Kanis JA, Odén A, et al. Body mass index as a predictor of fracture risk: a meta-analysis. *Osteoporos Int.* 2005;16(11):1330–1338. doi:10.1007/s00198-005-1863-y
119. Beals KA, Meyer NL. Female athlete triad update. *Clin Sports Med.* 2007;26(1):69–89. doi:10.1016/j.csm.2006.11.002
120. Giangregorio LM, Papaioannou A, Macintyre NJ, et al. Too Fit To Fracture: exercise recommendations for individuals with osteoporosis or osteoporotic vertebral fracture. *Osteoporos Int.* 2014;25(3):821–835. doi:10.1007/s00198-013-2523-2
121. Curry SJ, Krist AH, Owens DK, et al. Screening for osteoporosis to prevent fractures: US Preventive Services Task Force recommendation statement. *JAMA.* 2018;319(24):2521–2531. doi:10.1001/jama.2018.7498
122. Viswanathan M, Reddy S, Berkman N, et al. Screening to prevent osteoporotic fractures: updated evidence report and systematic review for the US Preventive Services Task Force. *JAMA.* 2018;319(24):2532–2551. doi:10.1001/jama.2018.6537

123. Camacho PM, Petak SM, Binkley N, et al. American Association of Clinical Endocrinologists/American College of Endocrinology clinical practice guidelines for the diagnosis and treatment of postmenopausal osteoporosis—2020 update. *Endocr Pract.* 2020;26(suppl 1):1–46. doi:10.4158/gl-2020-0524suppl
124. Buckley L, Guyatt G, Fink HA, et al. 2017 American College of Rheumatology guideline for the prevention and treatment of glucocorticoid-induced osteoporosis. *Arthritis Rheumatol.* 2017;69(8):1521–1537. doi:10.1002/art.40137
125. Centers for Disease Control and Prevention. Interventions. Updated January 20, 2023. Available at: https://www.cdc.gov/falls/programs/index.html. Accessed January 30, 2023.
126. Hawarden A, Jinks C, Mahmood W, et al. Public priorities for osteoporosis and fracture research: results from a focus group study. *Arch Osteoporos.* 2020;15(1):89. doi:10.1007/s11657-020-00766-9
127. Hampson G, Stone M, Lindsay JR, Crowley RK, Ralston SH. Diagnosis and management of osteoporosis during COVID-19: systematic review and practical guidance. *Calcif Tissue Int.* 2021;109(4):351–362. doi:10.1007/s00223-021-00858-9
128. Izmirly PM, Parton H, Wang L, et al. Prevalence of systemic lupus erythematosus in the United States: estimates from a meta-analysis of the Centers for Disease Control and Prevention national lupus registries. *Arthritis & Rheumatol.* 2021;73(6):991–996. doi:10.1002/art.41632
129. Centers for Disease Control and Prevention. Systemic lupus erythematosus (SLE). Updated July 5, 2022. Available at: https://www.cdc.gov/lupus/facts/detailed.html. Accessed January 31, 2023.
130. Kwon YC, Chun S, Kim K, Mak A. Update on the genetics of systemic lupus erythematosus: genome-wide association studies and beyond. *Cells.* 2019;8(10):1180. doi:10.3390/cells8101180
131. Petri M, Kim MY, Kalunian KC, et al. Combined oral contraceptives in women with systemic lupus erythematosus. *N Engl J Med.* 2005;353(24):2550–2558. doi:10.1056/nejmoa051135
132. Costenbader KH, Karlson EW. Cigarette smoking and systemic lupus erythematosus: a smoking gun? *Autoimmunity.* 2005;38(7):541–547. doi:10.1080/08916930500285758
133. Moulton VR, Suarez-Fueyo A, Meidan E, Li H, Mizui M, Tsokos GC. Pathogenesis of human systemic lupus erythematosus: a cellular perspective. *Trends Mol Med.* 2017;23(7):615–635. doi:10.1016/j.molmed.2017.05.006
134. Izmirly PM, Ferucci ED, Somers EC, et al. Incidence rates of systemic lupus erythematosus in the USA: estimates from a meta-analysis of the Centers For Disease Control and Prevention national lupus registries. *Lupus Sci Med.* 2021;8(1). doi:10.1136/lupus-2021-000614
135. Rees F, Doherty M, Grainge M, Davenport G, Lanyon P, Zhang W. The incidence and prevalence of systemic lupus erythematosus in the UK, 1999–2012. *Ann Rheum Dis.* 2016;75(1):136–141. doi:10.1136/annrheumdis-2014-206334
136. Singh RR, Yen EY. SLE mortality remains disproportionately high, despite improvements over the last decade. *Lupus.* 2018;27(10):1577–1581. doi:10.1177/0961203318786436
137. Manzi S, Meilahn EN, Rairie JE, et al. Age-specific incidence rates of myocardial infarction and angina in women with systemic lupus erythematosus: comparison with the Framingham Study. *Am J Epidemiol.* 1997;145(5):408–415. doi:10.1093/oxfordjournals.aje.a009122

138. Choi HS, Han KD, Jung JH, et al. The risk of end-stage renal disease in systemic lupus erythematosus: a nationwide population-based study in Korea. *Medicine (Baltimore).* 2019;98(28):e16420. doi:10.1097/md.0000000000016420
139. Yen EY, Singh RR. Brief report: lupus—an unrecognized leading cause of death in young females: a population-based study using nationwide death certificates, 2000–2015. *Arthritis Rheumatol.* 2018;70(8):1251–1255. doi:10.1002/art.40512
140. Bernatsky S, Boivin JF, Joseph L, et al. Mortality in systemic lupus erythematosus. *Arthritis Rheum.* 2006;54(8):2550–2557. doi:10.1002/art.21955
141. Carter EE, Barr SG, Clarke AE. The global burden of SLE: prevalence, health disparities and socioeconomic impact. *Nature Rev Rheumatol.* 2016;12(10):605–620. doi:10.1038/nrrheum.2016.137
142. Anandarajah AP, Luc M, Ritchlin CT. Hospitalization of patients with systemic lupus erythematosus is a major cause of direct and indirect healthcare costs. *Lupus.* 2017;26(7):756–761. doi:10.1177/0961203316676641
143. Carls G, Li T, Panopalis P, et al. Direct and indirect costs to employers of patients with systemic lupus erythematosus with and without nephritis. *J Occup Environ Med.* 2009;51(1):66–79. doi:10.1097/jom.0b013e31818a405a
144. Williams EM, Bruner L, Adkins A, et al. I too, am America: a review of research on systemic lupus erythematosus in African-Americans. *Lupus Sci Med.* 2016;3(1):e000144. doi:10.1136/lupus-2015-000144
145. The Lupus Initiative. Health disparities in lupus. Available at: https://thelupusinitiative.org/schools-library/health-disparities. Accessed January 31, 2023.
146. 2019 ACR/ARP annual meeting abstract supplement. *Arthritis Rheumatol.* 2019;71(suppl 10):1–5362. doi:10.1002/art.41108
147. Lim SS, Helmick CG, Bao G, et al. Racial disparities in mortality associated with systemic lupus erythematosus—Fulton and Dekalb Counties, Georgia, 2002–2016. *MMWR Morb Mortal Wkly Rep.* 2019;68(18):419–422. doi:10.15585/Mmwr.Mm6818a4
148. Gianfrancesco MA, Dall'era M, Murphy LB, et al. Mortality among minority populations with systemic lupus erythematosus, including Asian and Hispanic/Latino Persons—California, 2007–2017. *MMWR Morb Mortal Wkly Rep.* 2021;70(7):236–239. doi:10.15585/Mmwr.Mm7007a2
149. Buyon JP, Petri MA, Kim MY, et al. The effect of combined estrogen and progesterone hormone replacement therapy on disease activity in systemic lupus erythematosus: a randomized trial. *Ann Intern Med.* 2005;142(12 pt 1):953-962. doi:10.7326/0003-4819-142-12_Part_1-200506210-00004
150. Solhjoo M, Goyal A, Chauhan K. *Drug-Induced Lupus Erythematosus.* Treasure Island, FL: Statpearls Publishing; 2022.
151. Wichainun R, Kasitanon N, Wangkaew S, Hongsongkiat S, Sukitawut W, Louthrenoo W. Sensitivity and specificity of ANA and anti-dsDNA in the diagnosis of systemic lupus erythematosus: a comparison using control sera obtained from healthy individuals and patients with multiple medical problems. *Asian Pac J Allergy Immunol.* 2013;31(4):292–298. doi:10.12932/Ap0272.31.4.2013

152. Slater CA, Davis RB, Shmerling RH. Antinuclear antibody testing: a study of clinical utility. *Arch Intern Med.* 1996;156(13):1421–1425.
153. Hochberg MC. Updating the American College of Rheumatology revised criteria for the classification of systemic lupus erythematosus. *Arthritis Rheum.* 1997;40(9):1725. doi:10.1002/art.1780400928
154. Petri M, Purvey S, Fang H, Magder LS. Predictors of organ damage in systemic lupus erythematosus: the Hopkins Lupus Cohort. *Arthritis Rheum.* 2012;64(12):4021–4028. doi:10.1002/Art.34672
155. Aringer M, Costenbader K, Daikh D, et al. 2019 European League Against Rheumatism/American College of Rheumatology classification criteria for systemic lupus erythematosus. *Arthritis Rheumatol.* 2019;71(9):1400–1412. doi:10.1002/Art.40930
156. Johnson SR, Khanna D, Daikh D, et al. Use of consensus methodology to determine candidate items for systemic lupus erythematosus classification criteria. *J Rheumatol.* 2019;46(7):721–726. doi:10.3899/Jrheum.180478
157. Alarcón GS, McGwin G, Bertoli AM, et al. Effect of hydroxychloroquine on the survival of patients with systemic lupus erythematosus: data from Lumina, a multiethnic US cohort (Lumina L). *Ann Rheum Dis.* 2007;66(9):1168–1172. doi:10.1136/Ard.2006.068676
158. Fasano S, Pierro L, Pantano I, Iudici M, Valentini G. Longterm hydroxychloroquine therapy and low-dose aspirin may have an additive effectiveness in the primary prevention of cardiovascular events in patients with systemic lupus erythematosus. *J Rheumatol.* 2017;44(7):1032–1038. doi:10.3899/Jrheum.161351
159. Ruiz-Irastorza G, Crowther M, Branch W, Khamashta MA. Antiphospholipid syndrome. *Lancet.* 2010;376(9751):1498–509. doi:10.1016/S0140-6736(10)60709-X
160. Melles RB, Marmor MF. The risk of toxic retinopathy in patients on long-term hydroxychloroquine therapy. *JAMA Ophthalmol.* 2014;132(12):1453–1460. doi:10.1001/jamaophthalmol.2014.3459
161. Feldman CH, Collins J, Zhang Z, et al. Dynamic patterns and predictors of hydroxychloroquine nonadherence among Medicaid beneficiaries with systemic lupus erythematosus. *Semin Arthritis Rheum.* 2018;48(2):205–213. doi:10.1016/j.semarthrit.2018.01.002
162. Morand EF, Furie R, Tanaka Y, et al. Trial of anifrolumab in active systemic lupus erythematosus. *N Engl J Med.* 2019;382(3):211–221. doi:10.1056/Nejmoa1912196
163. Rovin BH, Teng YKO, Ginzler EM, et al. Efficacy and safety of voclosporin versus placebo for lupus nephritis (AURORA 1): a double-blind, randomised, multicentre, placebo-controlled, phase 3 trial. *Lancet.* 2021;397(10289):2070–2080. doi:10.1016/S0140-6736(21)00578-X
164. Fanouriakis A, Kostopoulou M, Alunno A, et al. 2019 update of the EULAR recommendations for the management of systemic lupus erythematosus. *Ann Rheum Dis.* 2019;78(6):736–745. doi:10.1136/annrheumdis-2019-215089

22

Chronic Liver Disease

Adnan Said, MD, MS, and Siddique Akram, MD

LEARNING OBJECTIVES

After completing this chapter, readers should be able to

1. Identify the different types of liver disease and their health effects.
2. Describe the trends in liver disease over the past two decades.
3. Understand which populations are at higher risk of liver disease and why.
4. Understand how to best reduce the risk of liver disease in specific populations.

INTRODUCTION

Liver disease is a term that encompasses a broad range of diagnoses and presentations. This ranges from mild liver test abnormalities in asymptomatic individuals at one end of the spectrum to end-stage liver disease with cirrhosis. Liver conditions can present as acute and fulminant disease with rapid liver failure or as chronic liver disease that slowly progresses over decades. Commonly used liver tests include measurement of serum liver enzymes (aspartate transaminase and alanine transaminase) that signify inflammation of the liver (i.e., hepatitis) and bilirubin levels that are an indicator of liver function and the severity of liver disease. Complications of advanced liver disease, such as cirrhosis, include gastrointestinal bleeding, accumulation of fluid in the abdominal cavity (ascites), and decreased cognitive function and neuromuscular function. The causes, consequences, and populations at high risk for liver disease are summarized in Figure 22-1 and described in detail in this chapter.

Significance

Chronic liver disease is a significant, important drain on global health care resources with approximately 4.5 million people with diagnosed liver disease in the United States, according to the 2017 National Vital Statistics Report by the Centers for Disease Control and Prevention (CDC). Globally, an estimated 1.5 billion persons were documented to have chronic liver disease in 2017.[1] The main etiologies of chronic liver disease include chronic hepatitis B, hepatitis C viral infection, alcohol-related liver disease, and

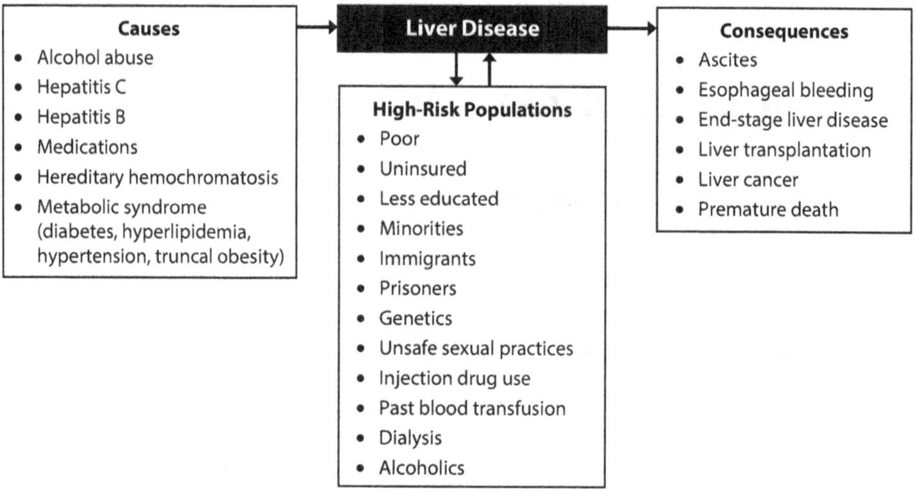

Figure 22-1. Liver Disease: Causes, Consequences, and High-Risk Populations

nonalcoholic fatty liver disease (NAFLD). Over the past two decades drastic changes in liver disease epidemiology and management have occurred, with the rise of the global epidemic of obesity in addition to the development of new antiviral regimens.[2] In this milieu, hepatitis B virus (HBV) can be prevented with vaccines and suppressed effectively with oral antiviral regimens in the chronic stage. Hepatitis C virus (HCV) can be cured with highly effective antiviral treatment regimens.[3] Moreover, liver transplantation has become a widely accepted procedure for patients with end-stage liver disease. The obesity epidemic in combination with metabolic syndrome (diabetes, hyperlipidemia, hypertension, and truncal obesity) has led to the continued increase in NAFLD, which is now the most common chronic liver disease in the United States and increasing worldwide as well.

Prevention of liver disease is integral to minimizing the burden of advanced liver disease. Development of the hepatitis B vaccine is one of the most important medical advances in this field. However, stigmatization of patients with alcoholism and viral hepatitis is an impediment to this goal. Patients with liver disease often are socially disadvantaged and have poor access to health care. Services to prevent and treat alcoholism and reduce the transmission of viral hepatitis have improved over the past two decades, but they need further support and dissemination. Obesity reduction through both individual practices and societal changes is needed to combat the increase in obesity-related liver disease.

Social and economic policies in the United States during the past century have played a significant role in the incidence of chronic liver disease. Liver-related mortality was high before the 1920s, plummeted during Prohibition, rose again during the Depression, with persistent increases through the time of World War II, and peaked in the early 1970s.[4]

Table 22-1. Trends in Age-Adjusted Mortality Rates for Liver Diseases

Year	Liver Cancer (*ICD-10*: C22.0)	Viral Hepatitis (*ICD-10*: B15–B19)	All Other Liver Disease (*ICD-10*: K70–K76)
1980	1.2	0.4	16.5
1985	1.4	0.4	13.9
1990	1.7	0.7	12.6
1995	1.9	1.3	11.3
2000	1.9	1.9	12.0
2005	2.1	1.8	11.9
2010	2.4	2.1	12.6
2014	2.5	2.1	13.8
2016	2.7	1.6	14.1
2018	2.8	1.2	14.4
2020	2.8	0.9	16.8

Source: Based on CDC WONDER.[7]

Note: International Classification of Diseases, Ninth Revision (*ICD-9*) codes were used from 1980–1995 and *International Classification of Diseases,* Tenth Revision (*ICD-10*) codes from 1999–2020, when abstracting data from CDC WONDER.

Between 1981 and 2010, age-adjusted death rates from chronic liver disease and liver cancer increased significantly. From 2006 to 2010, the average annual percentage change in death rates increased 1.5% for chronic liver disease and 2.6% for liver cancer.[5] In the United States in 2019, chronic liver disease and cirrhosis was the ninth leading cause of death for males (1.9% of deaths), but it was not in the top ten for females.[6] Trends for chronic liver disease mortality in the United States, including viral hepatitis, liver cancer, and other causes, from 1980 to 2014 are detailed in Table 22-1.[7]

Worldwide, liver disease accounts for approximately two million deaths per year: one million from complications associated with liver disease, and one million from viral hepatitis and hepatocellular carcinoma. Cirrhosis is currently the 11th most common cause of deaths worldwide and liver cancer is 16th—combined, cirrhosis and liver cancer account for 3.5% of all deaths globally.[2]

The morbidity from liver disease is just as important, given the effects on quality of life as well as the economic consequences. For instance, the health care costs associated with hospitalized patients with cirrhosis is increasing, with an increased number of admissions and a longer length of stay in both decompensated cirrhosis and compensated cirrhosis groups. Hospitalization costs for patients with cirrhosis increased 30.2% from 2008 ($5.7 billion) to 2014 ($7.4 billion) based on National Inpatient Sample data.[8]

Data from the Global Burden of Diseases Study revealed that from 1996 to 2016 there was a 4.3% per year increase in overall health care spending for patients with chronic liver diseases or cirrhosis, driven by a 17.8% per year (95% CI, 14.5%–21.6%) increase in price and intensity of hospital-based services. This is driven disproportionately by acute management, as is evidenced by the fact that over 60% of total expenditures are attributable to inpatient care.[9]

Causes

Liver disease can be attributed to a multitude of causes. Chronic liver disease is defined arbitrarily as liver disease that persists beyond six months from onset, and studies have demonstrated that up to 56% of people with chronic liver disease may be completely asymptomatic.[10] This is an important factor to consider when one is studying the occurrence of new cases as well as the overall prevalence.

The most prevalent causes in the population include NAFLD, alcoholic liver disease, viral hepatitis, hepatocellular carcinoma, and medication-related liver disease, and less commonly genetic conditions such as hereditary hemochromatosis, which leads to liver damage from iron overload. Data from the National Health and Nutrition Examination Survey (NHANES) illustrate some key emerging trends between 1988 and 2016. During this period the prevalence of hepatitis B and alcoholic liver disease remained stable, but the prevalence of chronic hepatitis C was reduced by nearly 50%: 1.6% in 1988 to 1994 to 0.9% in 2013 to 2016. Rates of NAFLD, in contrast, increased from 20% (1988–1994) to 31.9% (2013–2016).[11] NAFLD was the only liver disease with consistently increasing prevalence. Multivariable regression revealed that obesity and type 2 diabetes mellitus were the major independent predictors of NAFLD and both increased in prevalence over the study period.[3] The attributable risk for chronic liver disease and cirrhosis in the US population is detailed from various sources in Tables 22-2 and 22-3.[12,13]

Table 22-2. Primary Causes of Chronic Liver Disease

Factor	Attributable Risk for Chronic Liver Disease	Attributable Risk for Cirrhosis
Alcohol	20%	50%
Hepatitis C and alcohol	10%	10%
Hepatitis C	15%	10%
Hepatitis B	3%	5%
Non-alcoholic fatty liver disease (NAFLD)	35%	10%
Unknown	17%	15%
Total	100%	100%

Source: Based on Singh and Hoyert[12] and WHO.[13]

Table 22-3. Causes of Cirrhosis

Factor	Population Exposed	Relative Risk	Population-Attributable Risk
Alcohol	15 million	4-20	13%-50%
Hepatitis C	3.5 million	10-30	8%-25%
Hepatitis B	1 million	2.5-20	1%-7%
Metabolic syndrome	25 million	2-6	8%-20%

Note: Authors' estimates.

ALCOHOLIC LIVER DISEASE

Significance

Chronic heavy alcohol use can lead to liver disease that manifests as fatty liver disease, alcohol-induced hepatitis, or cirrhosis, conditions that can overlap. Alcohol-induced fatty liver can be seen in up to 90% of alcoholics.[14] It develops rapidly, in some studies after a weekend of bingeing. With alcohol cessation, it resolves quickly as well, within two weeks in some studies.[15] Alcohol-induced fatty liver can progress to cirrhosis in 10% to 15% of patients over long-term follow-up of 10 years or more.[16] The risk increases with the amount of alcohol consumed over this duration.

With alcohol-induced hepatitis, the clinical spectrum ranges from a self-limited disorder to a severe life-threatening illness with liver failure. With longitudinal follow-up, the risk of developing cirrhosis can be as high as 70% in patients with alcohol-induced hepatitis.[17] With cessation of alcohol intake, the changes of alcohol-induced hepatitis can be reversible except in the most severe cases.

Descriptive Epidemiology

Rates of alcoholic liver disease in populations are closely linked to per capita consumption of alcohol in those populations. In an examination of trends in chronic liver disease mortality and socioeconomic determinants in the United States from 1935 to 1996, alcohol use, unemployment, and minority concentration were closely linked to liver disease mortality. A 10% decrease in per capita alcohol consumption has been associated with a 2.5% reduction in cirrhosis mortality with a lag time as short as one year.[12] In a European study, a one-liter increase in alcohol consumption per capita was associated with a 14% increase in cirrhosis mortality for men and 8% for women.[18]

Along with alcohol consumption rates, death rates from alcohol-induced cirrhosis increased after Prohibition in the United States from the 1930s to 1973, a peak of 14.9 deaths per 100,000 population.[4] Alcohol-related deaths have declined from the 1970s in the United States. From 1973 to 1997 age-adjusted death rates from cirrhosis and chronic liver disease decreased at an average annual rate of 3.0% for the entire population, by 2.6% for White men, 3.0% for White women, 4.1% for African American men, and 4.8% for African American women. However, subsequently the US mortality rate from any cause of cirrhosis increased by 8.2% between 2000 and 2013, from 9.7 to 10.5 deaths per 100,000. Based on the cause of the cirrhosis, the mortality increase over time was higher for alcohol-related cirrhosis, with an 18.6% increase from 4.3 to 5.1 deaths per 100,000 people.[19]

Despite stable consumption rates, alcoholic liver disease–induced mortality has increased in the United Kingdom and other parts of Northern Europe. In England, the rate of alcohol-induced cirrhosis death increased from 2.8 per 100,000 in 1993 to 8.0 per 100,000 in 2000. These increases were seen in all ethnic groups, but the mortality rate in Asian men was 3.8 times that of White men.[20] In parts of Asia, including Japan, Korea, and China, the consumption of alcohol has increased steadily from the 1960s and the proportion of liver disease attributed to alcohol has increased commensurately.[21] In Japan, the proportion of all liver disease from alcohol increased from 5.1% in 1968 to 14.1% by 1986.[22]

Causes

The risk of alcohol-induced cirrhosis rises with the amount of alcohol consumed. The risk is increased with sustained intake of greater than 60 grams per day in men and greater than 20 grams per day in women, but the risk varies considerably (one drink is 8–12 g in the US). Only 6% to 40% of people drinking to this level will eventually develop cirrhosis. The risk also increases with lifetime alcohol use (100 kg in the Dionysos Italian population study).[23] The risk of death after alcohol-induced cirrhosis is diagnosed is much higher with continued drinking but improves significantly with abstinence. With continued drinking, the five-year survival in patients with alcohol-induced cirrhosis is less than 30%, but more than 60% with abstinence and more than 90% if they have compensated cirrhosis.[24]

The wide variability in the risk of cirrhosis with alcohol intake depends on incompletely understood genetic factors, including polymorphisms in genes that influence alcohol metabolism and absorption, coexistence of other liver injurious agents (e.g., hepatitis C), iron overload (as seen in genetic hemochromatosis), and sex differences. Although alcohol abuse and cirrhosis-related deaths predominate in men worldwide, including the United States, there is a growing proportion of women among heavy drinkers.[25] Women have a higher susceptibility to alcohol compared with men. The risk of cirrhosis develops with lower rates of drinking in women (20–60 g/day) compared with men (40–80 g/day) and cirrhosis develops with shorter duration of alcohol abuse in women. Multiple mechanisms are thought to underlie this susceptibility, including variations in alcohol distribution and levels in blood, gastric enzyme activity, first-pass metabolism, and sex hormone differences in endotoxin after exposure to alcohol.[26]

Ethnic differences in alcohol use and alcohol-induced liver disease exist, with the highest rates of alcoholic liver disease in Hispanic men, followed by Black men and White men.[27] Part of this may be explained by continued high rates of heavy drinking in Hispanic populations compared with other ethnic groups.[27] Differences in genetic predisposition, socioeconomic status, nutrition, and access to health care may all play a role, but this has not been clarified.

Alcohol use is common in patients with HCV infection, with some studies suggesting that as many as 60% to 70% of hepatitis C–infected individuals consume as much as 40 grams of alcohol per day.[28] The association of alcohol abuse and hepatitis C infection is associated with higher rates of progression to cirrhosis, liver cancer, and cirrhosis-related death. Some studies suggest that the association may be synergistic.[29] Alcoholics with hepatitis C infection are at higher risk of cirrhosis than alcoholics not infected with hepatitis C.[30] Conversely, of patients infected with hepatitis C, those who consume alcohol heavily (>50 g/day) have a higher risk of progression to cirrhosis than nondrinkers.[29] Even smaller amounts of alcohol use (30 g/day) have been shown to promote fibrosis of the liver in patients with chronic hepatitis C infection.[31]

The contributing role of diabetes and obesity—which themselves are risk factors for liver disease—needs further clarification in alcohol-induced liver disease. Some studies have not shown these to be independent risk factors whereas others have.[23,32] Obesity-related fatty liver disease may proceed along the same pathophysiologic pathways of liver injury as alcohol, and the combination may have synergistic effects on liver damage. There may also be a dose-dependent effect of alcohol on NAFLD, with small doses of alcohol protecting against progressive liver disease and increased consumption leading to the development of more advanced liver disease.[33,34] The association of diet, particularly the consumption of pork products with beer drinking, has been associated with liver disease in drinkers.[35] Other studies have found protective effects of coffee drinking.[36]

Interventions

See Chapter 10: Alcohol Use.

HEPATITIS A

The hepatitis A virus (HAV) is an RNA virus that spreads by fecal–oral contact from contaminated food and water as well by person-to-person contact. It occurs in both sporadic cases and in epidemic outbreaks (60% of US cases). Contaminated food, particularly shellfish, is a usual source of contamination. Susceptible individuals are at risk for epidemic outbreaks such as one that occurred in Shanghai from contaminated clams involving 290,000 people.[37] It has also been spread by contaminated green onions imported from Mexico and strawberries from Guatemala.[38]

Significance

Hepatitis A causes an acute illness. The likelihood of developing symptomatic disease is age-dependent, with more than 70% of children being asymptomatic and most adults and adolescents (>70%) developing symptomatic disease.[39] The symptoms are nonspecific and may include aches, fever, abdominal pain, and jaundice. The incubation period can last from 15 to 49 days; jaundice usually lasts one to three months.

Hepatitis A does not lead to chronic hepatitis except for very rare cases of relapsing forms, which ultimately resolve as well. Development of severe acute liver failure is also rare (1%) but more likely to occur in adults than children and in those adults with underlying chronic liver disease such as from hepatitis C.[40] Diagnosis is made by detection of serum hepatitis A antibody (hepatitis A immunoglobulin [Ig] M subtype) that is positive by the onset of symptoms and detectable up to six months after onset of illness. After recovery, the individual usually develops lifelong hepatitis A antibody IgG subtype rendering immunity from further attacks.[41]

Descriptive Epidemiology

The incidence of hepatitis A is much higher in developing countries and occurs earlier in childhood (95% are immune by adulthood), whereas in Europe and the United States, infection rates in children are lower and adult symptomatic infection is not uncommon, although it is decreasing. It is estimated that 33% of the US population has been infected with HAV.[42] There is no chronic infection, and these individuals are now immune to hepatitis A.

The incidence of hepatitis A in the United States has steadily decreased from the 1970s. The incidence was 28 cases per 100,000 in 1970, decreased to 13 per 100,000 by 1980, and remained steady until 1990. This decrease was likely secondary to improved food handling and processing as well as epidemic management. Since vaccination became available in 1995, hepatitis A rates have declined by 95% in the United States. In 2013 only 1,781 acute asymptomatic cases were reported, with 3,473 estimated new infections occurring. From 2015 to 2019, however, the United States experienced multistate increases in hepatitis A outbreaks primarily caused by person-to-person spread among adults who experience homelessness or use drugs. From 2019 to 2020 there was a 47% decrease in incidence. In 2020 several states declared an end to outbreaks, while only two states reported new outbreaks. Despite the reduction from 2019 to 2020, hepatitis A rates in 2020 remained seven times higher than in 2015 (Figure 22-2).[43] In the United States person-to-person transmission has become more common than transmission from contaminated food or water, although sporadic outbreaks caused by single contaminated food sources also have occurred. Higher risk groups for person-to-person transmission include incarcerated persons, men who

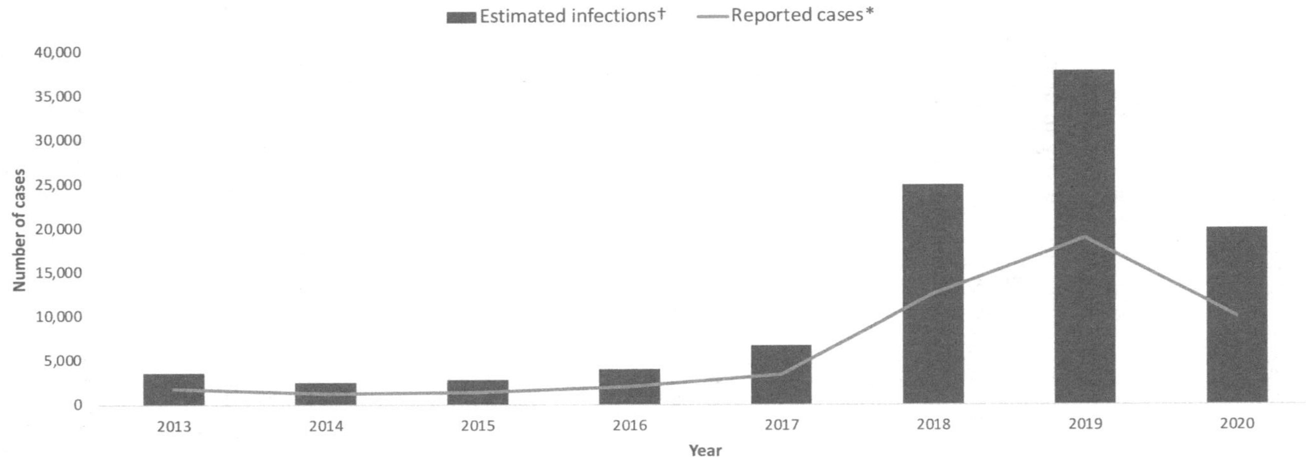

Hepatitis A	2013	2014	2015	2016	2017	2018	2019	2020
Reported cases*	1,781	1,239	1,390	2,007	3,366	12,474	18,846	9,952
Estimated infections†	3,600	2,500	2,800	4,000	6,700	24,900	37,700	19,900

*Reported confirmed cases. For the case definition, see https://ndc.services.cdc.gov/conditions/hepatitis-a-acute/.

† The number of estimated viral hepatitis infections was determined by multiplying the number of reported cases that met the classification criteria for a confirmed case by a factor that adjusted for underascertainment and underreporting. The 95% bootstrap confidence intervals for the estimated number of infections are displayed in the Appendix.

Source: Reprinted from CDC.[43]

Figure 22-2. Number of Reported Cases of Hepatitis A Virus Infection and Estimated Infections: United States, 2013–2020

have sex with men, and intravenous drug users in homeless populations, as well as persons with chronic liver disease or cirrhosis. In 2020, 84% of cases occurred among non-Hispanic White populations and rates were highest in people 30 to 39 years of age. From 2016 to 2020 there were 46,645 cases reported in the United States, with 736 resulting in death.[43]

Causes

Risk factors associated with higher rates of hepatitis A included household crowding and poverty. International travel is a risk factor as well, particularly to areas where hepatitis A is endemic, such as Mexico and Central and South America. Other risk factors include sexual and household contact with another person with hepatitis A and as noted, transmission in men who have sex with men and among those who use illicit drugs.[44]

Interventions

Hepatitis A infection can be prevented by improved sanitary conditions, including treatment of water, avoidance of contaminated shellfish and food, and hand washing. Source determination and vaccination of exposed susceptible individuals are key to controlling epidemics.

Eventually, vaccination of children should decrease incidence further. Immunization for hepatitis A is now recommended universally for all children aged 12 to 23 months and those at higher risk of transmission (e.g., travelers to endemic areas, men who have sex with men, intravenous and nonintravenous drug users). A highly effective vaccine has been available since 1996 (Figure 22-3).[45]

HEPATITIS B

Hepatitis B is a DNA virus belonging to the hepadnaviridae family and is extremely prevalent globally. The hepatitis B virus (HBV) is spread by parenteral exposure to blood and other body fluids. Because of a large prevalence in developing countries such as China (10%–20%), it is efficiently spread to neonates by vertical transmission (mother to child at birth), which is the main modality of transmission in the developing world.[46] In the United States, with a lower prevalence (est. 730,000 million cases, or 0.28% of the population) and better access to perinatal care and childhood immunization, vertical transmission is less common than adult-to-adult transmission through sexual contact or illicit drug use. In the era of universal vaccination in the United States (since 1991), the incidence of chronic HBV infection has declined in children, but not in adults older than 50 years of age.[47]

Children
All children aged 12–23 mo
Unvaccinated children and adolescents aged 2–18 y

People at increased risk for HAV infection
International travelers
Men who have sex with men
People who use injection or noninjection drugs (i.e., all those who use illegal drugs)
People with occupational risk for exposure
People who anticipate close personal contact with an international adoptee
People experiencing homelessness

People at increased risk for severe disease from HAV infection
People with chronic liver disease
People with human immunodeficiency virus infection

Other people recommended for vaccination
Pregnant women at risk for HAV infection or severe outcome from HAV infection
Any people who requests vaccination

Vaccination during outbreaks
Unvaccinated people in outbreak settings who are at risk for HAV infection or at risk for severe disease from HAV

Implementation strategies for settings providing services to adults
People in settings that provide services to adults in which a high proportion of those people have risk factors for HAV infection

Hepatitis A vaccination is no longer recommended by ACIP
People who receive blood products for clotting disorders (e.g., hemophilia)

Source: Adapted from Nelson et al.[45]
Note: ACIP = Advisory Committee on Immunization Practices; HAV = hepatitis A virus. For further information, see the "Recommendations for Hepatitis A Vaccine and Immune Globulin for Preexposure Prophylaxis" section of Nelson et al.[45]

Figure 22-3. Prevention of Hepatitis A Virus Infection: Recommendations of the Advisory Committee on Immunization Practices, United States, 2020

According to data from NHANES 1999 to 2006, the prevalence of markers of active or past infection from hepatitis B was higher among non-Hispanic Blacks (12.2%) and persons of "other" race/ethnicity (13.3%) than it was among non-Hispanic Whites (2.8%) or Mexican Americans (2.9%), and it was higher among foreign-born participants (12.2%) than it was among US-born participants (3.5%). Prevalence among

US-born children aged 6 to 19 years (0.5%) did not differ by race or ethnicity. Disparities between US-born and foreign-born children were smaller between 1999 and 2006 (0.5% vs. 2.0%) than 1988 to 1994 (1.0% vs. 12.8%). Among children aged 6 to 19 years, 56.7% had markers of vaccine-induced immunity. According to data from CDC in 2020, the prevalence of *acute* hepatitis B infection was higher among non-Hispanic Blacks (0.7%) and non-Hispanic Whites (0.7%) than it was among Hispanics (0.3%) and Asians/Pacific Islanders (0.2%).[43]

Significance

In children and neonates, acute infection is clinically silent in the majority. In adults, acute infection is symptomatic in 30% to 50% of the population. Hepatitis B virus acute infection has an incubation period of one to four months. Symptoms during the prodromal phase may be vague but include fatigue, aches, malaise, and abdominal pain. Jaundice can occur and can last from 4 to 12 weeks.[48]

With chronic infection, the risk of developing cirrhosis and hepatocellular carcinoma increases with longer duration of infection. In endemic countries, the risk is highest in men older than 40 years of age.[48] Increased risk of progressive liver disease also depends on the interaction between the host immune system and the virus. The risk is higher in those individuals with high levels of chronic viral replication and high levels of the virus in the blood. The risk is reduced considerably in those individuals in whom the immune system successfully suppresses viral replication.[49]

Increased risk of progressive liver disease leading to cirrhosis and hepatocellular carcinoma also occurs with concurrent tobacco and alcohol use. The lifetime risk of cirrhosis and hepatocellular carcinoma is higher in individuals from endemic areas likely because of longer durations of infection.[49]

Descriptive Epidemiology

High rates of vertical transmission (i.e., from mother to child) in developing countries result in high prevalence because of the high chances of developing chronic infection after exposure at this stage of life. In the United States, where most of the transmission is in adults, the lower rate of chronicity results in lower prevalence rates. The incidence of acute hepatitis B remained steady in the United States between 2013 and 2019 (1.1 case/100,000).[43] An estimated 880,000 to 1.89 million individuals are living with chronic HBV in the United States.

Foreign-born persons account for 69% of the chronic HBV in the United States.[50] Prevalence rates are highest in Asians (99% born outside the US) and Alaska Natives, and they are higher in incarcerated, homeless, and institutionalized individuals. According to an analysis of the national death registry, the age-adjusted mortality rate for hepatitis B–related illness increased throughout the 1980s and early 1990s from 0.2 per 100,000 to 0.8 per 100,000. This increase was followed by a relative plateau and then a decline starting in 1999. As of 2018, the mortality rate was approximately 0.43 per 100,000.[7]

Globally, hepatitis B is a huge issue, with 2 billion people who have been infected worldwide, 240 million chronic carriers of HBV, and about 800,000 deaths from associated liver disease, including liver cancer and cirrhosis. The figure of 240 million chronic HBV carriers is a reduction from previously published rates of 350 to 400 million. This reduction is primarily observed in younger age groups and is a function of availability of better population-based data; population-wide vaccination against hepatitis B in newborns, young children, and adolescents; and improved screening of blood products and safer injection procedures.[51] The prevalence rates vary greatly, from below 2% in tropical areas as well as in Latin America, North America, and Western Europe, to rates as high as 8.6% in East Asia.[52]

The incidence of hepatitis B in the United States has decreased after peaking in the 1980s (Figure 22-4).[53] The incidence of HBV was 4.1 per 100,000 in the United States in 1970, peaked in 1980 to 8.4 in 100,000, and remained at 8.5 in 100,000 by 1990. Between 1995 and 2013 the incidence of acute hepatitis B declined by 79% to 1.0 in 100,000, the lowest ever reported. In the United States, 78,000 estimated new infections occurred in 2001, and this had dropped to 18,760 by 2012 and to 2,157 by 2020.[43]

Declines were reported in all age groups but were most steep in children. In 2020, the highest rates of acute hepatitis B were in persons aged 40 to 49 years

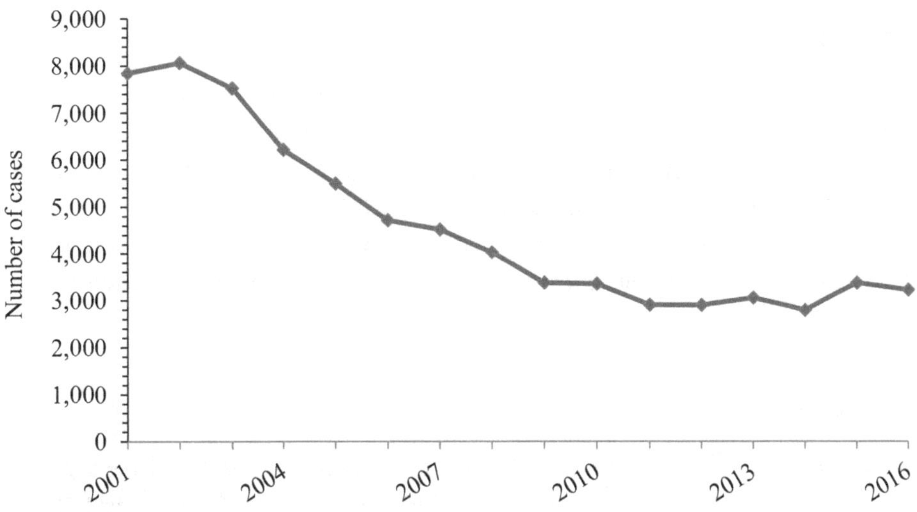

Source: Adapted from CDC.[53]

Figure 22-4. Reported Number of Acute Hepatitis B Cases: United States, 2001–2016

(1.7/100,000 population) and the lowest among adolescents and children younger than 19 years of age (0.0/100,000).[43] Universal hepatitis B vaccination has resulted in these reduced rates in children. High rates for hepatitis B continue among adults, however, particularly men aged 30 to 59 years, emphasizing the need to identify and vaccinate high-risk adults.

The rates for HBV infection in male individuals still predominated compared with female individuals (0.8 vs. 0.5/100,000 in 2020). The rates of hepatitis B declined for all races and ethnicities from 2000 to 2020. Rates were highest for non-Hispanic Blacks and non-Hispanic Whites in 2020 (both at 0.7/100,000) followed by Native Americans (0.4/100,000), Hispanics (0.3/100,000), and Asians/Pacific Islanders (0.2/100,000).

The reduction in incidence in the United States is likely the reason for the reduction in global acute hepatitis B infections. The reasons for this decline in incidence include a combination of universal vaccination of neonates and adolescents (<18 years) and recommendation of vaccination of high-risk adults. Safer needle use practices in injection drug users as well as continued screening of blood products has also contributed to the reduction in adult-to-adult transmission.[43]

Despite the decrease in incidence and prevalence of hepatitis B, the burden of disease has not decreased. The number of hospitalizations for hepatitis B–related liver disease in the United States increased fourfold between 1990 and 2006.[54] This increased morbidity may be attributable to increased access to health care or increased numbers of patients with hepatitis B developing cirrhosis and liver cancer from chronic infection, as well as an increased influx of immigrants with hepatitis B infection. It is estimated that 40,000 immigrants with HBV infection are admitted annually to the United States.[55]

Causes

Reported risk factors in the United States include sexual contact (32% multiple sex partners, 10% sexual contact with a person known to have hepatitis B, 13% men who have sex with men), and injection drug use (15%). Hemodialysis was a risk factor in 0.3%, blood transfusion in 0.2%, and occupational exposure in 0.8% (Figure 22-5).[56]

The risk of developing chronic infection depends on the age at which exposure occurs. Neonatal transmission results in chronic infection in 90% of unvaccinated children.[57] In adults, however, acute infection results in chronic infection in only 5%.[55]

Interventions

Hepatitis B is a vaccine-preventable disease. The vaccine has been available since the early 1980s, and the recent vaccine is more than 95% effective.[58] The World Health Organization has recommended universal childhood vaccination worldwide. So far, 158 countries have incorporated hepatitis vaccination in routine immunization, but

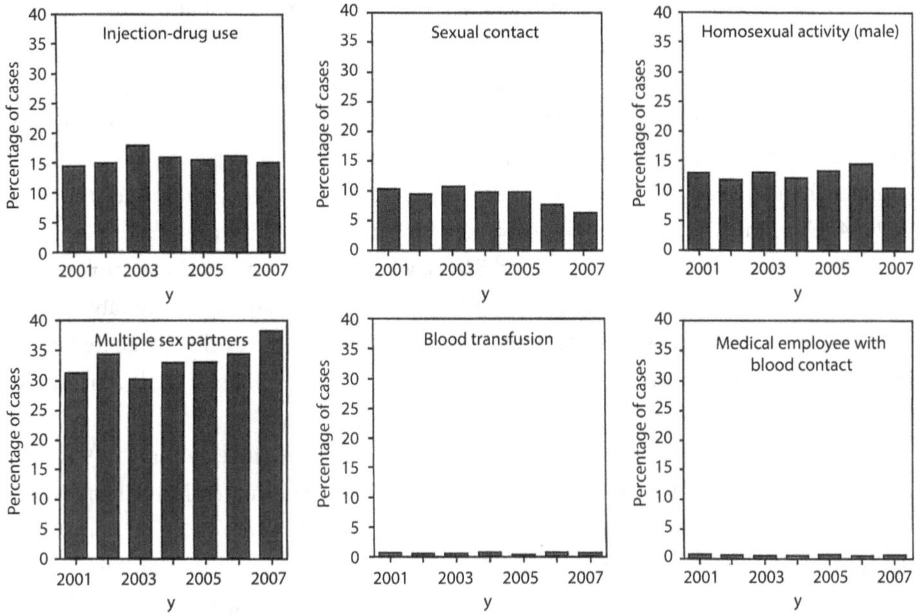

Source: Adapted from CDC.[53]

Note: The percentage of cases among persons in which a specific risk factor was reported was calculated based on the total number of persons for whom any information for that exposure was reported. Multiple risk factors may be reported for a single case.

Figure 22-5. Trends in Selected Epidemiological Characteristics Among Patients With Acute Hepatitis B by Year: United States, 2001–2007

coverage is far from universal with 60% coverage.[13] A comprehensive strategy to eliminate HBV transmission has been introduced in the United States since 1991, and was updated in 2006. Since 1991, vaccination has been recommended universally for all infants born in the United States as well for children younger than 18 years of age as a catch-up program.[59]

In addition, all women seeking prenatal care are screened for HBV infection; for women with hepatitis B, their infants are vaccinated and given prophylaxis with hepatitis B immunoglobulin at birth. Efficacy of this regimen is greater than 95%. For adults at high risk, screening and vaccination are recommended. Those at risk include users of illicit drugs, individuals with multiple sexual partners, sexual partners of persons with HBV infection, solid organ recipients, dialysis patients, and health care workers, among others.

In the United States, 56% of individuals attending dialysis were vaccinated against HBV in 2002 (47% in 1997), as well as 90% of dialysis staff. Hepatitis B incidence in 2002 was only 0.12% in dialysis center patients, compared with 1974, when the incidence of hepatitis B among dialysis patients was 6.2%, and selected hemodialysis centers reported rates as high as 30%.[60] This decline began in 1982, when HBV vaccination was first recommended for dialysis patients.

The efficacy of childhood vaccination is already seen in countries with a high rate of vertical and early childhood transmission. In Taiwan, for example, where universal neonatal vaccination was introduced in 1986, the prevalence of hepatitis B in children younger than 15 years of age was 9.8% before this implementation, but reduced to 1.2% in 2004.[61] The rate of hepatocellular carcinoma in children in Taiwan has also decreased by a third over this period. In the United States, where HBV transmission occurs mostly in adults, the results of universal childhood vaccination will have a considerably longer lag time before the benefits of vaccination are seen, although the decline in acute hepatitis B rates in children born in the United States over the past 15 years is likely attributable to universal vaccination.

Hepatitis B–specific antiviral agents have been available since the late 1990s, and with high potency and low levels of resistance since 2006. The currently available agents are effective in suppressing viral replication, but are not able to eradicate the virus from the human host. As a result, these must be taken daily and often for long durations to suppress the virus. In individuals with evidence of chronic liver damage and viral replication, these agents are used to decrease the risk of progression to cirrhosis and liver cancer.[62]

HEPATITIS C

Hepatitis C is an RNA virus belonging to the flaviviridae family that infects the liver. Hepatitis C virus (HCV) is spread parenterally by breach of mucosal membranes and is efficiently spread by illicit drug use, including injection drugs and intranasal cocaine, and somewhat less efficiently by sexual transmission. A surge in incidence of hepatitis C occurred in the 1970s and 1980s because of transmission of the virus by these routes as well as by blood transfusion.[63] Before the discovery of the hepatitis C viral genome in 1989, the safety of the blood supply was based on testing for elevated liver enzymes, and because chronic hepatitis C (called "non-A non-B hepatitis" before 1989) is often associated with normal liver enzymes, transfusion-associated transmission was not uncommon. With the discovery of the HCV genome in 1989 and the development of an accurate antibody test thereafter, the blood supply has become very safe, with the risk of transfusion-related hepatitis C estimated to be about 1 per 100,000 to 1 per 1,000,000 units transfused (Figure 22-6).[64]

Significance

After exposure to HCV, chronic infection occurs in 70% to 85%, with a minority clearing the virus within six months of exposure. Overall progression to cirrhosis is estimated to

Reported Acute (New) Cases of HCV								
2005	2006	2007	2008	2009	2010	2011	2012	2013
694	802	849	878	781	853	1,230	1,778	2,138

Estimated Actual New Cases of HCV (Range)		
2011[a]	2012[a]	2013[a]
16,500 (7,200–43,400)	24,700 (19,600–84,400)	29,700 (23,500–101,400)

Estimated No. of Chronic Cases	No. of Death Certificates Listing HCV as a Cause of Death			
	2010	2011	2012	2013[b]
2.7–3.9 million	16,627[c]	17,721[c]	18,650[c]	19,368[c]

Source: Adapted from CDC.[53]

Note: HCV = hepatitis C virus.

[a]Actual acute cases estimated to be 13.9 times the number of reported cases in any year.

[b]Underlying or contributing cause of death in most recent year available (2013).

[c]Current information indicates these represent a fraction of deaths attributable in whole or in part to chronic hepatitis C.

Figure 22-6. Burden of Hepatitis C: United States

occur in 10% to 20% of hepatitis C–infected patients over their lifetime.[65] Higher rates are seen with steady alcohol intake, in male individuals, and with longer duration of infection, as well as in individuals infected at older age (>40 years).[66] On average, it takes 20 years from initial HCV infection to develop cirrhosis in these patients. Hepatocellular carcinoma develops at the rate of 1% per year in those with cirrhosis.

Although researchers projected a decline in the prevalence of infection in the United States from a peak of 2.7% in the 1990s to 1% by 2030,[67] the number of acute hepatitis C cases in the United States increased gradually between 2010 and 2019, mostly as a result of the opioid epidemic. The number of acute infections increased from 0.3 per 100,000 in 2008 to 1.3 cases per 100,000 by 2019, with an estimated 57,500 acute infections in 2019.[43] The burden of disease attributable to hepatitis C is still rising because of the disease's chronicity and the lag time from acquisition of infection to development of clinically significant liver disease. The death rate from hepatitis C has increased from 0.4 deaths per 100,000 in 1982 to a peak of 4.4 per 100,000 in 2016, with a decline to 3.3 by 2019. Mortality rates were highest among persons aged 55 to 74 years, compared with other age categories, and deaths in this age group accounted for 76% of all hepatitis C–associated deaths reported during 2019. Non-Hispanic Whites accounted for 64% of all hepatitis C–associated deaths; however, the mortality rates among American Indian/Alaska Natives and non-Hispanic Blacks were 2.8 times and

1.8 times, respectively, the mortality rate among non-Hispanic Whites.[43] Some of the recent decline may be attributable to the availability of highly effective antiviral therapy for hepatitis C since 2013.[68]

Morbidity and health care costs for hepatitis C increased over the last two decades, with an early decline in liver transplants seen since the advent of the highly effective antiviral era. Between 1991 and 2013, the proportion of liver transplants related to hepatitis C increased from 12% to 40%, but have subsequently declined to 23.6% of all liver transplants in the United States.[69] Galbraith et al.[70] analyzed data from the National Ambulatory Medical Care Survey, the National Hospital Ambulatory Medical Care Survey, and the Nationwide Inpatient Sample. They found that individuals with HCV infection were responsible for more than 2.3 million outpatient, 73,000 emergency department, and 475,000 inpatient visits annually. Baby boomers accounted for 72%, 68%, and 71% of care episodes in these settings, respectively. Whereas the number of outpatient visits remained stable during the study period, inpatient admissions among hepatitis C–infected baby boomers increased by greater than 60%. Inpatient stays totaled 2.8 million days and cost more than $15 billion annually. Non-White, uninsured individuals, and those receiving publicly funded health insurance were disproportionately affected in all health care settings.[70] Hepatitis C also has a profound effect on quality of life in patients referred to health centers, some of which is related to concurrent comorbid illnesses such as depression.[71]

The increase in incidence of hepatocellular carcinoma in recent years is in large part attributable to the hepatitis C epidemic.[72] Currently, most patients estimated to have HCV infection do not have adequate access to health care and do not know that they have the disease. As the proportion of those with cirrhosis increases and becomes clinically apparent, the burden on the health care system is expected to increase.

Descriptive Epidemiology

Hepatitis C is a reportable disease, but there is significant underreporting despite active surveillance programs. The reasons for this are varied, but a large part of the problem is that acute HCV is overwhelmingly asymptomatic and goes unnoticed. Furthermore, populations at risk for HCV are socially and economically disadvantaged and often do not seek or have access to health care. Furthermore, national surveys such as NHANES exclude populations with high prevalence of the disease, such as incarcerated individuals and the homeless. Health care provider underreporting of diagnosed cases also occurs.

Hepatitis C leads to chronic disease, with spontaneous clearance occurring in only 15% to 30% of cases after exposure. Therefore, the prevalence of the virus is high, with an estimated 2.5 to 3.5 million cases in the United States.[73] The prevalence of infection is higher in men, who are 30% more likely to be infected than women. The incidence of acute HCV has more than doubled since 2013, a 124% increase, and it increased 15% from 2019. The rates of acute HCV also increased in 2020, particularly among those 20 to 39 years of age, a rise consistent with the age groups most affected by the nation's opioid crisis.[43] Among the reported acute HCV cases that included risk information for injection drug use, 66% reported injection drug use. American Indians and Alaskan Natives are the racial/ethnic group with the highest rates of reported acute hepatitis C infection at 2.1 reported cases per 100,000, followed by non-Hispanic Whites at 1.6 per 100,000 and non-Hispanic Blacks at 1.1 per 100,000. Males also have a higher rate of newly reported chronic hepatitis C than do women. Both males and females showed a biphasic pattern of newly reported chronic HCV infections with infections rising through the late teens and twenties, decreasing through the thirties, and rising again in the fifties before declining for the remaining years.[43] HCV prevalence is higher in certain groups, including 8.4% of veterans (but lower in currently active duty military personnel),[74] 4% to 36% of the homeless,[75] and 10.7% of incarcerated individuals.[76]

At the peak of the hepatitis C epidemic in the mid-1980s, between 180,000 and 230,000 new cases were occurring yearly in the United States.[77] Since then the incidence declined to an estimated 29,000 new infections each year in the United States by 2013, and then subsequently increased to 57,000 new infections by 2019—as noted earlier, an increase attributable to the opioid epidemic (see Figure 22-7).[43]

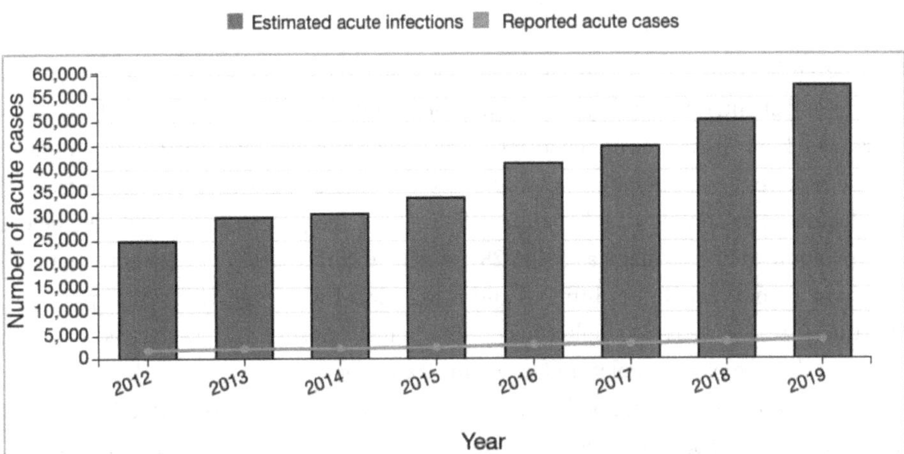

	2012	2013	2014	2015	2016	2017	2018	2019
Reported acute cases	1,778	2,138	2,194	2,436	2,967	3,216	3,621	4,136
Estimated acute infections	24,700	29,700	30,500	33,900	41,200	44,700	50,300	57,500

Source: Adapted from CDC.[53]

Figure 22-7. Incidence of Reported Acute Hepatitis C by Year, United States, 2012–2019

The initial decrease in HCV incidence was multifactorial. Declines in transfusion-related hepatitis C started occurring after the introduction of the 1985 guidelines for selecting safer blood donors and fell sharply with the introduction of HCV antibody testing of donated blood products starting in 1989. Safer injection drug needle practices and tattoo needle practices introduced to reduce HIV have also contributed to the reduced incidence. Declines have occurred in all groups. Persons aged 25 to 39 years had the highest incidence but also had the greatest declines, with a 92% decline in incidence of hepatitis C infection from 1992 to 2005.[78] The recent increase in incidence of HCV since 2010 is largely attributable to the opioid epidemic, and higher incidence was seen in those aged 20 to 39 and in males, non-Hispanic Whites, and American Indians/Alaska Natives.[43]

Causes

Several large population studies have identified risk factors for HCV infection. Risk factors included illicit drug use and number of sexual partners, as well as weaker associations with socioeconomic markers such as poverty index, educational level, and marital status.[79] Other population-based studies have found similar risk factors, with injection drug use being the strongest risk factor.[80] Other risk factors include blood transfusion or organ transplant before 1992, hemodialysis, and high-risk sexual behavior.[63,81]

Dialysis remains a risk factor despite universal infection control practices. HCV antibody was found in 6.9% of dialysis recipients in the United States in 2015. This is a decline of 40% from 11.5% in 2001 to 2015.[82] HCV testing was done in 2002 in 64% of centers. Routine HCV testing with anti-HCV antibody was recommended routinely every six months and at entry. Using disposable equipment in the dialysis machines has been associated with lower incidence of hepatitis C as well as having dedicated medication rooms.[82]

The incarcerated population has a high incidence and prevalence of HCV infection. Risk factors in prison for viral hepatitis include illicit drug use in more than 50% before incarceration, and in as many as 3% to 28% during incarceration.[84] Sexual activity in jail occurs in as many as 30% of inmates and is associated with high-risk sexual practices. Hepatitis C incidence is also higher in certain populations such as the veterans of foreign wars and the homeless population (see Figure 22-8).

Screening for HCV infection because of these risk factors was not very effective for a multitude of reasons, including both patient and provider factors. Because hepatitis C rates are higher in the baby boomer population (born 1945–1965) in the United States, CDC has endorsed screening for this birth cohort since 2012—regardless of risk factors. Since 2018, CDC has endorsed universal screening of all US adults (>18) irrespective of risk factors.[43]

Increase in progression toward severe liver disease has been shown with chronic alcohol intake, particularly moderate-to-severe alcohol intake (50 g/day).[85] Older age at

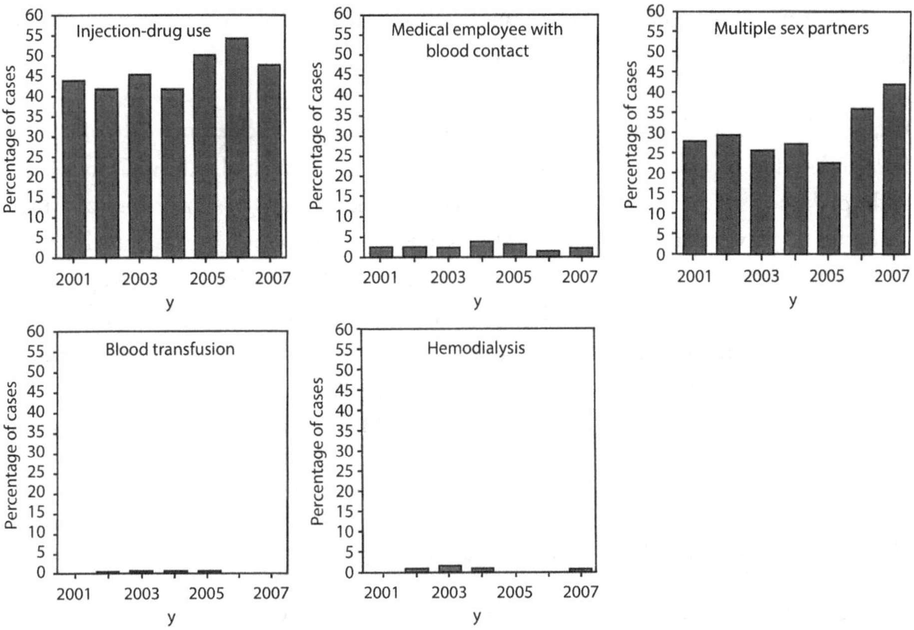

Source: Adapted from CDC.[53]

Note: The percentage of cases among persons in which a specific risk factor was reported was calculated based on the total number of persons for whom any information for that exposure was reported. Multiple risk factors may be reported for a single case.

Figure 22-8. Trends in Selected Epidemiological Characteristics Among Patients With Acute Hepatitis C by Year: United States, 2001–2007

infection has also been associated with increased risk of progressive liver disease. Given the propensity of obesity and metabolic syndrome to independently cause liver disease, the coexistence of obesity and metabolic syndrome with hepatitis C has been investigated in preliminary studies. There is some evidence that with increased body mass index and features of metabolic syndrome (diabetes, hypertension, hyperlipidemia, and truncal obesity), liver disease progresses more rapidly in patients with hepatitis C.[85] In a large meta-analysis, steatosis (or fat in the liver) was independently associated with increased fibrosis and liver damage in hepatitis C. In some analyses, male sex has been associated with increased fibrosis as well.[86]

Interventions

No vaccine is currently available for HCV. National recommendations issued in 1998 for prevention and control of HCV infection include the screening and testing of blood donors, viral inactivation of plasma products, and risk reduction counseling to reduce transmission in injection drug users and in those at high risk of sexual transmission (multiple sexual partners). Also recommended is application of these measures in health care settings (infection control practices, dialysis).

Historically, treatment for hepatitis C was with injectable interferon and oral ribavirin, antiviral agents that are associated with an average viral clearance rate of 10% to 50% and had to be taken for 24 to 48 weeks.[87] The treatment can be difficult to tolerate and uptake was poor.[88] Since 2011, the therapy for hepatitis C has improved considerably with the advent of direct-acting antiviral agents. These are all oral agents that work by directly suppressing one of the viral enzymes involved in hepatitis C replication. Response "cure" rates are greater than 90% with therapies as short as 8 to 12 weeks in most patients. Therapies are also well tolerated, with few drug interactions. Currently, given the high cost of the medications, access is limited even for individuals with insurance, though increased market competition should improve access to these medications.[89]

NONALCOHOLIC FATTY LIVER DISEASE

Nonalcoholic fatty liver disease (NAFLD) is a chronic liver disease characterized by fat infiltration in the liver (steatosis) and consequent liver injury of varying degree and severity. NAFLD has emerged as the most prevalent cause of chronic liver disease worldwide and is on track to become the leading cause for end-stage liver disease and liver transplantation. The average global prevalence is 25%, ranging from 13.5% in Africa to 31.8% in the Middle East—differences that are likely driven by physical activity, body fat distribution, socioeconomic status, and diet.[90]

Significance

Although many patients have a benign course of bland fat deposition in the liver (fatty liver disease), there is a subset of patients who will develop inflammation and fibrosis, called nonalcoholic steatohepatitis. Recent data suggest that the risk of liver-related mortality in NAFLD increases exponentially with increased stage of fibrosis.[91] These patients are at risk of progression to cirrhosis, liver failure, and hepatocellular carcinoma.[90]

NAFLD is closely associated with metabolic syndrome (truncal obesity, insulin resistance, hyperlipidemia, hypertension).[92] The natural history of the condition remains poorly understood. Adams et al.[93] published accounts of 420 patients diagnosed in Olmsted County, Minnesota, between 1980 and 2000 who were followed for a mean of 7.6 years culminating in 3,192 person-years of follow-up. Of these patients, 5% developed cirrhosis over this relatively short follow-up and 3.1% developed liver-related complications. The mortality was 13% during the follow-up, significantly higher than that in the general population (standardized mortality ratio, 1.34; 95% confidence interval [CI], 1.003–1.76; $p = .03$).[93] A longitudinal study describing 129 patients with biopsy-proven

NAFLD were compared with a matched reference population over 13.7 years. Of those patients with more advanced proven NAFLD, 5.4% were found to have end-stage liver disease as well as an increased mortality related to cardiovascular and liver-related causes. During the follow-up period, 69 of 88 patients (78%) developed diabetes or impaired glucose tolerance and 41% had progression of liver fibrosis. Those who had progressive liver damage were more likely to have had a significant amount of weight gain and were more insulin-resistant.[94]

Although most individuals with NAFLD do not progress to end-stage liver disease, given the high prevalence and increasing incidence of NAFLD, it is now the second most common indication for liver transplantation in the United States as well as the second most common cause of liver cancer. In the next decade, NAFLD is expected to surpass viral hepatitis as the most common indication for liver transplantation and cause of liver cancer in the United States.[92,95] In an international study of nonalcoholic steatohepatitis–related cirrhosis, the risk of mortality was like that in patients with hepatitis C–related cirrhosis.[96]

Descriptive Epidemiology

Longitudinal studies of NAFLD in the general US population have demonstrated an increased prevalence over 20 years from 5.5% in 1988 to 11% in 2008, while other chronic liver disease prevalence remained unchanged during this period.[97] NAFLD accounted for 75% of chronic liver disease in the general population by 2008.

NAFLD is known to be correlated with several metabolic conditions, including type 2 diabetes, obesity, hypertension, and hyperlipidemia, which have increased in parallel over this time period as well.[92] A meta-analysis estimated the global prevalence of NAFLD in patients with diabetes to be 55.5% (95% CI, 47.3–63.7), with a regional prevalence of 51.8% in the United States.[98]

US data on incidence of NAFLD is limited. Kanwal et al. have reported that the annual incidence of NAFLD based on liver enzyme levels in US veterans younger than 45 years of age increased from 2.3% in 2003 to 4.3% in 2011.[99] One of the few reported studies regarding incidence is a prospective, observational study from Japan. Using alanine transaminase (ALT) levels and ultrasonography of the liver in patients without significant alcohol use, they found that at baseline 812 of 4,401 (18%) participants had NAFLD. During the mean follow-up period of 414 days, the authors observed 308 new cases (10%) of NAFLD among 3,147 participants who had been disease-free at baseline.[100]

The determination of prevalence, while still laden with challenges, has proved more feasible. Studies have been difficult, however, because definitive diagnosis requires an invasive liver biopsy. As a result, most studies have elected to use either serum liver chemistries or radiologic imaging as surrogate diagnostic tools.

Published reports have stated NAFLD to be present in 27% to 56% of the North American population. A study that examined the US population from NHANES data from 2017 to 2018 found the prevalence of NAFLD to be 56% based on results from mobile imaging using a controlled attenuation parameter with Fibroscan, a tool for fatty liver estimation, but 12% utilizing elevated liver enzymes as the criterion.[11] Thus, the detection of NAFLD by imaging in recent years has increased sensitivity for detection (perhaps at the cost of specificity), as many patients with hepatic steatosis have normal liver enzymes and may have been overlooked in prior studies utilizing only elevated liver enzymes to make the diagnosis. In a study of 2,287 participants of the Dallas Heart Study, Browning et al.[101] evaluated for liver steatosis (fat) by proton nuclear magnetic resonance spectroscopy and found 31% to meet their criteria for diagnosis of NAFLD. Of these patients, 79% were found to have a normal ALT level.[101] The average prevalence of NAFLD has been reported to vary from a low of 13.5% in Africa to a high of 31.8% and 30.5% in the Middle East and South America, respectively, with both North American and European prevalence averaging around 24% (see Table 22-4).[98]

Increasingly, the pediatric population is being identified as part of this epidemic. A report was published by Schwimmer et al.[102] in which autopsy specimens were reviewed in 742 pediatric victims of accidental death between the ages of 2 and 19 years. They found a 9.6% rate of fatty liver in these patients, with a pronounced age-related distribution of hepatic steatosis ranging from 0.7% for age 2 to 4 years to up to 17.3% for age 15 to 19 years. The highest rate of fatty liver was seen in obese children (38%).[102] In a systematic review the pooled mean prevalence of NAFLD was found in 7.6% of the general pediatric population globally and in 34% of children from obesity clinics.[103]

NAFLD affects persons of all ages and sexes. Among both children and adults, NAFLD increases with age, with highest occurrences in the fifth and sixth decades. Data from

Table 22-4. NAFLD Prevalence by Region

Region	N	Prevalence (%)	95% CI (%)	I^2 (%)
Africa	2	13.48	(5.69-28.69)	84.37
Asia	14	27.37	(23.29-31.88)	99.17
Europe	11	23.71	(16.12-33.45)	98.78
Middle East	3	31.79	(13.48-58.23)	99.14
North America	13	24.13	(19.73-29.15)	99.19
South America	2	30.45	(22.74-39.44)	69.10
Overall	45	25.24	(22.1-28.65)	99.07

Source: Younossi et. al.[98] Reprinted with permission of Wolters Kluwer Health.

Note: CI = confidence interval; NAFLD = nonalcoholic fatty liver disease. Estimates were based on imaging studies. The I^2 statistic describes the percentage of variation across studies that is due to heterogeneity rather than chance.

NHANES III showed that NAFLD based on elevated ALT levels peaked in the fifth decade among men and in the sixth decade among women. Early descriptions of persons with NAFLD showed a female preponderance to the condition; however, more recent studies in Japanese, Italian, and US populations have consistently found men to be at increased risk.[92]

Ethnic variation has been demonstrated repeatedly, with the Hispanic population being at the highest risk of fatty liver disease and Blacks being at the lowest risk when compared with non-Hispanic Whites. Asians also appear to be at decreased risk, although this is applicable to Asians of East Asian descent and not from the Indian subcontinent, where the prevalence is higher. A cross-sectional study of newly diagnosed cases of NAFLD in the Chronic Liver Disease Surveillance Study was performed. Of the 742 persons evaluated, 159 (21.4%) had definite or probable NAFLD, with the following breakdown: Whites, 45%; Hispanics, 28%; Asians, 18%; African Americans, 3%; and other races, 6%. Clinical correlates of NAFLD (obesity, hyperlipidemia, diabetes) were similar among racial/ethnic groups, except that body mass index was lower in Asians compared with other groups. Compared with the base population, Hispanics with NAFLD were overrepresented (28% vs. 10%) and Whites were underrepresented (45% vs. 59%).[104] A single nucleotide polymorphism in a gene that regulates lipid metabolism in the liver (*PNPLA3*) has been repeatedly reported to account for most of the ethnic variation in the prevalence of NAFLD.[105]

These racial/ethnic differences are partly attributable to true genetic differences in risk of NAFLD and partly influenced by cultural susceptibility in diet and lifestyle patterns. However, referral patterns and health care availability may influence results. The NHANES general population studies avoid many biases that studies in certain populations may encounter. They, too, found Hispanics to have a higher prevalence of NAFLD independent of body mass index, demographic factors, and metabolic factors, compared with non-Hispanic Whites, while Blacks continued to demonstrate less NAFLD after adjustment for these factors.[106] NAFLD is also more prevalent in individuals with obesity (prevalence >75%) and those with diabetes (prevalence 60%–70%).[107]

Causes

NAFLD is associated with metabolic syndrome, with diabetes, insulin resistance, and truncal obesity being the most closely linked correlates.[100] Other common associations include hyperlipidemia and hypertension, as well as sleep apnea. Secondary causes of fatty liver disease include medications (such as steroids and tamoxifen), hepatitis viruses such as hepatitis C, surgical procedures that lead to rapid and excessive weight loss, and total parenteral nutrition. Gholam et al.[108] published a paper that identified NAFLD in 89% of severely obese patients. The presence of nonalcoholic steatohepatitis and fibrosis (signifying more advanced liver damage from NAFLD) was significantly less at 36% and 25%, respectively. In further subgroup analysis, hyperlipidemia—particularly low high-density lipoprotein cholesterol—hyperglycemia, and insulin resistance were strongly associated with NAFLD.[108]

Diabetes is known to be commonly linked with central obesity. Several studies have found the risk of diabetes in causing NAFLD to be independent of the degree of obesity.[109] Insulin resistance itself is believed to be centrally related to the pathogenesis of NAFLD. Other associations with NAFLD include sleep apnea and hypothyroidism.

Interventions

Currently there are no US Food and Drug Administration–approved therapies for NAFLD, although several agents are in Phase 3 development. The American Association for the Study of Liver Disease 2018 guidelines recommend weight loss of 7% to 10% of body weight (through both a hypocaloric diet and exercise) as therapy for NAFLD. In individuals with the progressive form of NAFLD (nonalcoholic steatohepatitis) that is biopsy-proven, agents such as vitamin E and pioglitazone can be considered, though no long-term trials currently exist to support their use.[110] In selected individuals with progressive liver disease who are unable to lose weight with diet and exercise, weight loss surgeries (bariatric surgery) may be an option for treatment.

As described previously, the potential for advanced liver disease in the form of cirrhosis and hepatocellular carcinoma is present in those patients with NAFLD. Determining those at increased risk for progressive damage in NAFLD (nonalcoholic steatohepatitis), as opposed to those with merely benign fatty liver disease, is of utmost importance in determining prognosis and prioritizing treatment. Noninvasive markers in the determination of these two groups are also of utmost importance, given the magnitude of this condition in the otherwise healthy population. As society continues the trend toward obesity, so too will the trend of NAFLD continue to rise, including the diagnosis of cirrhosis and associated hepatocellular carcinoma. Thus, many relatively new and evolving issues regarding NAFLD will remain significant in the coming years. In addition, patients with NAFLD have an increased risk of cardiovascular disease beyond that predicted by the presence of the underlying metabolic syndrome. Optimizing management of underlying metabolic conditions (diabetes, hypertension, hyperlipidemia) and prevention of cardiovascular disease are critical in reducing morbidity and mortality in this population.

HEPATOCELLULAR CARCINOMA

Worldwide, liver cancers are the fourth most common cause of cancer-related death and rank sixth in terms of cancer incidence.[111] Liver cancer is a bigger problem in less developed regions, where 83% of the estimated 782,000 new cancer cases worldwide occurred in 2012—of these, 50% were in China alone. It is the fifth most common cancer in men (554,000 cases, 7.5% of the total) and the ninth in women (228,000 cases, 3.4%).[112]

Significance

Hepatocellular carcinoma is rapidly fatal in most patients, since it is often found at late stages of the disease because of low screening rates in underlying conditions like cirrhosis and chronic hepatitis B; consequently, the prevalence, incidence, and mortality rates are very similar. With a five-year survival of 18%, liver cancer is among the most lethal cancers—second only to pancreatic cancer.[113]

Descriptive Epidemiology

Hepatocellular carcinoma is more common in men than women worldwide. The gender disparity is noted to be more pronounced in endemic areas (2.1–5.7:1 male-to-female ratio), whereas intermediate- and low-incidence areas have progressively lower ratios.[114] Although not fully understood, these differences are theorized to be related to variations in viral hepatitis, alcohol abuse, toxins, and the trophic effect of androgens.

The hepatocellular carcinoma incidence in the United States is low compared with that in other countries in the developing world. However, there has been an increase in incidence over the past few decades, from 1.4 per 100,000 in 1976 to 1980 to 3.2 per 100,000 in 2006 and 8.4 per 100,000 in 2019, and estimates show a continued increase (Figure 22-9). In the United States, the rate of death from liver cancer increased by 43% from 2000 to 2016.[115]

Men are more likely to develop hepatocellular carcinoma than women in all parts of the world (2–5 times more frequent in men).[116] The US incidence is highest in White Hispanics (13.2/100,000), followed by Asians (11.4/100,000) and then Native Americans (10.5/100,000), Blacks (9.6/100,000), and non-Hispanic Whites (7.8/100,000). Parallel to these increases has been a 43% increase in mortality from primary liver cancers.[72]

Geographic distributions are associated with significant variety among the incidence rates of this cancer, even showing variation between ethnicities and regions within the same country. The age-adjusted incidence rates for hepatocellular carcinoma in developed versus developing countries is 8.7 for males and 2.9 for females per 100,000 compared with 17.4 for males and 6.8 for females per 100,000, respectively.[112] Some Asian and African regions have extraordinarily high rates, such as Mongolia (78/100,000) and The Gambia (40/100,000).[117,118] In Australia, Europe, and the Americas, the rates are far less than 10 per 100,000 and with much less regional variability.[119]

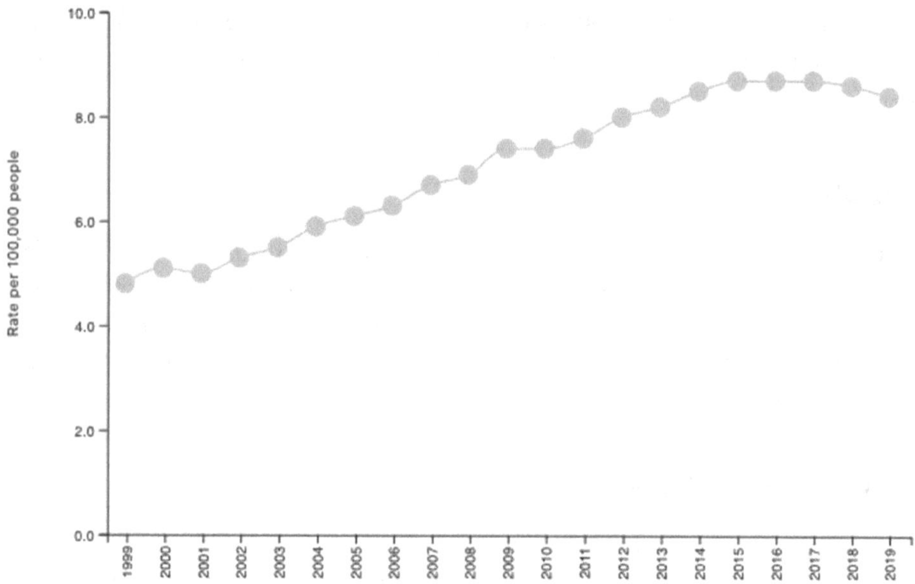

Source: Adapted from CDC WONDER.[7]

Note: Age was adjusted to the 2000 US standard population. There were 48,596 cases overall.

Figure 22-9. Hepatocellular Carcinoma Incidence Rate: United States, 1999–2019

Causes

The vast majority of hepatocellular carcinoma occurs in the setting of chronic liver disease and cirrhosis. Overall, 75% to 80% of hepatocellular carcinoma can be related to persistent viral infections with either HBV (50%–55%) or HCV (25%–30%), which is further supported by the strong geographical correlation between the incidence of hepatocellular carcinoma and known prevalence of these viral infections. The risk associated with hepatitis B appears to be more profound in endemic regions where transmission often occurs vertically (at childbirth) and, consequently, longer duration of infection is seen. In areas such as the United States, where most HBV transmission occurs later in life through sexual transmission, the risk of hepatocellular carcinoma is much less.[119]

The risk of hepatitis C–related liver disease leading to hepatocellular carcinoma is high in the United States because of the maturing of the hepatitis C epidemic of the 1970s and 1980s, leading to increased rates of hepatitis C–related cirrhosis at the current time. Any condition that can lead to cirrhosis is considered a risk for hepatocellular carcinoma. Alcohol either alone or in combination with viral hepatitis leading to cirrhosis is a risk, though it is unclear whether alcohol is itself carcinogenic in addition to increasing the risk of cirrhosis. Iron overload, autoimmune diseases, and nonalcoholic steatohepatitis are known to lead to hepatocellular carcinoma in individuals at the stage of cirrhosis and in the US nonalcoholic steatohepatitis–related cirrhosis is a rapidly increasing underlying cause of hepatocellular carcinoma. Rarer and debated causes include exposure in parts of Africa to aflatoxin, a mycotoxin that may contaminate the diet; betel nut chewing, which is widespread in Asia; and tobacco use, which has been demonstrated in some studies to be a risk factor.

Interventions

Protective measures include the prevention and treatment of diseases that cause cirrhosis with the goal to delay or avoid the development of cirrhosis. Recent observational studies have also suggested that coffee may be protective, and a meta-analysis performed by Larsson and Wolk[120] showed a 43% reduction of liver cancers occurred possibly because of coffee's antioxidant properties. Association of hepatocellular carcinoma with red meat and saturated fat has been reported in epidemiologic studies along with a reduced risk with consumption of fish, white meat, and vegetables.[121] A remarkable decrease in HBV infections has occurred with the introduction of the universal childhood vaccine in 1984; the expectation is that there will be a long-term effect on the hepatocellular carcinoma rates. Results from Taiwan have shown that hepatocellular carcinoma incidence rate in children aged 6 to 14 years old fell from 0.52 to 0.54 to 0.13 to 0.20 per 100,000 (relative risk [RR] = 0.25–0.36).[122]

Recent advances in treatment options have brought a new perspective to this condition traditionally considered a terminal illness with very poor outcomes, few treatment options, and a life expectancy of six months or less. Such advances include surgical resection, local ablation with alcohol, radiofrequency, chemoembolization, and liver transplantation. Recent studies have shown hepatocellular carcinoma to be the leading cause of mortality from cirrhosis, as opposed to liver failure or nonmalignant liver-related conditions.[123] In response, health care providers have developed surveillance and treatment protocols that have dramatically improved survival in those patients diagnosed in the early stages of hepatocellular carcinoma. Prevention of chronic liver disease, such as with hepatitis B vaccination and reducing alcoholism and transmission of hepatitis C, is still the most cost-effective way to deal with hepatocellular carcinoma. In Western countries, NAFLD will soon become a leading cause of liver cancer, and so lifestyle changes will become increasingly important.[111]

HEMOCHROMATOSIS

Other causes of chronic liver disease include genetic conditions such as metabolic liver disease from increased iron deposition in the liver and organs, known as hemochromatosis, or from copper accumulation in the liver in Wilson's disease; from cholestatic disorders such as primary biliary cirrhosis and primary sclerosing cholangitis; and from autoimmune disorders and drug-related liver disease. Hereditary hemochromatosis is an autosomal recessive disorder with a prevalence of 1 in 200 to 1 in 250 in White populations in the United States and Europe. Hereditary hemochromatosis is among the most common genetic disorders in people of Northern European descent.[124] The most common genetic mutation is the *C282Y* mutation, which results in excessive absorption of iron from the gut.

Significance

Organ iron overload can in time lead to cirrhosis, heart failure, diabetes, and hypogonadism. Organ damage is delayed in women compared with men because of menstrual iron loss.

Descriptive Epidemiology

Despite the presence of the mutation for hemochromatosis, the penetrance is variable. In a large study in California that used data from the Kaiser Permanente health clinic of 41,038 individuals, 152 were homozygous for the *C282Y* mutation. Of these 152, only one had clinically evident disease.[125]

The yield of severe liver disease was similarly low in the Hemochromatosis and Iron Overload Screening Study, which screened 101,168 primary care participants for iron overload. In that study 333 *C282Y* homozygotes were detected; 75 had been previously diagnosed. Of the 302 *C282Y* homozygotes that underwent additional testing, 16% and 12% had increased levels of alanine transaminase (ALT) and aspartate transaminase (AST), respectively, compared with 11% and 8%, respectively, in controls. Of the 11 centrally reviewed liver biopsies, all showed increased liver iron concentrations, but only 2 had stage 3 or 4 fibrosis.[126]

Interventions

On the basis of these large population studies, the US Preventive Services Task Force recommended against the use of routine genetic screening for hereditary hemochromatosis in the asymptomatic general population. Screening of family members of an individual with hemochromatosis is effective because of higher pretest probability and should be performed with genetic testing if the proband is available.

DISCUSSION QUESTIONS

1. Identify two or three risk factors for liver disease and discuss how you might design an intervention to address these factors in a defined population.

2. What is NAFLD? How might you go about addressing the rising prevalence of this disease in the United States and around the world?
3. Discuss the major risk factors for hepatocellular carcinoma (liver cancer) and why most liver cancer is found at an advanced stage, with low five-year survival. How might you improve this with screening or risk factor identification?

REFERENCES

1. Moon AM, Singal AG, Tapper EB. Contemporary epidemiology of chronic liver disease and cirrhosis. *Clin Gastroenterol Hepatol.* 2020;18(12):2650–2666. doi:10.1016/j.cgh.2019.07.060
2. Asrani SK, Devarbhavi H, Eaton J, Kamath PS. Burden of liver diseases in the world. *J Hepatol.* 2019;70(1):151–171. doi:10.1016/j.jhep.2018.09.014
3. Younossi ZM, Stepanova M, Younossi Y, et al. Epidemiology of chronic liver diseases in the USA in the past three decades. *Gut.* 2020;69(3):564–568. doi:10.1136/gutjnl-2019-318813
4. Terris M. Epidemiology of cirrhosis of the liver: national mortality data. *Am J Public Health Nations Health.* 1967;57(12):2076–2088. doi:10.2105/ajph.57.12.2076
5. Kim Y, Ejaz A, Tayal A, et al. Temporal trends in population-based death rates associated with chronic liver disease and liver cancer in the United States over the last 30 years. *Cancer.* 2014;120(19):3058–3965. doi:10.1002/cncr.28843
6. Heron M. Deaths: leading causes for 2019. *Natl Vital Stat Rep.* 2021;70(9):1–114.
7. Centers for Disease Control and Prevention. WONDER online databases. Available at: https://wonder.cdc.gov. Accessed March 31, 2023.
8. Desai AP, Mohan P, Nokes B, et al. Increasing economic burden in hospitalized patients with cirrhosis: analysis of a national database. *Clin Transl Gastroenterol.* 2019;10(7):e00062. doi:10.14309/ctg.0000000000000062
9. Ma C, Qian AS, Nguyen NH, et al. Trends in the economic burden of chronic liver diseases and cirrhosis in the United States: 1996–2016. *Am J Gastroenterol.* 2021;116(10):2060–2067. doi:10.14309/ajg.0000000000001292
10. Zaman SN, Johnson PJ, Williams R. Silent cirrhosis in patients with hepatocellular carcinoma. Implications for screening in high-incidence and low-incidence areas. *Cancer.* 1990;65(7):1607–1610. doi:10.1002/1097-0142(19900401)65:7<1607::aid-cncr2820650726>3.0.co;2-2
11. Zhang X, Heredia NI, Balakrishnan M, Thrift AP. Prevalence and factors associated with NAFLD detected by vibration controlled transient elastography among US adults: results from NHANES 2017–2018. *PLoS One.* 2021;16(6):e0252164. doi:10.1371/journal.pone.0252164
12. Singh GK, Hoyert DL. Social epidemiology of chronic liver disease and cirrhosis mortality in the United States, 1935–1997: trends and differentials by ethnicity, socioeconomic status, and alcohol consumption. *Hum Biol.* 2000;72(5):801–820.
13. World Health Organization. Immunization analysis and insights. https://www.who.int/teams/immunization-vaccines-and-biologicals/immunization-analysis-and-insights/surveillance. Accessed March 31, 2023.
14. Schiff ER, Maddrey WC, Reddy KR. *Schiff's Diseases of the Liver.* 12th ed. Oxford, UK: Wiley-Blackwell; 2018.

15. Thaler H. Alcohol consumption and diseases of the liver. *Nutr Metab.* 1977;21(1–3):196–193.
16. Sørensen TI, Orholm M, Bentsen KD, Høybye G, Eghøje K, Christoffersen P. Prospective evaluation of alcohol abuse and alcoholic liver injury in men as predictors of development of cirrhosis. *Lancet.* 1984;2(8397):241–244. doi:10.1016/s0140-6736(84)90295-2
17. Diehl AM. Alcoholic liver disease: natural history. *Liver Transpl Surg.* 1997;3(3):206–211.
18. Ramstedt M. Population drinking and liver cirrhosis mortality: is there a link in Eastern Europe? *Addiction.* 2007;102(8):1212–1223. doi:10.1111/j.1360-0443.2007.01872.x
19. Singal AK, Salameh H, Kamath PS. Prevalence and in-hospital mortality trends of infections among patients with cirrhosis: a nationwide study of hospitalised patients in the United States. *Aliment Pharmacol Ther.* 2014;40(1):105–112. doi:10.1111/apt.12797
20. Fisher NC, Hanson J, Phillips A, Rao JN, Swarbrick ET. Mortality from liver disease in the West Midlands, 1993–2000: observational study. *BMJ.* 2002;325(7359):312–313. doi:10.1136/bmj.325.7359.312
21. Park SC, Oh SI, Lee MS. Korean status of alcoholics and alcohol-related health problems. *Alcohol Clin Exp Res.* 1998;22(S3 pt 1):170s–172s. doi:10.1111/acer.1998.22.s3_part1.170s
22. Hasumura Y, Takeuchi J. Alcoholic liver disease in Japanese patients: a comparison with Caucasians. *J Gastroenterol Hepatol.* 1991;6(5):520–527. doi:10.1111/j.1440-1746.1991.tb00898.x
23. Bellentani S, Saccoccio G, Costa G, et al. Drinking habits as cofactors of risk for alcohol induced liver damage. The Dionysos Study Group. *Gut.* 1997;41(6):845–850. doi:10.1136/gut.41.6.845
24. Mandayam S, Jamal MM, Morgan TR. Epidemiology of alcoholic liver disease. *Semin Liver Dis.* 2004;24(3):217–232. doi:10.1055/s-2004-832936
25. Blume SB. Women and alcohol: a review. *JAMA.* 1986;256(11):1467–1470.
26. Parlesak A, Schäfer C, Schütz T, Bode JC, Bode C. Increased intestinal permeability to macromolecules and endotoxemia in patients with chronic alcohol abuse in different stages of alcohol-induced liver disease. *J Hepatol.* 2000;32(5):742–747. doi:10.1016/s0168-8278(00)80242-1
27. Stinson FS, Grant BF, Dufour MC. The critical dimension of ethnicity in liver cirrhosis mortality statistics. *Alcohol Clin Exp Res.* 2001;25(8):1181–1187.
28. Loguercio C, Di Pierro M, Di Marino MP, et al. Drinking habits of subjects with hepatitis C virus-related chronic liver disease: prevalence and effect on clinical, virological and pathological aspects. *Alcohol Alcohol.* 2000;35(3):296–301. doi:10.1093/alcalc/35.3.296
29. Corrao G, Aricò S. Independent and combined action of hepatitis C virus infection and alcohol consumption on the risk of symptomatic liver cirrhosis. *Hepatology.* 1998;27(4):914–919. doi:10.1002/hep.510270404
30. Ostapowicz G, Watson KJ, Locarnini SA, Desmond PV. Role of alcohol in the progression of liver disease caused by hepatitis C virus infection. *Hepatology.* 1998;27(6):1730–1735. doi:10.1002/hep.510270637
31. Westin J, Lagging LM, Spak F, et al. Moderate alcohol intake increases fibrosis progression in untreated patients with hepatitis C virus infection. *J Viral Hepat.* 2002;9(3):235–241. doi:10.1046/j.1365-2893.2002.00356.x
32. Naveau S, Giraud V, Borotto E, Aubert A, Capron F, Chaput JC. Excess weight risk factor for alcoholic liver disease. *Hepatology.* 1997;25(1):108–111. doi:10.1002/hep.510250120

33. Dunn W, Sanyal AJ, Brunt EM, et al. Modest alcohol consumption is associated with decreased prevalence of steatohepatitis in patients with non-alcoholic fatty liver disease (NAFLD). *J Hepatol.* 2012;57(2):384–391. doi:10.1016/j.jhep.2012.03.024
34. Raynard B, Balian A, Fallik D, et al. Risk factors of fibrosis in alcohol-induced liver disease. *Hepatology*. 2002;35(3):635–638. doi:10.1053/jhep.2002.31782
35. Bode C, Bode JC, Erhardt JG, French BA, French SW. Effect of the type of beverage and meat consumed by alcoholics with alcoholic liver disease. *Alcohol Clin Exp Res.* 1998;22(8):1803–1805.
36. Ruhl CE, Everhart JE. Coffee and tea consumption are associated with a lower incidence of chronic liver disease in the United States. *Gastroenterology*. 2005;129(6):1928–1936. doi:10.1053/j.gastro.2005.08.056
37. Tang YW, Wang JX, Xu ZY, Guo YF, Qian WH, Xu JX. A serologically confirmed, case-control study, of a large outbreak of hepatitis A in China, associated with consumption of clams. *Epidemiol Infect.* 1991;107(3):651–657. doi:10.1017/s0950268800049347
38. Wheeler C, Vogt TM, Armstrong GL, et al. An outbreak of hepatitis A associated with green onions. *N Engl J Med.* 2005;353(9):890–897. doi:10.1056/NEJMoa050855
39. Tong MJ, el-Farra NS, Grew MI. Clinical manifestations of hepatitis A: recent experience in a community teaching hospital. *J Infect Dis.* 1995;171(suppl 1):S15–S18. doi:10.1093/infdis/171.supplement_1.s15
40. Vento S, Garofano T, Renzini C, et al. Fulminant hepatitis associated with hepatitis A virus superinfection in patients with chronic hepatitis C. *N Engl J Med.* 1998;338(5):286–290. doi:10.1056/nejm199801293380503
41. Koff RS. Clinical manifestations and diagnosis of hepatitis A virus infection. *Vaccine.* 1992;10(suppl 1):S15–S17. doi:10.1016/0264-410x(92)90533-p
42. Fiore AE, Wasley A, Bell BP. Prevention of hepatitis A through active or passive immunization: recommendations of the Advisory Committee on Immunization Practices (ACIP). *MMWR Recomm Rep.* 2006;55(Rr-7):1–23.
43. Centers for Disease Control and Prevention. Number of reported cases of hepatitis A virus infection and estimated infections. United States, 2013–2020. Available at: https://www.cdc.gov/hepatitis/statistics/2020surveillance/data/pdf/CDCViralHep_2020_SurvData_508.pdf. Accessed April 4, 2023.
44. Jacobsen KH, Koopman JS. Declining hepatitis A seroprevalence: a global review and analysis. *Epidemiol Infect.* 2004;132(6):1005–1022. doi:10.1017/s0950268804002857
45. Nelson NP, Weng MK, Hofmeister MG, et al. Prevention of hepatitis A virus infection in the United States: recommendations of the Advisory Committee on Immunization Practices, 2020. *MMWR Recomm Rep.* 2020;69(RR-5):1–38. doi:10.15585/mmwr.rr6905a1
46. Alter MJ, Hadler SC, Margolis HS, et al. The changing epidemiology of hepatitis B in the United States. Need for alternative vaccination strategies. *JAMA*. 1990;263(9):1218–1222.
47. Wasley A, Kruszon-Moran D, Kuhnert W, et al. The prevalence of hepatitis B virus infection in the United States in the era of vaccination. *J Infect Dis.* 2010;202(2):192–201. doi:10.1086/653622
48. Liaw YF, Tsai SL, Sheen IS, et al. Clinical and virological course of chronic hepatitis B virus infection with hepatitis C and D virus markers. *Am J Gastroenterol.* 1998;93(3):354–359. doi:10.1111/j.1572-0241.1998.00354.x

49. Chen CJ, Yang HI, Su J, et al. Risk of hepatocellular carcinoma across a biological gradient of serum hepatitis B virus DNA level. *JAMA*. 2006;295(1):65–73. doi:10.1001/jama.295.1.65
50. Wong RJ, Brosgart CL, Welch S, et al. An updated assessment of chronic hepatitis B prevalence among foreign-born persons living in the United States. *Hepatology*. 2021;74(2): 607–626. doi:10.1002/hep.31782
51. Lavanchy D, Kane M. Global epidemiology of hepatitis B virus infection. In: Liaw YF, Zoulim F, eds. *Hepatitis B Virus in Human Diseases*. Springer International Publishing; 2016:187–203.
52. Ott JJ, Stevens GA, Groeger J, Wiersma ST. Global epidemiology of hepatitis B virus infection: new estimates of age-specific HBsAg seroprevalence and endemicity. *Vaccine*. 2012;30(12): 2212–2219. doi:10.1016/j.vaccine.2011.12.116
53. Centers for Disease Control and Prevention. Surveillance for viral hepatitis—United States, 2016. Updated April 16, 2018. Available at: https://www.cdc.gov/hepatitis/statistics/2016surveillance/index.htm. Accessed January 31, 2023.
54. Kim WR. Epidemiology of hepatitis B in the United States. *Hepatology*. 2009;49(5 suppl): S28–S34. doi:10.1002/hep.22975
55. Mast EE, Weinbaum CM, Fiore AE, et al. A comprehensive immunization strategy to eliminate transmission of hepatitis B virus infection in the United States: recommendations of the Advisory Committee on Immunization Practices (ACIP) Part II: immunization of adults. *MMWR Recomm Rep*. 2006;55(Rr-16):1–33; quiz CE1-4.
56. Wasley A, Miller JT, Finelli L. Surveillance for acute viral hepatitis—United States, 2005. *MMWR Surveill Summ*. 2007;56(3):1–24.
57. Stevens CE, Beasley RP, Tsui J, Lee WC. Vertical transmission of hepatitis B antigen in Taiwan. *N Engl J Med*. 1975;292(15):771–774. doi:10.1056/nejm197504102921503
58. Lai CL, Wong BC, Yeoh EK, Lim WL, Chang WK, Lin HJ. Five-year follow-up of a prospective randomized trial of hepatitis B recombinant DNA yeast vaccine vs. plasma-derived vaccine in children: immunogenicity and anamnestic responses. *Hepatology*. 1993;18(4):763–767. doi:10.1002/hep.1840180403
59. Hepatitis B virus: a comprehensive strategy for eliminating transmission in the United States through universal childhood vaccination. Recommendations of the Immunization Practices Advisory Committee (ACIP). *MMWR Recomm Rep*. 1991;40(Rr-13):1–25.
60. Centers for Disease Control and Prevention. 2016 update to the 2001 CDC hemodialysis recommendations. Updated November 17, 2017. Available at: https://www.cdc.gov/dialysis/guidelines/index.html. Accessed January 31, 2023.
61. Ni YH, Huang LM, Chang MH, et al. Two decades of universal hepatitis B vaccination in Taiwan: impact and implication for future strategies. *Gastroenterology*. 2007;132(4):1287–1293. doi:10.1053/j.gastro.2007.02.055
62. Terrault NA, Bzowej NH, Chang KM, Hwang JP, Jonas MM, Murad MH. AASLD guidelines for treatment of chronic hepatitis B. *Hepatology*. 2016;63(1):261–283. doi:10.1002/hep.28156
63. Alter HJ, Purcell RH, Shih JW, et al. Detection of antibody to hepatitis C virus in prospectively followed transfusion recipients with acute and chronic non-A, non-B hepatitis. *N Engl J Med*. 1989;321(22):1494–1500. doi:10.1056/nejm198911303212202
64. Pomper GJ, Wu Y, Snyder EL. Risks of transfusion-transmitted infections: 2003. *Curr Opin Hematol*. 2003;10(6):412–418. doi:10.1097/00062752-200311000-00003

65. Freeman AJ, Dore GJ, Law MG, et al. Estimating progression to cirrhosis in chronic hepatitis C virus infection. *Hepatology*. 2001;34(4 pt 1):809–816. doi:10.1053/jhep.2001.27831
66. Poynard T, Bedossa P, Opolon P. Natural history of liver fibrosis progression in patients with chronic hepatitis C. The OBSVIRC, METAVIR, CLINIVIR, and DOSVIRC groups. *Lancet*. 1997;349(9055):825–832. doi:10.1016/s0140-6736(96)07642-8
67. Armstrong GL, Alter MJ, McQuillan GM, Margolis HS. The past incidence of hepatitis C virus infection: implications for the future burden of chronic liver disease in the United States. *Hepatology*. 2000;31(3):777–782. doi:10.1002/hep.510310332
68. Kalidindi Y, Jung J, Feldman R, Riley T, III. Association of direct-acting antiviral treatment with mortality among Medicare beneficiaries with hepatitis C. *JAMA Netw Open*. 2020;3(7):e2011055. doi:10.1001/jamanetworkopen.2020.11055
69. Parrish NF, Feurer ID, Matsuoka LK, Rega SA, Perri R, Alexopoulos SP. The changing face of liver transplantation in the United States: the effect of HCV antiviral eras on transplantation trends and outcomes. *Transplant Direct*. 2019;5(3):e427. doi:10.1097/txd.0000000000000866
70. Galbraith JW, Donnelly JP, Franco RA, Overton ET, Rodgers JB, Wang HE. National estimates of healthcare utilization by individuals with hepatitis C virus infection in the United States. *Clin Infect Dis*. 2014;59(6):755–764. doi:10.1093/cid/ciu427
71. Hussain KB, Fontana RJ, Moyer CA, Su GL, Sneed-Pee N, Lok AS. Comorbid illness is an important determinant of health-related quality of life in patients with chronic hepatitis C. *Am J Gastroenterol*. 2001;96(9):2737–2744. doi:10.1111/j.1572-0241.2001.04133.x
72. El-Serag HB. Epidemiology of viral hepatitis and hepatocellular carcinoma. *Gastroenterology*. 2012;142(6):1264–1273.e1. doi:10.1053/j.gastro.2011.12.061
73. Edlin BR, Eckhardt BJ, Shu MA, Holmberg SD, Swan T. Toward a more accurate estimate of the prevalence of hepatitis C in the United States. *Hepatology*. 2015;62(5):1353–1363. doi:10.1002/hep.27978
74. Backus LI, Belperio PS, Loomis TP, Yip GH, Mole LA. Hepatitis C virus screening and prevalence among US veterans in Department of Veterans Affairs care. *JAMA Intern Med*. 2013; 173(16):1549–1552. doi:10.1001/jamainternmed.2013.8133
75. Beijer U, Wolf A, Fazel S. Prevalence of tuberculosis, hepatitis C virus, and HIV in homeless people: a systematic review and meta-analysis. *Lancet Infectious Dis*. 2012;12(11):859–870.
76. Hofmeister MG, Rosenthal EM, Barker LK, et al. Estimating prevalence of hepatitis C virus infection in the United States, 2013–2016. *Hepatology*. 2019;69(3):1020–1031. doi:10.1002/hep.30297
77. Williams I. Epidemiology of hepatitis C in the United States. *Am J Med*. 1999;107(6b):2s–9s. doi:10.1016/s0002-9343(99)00373-3
78. Wasley A, Finelli L, Miller JT. Surveillance for acute viral hepatitis, United States, 2005. *MMWR Surveill Summ*. 2007;56(SS-3). Available at: https://stacks.cdc.gov/view/cdc/6820. Accessed January 31, 2023.
79. Alter MJ, Kruszon-Moran D, Nainan OV, et al. The prevalence of hepatitis C virus infection in the United States, 1988 through 1994. *N Engl J Med*. 1999;341(8):556–562. doi:10.1056/nejm199908193410802
80. Garfein RS, Vlahov D, Galai N, Doherty MC, Nelson KE. Viral infections in short-term injection drug users: the prevalence of the hepatitis C, hepatitis B, human immunodeficiency, and

human T-lymphotropic viruses. *Am J Public Health.* 1996;86(5):655–661. doi:10.2105/ajph.86.5.655

81. Geerlings W, Tufveson G, Ehrich JH, et al. Report on management of renal failure in Europe, XXIII. *Nephrol Dial Transplant.* 1994;9(suppl 1):6–25.
82. Jadoul M, Bieber BA, Martin P, et al. Prevalence, incidence, and risk factors for hepatitis C virus infection in hemodialysis patients. *Kidney Int.* 2019;95(4):939–947. doi:10.1016/j.kint.2018.11.038
83. Finelli L, Miller JT, Tokars JI, Alter MJ, Arduino MJ. National surveillance of dialysis-associated diseases in the United States, 2002. *Semin Dial.* 2005;18(1):52–61. doi:10.1111/j.1525-139X.2005.18108.x
84. Weinbaum C, Lyerla R, Margolis HS. Prevention and control of infections with hepatitis viruses in correctional settings. *MMWR Recomm Rep.* 2003;52(RR-1):1–36; quiz CE1-4.
85. Zarski JP, Mc Hutchison J, Bronowicki JP, et al. Rate of natural disease progression in patients with chronic hepatitis C. *J Hepatol.* 2003;38(3):307–134. doi:10.1016/s0168-8278(02)00387-2
86. Leandro G, Mangia A, Hui J, et al. Relationship between steatosis, inflammation, and fibrosis in chronic hepatitis C: a meta-analysis of individual patient data. *Gastroenterology.* 2006;130(6):1636–1642. doi:10.1053/j.gastro.2006.03.014
87. Fried MW, Shiffman ML, Reddy KR, et al. Peginterferon alfa-2a plus ribavirin for chronic hepatitis C virus infection. *N Engl J Med.* 2002;347(13):975–982. doi:10.1056/NEJMoa020047
88. Younossi Z, Kallman J, Kincaid J. The effects of HCV infection and management on health-related quality of life. *Hepatology.* 2007;45(3):806–816. doi:10.1002/hep.21565
89. Davies S, Greenwald R, Harvey J, Raymond D, Simmons A. Center for Health Law and Policy Innovation & National Viral Hepatitis Roundtable, Hepatitis C: state of Medicaid access, 2022 national summary report. Available at: https://stateofhepc.org. Accessed January 23, 2023.
90. Powell EE, Wong VW, Rinella M. Non-alcoholic fatty liver disease. *Lancet.* 2021;397(10290): 2212–2224. doi:10.1016/s0140-6736(20)32511-3
91. Angulo P, Kleiner DE, Dam-Larsen S, et al. Liver fibrosis, but no other histologic features, is associated with long-term outcomes of patients with nonalcoholic fatty liver disease. *Gastroenterology.* 2015;149(2):389–397.e10. doi:10.1053/j.gastro.2015.04.043
92. Younossi Z, Anstee QM, Marietti M, et al. Global burden of NAFLD and NASH: trends, predictions, risk factors and prevention. *Nature Rev Gastroenterol Hepatol.* 2018;15(1):11–20. doi:10.1038/nrgastro.2017.109
93. Adams LA, Lymp JF, St Sauver J, et al. The natural history of nonalcoholic fatty liver disease: a population-based cohort study. *Gastroenterology.* 2005;129(1):113–121. doi:10.1053/j.gastro.2005.04.014
94. Ekstedt M, Franzén LE, Mathiesen UL, et al. Long-term follow-up of patients with NAFLD and elevated liver enzymes. *Hepatology.* 2006;44(4):865–873. doi:10.1002/hep.21327
95. Younossi ZM, Otgonsuren M, Henry L, et al. Association of nonalcoholic fatty liver disease (NAFLD) with hepatocellular carcinoma (HCC) in the United States from 2004 to 2009. *Hepatology.* 2015;62(6):1723-1730. doi:10.1002/hep.28123
96. Yatsuji S, Hashimoto E, Tobari M, Taniai M, Tokushige K, Shiratori K. Clinical features and outcomes of cirrhosis due to non-alcoholic steatohepatitis compared with cirrhosis caused by

chronic hepatitis C. *J Gastroenterol Hepatol.* 2009;24(2):248–254. doi:10.1111/j.1440-1746.2008.05640.x

97. Younossi ZM, Stepanova M, Afendy M, et al. Changes in the prevalence of the most common causes of chronic liver diseases in the United States from 1988 to 2008. *Clin Gastroenterol Hepatol.* 2011;9(6):524–530.e1; quiz e60. doi:10.1016/j.cgh.2011.03.020
98. Younossi ZM, Koenig AB, Abdelatif D, Fazel Y, Henry L, Wymer M. Global epidemiology of nonalcoholic fatty liver disease—meta-analytic assessment of prevalence, incidence, and outcomes. *Hepatology.* 2016;64(1):73–84. doi:10.1002/hep.28431
99. Kanwal F, Kramer JR, Duan Z, Yu X, White D, El-Serag HB. Trends in the burden of nonalcoholic fatty liver disease in a United States cohort of veterans. *Clin Gastroenterol Hepatol.* 2016;14(2):301–308.e1–e2. doi:10.1016/j.cgh.2015.08.010
100. Hamaguchi M, Kojima T, Takeda N, et al. The metabolic syndrome as a predictor of nonalcoholic fatty liver disease. *Ann Intern Med.* 2005;143(10):722–728. doi:10.7326/0003-4819-143-10-200511150-00009
101. Browning JD, Szczepaniak LS, Dobbins R, et al. Prevalence of hepatic steatosis in an urban population in the United States: impact of ethnicity. *Hepatology.* 2004;40(6):1387–1395. doi:10.1002/hep.20466
102. Schwimmer JB, Deutsch R, Kahen T, Lavine JE, Stanley C, Behling C. Prevalence of fatty liver in children and adolescents. *Pediatrics.* 2006;118(4):1388–1393.
103. Anderson EL, Howe LD, Jones HE, Higgins JP, Lawlor DA, Fraser A. The prevalence of non-alcoholic fatty liver disease in children and adolescents: a systematic review and meta-analysis. *PLoS One.* 2015;10(10):e0140908. doi:10.1371/journal.pone.0140908
104. Weston SR, Leyden W, Murphy R, et al. Racial and ethnic distribution of nonalcoholic fatty liver in persons with newly diagnosed chronic liver disease. *Hepatology.* 2005;41(2):372–379. doi:10.1002/hep.20554
105. Romeo S, Kozlitina J, Xing C, et al. Genetic variation in PNPLA3 confers susceptibility to nonalcoholic fatty liver disease. *Nat Genet.* 2008;40(12):1461–1465. doi:10.1038/ng.257
106. Ruhl CE, Everhart JE. Epidemiology of nonalcoholic fatty liver. *Clinics in liver disease.* 2004;8(3):501–519.
107. Fazel Y, Koenig AB, Sayiner M, Goodman ZD, Younossi ZM. Epidemiology and natural history of non-alcoholic fatty liver disease. *Metabolism.* 2016;65(8):1017–1025. doi:10.1016/j.metabol.2016.01.012
108. Gholam PM, Flancbaum L, Machan JT, Charney DA, Kotler DP. Nonalcoholic fatty liver disease in severely obese subjects. *Am J Gastroenterol.* 2007;102(2):399–408. doi:10.1111/j.1572-0241.2006.01041.x
109. Ogden CL, Yanovski SZ, Carroll MD, Flegal KM. The epidemiology of obesity. *Gastroenterology.* 2007;132(6):2087–2102.
110. Chalasani N, Younossi Z, Lavine JE, et al. The diagnosis and management of nonalcoholic fatty liver disease: practice guidance from the American Association for the Study of Liver Diseases. *Hepatology.* 2018;67(1):328–357.
111. Villanueva A. Hepatocellular carcinoma. *N Engl J Med.* 2019;380(15):1450–1462. doi:10.1056/NEJMra1713263

112. International Agency for Research on Cancer. Liver cancer: estimated incidence, mortality and prevalence worldwide in 2012. 2012. Available at: https://publications.iarc.fr/Databases/Iarc-Cancerbases/GLOBOCAN-2012-Estimated-Cancer-Incidence-Mortality-And-Prevalence-Worldwide-In-2012-V1.0-2012. Accessed January 31, 2023.
113. Jemal A, Ward EM, Johnson CJ, et al. Annual report to the nation on the status of cancer, 1975–2014, featuring survival. *J Natl Cancer Inst.* 2017;109(9). doi:10.1093/jnci/djx030
114. Bosch FX, Ribes J, Cléries R, Díaz M. Epidemiology of hepatocellular carcinoma. *Clin Liver Dis.* 2005;9(2):191–211, v. doi:10.1016/j.cld.2004.12.009
115. Xu J. Trends in liver cancer mortality among adults aged 25 and over in the United States, 2000–2016. *NCHS Data Brief.* 2018;(314):1–8.
116. Jemal A, Bray F, Center MM, Ferlay J, Ward E, Forman D. Global cancer statistics. *CA Cancer J Clin.* 2011;61(2):69–90. doi:10.3322/caac.20107
117. Baatarkhuu O, Gerelchimeg T, Munkh-Orshikh D, Batsukh B, Sarangua G, Amarsanaa J. Epidemiology, genotype distribution, prognosis, control, and management of viral hepatitis B, C, D, and hepatocellular carcinoma in Mongolia. *Euroasian J Hepatogastroenterol.* 2018;8(1):57–62. doi:10.5005/jp-journals-10018-1260
118. Mak D, Kramvis A. Epidemiology and aetiology of hepatocellular carcinoma in Sub-Saharan Africa. *Hepatoma Res.* 2021;7:39.
119. McGlynn KA, Petrick JL, El-Serag HB. Epidemiology of hepatocellular carcinoma. *Hepatology.* 2021;73:4–13.
120. Larsson SC, Wolk A. Coffee consumption and risk of liver cancer: a meta-analysis. *Gastroenterology.* 2007;132(5):1740–1745.
121. Bamia C, Lagiou P, Jenab M, et al. Fruit and vegetable consumption in relation to hepatocellular carcinoma in a multi-centre, European cohort study. *Br J Cancer.* 2015;112(7):1273–1282.
122. Chang M-H. Cancer prevention by vaccination against hepatitis B. *Cancer Prev II.* 2009;181:85–94.
123. Benvegnu L, Gios M, Boccato S, Alberti A. Natural history of compensated viral cirrhosis: a prospective study on the incidence and hierarchy of major complications. *Gut.* 2004;53(5):744–749.
124. Kowdley KV, Brown KE, Ahn J, Sundaram V. ACG clinical guideline: hereditary hemochromatosis. *Am J Gastroenterol.* 2019;114(8):1202–1218. doi:10.14309/ajg.0000000000000315
125. Beutler E, Felitti VJ, Koziol JA, Ho NJ, Gelbart T. Penetrance of 845G→ A (C282Y) HFE hereditary haemochromatosis mutation in the USA. *Lancet.* 2002;359(9302):211–218.
126. Adams PC, Reboussin DM, Barton JC, et al. Hemochromatosis and iron-overload screening in a racially diverse population. *N Engl J Med.* 2005;352(17):1769–1778.

23

Chronic Kidney Disease

Tripti Singh, MD, and Brad C. Astor, PhD, MPH

LEARNING OBJECTIVES

After completing this chapter, readers should be able to

1. Identify the populations at high risk for developing chronic kidney disease.
2. Identify the modifiable and nonmodifiable risk factors for progression of chronic kidney disease.
3. Identify the targets of treatment in slowing down the progression of chronic kidney disease.

INTRODUCTION

Chronic kidney disease (CKD) is a term applied to a variety of disorders that cause progressive kidney damage resulting in decreased kidney function. These disorders include sequelae of chronic conditions like diabetes mellitus or hypertension, genetic disorders that may manifest at any age (e.g., autosomal dominant polycystic kidney disease), glomerulonephritis, infections (e.g., HIV/AIDS, hepatitis C), toxicity from medications (e.g., nonsteroidal anti-inflammatory drugs), and disorders of organs outside the kidneys (e.g., prostate, urinary bladder, uterus) that result in blockage of urine flow.

Chronic kidney disease can progress to end-stage kidney disease (ESKD), requiring kidney transplantation or maintenance dialysis treatment for survival. Earlier stages of CKD, however, are much more common than ESKD and are associated with elevated risk of death, cardiovascular events, and other conditions.[1] Primary prevention, early detection, and interventions limiting progression of CKD are needed to reduce these outcomes. In this chapter, we discuss the significance, causes, and consequences of CKD (Figure 23-1).

End-Stage Kidney Disease

When Congress extended Medicare coverage in 1973 to all Americans with ESKD, regardless of age, it provided coverage for 10,000 patients to receive dialysis. Since that

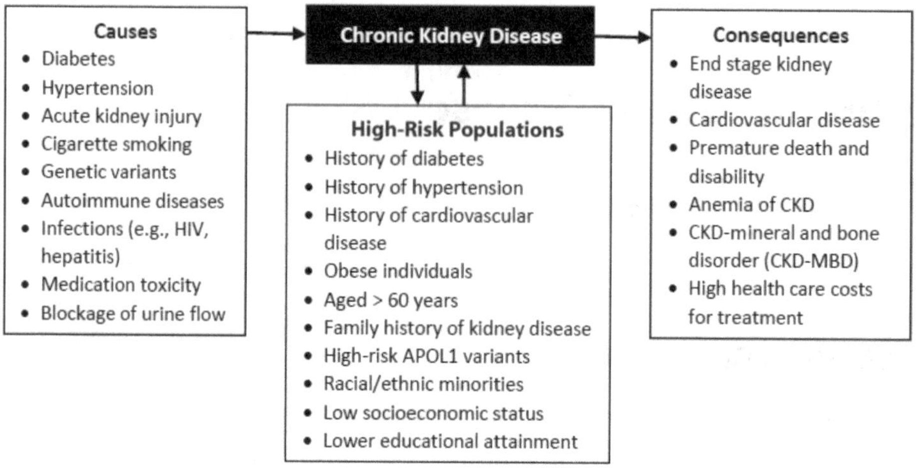

Figure 23-1. Chronic Kidney Disease (CKD): Causes, Consequences, and High-Risk Populations

time the number of individuals with ESKD in the United States has grown to more than 800,000.[2] The growing number of patients treated for ESKD represents an enormous burden in terms of economic cost, with total Medicare-related expenditures estimated at $51 billion in 2019. This is approximately 7.2% of Medicare fee-for-service expenditures for 1% of the US Medicare fee-for-service population. Approximately 30% of individuals with ESKD have a functioning kidney transplant, while the remaining 70% receive some form of dialysis, in which the blood-filtering function of the kidneys is performed by an external machine (in the case of hemodialysis) or the peritoneum (in the case of peritoneal dialysis). The large majority (87%) of these individuals receive in-center hemodialysis, while 11% receive peritoneal dialysis and 2% receive home hemodialysis. A 2019 presidential executive order, Advancing American Kidney Health, aimed to significantly increase the proportion of patients receiving transplantation and home hemodialysis.[3]

Chronic Kidney Disease

While ESKD represents the most severe form and confers a large burden, there are far more individuals with less severe CKD, as a minority of patients with CKD survive long enough to reach ESKD. An estimated 37 million adults in the US (15% of the population) have some form of CKD.[4] Chronic kidney disease is defined and classified into stages depending on two markers of kidney health: kidney function and kidney damage.[1] Kidney function is evaluated by measuring or estimating the glomerular filtration rate (GFR), whereas kidney damage is evaluated by measuring urinary excretion of albumin (albuminuria) or total protein (proteinuria) (Figure 23-2).[1]

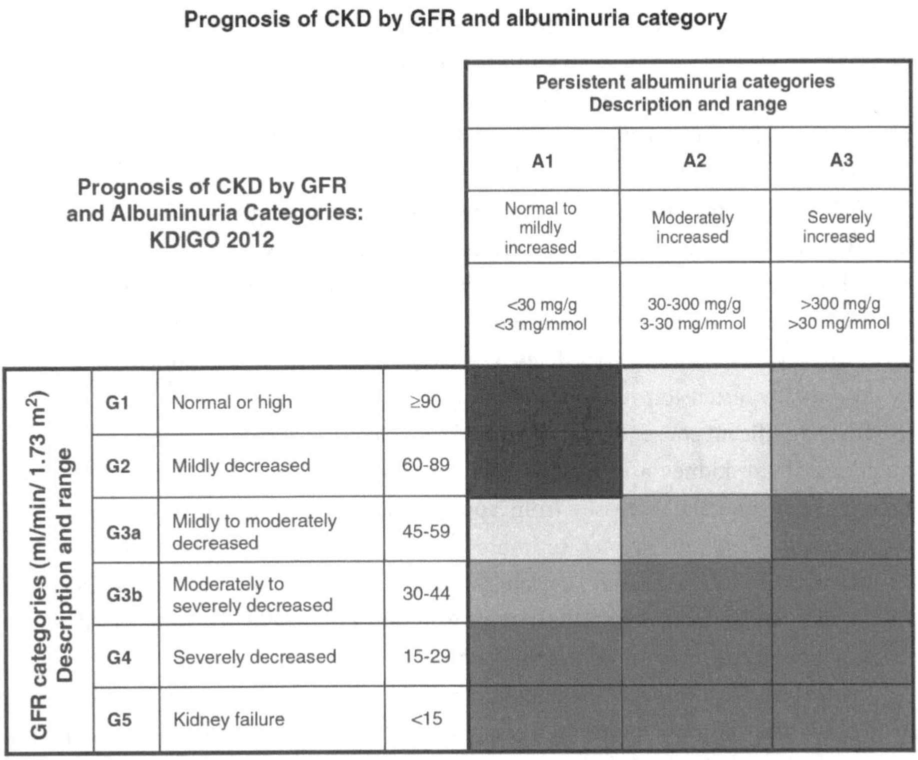

Dark gray: low risk (if no other markers of kidney disease, no CKD); light grey: moderately increased risk; medium light gray: high risk; medium dark gray: very high risk.

Source: Reprinted with permission of KDIGO.[1]

Note: CKD = chronic kidney disease; GFR = glomerular filtration rate. CKD is defined as abnormalities of kidney structure or function, present for more than 3 months, with implications for health. The disease is classified based on cause, GFR category, and albuminuria category (CGA).

Figure 23-2. Current KDIGO Chronic Kidney Disease Nomenclature

As many individuals with CKD do not develop symptoms until they have a significant decline in kidney function, the epidemic of CKD is largely a silent one. Data from the 2009 to 2012 National Health and Nutritional Examination Survey (NHANES), revealed that fewer than 10% of patients with CKD Stage 1 to 3 are aware of their kidney disease.[5]

PUBLIC HEALTH IMPACT

Mortality rates among patients with ESKD aged 66 to 74 years treated with dialysis are more than 10 times higher for men and approximately 15 times higher for women than for their counterparts without ESKD.[6] Individuals with a functioning kidney transplant have much better survival than those on dialysis. The number of kidney transplants, however, is limited by the availability of organs from living and deceased donors. Cardiovascular disease remains the leading cause of death in both kidney transplant recipients and patients receiving chronic dialysis.

Analyses from the international Chronic Kidney Disease Prognosis Consortium (CKD-PC) and others have shown that both lower estimated glomerular filtration rate (eGFR) and higher albuminuria, well before a diagnosis of ESKD, are strongly associated with all-cause and cardiovascular mortality,[7] ESKD,[8] acute kidney injury,[9] and progressive CKD in both general and high-risk populations, independent of each other and of other cardiovascular risk factors. These associations are consistent in subgroups defined by sex, race, hypertension, and diabetes.

Other significant consequences of CKD derive from the loss of endocrine or exocrine functions of the kidney and include anemia, as well as mineral and bone disorders. Prevalence of anemia increases from approximately 4% in those with an eGFR of 90 mL/min/1.73 m^2 or greater to more than 50% in those with eGFR less than 30 mL/min/1.73 m^2.[10] Anemia is strongly associated with quality of life in CKD and ESKD and can be treated effectively with iron and erythropoietin stimulating agents (ESAs), though care is required to avoid complications.[11]

Changes in bone mineral metabolism and disturbances of calcium and phosphate hemostasis also become more prevalent as CKD worsens. The term *chronic kidney disease–mineral and bone disorder* (CKD-MBD) is used to refer to these multiple abnormalities.[12] Clinical monitoring and treatments to achieve target serum concentrations of calcium, phosphate, and parathyroid hormone are major concerns in ESKD, especially for those patients on chronic dialysis, but these abnormalities are also of importance in earlier stages of CKD.

DESCRIPTIVE EPIDEMIOLOGY

The prevalence of CKD and ESKD increases significantly with age. In patients aged 65 years and older, CKD is present in approximately 38% of the population (Table 23-1).[2] While CKD is slightly more common in women than in men (14.3% vs. 12.4%), ESKD is more common in men than in women.[2] This relative difference has grown over the last two decades and continues to increase. Similarly, the prevalence of early kidney disease is comparable across racial and ethnic groups, but the prevalence of ESKD is much greater among minority populations.[13] The prevalence of ESKD in Blacks is roughly 3.4 times higher than in Whites.[2] This difference is largely attributed to higher rates and earlier onset of diabetes and hypertension in this population. ESKD prevalence also is significantly higher in Native Americans and Hispanics than in non-Hispanic Whites.[2]

Table 23-1. Chronic Kidney Disease and End-Stage Kidney Disease Prevalence by Age, Gender, and Race/Ethnicity

Characteristic	CKD		ESKD	
	Prevalence, %	Prevalence Ratio	Prevalence (Million)	Prevalence Ratio
18–44 y	6.0	Reference	88.4	1
45–64 y	12.4	2.07	4,157.3	47.03
≥65 y	38.1	6.35	~7,300	~82.58
Men	12.4	Reference	2,834.5	Reference
Women	14.3	1.15	1,975.5	0.70
Non-Hispanic White	12.7	Reference	1,703.5	Reference
Non-Hispanic Black	16.3	1.28	5854.8	3.44
Non-Hispanic Asian	12.9	1.02	2,275.3	1.34
Hispanic	13.6	1.07	~2600	~1.54

Note: CKD = chronic kidney disease; ESKD = end-stage kidney disease.

Socioeconomic factors also affect the prevalence of CKD. Analyses of NHANES data from 2015 to 2016 found a higher prevalence of CKD among individuals with lower income (14.3%) versus higher income (9.4%) and lower formal education (15.2% among those with less than a high school education) versus higher formal education (13.4% among those with at least some college).[14] The association with income is present in within-race analyses, with a greater prevalence among lower-income African Americans compared with those at higher income levels.[15]

Geographic Distribution

The incidence of ESKD is noticeably higher in areas of the Southeast, the Mid-Atlantic, the lower Mississippi River valley, and some areas of the Southwest (Figure 23-3).[2] The incidence is lower in the Mountain West.

Time Trends

The incidence of ESKD, adjusted for age and sex, has decreased over the last two decades for all racial groups (Figure 23-4).[2] This decrease is most noticeable in racial minorities, who continue to have much higher incidence than Whites. Despite the decreasing adjusted incidence, the overall prevalence of ESKD continues to grow substantially, from 697 per million in 1990 to 2,302 per million in 2019 as a result of the aging of the population and improved survival of those with ESKD.

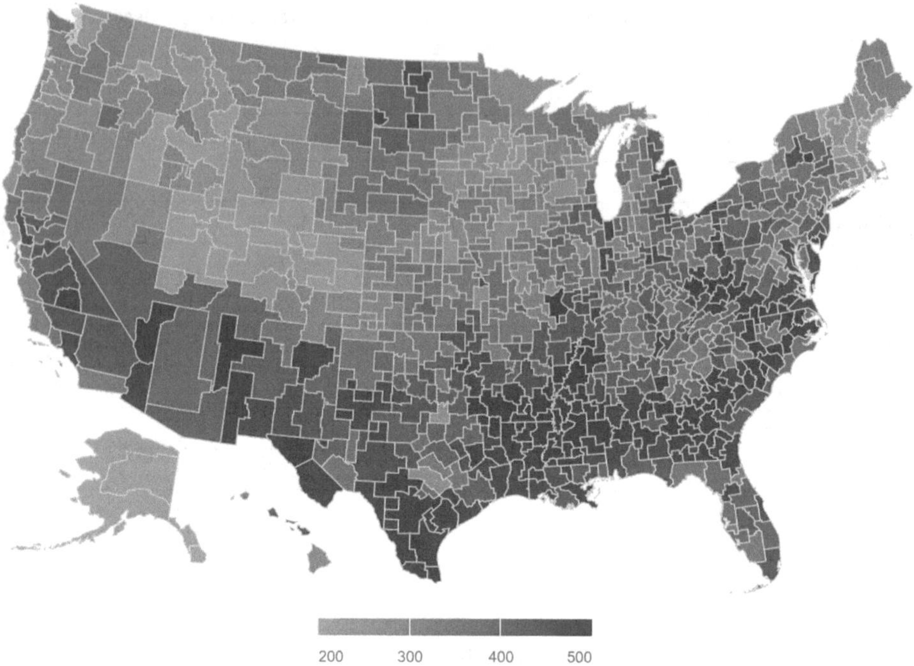

Source: Reprinted from US Renal Data System.[2]

Figure 23-3. Incidence of End-Stage Kidney Disease by Health Service Area

CAUSES

The major causes of ESKD in the United States are diabetes mellitus and hypertension. Diabetes is listed as the primary cause of ESKD in approximately 39% of cases, and hypertension listed in approximately 28% of cases.[2] Up to 40% of patients with type 1 diabetes and 5% of patients with type 2 diabetes develop kidney failure from diabetic nephropathy. Kidney damage in patients with diabetes is a consequence of high blood sugar levels leading to advanced glycation end product formation and damage to the glomeruli. Kidney damage is one component of the microvascular disease seen in patients with diabetes mellitus who develop other complications, such as diabetic retinopathy and neuropathy. Increased albumin excretion in the urine is the earliest manifestation of diabetic kidney disease. Hypertension is both a cause and a consequence of chronic kidney disease and is associated with progression of CKD.

Another leading cause of ESKD is glomerulonephritis, listed as the primary cause of 15% of ESKD cases. Glomerulonephritis is commonly a consequence of autoimmune diseases, including systemic lupus erythematosus (i.e., lupus nephritis) or IgA nephropathy.

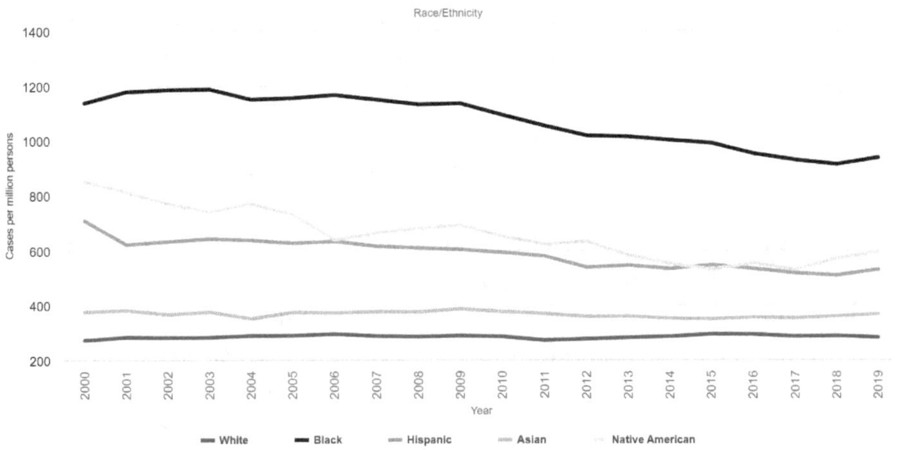

Source: Reprinted from US Renal Data System.[2]

Figure 23-4. Adjusted Incidence of End-Stage Kidney Disease by Patient Characteristics

An increased risk of many types of nondiabetic kidney disease has been attributed to genetic variants in the apoL1 (APOL1) gene, found only in individuals with recent African ancestry.[16] These high-risk alleles are strongly associated with hypertensive-related kidney disease, focal segmental glomerulosclerosis, and HIV-associated nephropathy. The effect of carrying two APOL1 risk alleles explains an estimated 18% of focal segmental glomerulosclerosis and 35% of HIV-associated nephropathy.[17] Approximately 13% of African Americans have two high-risk alleles.[18]

Individuals with family members with kidney failure are at significantly greater risk of CKD.[4] Heritability of ESKD has been estimated at 60% and heritability for eGFR is estimated to be 41% in Northern European populations.[19,20] A first-degree relative with CKD is associated with a three fold higher risk of CKD.

Metabolic acidosis also is noted as a risk factor for CKD and associated with progression to ESKD.[21] Serum bicarbonate often decreases with decreasing kidney function because of reduced acid excretion, leading to net acid accumulation. Recent studies have also found that acid retention is associated with increased risk of CKD progression and ESKD even before overt clinical metabolic acidosis.[22]

Modifiable Risk Factors

The primary modifiable risk factors for development and progression of CKD are hyperglycemia, high blood pressure, and smoking. Intensive glycemic control in diabetes can help prevent the development of albuminuria and slow the progression of established diabetic nephropathy. The presence of inadequately controlled blood pressure in the setting of CKD from any cause has an additive impact on disease progression. Aggressive blood pressure control is recommended for all individuals with CKD regardless of etiology. Tobacco use is also associated with the development of proteinuria and more rapid progression of CKD.[23]

As obesity is often upstream from developing diabetes and hypertension, reducing obesity is critical to reducing the burden of CKD. A meta-analysis of over 5 million participants in 39 studies found a nearly linear association of greater adiposity above a body mass index (BMI) of 25 kg/m^2 and decline in eGFR over eight years of follow-up after adjustment for age, sex, race, and current smoking. Body mass indices of 30, 35, and 40 were associated with 18%, 69%, and 102% higher risk of GFR decline, respectively, compared with a BMI of 25. This association was similar in those without hypertension and even somewhat stronger among individuals without diabetes.[24]

Acute kidney injury (AKI), an abrupt and usually reversible decline in kidney function, is relatively common in hospitalized patients, especially in intensive care units. A meta-analysis based on 154 studies estimated the overall incidence of AKI during hospitalization as 22%.[25] Hospitalized patients with AKI have a 2.7 times higher risk of new or progressive CKD and 4.8 times higher risk of ESKD than do their counterparts without AKI. These risks are greater with higher AKI stage. Interventions to prevent or reduce severity of hospital-based and community-acquired AKI may have significant impacts on CKD.

EVIDENCE-BASED INTERVENTIONS

Prevention

Diabetes mellitus and hypertension together account for nearly two-thirds of prevalent ESKD cases in the United States.[2] As such, prevention, early identification, risk factor modification, and treatment of diabetes mellitus and hypertension may have a significant impact on incidence of CKD. Effective control of diabetes has been shown to decrease the rate of heart disease, peripheral vascular disease, and CKD.

Another essential step for prevention of CKD is to increase public awareness. In a study of 29,144 participants with CKD, only 6,751 (23%) reported that they were aware of their disease.[26] A greater emphasis should be placed on prevention of CKD in medical school curricula and by those training allied health personnel, and student clerkships in medical schools should increase the emphasis on continuity of patient care. Public health and preventive medicine programs should include training in development of community-based programs for managing the broad epidemic of CKD. On an individual level, physicians and other health care workers need adequate training in how to diagnose CKD early in its course.

Screening: Who

The complex care that must be provided for patients with CKD cannot be overemphasized. However, the ability of the current US health care system to appropriately manage all of the individuals identified with CKD via effective screening programs remains unclear. All patients should be assessed as a part of their health examinations to determine whether they are at increased risk of CKD.

A recommendation for CKD screening is currently being considered by the US Preventive Services Task Force.[27] At this time, screening for CKD is recommended only for high-risk individuals (Figure 23-1). Screening programs in communities with high-risk populations are effective in detecting previously unidentified people with CKD. An example of such an approach is the Kidney Early Evaluation Program (KEEP), a free kidney disease–screening program designed to detect CKD and promote follow-up evaluation with clinicians to improve outcomes. This program screens individuals with diabetes or hypertension and those with a first-degree relative with diabetes, hypertension, or kidney disease, estimated to include 93% of individuals with CKD.[28]

Screening: How

All patients who have risk factors for CKD should be screened with a blood test for creatinine to estimate GFR and a urine test for protein excretion, preferably by measuring the urinary albumin-to-creatinine ratio.[1] Chronic kidney disease is diagnosed in any individual who has an eGFR below 60 mL/min/1.73 m^2 for a period of at least three months. In addition, CKD is diagnosed in patients with any level of eGFR in the presence of structural (e.g., polycystic kidney disease) or functional (e.g., proteinuria, albuminuria) damage that persists for more than three months (Figure 23-2).

As creatinine is affected by muscle mass, GFR is most often estimated using an equation that takes into consideration the age and sex of the patient. The American Society of Nephrology recommended in 2021 that the new eGFR 2021 CKD-Epi equation, without consideration of race, should be used by US laboratories.[29] The use of an equation with both creatinine and cystatin C results in slightly more accurate estimation of GFR without race.[30] It must be pointed out that the formula for estimating GFR is unreliable in the hospitalized patient or in the setting of acute kidney injury, when serum creatinine levels can fluctuate daily because of such factors as changes in volume status and disturbances of cardiac function.

Urinary protein excretion should be quantified by measurement of total protein or albumin, the most abundant protein in urine, preferably in an early morning specimen. It is recommended that the ratio of albumin to creatinine excreted be used to estimate albuminuria.[1] It is noted that 24-hour urine collections are cumbersome and may actually be inaccurate because of missed collections. Albuminuria of less than 30 milligrams per gram of creatinine is considered to be in the normal or mildly increased range of albumin excretion, moderately increased albuminuria is defined as an albumin excretion of 30 to 300 milligrams of albumin per gram of creatinine, and severely increased albuminuria is defined as an albumin excretion of greater than 300 milligrams of albumin per gram of creatinine. However, even low levels of urinary albumin excretion in patients with diabetes may be associated with an increased incidence of cardiovascular disease.

Treatment

In a patient in the early stages of CKD, greater emphasis should be placed on diagnosing and managing the conditions causing CKD. In a patient in advanced stages of CKD, the care shifts to preventing and managing the complications of CKD. Early referral of patients with advanced CKD (Stage 4 and 5) to a kidney specialist is recommended to facilitate planning and education for transition to dialysis and kidney transplantation.[1] Despite these guidelines, in the United States timely referral to a kidney specialist remains a challenge. A retrospective longitudinal cohort study of more than 12,500 older veterans with diabetes found that nearly half the patients had CKD and only 7.2% had a nephrology visit during the five-year study period. Even among those with Stage 4 CKD, only 32% had been seen in the nephrology clinic.[31] An estimated 19% of patients with incident ESKD in 2019 also had no pre-ESKD nephrology care.[2]

Diabetes Control in Chronic Kidney Disease

Intensive glycemic control was associated with a 67% risk reduction for a doubling of plasma creatinine levels at nine years in the UK Prospective Diabetes Study (UKPDS).[32] The current Kidney Disease: Improving Global Outcomes (KDIGO) guidelines recommend a target hemoglobin A1c of 6.5% to 8% to prevent or delay progression of the CKD.[1] Metformin and sodium glucose co-transporter 2 inhibitor (SGLT2i) should be used as first-line agents in patients with type 2 diabetes mellitus and an eGFR higher than 30mL/min. A meta-analysis of RCTs showed that SGLT2i substantially reduces the risk of dialysis, transplantation, or death from kidney disease (risk ratio [RR] 0.67; 95% confidence interval [CI], 0.52–0.86) and the risk of ESKD (RR 0.65; 95% CI, 0.53–0.81).[33]

Blood Pressure Control in Chronic Kidney Disease

Blood pressure should be closely monitored, as elevated blood pressure is very common in CKD patients and is a risk factor for further progression of kidney damage. Clinical guidelines have set target blood pressure values for patients with CKD at less than 120/80 mm Hg if tolerated by the patient.[1] However, it is recommended for clinicians to apply this recommendation based on patient factors, as the tight control of blood pressure is associated with increased risk of falls. Renin-angiotensin blocking agents should be the first-line drugs in patients with severely increased albuminuria.

Proteinuria in Chronic Kidney Disease

As mentioned previously, increased urinary albumin (or protein) excretion is an important risk factor for progression of CKD. Reduction of proteinuria has been associated with a decreased risk of death and development of ESKD in patients with both diabetic and nondiabetic CKD. The most common treatments for albuminuria reduction are the use of drugs such as angiotensin-converting enzyme (ACE) inhibitors or angiotensin receptor blockers (ARBs). Studies with ARBs in patients with type 2 diabetes have shown that the reduction in albuminuria at six months strongly predicts a decrease in adverse renal and cardiovascular outcomes.[34] This improvement in outcomes was independent of the blood pressure–lowering effects of these medications. Patients with hypertension, CKD, and cardiovascular disease also have improved cardiovascular outcomes with a reduction in proteinuria.[35] Reducing albuminuria via treatment with drugs to block the renin-angiotensin system in patients with CKD is recommended even if the blood pressure is at goal.

In some patients with diabetic kidney disease, proteinuria persists despite them being on the maximal dosage of ACE inhibitors or ARBs. Combining ACE inhibitors with ARBs is not recommended, however, because of an increased risk of hyperkalemia and mortality.[36] Addition of a selective mineralocorticoid antagonist (MRA; e.g., finerenone) to ACE inhibitor or ARB therapy in patients with chronic kidney disease from diabetes has been shown to slow the progress of CKD and cardiovascular events compared with placebo.[37] Addition of MRA, however, was associated with a higher risk of hyperkalemia (2.9% with MRA vs. 0.9 % with placebo).

Dietary sodium restriction of less than 2,000 mg per day or sodium chloride less than 5,000 mg per day is recommended in patients with chronic kidney disease, hypertension, or proteinuria.[1] Acidemia is often seen in patients with advanced CKD, and recent evidence suggests that treating such patients with low acid diet (low animal protein) and high basic diet (increased fruits and vegetables) and oral bicarbonate therapy to bring their sodium bicarbonate to a level greater than or equal to 23 milliequivalents (mEq) per liter slows the progression of CKD and decreases the risk of developing ESKD.[38]

A meta-analysis of 18 randomized clinical trials showed that lipid-lowering therapy in patients with CKD decreases the risk of cardiac mortality (RR = 0.82).[39] KDIGO guidelines recommend initiation of treatment with a statin in patients with CKD who are not yet on dialysis.[40]

Anemia is a common complication of CKD. Persistent hemoglobin levels less than 11 grams per deciliter are associated with an increased risk of death.[41] KDIGO guidelines recommend initiating treatment with erythropoietin-stimulating agents once the hemoglobin concentration is below 10 grams per deciliter in dialysis patients.

These measures to limit progressive kidney damage are important, but patients diagnosed with CKD also require regular follow-up and need to avoid exposure to nephrotoxic medications and therapeutic and diagnostic agents, including nonsteroidal anti-inflammatory drugs and iodinated radio-contrast agents used in diagnostic procedures.[42] Preventive goals and treatment strategies specific to patients with CKD can differ from those for the general population; for example, it is recommended that all patients with CKD be vaccinated against hepatitis B.[1]

MOVING FORWARD

Medications made available in the last five years can slow the progression of CKD and decrease morbidity and mortality in patients with CKD. These include SGLT2i and selective MRA. Given the high prevalence and increasing incidence of CKD, there remains a need for newer therapies and medication to prevent CKD and decrease the resulting morbidity and mortality. Diagnosis and management of CKD needs to be a central part of future public health planning in the management of the patient with chronic noncommunicable diseases.

Primary care physicians and other health care providers have an increasingly vital role to play for the patient with CKD, as it is not possible for the current number of nephrologists to directly manage the ongoing care for the expected increase in the number of patients with CKD. Appropriate guidelines and intervention programs are being developed for a simplified and streamlined program to include primary care physicians as well as ancillary health care personnel in CKD management. Pilot clinical programs have shown that such shared care programs are effective in caring for patients with CKD and in preserving kidney function when compared with traditional nephrology-based patient care.[43]

Additional research needs to be done on the detection, management, and most important, prevention of CKD. Interventions directed at the consumer level could include measures to improve the health literacy of the population, empowering patients to be responsible for their own health, and to be actively involved in decision-making.

Basic research aimed at understanding the progressive nature of CKD and pathophysiologic processes responsible for tissue damage should be prioritized. Finally, the importance of translational research—applying discoveries generated during research in the laboratory and preclinical studies to studies in human participants with the disease and using methods aimed at enhancing the adoption of best practices in the community—is now being recognized. Clinical and translational science awards initiated by the National Institutes of Health and development of public–private biomedical research partnerships with the pharmaceutical industry appear to be promising.[44] Clearly, easing the substantial social and economic burden that CKD imposes on the individual and on society will require a multifaceted strategy to manage the growing epidemic in the complex population that comprises those with CKD.

Risk factor reduction is likely to have the most significant impact on preventing CKD in the population. Diabetes and hypertension account for a significant majority of US cases of ESKD and likely also account for most cases of earlier stages of CKD.[2] As both of these conditions may result from obesity and physical inactivity, interventions to reduce these upstream factors would also likely have benefits for reducing CKD. Population-based efforts targeting early detection of diabetes and hypertension and improved control of blood glucose and blood pressure also would benefit kidney organ damage from these conditions.

DISCUSSION QUESTIONS

1. You are asked to advise on the best allocation of resources to alleviate complications from chronic kidney disease. What factors must be considered when deciding between allocating more resources for treating patients on chronic dialysis versus those at high risk of progression from CKD to ESKD?
2. The best treatment for ESKD currently available is kidney transplantation. The availability of transplantation, however, is limited by the lack of organ donors. This is especially true in racial minorities. Why do you think this is, and what could be done to increase organ donation?
3. What factors do you think explain the apparent discrepancies between the prevalence of CKD (slightly higher in women than men) and the prevalence of ESKD (significantly higher in men than women)?
4. What factors do you think explain the decreasing incidence of ESKD and the increasing prevalence of ESKD?

REFERENCES

1. Kidney Disease: Improving Global Outcomes (KDIGO). KDIGO 2012 clinical practice guideline for the evaluation and management of chronic kidney disease. *Kidney Int Suppl.* 2013;3(1):1–150.
2. US Renal Data System. *2021 USRDS Annual Data Report: Epidemiology of Kidney Disease in the United States*. Bethesda, MD: National Institutes of Health, National Institute of Diabetes and Digestive and Kidney Diseases; 2021.
3. Lentine KL, Mannon RB. The Advancing American Kidney Health (AAKH) executive order: promise and caveats for expanding access to kidney transplantation. *Kidney360.* 2020;1(6): 557–560.
4. Centers for Disease Control and Prevention. Chronic Kidney Disease (CKD) Surveillance System. Updated September 10, 2021. Available at: https://nccd.cdc.gov/CKD. Accessed February 1, 2023.

5. Chu CD, McCulloch CE, Banerjee T, et al. CKD Awareness among US adults by future risk of kidney failure. *Am J Kidney Dis.* 2020;76(2):174–183.
6. Foley RN, Parfrey PS, Sarnak MJ. Clinical epidemiology of cardiovascular disease in chronic renal disease. *Am J Kidney Dis.* 1998;32(5 suppl 3):S112–S119.
7. Chronic Kidney Disease Prognosis Consortium et al. Association of estimated glomerular filtration rate and albuminuria with all-cause and cardiovascular mortality in general population cohorts: a collaborative meta-analysis. *Lancet.* 2010;375:2073–2081.
8. Fox CS, Matsushita K, Woodward M, et al. Associations of kidney disease measures with mortality and end-stage renal disease in individuals with and without diabetes: a meta-analysis. *Lancet.* 2012;380(9854):1662–1673.
9. Grams ME, Sang Y, Ballew SH, et al. A meta-analysis of the association of estimated GFR, albuminuria, age, race, and sex with acute kidney injury. *Am J Kidney Dis.* 2015;66(4): 591–601.
10. Inker LA, Coresh J, Levey AS, Tonelli M, Muntner P. Estimated GFR, albuminuria, and complications of chronic kidney disease. *J Am Soc Nephrol.* 2011;22:2322–2331.
11. Kliger AS, Foley RN, Goldfarb DS, et al. KDOQI US commentary on the 2012 KDIGO Clinical Practice Guideline for Anemia in CKD. *Am J Kidney Dis.* 2013;62(5):849–859.
12. Uhlig K, Berns JS, Kestenbaum B, et al. KDOQI US commentary on the 2009 KDIGO Clinical Practice Guideline for the Diagnosis, Evaluation, and Treatment of CKD–Mineral and Bone Disorder (CKD-MBD). *Am J Kidney Dis.* 2010;55(5):773–799.
13. Martins D, Agodoa L, Norris K. Chronic kidney disease in disadvantaged populations. *Int J Nephrol.* 2012;2012:1–6.
14. Vart P, Powe NR, McCulloch CE, et al. National trends in the prevalence of chronic kidney disease among racial/ethnic and socioeconomic status groups, 1988-2016. *JAMA Netw Open.* 2020;3(7):e207932.
15. Peralta CA, Ziv E, Katz R, et al. African ancestry, socioeconomic status, and kidney function in elderly African Americans: a genetic admixture analysis. *J Am Soc Nephrol.* 2006;17(12): 3491–3496.
16. Friedman DJ, Kozlitina J, Genovese G, Jog P, Pollak MR. Population-based risk assessment of APOL1 on renal disease. *J Am Soc Nephrol.* 2011;22:2098–2105.
17. Friedman DJ, Pollak MR. APOL1 nephropathy: from genetics to clinical applications. *Clin J Am Soc Nephrol.* 2021;16:294–303.
18. Grams ME, Rebholz CM, Chen Y, et al. Race, APOL1 risk, and eGFR decline in the general population. *J Am Soc Nephrol.* 2016;27(9):2842–2850.
19. Akrawi DS, PirouziFard MN, Fjellstedt E, et al. Heritability of end-stage renal disease: a Swedish adoption study. *Nephrology.* 2018;138(2):157–165.
20. Zhang J, Thio CHL, Gansevoort RT, Snieder H. Familial aggregation of CKD and heritability of kidney biomarkers in the general population: the Lifelines Cohort Study. *Am J Kidney Dis.* 2021;77:869–878.
21. Melamed ML, Raphael KL. Metabolic acidosis in CKD: a review of recent findings. *Kidney Med.* 2021;3:267–277.
22. Raphael KL, Carroll DJ, Murray J, Greene T, Beddhu S. Urine ammonium predicts clinical outcomes in hypertensive kidney disease. *J Am Soc Nephrol.* 2017;28:2483–2490.

23. Orth SR. Smoking in chronic kidney disease. In: Turner NN, et al., eds. *Oxford Textbook of Clinical Nephrology: Three-Volume Pack*. 4th ed. Oxford, UK; Oxford Academic; 2015. doi:10.1093/med/9780199592548.003.0103
24. Chang AR, Grams ME, Ballew SH, et al. Adiposity and risk of decline in glomerular filtration rate: meta-analysis of individual participant data in a global consortium. *BMJ*. 2019;10(364): k5301. doi:10.1136/bmj.k5301
25. Susantitaphong P, Cruz DN, Cerda, J, et al. World incidence of AKI: a meta-analysis. *Clin J Am Soc Nephrol*. 2013;8(9):1482–1493.
26. Shah A, Fried LF, Chen SC, et al. Associations between access to care and awareness of CKD. *Am J Kidney Dis*. 2012;59(3 suppl 2):S16–S23.
27. Seaborg E. US Preventive Services Task Force will consider CKD screening recommendation. *KidneyNews Online*. 2022;14(4):1–8. Available at: https://www.kidneynews.org/view/journals/kidney-news/14/4/article-p1_1.xml. Accessed February 1, 2023.
28. Vassalotti JA, Li S, McCullough PA, Bakris GL. Kidney early evaluation program: a community-based screening approach to address disparities in chronic kidney disease. *Semin Nephrol*. 2019;30:66–73.
29. Delgado C et al. A unifying approach for GFR estimation: recommendations of the NKF-ASN Task Force on Reassessing the Inclusion of Race in Diagnosing Kidney Disease. *Am J Kidney Dis*. 2022;79(2):268–288.e1.
30. Inker LA, Eneanya, ND, Coresh J, et al. New creatinine- and cystatin C-based equations to estimate GFR without race. *N Engl J Med*. 2021;385(19):1737–1749.
31. Patel UD., Young EW, Ojo AO, Hayward RA. CKD progression and mortality among older patients with diabetes. *Am J Kidney Dis*. 2005;46:406–414.
32. Intensive blood-glucose control with sulphonylureas or insulin compared with conventional treatment and risk of complications in patients with type 2 diabetes (UKPDS 33). *Lancet*. 1998;352(9131):837–853.
33. Neuen BL, Young T, Heerspink HJL, et al. SGLT2 inhibitors for the prevention of kidney failure in patients with type 2 diabetes: a systematic review and meta-analysis. *Lancet Diabetes Endocrinol*. 2019;7(11):845–854.
34. de Zeeuw D, Remuzzi G, Parving HH, et al. Proteinuria, a target for renoprotection in patients with type 2 diabetic nephropathy: lessons from RENAAL. *Kidney Int*. 2004;65(6): 2309–2320.
35. Ibsen H, Olsen MH, Wachtell K, et al. Reduction in albuminuria translates to reduction in cardiovascular events in hypertensive patients: losartan intervention for endpoint reduction in hypertension study. *Hypertension*. 2005;45:198–202.
36. ONTARGET Investigators Yusuf S, Teo KK, Pague J, et al. Telmisartan, ramipril, or both in patients at high risk for vascular events. *N Engl J Med*. 2008;358(15):1547–1559.
37. Bakris GL, Agarwal R, Anker SD, et al. Effect of finerenone on chronic kidney disease outcomes in type 2 diabetes. *The N Engl J Med*. 2020;383(23):2219–2229.
38. de Brito-Ashurst I, Varagunam M, Raftery MJ, Yaqoob MM. Bicarbonate supplementation slows progression of CKD and improves nutritional status. *J Am Soc Nephrol*. 2009;20:2075–2084.
39. Upadhyay A, Earley A, Lamont JL, et al. Lipid-lowering therapy in persons with chronic kidney disease: a systematic review and meta-analysis. *Ann Intern Med*. 2012;157(4):251–262.

40. Sarnak MJ, Bloom R, Munter P, et al. KDOQI US commentary on the 2013 KDIGO Clinical Practice Guideline for Lipid Management in CKD. *Am J Kidney Dis.* 2015;65(3):354–366.
41. Coyne DW. The KDOQI US commentary on KDIGO anemia guideline and quality of life. *Am J Kidney Dis.* 2014;63:540.
42. Choudhury D, Luna-Salazar C. Preventive health care in chronic kidney disease and end-stage renal disease. *Nature Clin Pract Nephrol.* 2008;4:194–206.
43. Jones C, Roderick P, Harris S, Rogerson M. An evaluation of a shared primary and secondary care nephrology service for managing patients with moderate to advanced CKD. *Am J Kidney Dis.* 2006;47:103–114.
44. Zerhouni EA. Translational research: moving discovery to practice. *Clin Pharmacol Ther.* 2007;81(1):126–128. doi:10.1038/sj.clpt.6100029

24

Chronic Oral Diseases

Greg Nycz, BS, Ingrid Glurich, PhD, Russell Dunkel, DDS, Tena Springer, MA, Megan Ryan, DMD, and Neel Shimpi, PhD, MM, BDS

LEARNING OBJECTIVES

After completing this chapter, readers should be able to

1. Describe contributory factors to development of chronic oral conditions.
2. Understand consequences to chronicity of oral diseases.
3. Characterize risk factors for developing chronic oral conditions and those populations at highest risk.
4. Understand the basics of clinical management with respect to screening, intervention, and prevention.

INTRODUCTION

Oral disease, though largely preventable, continues to reach epidemic levels in the United States and globally.[1] Moreover, a growing evidence base delineating bidirectional interaction between oral diseases and systemic conditions supports a growing urgency for trans-professional training to increase visibility of oral disease in the public health realm. Gaps identified include a need for (1) increased professional health literacy and training on oral health and (2) improved policies addressing health care access for high-risk populations. This chapter adopts a case study format that focuses specifically on increasing awareness of two highly prevalent oral diseases that have continued to rank among the top 10 global chronic health conditions for decades: dental caries and periodontal disease (ranked 1 and 8, respectively).[1]

Dental caries occur when integrity of the protective enamel of the teeth is compromised, allowing bacterial access and subsequent onset of tooth decay resolvable only by professional intervention involving removal of decayed surfaces and subsequent tooth restoration to reinstate a protective surface. Consequences of dental caries span the age spectrum.

Poor oral hygiene promotes periodontal disease development, which arises due to infectious processes that stimulate local inflammation in the gums. While preventable in early stages with improved oral hygiene and removal of plaque by dental professionals, untreated periodontal disease advances and establishes chronicity, requiring clinical interventions for management. Periodontal disease prevalence increases with age.

The 2022 National Institutes of Health report *Oral Health in America*[2] reviewed progress made in the intervening years since publication of Surgeon General Satcher's report that first drew attention to the status of oral disease in America in 2000, proclaiming it the "silent epidemic" and delineating factors contributing to its persistence.[3] Healthy People 2030 developed objectives to advance oral health in response to identified areas requiring improvement.[4] Further, the guiding principles and objectives outlined by the World Health Organization (WHO) in 2021 for advancing oral health on a global scale through 2030 offer a strategic plan for addressing the persisting prevalence of these conditions and reducing collateral impact of oral disease on global health.[5]

CHRONIC ORAL DISEASES

The focus of this chapter is two of the most common chronic oral conditions: dental caries and periodontal diseases, and begins with a detailed description of each condition.

Dental Caries

Dental caries, or tooth decay, is defined as the localized destruction of susceptible dental hard tissues caused by acidic by-products from bacterial fermentation of dietary carbohydrates.[6] Although one of the most preventable oral conditions, untreated tooth decay of permanent and deciduous (primary) teeth has consistently been ranked among the most prevalent health conditions worldwide,[1] attributable in part to inadequate dental care access. Thus, dental caries prevention persists as a high-priority public health gap at a global scale. Dental caries is a multifactorial disease that affects 97% of the population across their life span and affects all age groups from birth through end of life.

Microbiological shifts in the mouth, salivary composition and flow, diet, and oral hygiene practices affect the balance between tooth demineralization and remineralization. Caries development results when healthy balances in the oral cavity are disrupted.

Early childhood cariogenesis is characterized by the presence of one or more decayed, missing, or restored teeth present in a child less than five years of age. Early childhood cariogenesis ranks as the most prevalent childhood disease[1] and arises mainly by transfer of cariogenic bacteria from mother to child after birth. Early childhood caries is a global concern because it affects deciduous dentition in infants and toddlers while also predisposing to risk for future cariogenesis in permanent dentition and, potentially, loss of teeth due to untreated dental caries as the child ages. Initially, white spot appearance along the gum margin of upper primary incisors heralds early decay onset and, if untreated, transitions to cavities, resulting in complete loss of the tooth crown.

Longitudinally over time, prevalence of dental caries among adults aged 20 through 64 has decreased slightly from 92% between 1999 through 2004 to 90% during 2011 through 2016.[7] As dental knowledge and treatment options have improved, along with increased life expectancy, a larger percentage of the population is maintaining their dentition later in life. This has led to increases in gingival recession and the presence of dental root caries, caused by decay at the root of the tooth. Increased gingival recession and declining physical and mental health that may decrease ability to conduct good oral hygiene over time converge to increase risk for root caries in aging populations.

Periodontal Diseases

Periodontal disease presents in multiple forms and thus represents a range of conditions, including aggressive, chronic, necrotizing, and juvenile onset (associated with genetic predisposition) and may arise from underlying systemic conditions (e.g., type 2 diabetes mellitus).[2] The condition is caused by a broad range of periodontal pathogens often producing disease through symbiotic relationships with other oral organisms. Periodontal pathogens are generally anaerobes or facultative anaerobes that lay down plaque biofilm as a protective barrier to create a reduced oxygen environment while protecting themselves from the host's immune attacks.

Periodontal disease arises as a result of infection and inflammation of structural tissue supporting the teeth, including the gums (gingival tissue), periodontal ligament, and bone. Gingivitis is a localized self-limited inflammation of the gums and may present with bleeding in response to slight mechanical trauma such as brushing teeth. Gingivitis, a precursor of periodontal disease, can be found in up to 90% of the population and is reversible with improved oral hygiene. However, without cleaning of the tooth surface by dental professionals and thorough daily oral hygiene, the condition can progress to periodontal disease, which may develop chronicity. Periodontal disease evolves as a result of escalation of inflammatory processes affecting the gums, driven by chronic infectious processes established by pathogenic microbes. These periodontal pathogens establish themselves by colonizing gingival tissue below the gum line along the tooth surface. Here, they produce protective layers of plaque, rendering them impervious to the body's defense mechanisms. If untreated, ever-deepening pockets form, separating the gums from the tooth surface, while also undermining the tooth's structural support. Ineffectual immune responses further escalate inflammation that promotes destruction of the periodontal ligament, ultimately resulting in bone destruction and tooth loss.

Notably, curtailment of periodontal disease parallels prophylactic approaches already outlined for caries prevention: proper oral hygiene and access to regular professional oral health maintenance as recommended by dental professionals based on assessment of gingival health. Most commonly, periodontal disease develops during adulthood and,

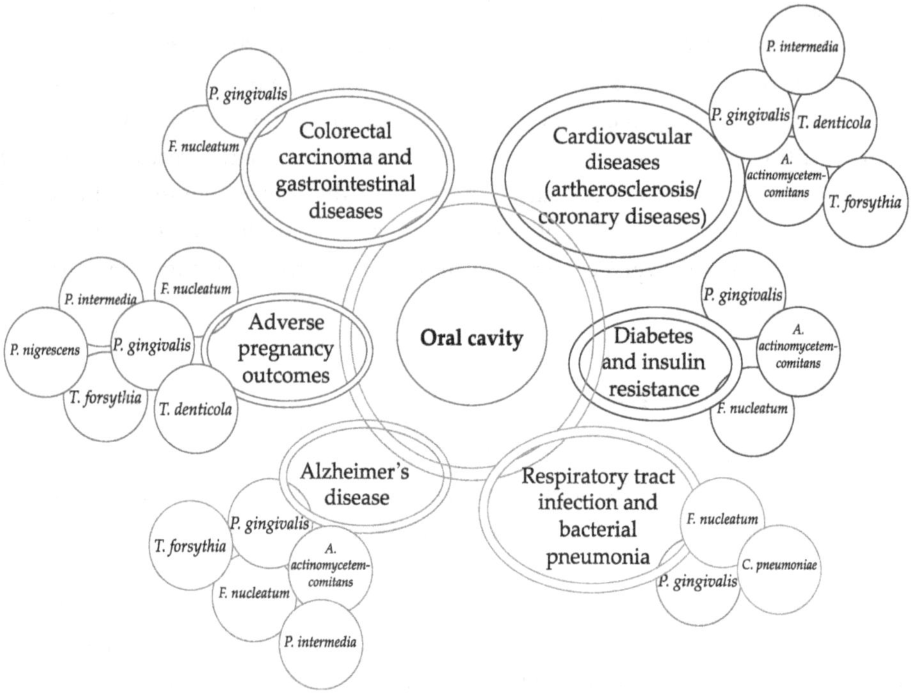

Note: Systemic inflammation promotes exacerbation of oral and systemic diseases.

Figure 24-1. Overview of Evidence-Based Support for Disease Association Between Oral Pathogens Associated With Periodontal Disease and Other Systemic Chronic Conditions

like dental caries, is highly associated with social determinants of health (SDOH), considered later in the chapter.

A substantive evidence base identifies inflammation as the common denominator driving association between periodontal disease and other chronic systemic diseases as shown in Figure 24-1.[8] Chronic infectious processes associated with periodontal disease escalate the cumulative systemic inflammatory burden, thereby sustaining or intensifying severity of oral and systemic diseases driven by inflammation. Since periodontal disease is also a highly preventable condition that has achieved epidemic status in the United States and other countries worldwide, containment of periodontal disease needs to be prioritized as a public health and policy focus.

Despite the oral-systemic connections, medical practitioners are not trained to evaluate periodontal disease severity when examining the oral cavity. In a recent study, less than 25% of primary care providers surveyed reported confidence in their ability to evaluate oral health status, and dental referrals were reported by only 32%.[9]

The need for improved interdisciplinary education and collaboration between medicine and dentistry to acknowledge and treat all diseases (both oral and systemic) with standardized assessment approaches is illustrated by the following scenario. Whereas a diabetic ulcer on the foot with a wound surface area measuring 3 to 4 cm^2 would be concerning and deserving of attention to a medical provider, the size of the wound associated with active inflammatory processes in the gums of the same patient with co-morbid chronic periodontal disease may achieve a surface area between 10 to 20 cm^2 depending on periodontal disease severity.[10] Notably, the periodontal wound is largely overlooked by medical providers, frequently with no triage to dental care offered to the patient. Moreover, both lesions would escalate systemic inflammation and further stimulate the host immune/inflammatory responses, driving other chronic conditions, as shown in Figure 24-1.

PUBLIC HEALTH IMPACT

Reducing prevalence of dental caries and periodontal disease represents a challenge that requires more prioritization by the public health and policy sectors because of high potential for achieving significant improvement in population health. For example, demonstration of significant reduction in caries risk among populations following exposure to fluoridated water has been a major success story for the dental public health arena.[6] Notably, access to care disparities, SDOH and socioeconomic risk factors have been recognized as key drivers of high caries prevalence across the global population. The siloed nature of medical and dental health care delivery, dating back to 1840 with the establishment of the first dental college,[11] has also contributed significantly to oral health disparities. The separation of oral care from that of the rest of the body has led to variability in clinical care delivery, including disparate designs in health records, with dental records capturing treatment versus diagnostic codes tracked in medicine. Dental payer structures also evolved autonomously, with dental coverage remaining a largely optional benefit.

Whereas dental cariogenesis is a multifactorial condition, it is largely preventable with the implementation of evidence-based approaches, including water fluoridation, timely application of varnishes or silver diamine fluoride to high-risk teeth, placement of sealants on permanent teeth of children and adolescents upon eruption, and emphasis on increasing oral health literacy of the population. Provision of appropriate equitable access to dental care for all segments of the population for preventive maintenance remains an unmet health priority. Concerted efforts are needed to improve oral health literacy to highlight the importance and benefits of sustained oral hygiene practices and regular access to preventive care during early childhood, beginning at one year of age, and throughout the lifespan for the entire global population.

From the public health perspective, Figure 24-2a highlights key person-level and health-related factors that must be strategically addressed, especially in the context of provision of care access for vulnerable populations, in order to mitigate negative downstream consequences, stem the tide of the current epidemic magnitude of both

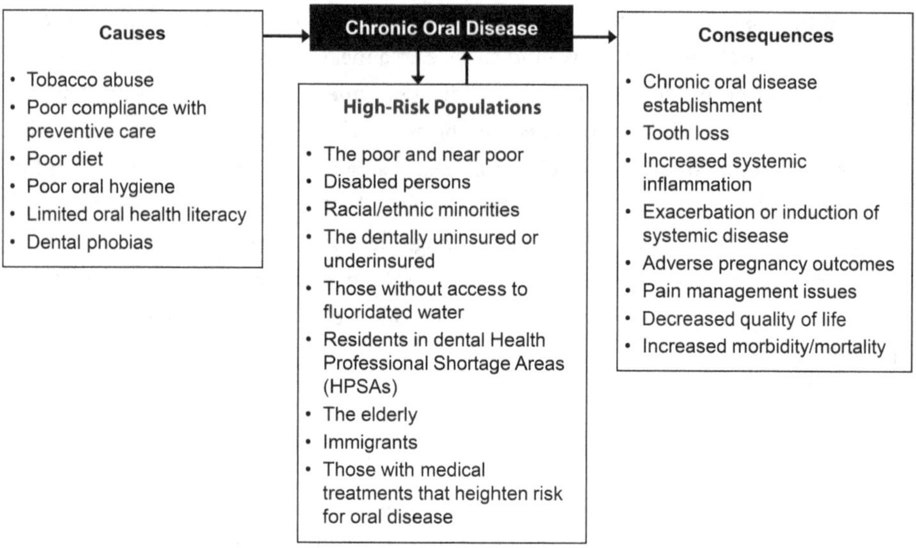

Figure 24-2a. Chronic Oral Diseases: Causes, Consequences, and High-Risk Populations

periodontal disease and dental caries, and alleviate current inequities observable in oral health outcomes in at-risk populations. Figure 24-2b further breaks down the impact of policy-based contributory factors and delineates the aggregate economic impact of oral diseases on a community cumulatively contributed by relevant risk factors listed in Figures 24-2a and 24-2b.

Collectively, failure to address these gaps in population health delivery continues to deprive segments of the population of appropriate access to care and drives up the cost of care. From a population-based perspective, increased focus on prevention versus treatment of established disease is needed for more cost-effective care delivery. Moreover, lack of appropriate and timely intervention that leads to disease onset and establishment of chronicity is associated with huge reductions in quality of life that come at a high societal cost.

Population health initiatives targeting improvement in access equity include expansion of the community health center dental infrastructure and creation of other dental safety net programs that have enabled more Medicaid beneficiaries and those living in, or near, poverty to gain access to subsidized oral health care. Operationalized by direct grants from Congress and states to support community health centers, the allocated funds provide subsidized access to millions of low-income Americans. Congress has allocated funding to community health centers, while the government's executive branch has issued expansion grants targeted to expand dental access infrastructure. Given the epidemic scope of oral disease, support to community health centers and safety net operations currently remains insufficient to stem the tide.

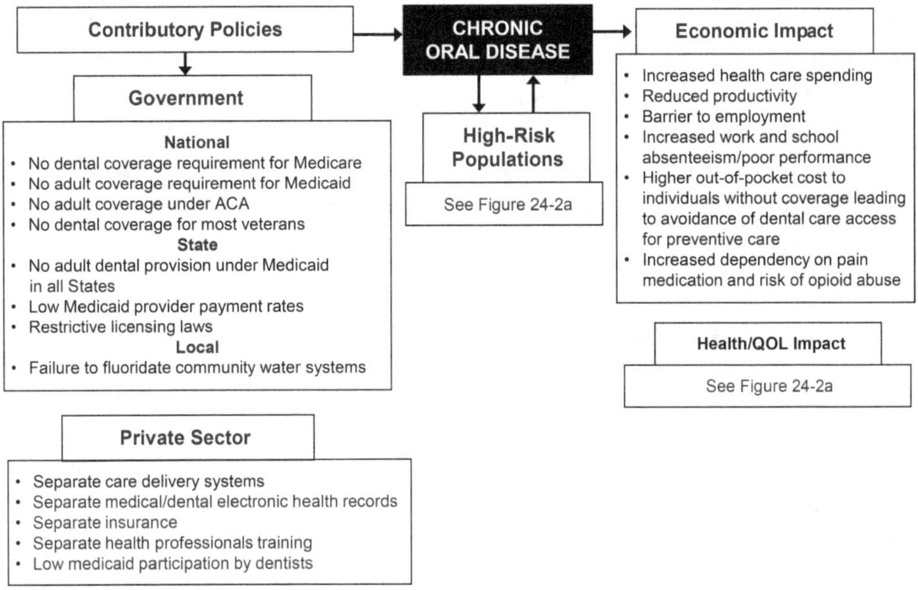

Note: ACA = Affordable Care Act (2010); QOL = quality of life.

Figure 24-2b. Upstream Contributory Policies and Economic/Health-Related Impact Relevant to Caries and Periodontal Disease

DESCRIPTIVE EPIDEMIOLOGY

Whereas dental caries and periodontal disease represent distinct oral diseases, shared risk factors continue to drive global prevalence of the two conditions. However, epidemiological aspects of periodontal disease and dental caries are distinct.

Dental Caries

Epidemiology

Computations by the Global Burden of Disease (GBD) 2019 ranked untreated dental caries as the most prevalent health condition in the world for both pediatric and adult populations, with age-adjusted estimates for prevalence exceeding 30%.[1] In adults, prevalence of untreated dental caries in permanent teeth was estimated at 2.0 billion (95% CI, 1.8–2.3 billion), translating to an age-standardized prevalence rate of 25,626 (95% CI, 22,281–29,372) per 100,000 person years.[1] The study further reported an "untreated caries rate in deciduous teeth" prevalence rate of 0.5 billion (95% CI, 0.4–1.6), with an age-standardized prevalence of 7,673 (95% CI, 6,113–9,340) for children aged 0 to 14 years, similarly placing this as the top-ranked condition across the countries and territories worldwide represented in the 2019 GBD super-region.[1] Between 1990 and 2019, global prevalence of untreated dental caries in permanent teeth and deciduous teeth decreased only marginally by 3.6% (95% CI, 2.6%–4.5%) and 3.0% (95% CI, 1.3%–4.9%), respectively. Despite a slight decrease in prevalence, the number of cases of dental caries in permanent teeth increased approximately 46% between 1990 and 2019, attributable to a 49% increase in population growth, while accounting for shifts in age structure over time. The same pattern, again attributable to population growth, was noted among caries rates in deciduous teeth.[1]

Geographic Distribution

Based on data collected between 2000 and 2016 by WHO, the median of diseased, missing, filled, teeth (DMFT) scores used to measure severity of dental caries lesions were nearly twice as high in middle- to low-income countries compared to high-income countries (DMFT scores of 3.9 and 4.1, vs. 2.0, respectively).[12] On a global scale, Wen et al.[1] also calculated a measure of the burden of untreated dental caries in permanent and deciduous dentition attributable to sociodemographic inequities. Their study reported 64.6 million (95% CI, 64.4–64.9 million) and 62.9 million (95% CI, 62.8–63.1 million) individuals with age-standardized untreated caries cases in permanent and deciduous teeth, respectively. Lack of treatment was associated with inequities attributable to sociodemographic variables. Moreover, sociodemographic inequities contributed to 3.2% and 12.1% dental caries prevalence in permanent and deciduous teeth, respectively.[1] Untreated caries in permanent teeth data for United States by state (2019) are summarized in Figure 24-3.[13]

Time Trends

Patterns in untreated caries rates over time in the United States between 1988 through 2018 broken out by race, ethnicity, and poverty level are shown in Figure 24-4.[14]

High-Risk Populations and Health Disparities

Notably, caries rates differ by gender, race/ethnicity, and poverty status across the age spectrum. In the United States, substantially higher rates of untreated caries are noted among Black, Asian, and Hispanic populations, and among populations in poverty compared with White, non-Hispanic populations or those with greater income.[14]

These populations are also disproportionately affected by other environmental factors, including residency in low-income housing often located in neighborhoods that are food deserts, resulting in exposure to unhealthy diets that contribute to unhealthy gums and teeth, especially when high in sugar content. Often, these populations lack affordable insurance and cannot afford dental care, and the Affordable Care Act did not mandate

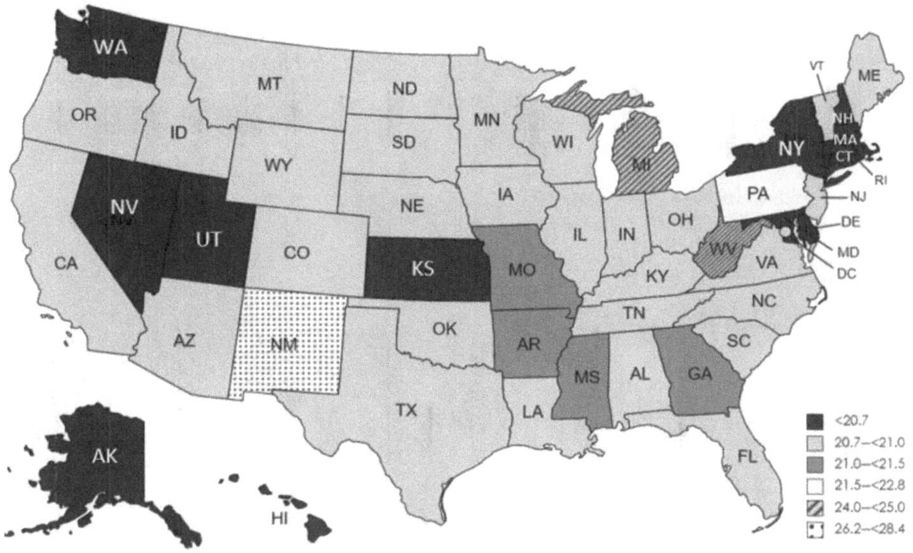

Source: Based on IHME.[13]

Note: DALY = disability-adjusted life years. Rates are for both sexes.

Figure 24-3. Age-Standardized DALY Rates per 100,000 of Caries in Permanent Teeth: United States, 2019

providing adult dental coverage. Whereas Medicaid does provide coverage for children, federal mandates for adult coverage under Medicaid are optional and determined independently at the state level. Moreover, because of traditionally poor reimbursement policies for Medicaid, many dentists do not participate and many more limit the number of Medicaid beneficiaries they will see in their practice.

In the United States and globally, SDOH have been identified as a major risk factor for oral health, including dental caries.[2] SDOH include low income, low level of education, marginalized and institutionalized populations, and special populations such as disabled people, and veterans who are ineligible to receive dental benefits from the United States Department of Veteran Affairs and lack access to care.

During years when individuals are employed, dental insurance coverage availability varies by employer. Private dental insurance can be costly, provides limited coverage annually, and is accepted selectively by some providers. This variability is especially true for younger adults in startup or lower-income jobs. While they may not meet poverty-level definitions, their income level precludes purchase of commercial insurance if not provided by their employer. By age 65, the number of adults with dental insurance coverage declines because these benefits are not provided through Medicare or other national initiatives. In addition, with increasing age, challenges with transportation or access to care arise when risk for institutionalization grows.

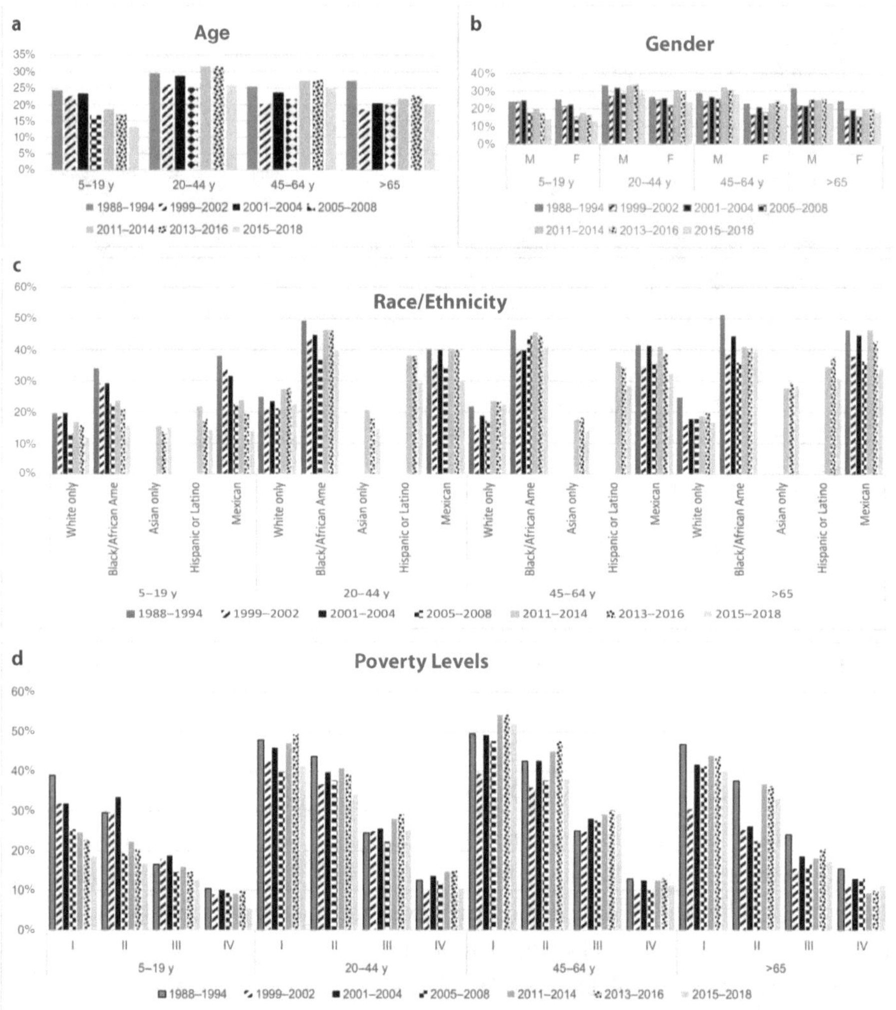

Note: level I = <100%; level II = 100%-199%; level III 200%-399%; level IV = ≥400%.

Figure 24-4. Longitudinal Patterns of Untreated Dental Caries by (a) Age, (b) Gender, (c) Race/Ethnicity, and (d) Poverty Levels: United States, 1988–2018

Periodontal Disease

Descriptive Epidemiology

Having achieved epidemic proportions, periodontal disease affected over a billion people worldwide by 2019.[1] Periodontal disease was globally ranked eighth among the top 10 level 4 conditions by the GBD in 2019 (Table 24-1).

Higher rank was achieved for periodontal disease at the extremes of countries stratified by sociodemographic indices (SDI) such that countries with the highest SDI

Table 24-1. Ranking of Periodontal Diseases and Dental Caries Among the Top 10 Global Burden of Disease Level 4 Diseases, 2019

	Dental Caries	Periodontal Disease
Total Cases (95% CI)	2,030,763,252 (1,767,921,269–2,325,620,589)	1,087,367,744 (827,508,090–1,356,867,505)
Global Rank	1	8
Countries scoring low SDI	1	6
Countries scoring mid SDI	2	8
Countries scoring high SDI	2	5

Source: Based on Wen et al.[1]

Note: CI = confidence interval; GBD = global burden of disease, level 4 diseases ranking scale; SDI = sociodemographic index. Two oral diseases, periodontal diseases (global rank 8), and dental caries in permanent teeth (global rank 1) were ranked among the top 10 GBD level 4 conditions in 2019. Notably, for the United States, which is classified among countries with a high SDI, periodontal diseases was ranked 5th among the top 10 conditions and 2nd for dental caries prevalence.

(periodontal disease rank 5) and lowest SDI (periodontal disease rank 6) achieved notably higher rankings than the global ranking (periodontal disease rank 8).

A study by the GBD collaborators[15] examined changes in ranking among the top 25 leading conditions and disability-adjusted life years (DALY) by age groups from 1990 to 2019. During that temporal window, periodontal disease advanced in ranking to the top 25 leading condition with advancing age across all three age ranges (Table 24-2). These data indicate an increase in the burden of oral disease globally.

Geographic Distribution

State-level rates of periodontal disease in adults aged 30 to 79 based on National Health and Nutrition Examination Survey (NHANES) data from 2009 to 2012 are shown in Figure 24-5.[16] Rates by state range from 33.7% to 68%.[16]

Estimated rates of all levels of periodontal disease (mild, moderate, severe), and severe periodontal disease only in the same demographic cohort range from 37.7% to 52.8% and 6.4% to 11.3%, respectively.[16] Among US states, 36% are associated with notably high prevalence rates, with southern states most strongly affected. States with highest prevalence include New Mexico, Texas, Louisiana, South Carolina, Florida, Mississippi, and Hawaii; followed by California, Nevada, Arizona, Alabama, Arkansas, Oklahoma, Tennessee, Georgia, South Carolina, North Carolina, and New York.[16]

Time Trends

Trends in periodontal disease prevalence over time are more challenging to interpret for several reasons.[17] First, the main source of surveillance data is derived from NHANES,

Table 24-2. Percent Change in Disability-Adjusted Life Years Rate, 1990–2019

Periodontal Disease Rank	Age Range, y		
	25–49	50–74	>75
1990 rank	32	28	23
2019 rank	25	24	22
Percentage of Change (95% CI) in DALY Rate			
1990–2019[a]	70.7% (66.4%–74.1%)	90.5% (86.0%–94.7%)	112.0% (106.4%–117.6%)
1990–2019[b]	2.8 (0.5% to 5.1%)	−7.4% (−9.6% to −5.1%)	−10.9% (−12.9% to −8.8%)

Source: Based on Abbafati et al.[15]

Note: CI = confidence interval; DALY = disability-adjusted life years. Conditions ranking among the top 25 leading conditions and disability-adjusted life years (DALY) by age groups from 1990–2019 include periodontal disease across all age groups.

[a]Rate is unadjusted.

[b]Rate is age-adjusted.

which began collecting and measuring data in 1960 and continues to measure trends over a four-year window. However, in an effort to improve survey validity, the survey has been modified over time. Second, periodontal assessment protocols have evolved over time, with changes including partial mouth evaluation of several quadrants or full mouth evaluation and new protocols for assessing periodontal pocket depth and clinical attachment loss at two or three sites. Notably, accuracy of the measures varied with the protocol applied.[17] Over time, changes in clinical definitions of periodontal disease have continued to evolve, including the definition of assessment criteria and periodontal measures.[18] As such, definitions of prevalence across time are not readily comparable.

Most recent data on periodontal disease prevalence that are broken out by race/ethnicity, age, gender, economic status, educational levels, insurance status, and affiliation with marginalized or special-needs populations reflect oral health disparities attributable to SDOH that are reminiscent of longitudinal trends found for dental caries. Despite evolution of the assessment criteria over time, statistically significant differences in the rate of periodontal disease prevalence trends over time were noted.[19]

Patterns noted are exemplified by those collected from the NHANES survey cohort for the cross-sectional time interval from 2009 to 2014, and are shown for race/ethnicity, sex, and age range in Table 24-3.[19] In this report,[19] the highest prevalence for periodontal disease was noted among Black non-Hispanic populations, Mexican Americans, other Hispanic ethnicities, and other races (Asian, Native American, and multiracial) compared with White, non-Hispanic populations. Higher prevalence rates also continue to be noted in males and individuals of older age (≥65 years).

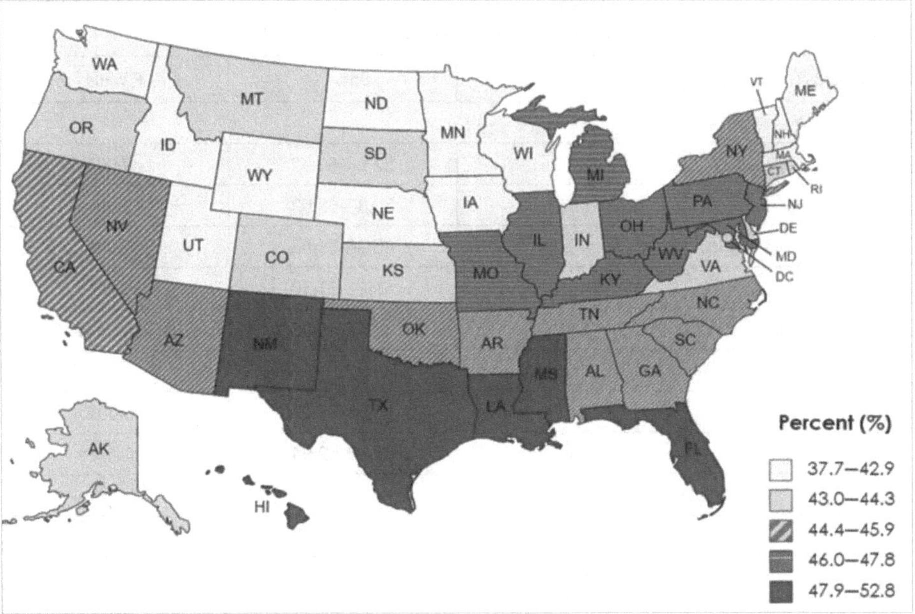

Source: Based on Eke et al.[16]

Figure 24-5. Prevalence of Periodontal Disease (All Levels) by State: United States, 2009-2012

Notably, a recent systematic review reported a positive effect associated with acculturation of ethnic minority and immigrant populations relative to a decrease in rates of periodontal disease and other oral health outcomes, oral health behaviors, and dental health literacy.[20] These pivotal findings point to several low-cost strategies that merit further exploration in stemming the epidemic tide achieved by preventable oral health disease.

CAUSES AND EVIDENCE-BASED INTERVENTIONS FOR ORAL DISEASES

Modifiable Risk Factors

Several key variables stand out as driving factors that have fueled the perfect storm for preventable oral health diseases to reach global epidemic proportions. These include poor health literacy of both patients and providers; risk factors that are largely behavioral, involving hygiene and diet; underappreciation of the importance of oral health to overall well-being and quality of life; and societal impacts, including the SDOH, poverty, and lack of targeted investment in addressing interventional strategies at a policy level.

Moreover, as insights into oral-systemic connectivity between chronic illnesses have gradually been discerned over the past few decades, the true impact of segregating medical and dental health care delivery has become more apparent. Critical changes that

Table 24-3. Prevalence of Severe and Non-Severe Periodontal Disease by Race/Ethnicity, Sex, and Age: National Health and Nutrition Examination Survey, United States, 2009–2014

Participants (n = 10,683)	%	95% CI	P Value
Race/Ethnicity			
Black (non-Hispanic)	56.6	52.68-60.52	<0.001
Mexican American	59.7	56.37-63.03	<0.001
Other Hispanic	48.5	45.36-51.63	<0.001
Other races	46.2	41.11-51.30	<0.05
White (non-Hispanic)	37.0	33.97-40.03	Reference
Sex			
Female	34.6	31.66-37.53	<0.001
Male	50.2	47.46-52.94	Reference
Age			
≥65 y	59.8	55.68-63.92	<0.001
45–64 y	46.0	42.87-49.13	<0.001
30–44 y	29.5	26.56-32.44	NA

Source: Based on Eke et al.[19]
Note: CI = confidence interval; NA = not applicable.

could address the core challenges facing dental public health and the current health care delivery infrastructure include: innovative, transformational changes in policy; an increase in health literacy; recognition and correction of prejudicial behavior largely driven by economic factors that require restructuring of health care delivery; and innovative changes to address workforce issues. Novel, creative models to correct lack of dental care access are beginning to emerge and are achieving positive outcomes in stemming the epidemic tide of oral disease. An ever-expanding evidence base continues to reveal the importance of oral health to overall health and societal consequences associated with the persistence of epidemic oral disease. Strong leadership from a motivated oral/dental public health sector is required to increase visibility and promote positive gains in population health, leveraged by emergent transformational initiatives, more integrated health care delivery models, and policies designed to correct identified deficits in the oral/dental health domain.

Risk factors for dental caries and periodontal disease across the age spectrum are summarized in Table 24-4. Notably, many risk factors for both dental caries and periodontal disease overlap. Collectively, these factors interact symbiotically and have given rise to two of the most globally pervasive epidemic chronic health conditions despite being nearly entirely preventable. Strikingly, the content of Table 24-4 reveals that nearly all the named variables represent *modifiable* risk factors.

Table 24-4. Risk Factors for Dental Caries and Periodontal Disease by Age Group

Risk Variable	Relevant Risk Factor for Age Group, y				
	0–5	6–12	13–20	21–64	≥65
Mother with untreated dental caries colonizes infant with cariogenic bacteria	C	NA	NA	NA	NA
Exposed to drinks with high sugar content with no cleaning of gums/teeth	C	C	NA	NA	NA
Live in families with low health literacy	C	C	C	P	P
Live in households that don't seek preventive dental care	C	C	C	C; P	C; P
Do not practice or learn good oral hygiene	C	C	C	C; P	C; P
Live in dental HPSAs	C	C	C	C; P	C; P
Live in households ≤ the poverty level	C	C	C	C; P	C; P
Family lacks dental insurance	C	C	C	C; P	C; P
Seek care in practices that limit access to Medicaid/Medicare populations	C	C	C	C; P	C; P
Encounter racial, ethnic, or other marginalized population in clinical setting	C	C	C	C; P	C; P
Live in area with no water fluoridation	C	C	C	C	C
Poor diet/inadequate intake of nutrients	C	C	C	C; P	C; P
Live in food deserts	C	C	C	C; P	C; P
Do not receive sealant placement in a timely manner	C	C	C	C	C
Presence of untreated caries	C	C	C	C	C
Early tooth loss from untreated caries or untreated PD	C	C	C	C; P	C; P
Smoking	NA	NA	C; P	C; P	C; P
Poor mental health that affects dental health (e.g., bulimia, depression, poor self-image), promotes lack of hygiene	NA	NA	C; P	C; P	C; P
Limited education	C	C	C	C; P	C; P
Employment with no dental insurance benefit	C	C	C; P	C; P	C; P
Above poverty level but low-income wage	C	C	C; P	C; P	C; P
History of caries	C	C	C	C	C
Lack of periodicity in seeking preventive dental care	C	C	C; P	C; P	C; P
Dental fear	C	C	C; P	C; P	C; P
No coverage for adult dental care	C	C	C; P	C; P	C; P
Institutionalization	C	C	C; P	C; P	C; P
Limited access because of physical disability	C	C	C; P	C; P	C; P
History of tooth loss	C	C	C; P	C; P	C; P

(Continued)

Table 24-4. (Continued)

Risk Variable	Relevant Risk Factor for Age Group, y				
	0–5	6–12	13–20	21–64	≥65
Lack of transportation	C	C	C; P	C; P	C; P
Declining physical or mental health	C	C	C; P	C; P	C; P
Uncontrolled diabetes, hyperglycemia, obesity, or other chronic illnesses that contribute to escalation of systemic inflammation	NA	NA	P	P	P

Source: Based on Eke et al.[19]

Note: C = dental caries risk; HSPA = health professional shortage area; NA = non-applicable; P = periodontal disease risk; PD = periodontal disease.

Population-Attributable Risk

Tooth loss has emerged as a major independent risk factor for many chronic health conditions, including stroke and cardiovascular disease, and the associated risk for mortality.[21] Notably, tooth loss is also an outcome associated with advanced dental caries and severe periodontal disease. Outcomes of a study that modeled population-attributable risk of the impact of periodontal disease and bone loss on tooth loss are shown in Table 24-5.[22] In this study, stepwise regression analysis was first undertaken to define sociodemographic variables most associated with tooth loss after modeling NHANES 2011 to 2018 (n = 15,161).[22]

Clinical Care Approaches: Screening, Treatment, and Prevention in the Context of the Current Value-Based Care Delivery Model

Both dental caries and periodontal disease are infectious, transmissible diseases of bacterial origin. Prevention, screening, and early treatment are key to ensuring the best oral health outcomes for all patients. Value-based oral health care focuses on improving oral health outcomes. Integration of dental and medical services focuses on prevention of oral health issues, and maintenance of good oral health is the focus in a value-based system. There is a need to shift from reactionary treatment-oriented approaches to caries, periodontal disease, and pain management to prophylactic interventions involving education, prevention, and early intervention to improve and/or maintain population oral health. Transdisciplinary approaches to care delivery with active participation by both medical and dental professionals are required to achieve this strategic approach to coordinated care delivery. Emphasis is placed on using patient-centered, culturally appropriate, and team-based approaches to ensure coordinated care delivery.[23] This is referred to as having a "patient-centered medical/dental home."[24] Clinically homed individuals have a primary care provider that assists in coordinating care delivery for their complex health

Table 24-5. Risk Modeling Outcomes and Determination of Attributable Risk of Periodontal Disease on Tooth Loss

Risk Variable	Attributable Risk (95% CI)	P Value
Socioeconomic		
Age, y		
20–44	Reference	
45–64	4.40 (2.3-6.5)	<0.001
≥65	10.41 (8.3-12.5)	<0.001
Sex		
Male	−0.48 (0.39–0.57)	<0.001
Female	Reference	
Race/Ethnicity		
Hispanic	−1.82 (1.79–1.85)	<0.001
White (non-Hispanic)	Reference	
Black (non-Hispanic)	0.47 (0.37–0.56)	0.003
Asian (non-Hispanic)	−1.09 (1.05–1.13)	<0.001
Other race/multiracial	1.15 (1.09–1.21)	0.001
Education Level		
< High school	4.22 (4.19–4.25)	<0.001
High school graduate	1.77 (1.74–1.80)	<0.001
> High school	Reference	
Monthly Income		
≤$2099	3.03 (2.99–3.07)	<0.001
$2100–$5399	1.59 (1.55–1.63)	<0.001
$5400–$8399	0.81 (0.77–0.86)	0.007
≥$8400	Reference	
Behavioral Risk		
Current smoking status		
Yes	2.87 (2.83–2.91)	<0.001
No	Reference	
Health-Related Risks: Diabetes and Periodontal Disease		
Diabetes		
Yes	1.85 (1.82–1.89)	<0.001
No	Reference	

(Continued)

Table 24-5. (Continued)

Risk Variable	Attributable Risk (95% CI)	P Value
	Periodontal Disease Associated Risk	
History of oral bone loss		
Yes	2.28 (2.24-2.322)	<0.001
No	Reference	
History of periodontal disease		
Yes	−1.47 (1.44-1.50)	
No	Reference	<0.001

Source: Based on Lee et al.[22]

Note: CI = confidence interval. These outcomes of attributable risk model 4 were adapted using National Health and Nutrition Examination Survey data (2011-2018). Attributable risk for tooth loss of 0.34 was determined following adjustment for periodontal disease-associated variables, including history of bone loss and history of gum disease.

care needs, especially when care delivery encompasses access to disparate health care delivery domains. Descriptions of clinical approaches and practice guidelines for prevention, screening, and intervention follow.

Dental Caries

Strong emphasis is placed on prevention and timely screening to reduce the risk of caries development. Treatment of caries includes both lesional restoration and promotion of protective/preventive factors including (1) behavior modification to decrease caries risk and (2) interventional strategies such as exposure to fluoridated drinking water and timely sealant placement or treatment with varnish or diamine silver fluoride to reduce risk and promote prevention. Early intervention and education set the groundwork for future success.

Notably, adults also benefit from topically applied (e.g., fluoridated toothpaste use or varnish application) and/or systemically ingested fluoride (e.g. fluoridated water), making topical and systemic fluoride exposure important throughout the life span. This benefit also extends to adults residing in nursing homes, long-term care facilities, or other institutional settings.

Another extremely successful caries prevention strategy is the use of dental sealants. Caries incidence on chewing surfaces of posterior dentition is often higher due to anatomic grooves (pits/fissures) that trap caries-causing bacteria. Sealing these grooves with resin-based or glass ionomer sealants decreases caries incidence.[25] Sealants can also inhibit caries progression with non-cavitated lesions. Since caries risk increases as children age, application of sealants at eruption of posterior permanent dentition is key to maximizing prevention benefits. A two-year follow-up study showed that sealant-treated teeth had a threefold lower rate of caries compared with untreated teeth, and that 79% of treated teeth were unaffected by caries.[25]

Since caries is a transmissible infectious disease, caries management in pregnant women is essential. Many pregnant women are at increased risk for dental caries contributed by a variety of factors, including behavioral changes. Women with high prevalence of cariogenic bacteria will transmit these bacteria to the mouth of their infants, thereby increasing caries risk for their infants. Many barriers to dental care exist during pregnancy, including changes in insurance coverage, myths around safety of dental treatment during pregnancy, and lack of understanding of dental health changes and the need for oral health care during pregnancy. Evidence-based screening, education, and treatment of dental caries during pregnancy is essential and often facilitated by the medical team. Oral health screening, discussions around the safety of dental care, and referral to a dental provider will aid the dental team in providing the most appropriate and effective oral health care possible. Evidence-based studies have routinely demonstrated the importance of clinical and radiographic dental exams during pregnancy, along with routine dental treatment.[26] Restoration of untreated caries, use of fluoride toothpaste and appropriate antimicrobial rinses (e.g., chlorhexidine), and education are key to decreasing caries risk for pregnant women and their children.

Caries screening involves clinical and radiographic examination at appropriate intervals based on caries risk assessment and oral health history. Caries risk assessment assigns a risk level for patient caries incidence/activity over a certain time period. Since cariogenesis is multifactorial, risk assessment is also multifactorial. Evaluations encompass assessment of demographic, social, and behavioral variables, in combination with clinical and radiographic examination, ultimately assigning a caries risk level (low, moderate, or high). Various surveys and screening tools exist to support risk assessment and allow dental teams to evaluate patient risk, develop a plan to reduce caries risk, and enhance protective factors while proactively monitoring successes and failures.

With knowledge gained from risk assessment and full examination, oral/dental health care providers can develop an individualized caries management plan. A management plan is of paramount importance in eliminating caries during pregnancy to ensure the oral health of both the mother and child and reduce risk for onset of early childhood caries following childbirth. Noncavitated lesions (incipient or initial lesions) often present without clinical evidence of cavitation. These lesions may reverse or arrest with chemical or mechanical intervention such as fluoride varnish, sealants, or silver diamine fluoride application. Silver diamine fluoride is typically used as a desensitizing agent but has increasingly been found to successfully arrest caries progression. Application of silver diamine fluoride is particularly useful in young children, special-needs patients who may not tolerate traditional dental treatments, and elderly patients experiencing an increased prevalence of root caries.

A cavitated lesion shows a disruption in the integrity of the tooth surface, and thus treatment options should be evaluated. Treatment options should include analysis of traditional restorative treatments, such as amalgam or composite restorations, along with nonsurgical treatment such as silver diamine fluoride application or use of glass ionomer cements. Restorations should restore form and function of dentition as well as allow for plaque control and management of caries risk moving forward.

Dental Root Caries

Risk assessments will provide assistance in determining prevention and treatment needs related to root caries. Prevention of root caries focuses on home care, dietary control, and fluoride and chlorhexidine use. Treatment options again include traditional restorations such as amalgam and composite. More recent approaches include atraumatic restorative treatment, which involves less invasive caries removal, such as with hand instruments, followed by silver diamine fluoride application and/or use of fluoride-releasing restorative materials such as resin-modified glass ionomers.

Periodontal Disease

Since the development of the Armitage 1999 periodontal classification,[18] national and global efforts have been directed to improve case definition. In 2018 the Armitage 1999 classification was further revised by the global joint efforts of the European Federation of Periodontology and the American Academy of Periodontology[18] as follows:

- Stage 0: Gingivitis
- Stage I: Initial
- Stage II: Moderate
- Stage III: Severe with potential for additional tooth loss
- Stage IV: Severe with significant potential for additional loss of dentition

The development of these new periodontal classification systems has improved the ability to identify the disease based on severity and complexity of management, thereby improving the grading that rates the risk of disease progression.

The evaluation and diagnosis assigned to each case type is based on the use of multiple clinical criteria, including: measurement of clinical attachment loss, periodontal probing (six measures per tooth), testing for bleeding on probing, checking for tooth mobility, and assessment of intraoral radiographs for bone loss. The approach to periodontal disease treatment and dental caries case management is reminiscent of medical diagnosis and treatment in assessing an individual patient's oral issues in the context of the patient's unique conditions. Patients presenting with minimal disease and risk generally have their treatment completed within a limited number of appointments and a routine or standardized post-treatment recall system. However, those individuals with more complex and extensive oral disease (such as rampant dental decay or moderate-to-severe periodontal disease) require more complex treatment planning and a customized system of recalls or post-case management protocols. Thus, treatment planning and postoperative assessment are tailored to each individual patient.

Periodontal disease treatment is focused on controlling bacterial plaque and eliminating or altering risk factors. The host response plays an essential role in periodontal disease pathogenesis and success of periodontal treatment. Periodontal disease emergence is facilitated by both patient-specific risk factors and inadequate oral hygiene. Contributory risk factors include modifiable variables, such as smoking, poor oral hygiene, poor diet, and certain non-modifiable risk factors, including age or underlying genetic predisposition.

Nonsurgical treatment is the first step in periodontal treatment and is customized to meet the unique needs of the individual. Treatment is initiated with a professional dental cleaning and patient education on oral hygiene self-care. The professional cleaning reduces bacterial risk factors that influence host response. Self-care is vital to controlling the bacterial challenge and sustaining oral health improvements. Modifiable risk factors are addressed to minimize their impact on oral health status. Follow-up periodontal maintenance appointments are necessary to monitor the periodontal status and prevent recurrence. Periodontal treatment is successful when disease progression is arrested and recurrence is prevented. If nonsurgical treatment does not achieve optimal periodontal health, surgical treatment may be recommended. When access to care is limited, the patient's ability to comply with the follow-up appointments may result in periodontal disease recurrence and, potentially, loss of teeth. Upstream factors shown in Table 24-3 that influence clinical outcomes may leverage negative outcomes by disrupting treatment processes and patient compliance. Limited or nonexistent insurance benefits for periodontal treatment are risk factors for increasing disease severity and eventual tooth loss as a clinical outcome. As with most chronic conditions where early detection and treatment improves likelihood of better outcomes, continued disease management is essential to sustain oral health and stabilize the disease state. The global success or failure of each individual patient's clinical outcomes depends on a multitude of factors, as summarized in Figure 24-6.

MOVING FORWARD

Considering the highly preventable nature of caries and periodontal disease in juxtaposition to the epidemic status of these conditions, reexamination of inadequacies in current care delivery models and public health policies relative to oral health care delivery is central to scaling improvement of population health in the oral health arena. Moreover, in the presence of oral disease, a growing evidence base supports risk for collateral extra-oral adverse health outcomes mediated by escalating pathological processes driven by oral-systemic interactions, including exacerbation of diabetes and other medical conditions. Therefore, opportunities for reintegrating oral health care and medicine would be important to identify, while simultaneously solving other issues related to segregation of the medical/dental care delivery domains, including separate insurance structures; lack of medical and dental electronic health record integration; limited integrated care delivery; and minimal transdisciplinary communication, training, and education.

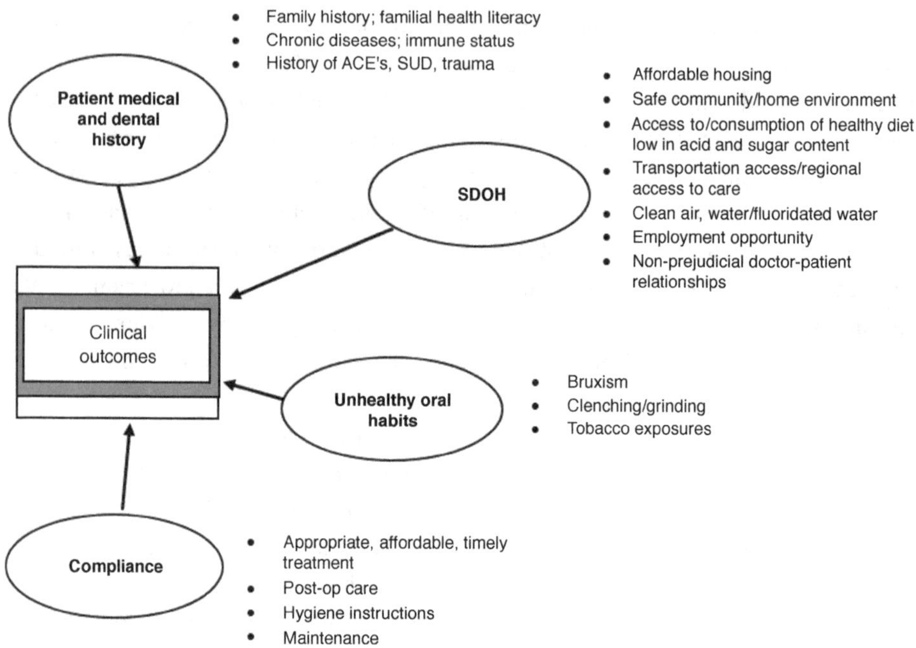

Note: ACEs = adverse childhood experiences; SDOH = social determinants of health; SUD = substance use disorder.

Figure 24-6. Factors Affecting Clinical Outcomes

Virtual exclusion of oral public health from the public health domain has inadvertently contributed to perpetuation of oral disease as the silent epidemic described by Dr. Satcher in 2000.[3] The follow-up report by the National Institutes of Health in 2022 noted only marginal improvements in the state of oral population health and attests to the need for promoting oral public health visibility.[2] The report further brings into focus major factors that present barriers or contribute to inequities in health care access.[2] How to begin strategically solving or mitigating the impact of these factors represents a major priority for the public health and policy sectors.

Since dental access is critical to prevention of dental caries and periodontal disease, solutions to address lack of dental access and prevalent workforce shortages need to be defined and addressed. Dental workforce shortages are projected to increase because the current dental workforce is skewed toward older age groups rapidly approaching retirement age. The training of new dental professionals is currently not keeping pace, particularly in dental Health Professional Shortage Areas. The need for workforce expansion, introduction of intermediate-level providers, and training of competent support staff is becoming increasingly more urgent, especially with the ever-growing challenges of providing oral health care delivery in rural and urban settings where aging populations and other under-resourced and vulnerable populations are more likely to be uninsured for dental services.

Poor oral health can be caused by various contributory factors, including limited access to dental services, low oral health literacy, and underlying personal and sociocultural values. Lack of patient health literacy can prevent patient engagement, resulting in negative health-related outcomes such as higher hospitalization rates, increased health care costs, and reduced quality of life. The creation of a collaborative approach with inputs from providers and patients will inform development of effective educational materials for patients.

An additional improvement that needs to be made is a more timely release of high-quality surveillance data for rates of dental disease. For example, reductions in rates for early childhood cariogenesis require reliable establishment of current rates and programs to improve oral health among pregnant women. Gaps in clinical care delivery surrounding caries reduction, prevention, and management include evaluation of comparative efficacy of use of silver diamine treatment versus fluoride to arrest decay. Sealant tracking also requires improvement. Tracking is largely conducted using paper records and not systematically quantified at a national level, with only some states reporting reliable data. Further, sealant programs are only available in certain designated public schools based on a defined census of low-income student populations. Thus, students in schools without such programs or those with a low likelihood of sealant placement due to domestic circumstances may be excluded. If caries development ensues, affected children experience pain that may affect the quality of their schoolwork and capacity for learning. In some instances, such infections proved fatal,[11] with morbidity and mortality documented across the entire life course.

Damage to teeth caused by dental disease also affects physical appearance and may further cause psychological disturbances in children and adults. Dental pain also affects the ability to chew and may therefore cause dietary insufficiency. In the context of pain management, guidelines for responsible strategic use of opioids and antibiotics in the dental clinical setting need to be created in light of the prevailing opioid crisis occurring in the United States and other countries worldwide.

Evidence-based demonstration of associations between oral and systemic diseases and new models for person-centered care delivery provide examples that emphasize a need for better integration of data associated with medical and dental care delivery. One such integrated model was developed at an integrated dental-medical clinical practice and involved pairing the large community practice with a dedicated research team engaged in translational research with the goal of increasing access to dental care for disparity populations. Initiatives include needs assessments and the creation of tools to support measurable improvements in health care delivery. Such translational models hold great promise for establishing cost-effective, high-quality, integrated oral and systemic health care delivery and are promoted through the adoption of value-based care, which evolved from the Triple Aim. The shift in emphasis to delivery of "value-based care-preventive medicine" includes incorporating evidence-based, quality-centric, and alternative models of care.

Innovations in Clinical Practice

Collaborative efforts between the clinical sector and translational researchers resulting from the requirement to emphasize value-based care have led to some innovations in clinical practice. Several examples of health informatics research initiatives that have been leveraged to improve patient outcomes and translated into the clinical care arena to further advance dental care and/or delivery of integrated care include:

- Clinical decision support tools to track sealant placement.[27]
- Clinical decision support systems in integrated electronic medical and dental records (iEHR) at point of care.[28]
- Development of quality metrics and dental quality dashboards.[29]
- Improved care and access by use of iEHR.[30]

Each of these initiatives is further detailed below.

Clinical Decision Support Tools for Sealant Placement Tracking

Because untreated dental caries remains a frequently observed disease among US children, use of clinical decision support systems for tracking sealant placement by dental hygienists during scheduled preventive care visits was shown to be highly effective in reducing the incidence of dental caries.[27]

Clinical Decision Support Systems in Integrated Medical-Dental Records for Use at Point of Care

Heightened systemic inflammation exacerbated by periodontal disease and diabetes may cause challenges in achieving glycemic control in individuals with diabetes and may also increase severity of periodontal disease. A study by Hegde et al.[28] described the development and integration of a clinical decision support tool into an integrated electronic medical-dental health record to flag at-risk patients with no glycemic assessment or dental examination for a period of 12 or more months to alert physicians and dentists of the need for referral.

Quality Metrics and Dental Quality Dashboards

Quality metrics have not been widely adopted in dental clinical practice to date. The study by Shimpi et al.[29] created a quality dental dashboard and capacity for tracking of benchmarked quality metrics. Outcomes included demonstration of improved care delivery, patient access, and health outcomes, as well as improvement in, or achievement of, metric benchmarks.

Improved Care and Access Mediated by an Integrated Medical-Dental Electronic Health Record

A Marshfield Clinic Health System study by Shimpi et al.[30] described how integrated care delivery was facilitated by iEHR and enabled exchange of medical and dental information electronically. The creation of a collaborative environment across disciplines by utilizing an iEHR supported provision of state-of-the-art, high-quality, holistic care to all segments of the population.

Other Strategic Initiatives

Several strategic initiatives are being advanced to expand oral public health. Several of these initiatives include (1) Healthy People 2030, which sets benchmarks for improvement surrounding key oral health outcomes in the context of population health[4]; (2) expansion of the quality initiative to encourage adoption of dental quality metrics by clinical practices as a standard of care in examining excellence of optimal health care delivery[31]; and (3) formulation of metrics to evaluate efficacy of value-based preventive care versus interventional treatment orientation in improving oral health outcomes. The strategic guiding principles and objectives issued in 2021 by WHO to decrease oral health disparity and reduce high prevalence of oral disease on a global scale through 2030[5] may also have high applicability in developed countries and should receive greater attention by the public health sector going forward.

The Primary Care Collaborative released a report in 2021 that comprehensively summarizes successful, innovative initiatives undertaken to date to improve oral health and primary care integration.[32] While the featured initiatives were largely undertaken independently by organizations across the country to address access issues and oral health disparities of their constituent populations, the initiatives hold promise for some creative and effective solutions. From a dental public health perspective, closer evaluation of these models for potential portability and scalability to other settings nationally is necessary to gauge whether improvements in care delivery initially achieved by these models might be replicable in other settings. Encouraging their promotion holds potential for achieving improved patient outcomes on a national scale.

DISCUSSION QUESTIONS

1. Describe some of the reasons oral disease traditionally has not been well integrated into the public health system, and discuss some ways dental health practitioners might be able to increase its visibility in the future.
2. What are some public health strategies to improve dental care access?
3. From a public health standpoint, does addressing oral disease differ from addressing other chronic diseases? If so, how?

REFERENCES

1. Wen PYF, Chen MX, Zhong YJ, Dong QQ, Wong HM. Global burden and inequality of dental caries, 1990 to 2019. *J Dent Res.* 2022;101(4):392–399. doi:10.1177/00220345211056247
2. National Institute of Dental and Craniofacial Research. Oral health in America: advances and challenges. 2021. Updated January 2023. Available at: https://www.nidcr.nih.gov/research/oralhealthinamerica. Accessed February 2, 2023.
3. National Institute of Dental and Craniofacial Research. 2000 surgeon general's report on oral health in America. Available at: https://www.nidcr.nih.gov/research/data-statistics/surgeon-general. Accessed February 2, 2023.
4. US Department of Health and Human Services. Healthy People 2030. Oral Health Workgroup. 2020. Available at: https://health.gov/healthypeople/about/workgroups/oral-health-workgroup. Accessed February 2, 2023.
5. World Health Organization. Draft global strategy on oral health. August 9, 2021. Available at: https://www.who.int/publications/m/item/who-discussion-paper-draft-global-strategy-on-oral-health. Accessed February 2, 2023.
6. Iheozor-Ejiofor Z, Worthington HV., Walsh T, et al. Water fluoridation for the prevention of dental caries. *Cochrane Database Syst Rev.* 2015;2015(6):CD010856. doi:10.1002/14651858.CD010856.PUB2
7. Centers for Disease Control and Prevention. Dental caries among adults and older adults. Available at: https://www.cdc.gov/oralhealth/publications/OHSR-2019-dental-carries-adults.html. Accessed February 2, 2023.
8. Surlari Z, Virvescu DI, Baciu ER, Vasluianu RI, Budală DG. The link between periodontal disease and oral cancer—a certainty or a never-ending dilemma? *Applied Sci.* 2021;11(24):12100. doi:10.3390/app112412100
9. Shimpi N, Schroeder D, Kilsdonk J, et al. Medical providers' oral health knowledgeability, attitudes, and practice behaviors: an opportunity for interprofessional collaboration. *J Evid Based Dent Pract.* 2016;16(1):19–29. doi:10.1016/j.jebdp.2016.01.002
10. Hujoel PP, White BA, García RI, Listgarten MA. The dentogingival epithelial surface area revisited. *J Periodontal Res.* 2001;36(1):48–55. doi:10.1034/J.1600-0765.2001.00011.X
11. Otto *M. Teeth: The Story of Beauty, Inequality, and the Struggle for Oral Health in America.* New York, NY: The New Press; 2017. Available at: https://thenewpress.com/books/teeth. Accessed February 2, 2023.
12. Frencken JE, Sharma P, Stenhouse L, et al. Global epidemiology of dental caries and severe periodontitis—a comprehensive review. *J Clin Periodontol.* 2017;44:94–105. doi:10.1111/jcpe.12677
13. Institute for Health Metrics and Evaluation. Caries of permanent teeth: level 4 cause. Available at: https://www.healthdata.org/results/gbd_summaries/2019/caries-permanent-teeth-level-4-cause. Accessed February 1, 2023.
14. Centers for Disease Control and Prevention, National Center for Health Statistics. Health, United States data finder: Table 28. 2019. Available at: https://www.cdc.gov/nchs/data/hus/2019/028-508.pdf. Accessed February 1, 2023.

15. Abbafati C, Abbas KM, Abbasi-Kangevari M, et al. Global burden of 369 diseases and injuries in 204 countries and territories, 1990–2019: a systematic analysis for the Global Burden of Disease Study 2019. *Lancet.* 2020;396(10258):1204–1222. doi:10.1016/S0140-6736(20)30925-9
16. Eke PI, Borgnakke WS, Genco RJ. Recent epidemiologic trends in periodontitis in the USA. *Periodontol 2000.* 2020;82(1):257–267. doi:10.1111/prd.12323
17. Eke PI, Thornton-Evans GO, Wei L, Borgnakke WS, Dye BA. Accuracy of NHANES periodontal examination protocols. *J Dent Res.* 2010;89(11):1208–1213. doi:10.1177/0022034510377793
18. Caton JG, Armitage G, Berglundh T, et al. A new classification scheme for periodontal and peri-implant diseases and conditions—introduction and key changes from the 1999 classification. *J Periodontol.* 2018;89(suppl 1):S1–S8. doi:10.1002/JPER.18-0157
19. Eke PI, Thornton-Evans GO, Wei L, Borgnakke WS, Dye BA, Genco RJ. Periodontitis in US adults: National Health and Nutrition Examination Survey 2009–2014. *J Am Dent Assoc.* 2018;149(7):576–588.e6. doi:10.1016/j.adaj.2018.04.023
20. Dahlan R, Badri P, Saltaji H, Amin M. Impact of acculturation on oral health among immigrants and ethnic minorities: a systematic review. *PLoS One.* 2019;14(2):e0212891. doi:10.1371/journal.pone.0212891
21. Liljestrand JM, Havulinna AS, Paju S, Männistö S, Salomaa V, Pussinen PJ. Missing teeth predict incident cardiovascular events, diabetes, and death. *J Dent Res.* 2015;94(8):1055–1062. doi:10.1177/0022034515586352
22. Lee H, Kim D, Jung A, Chae W. Ethnicity, social, and clinical risk factors to tooth loss among older adults in the US, NHANES 2011–2018. *Int J Environ Res Public Heal.* 2022;19(4):2382. doi:10.3390/IJERPH19042382
23. Centers for Disease Control and Prevention, Division for Heart Disease and Stroke Prevention. Policy resources on heart disease and stroke prevention. November 1, 2022. Available at: https://www.cdc.gov/dhdsp/policy_resources/index.htm. Accessed March 30, 2023.
24. Agency for Healthcare Research Quality. Defining the PCMH. Last reviewed August 2022. Available at: https://www.ahrq.gov/ncepcr/research/care-coordination/pcmh/define.html. Accessed March 30, 2023.
25. Canga M, Malagnino G, Malagnino VA, Malagnino I. Effectiveness of sealants treatment in permanent molars: a longitudinal study. *Int J Clin Pediatr Dent.* 2021;14(1):41–45. doi:10.5005/jp-journals-10005-1878
26. Favero V, Bacci C, Volpato A, Bandiera M, Favero L, Zanette G. Pregnancy and dentistry: a literature review on risk management during dental surgical procedures. *Dent J.* 2021;9(4):46. doi:10.3390/DJ9040046
27. Nycz G, Shimpi N, Glurich I, et al. Positioning operations in the dental safety net to enhance value-based care delivery in an integrated health-care setting. *J Public Health Dent.* 2020;8(suppl 2):S71–S76. doi:10.1111/jphd.12392
28. Hegde H, Shimpi N, Panny A, Glurich I, Christie P, Acharya A. Development of non-invasive diabetes risk prediction models as decision support tools designed for application in the dental clinical environment. *Inform Med Unlocked.* 2019;17:100254. doi:10.1016/j.imu.2019.100254

29. Shimpi N, Hegde H, Glurich I, Ryan M, Acharya A. Establishing a quality improvement culture within a large integrated medical-dental health system with a population based focus. *J Evid Based Dent Pract.* 2021;21(4):101589. doi:10.1016/J.JEBDP.2021.101589
30. Shimpi N, Glurich I, Acharya A. Integrated care case study: Marshfield Clinic Health System. In: Acharya A, Powell V, Torres-Urquidy MH, Posteraro RH, Thyvalikakath T, eds. *Integration of Medical and Dental Care and Patient Data.* 2nd ed. London, UK: Springer; 2019:315–326. doi:10.1007/978-3-319-98298-4_17
31. Dental Quality Alliance. *Quality Measurement in Dentistry: A Guidebook.* American Dental Association; 2019. Available at: www.ada.org/dqa. Accessed February 2, 2023.
32. Primary Care Collaborative. Innovations in oral health and primary care integration: alignment with the shared principles of primary care. January 2021. Available at: http://www.pcpcc.org/resource/OHPCintegrationreport. Accessed March 28, 2023.

Resources

These resources have been provided by chapter authors and selected by the editors to be helpful references for continued reading and study of many topics covered in this text.

Agency for Health Care Research and Quality, http://www.ahrq.gov

American Cancer Society, http://www.cancer.org

American College of Cardiology, http://www.acc.org

American Diabetes Association, http://www.diabetes.org

American Heart Association, https://www.heart.org/

American Society of Hypertension, http://www.ash-us.org

American Society of Addiction Medicine, http://www.asam.org

American Stroke Association, http://www.strokeassociation.org/STROKEORG

Behavioral Risk Factor Surveillance System, http://www.cdc.gov/BRFSS

Centers for Disease Control and Prevention (CDC), http://www.cdc.gov

CDC, Division for Heart Disease and Stroke Prevention, http://www.cdc.gov/DHDSP

CDC, National Center for Injury Prevention and Control, Web-based Injury Statistics Query and Reporting System (WISQARS), http://www.cdc.gov/injury/wisqars

CDC WONDER, http://wonder.cdc.gov

Centers for Medicare and Medicaid Services, http://www.cms.hhs.gov

Framingham Heart Study, http://www.framinghamheartstudy.org

Healthy People 2030, https://www.healthypeople.gov

Heart Failure Society of America, http://www.hfsa.org

National Alliance on Mental Illness, http://www.nami.org

National Cancer Institute, Cancer Information Service, http://www.cancer.gov

National Cancer Institute, Surveillance, Epidemiology, and End Results Program, http://seer.cancer.gov

National Heart, Lung, and Blood Institute, http://www.nhlbi.nih.gov

National Institute for Occupational Safety and Health, Sentinel Event Notification System for Occupational Risks (SENSOR), https://www.cdc.gov/niosh/topics/pesticides/overview.html

National Institute on Alcohol Abuse and Alcoholism (NIAAA), http://www.niaaa.nih.gov

National Institutes of Health, including the National Cancer Institute, the National Heart, Lung, and Blood Institute, and the National Institute on Drug Abuse, https://www.nih.gov

National Institute of Neurological Disorders and Stroke, http://www.ninds.nih.gov

National Notifiable Diseases Surveillance System, https://www.cdc.gov/nndss/index.html

National Registry of Evidence-Based Programs and Practices, https://www.samhsa.gov/resource-search/ebp

National Survey on Drug Use and Health, https://nsduhweb.rti.org/respweb/homepage.cfm

Physical Activity Guidelines for Americans, https://health.gov/our-work/nutrition-physical-activity/physical-activity-guidelines

Substance Abuse and Mental Health Services Administration (SAMHSA), http://www.samhsa.gov

Surgeon General's Report on Suicide Prevention (2012), http://www.surgeongeneral.gov/library/reports/national-strategy-suicide-prevention/index.html

The Community Guide: What Works to Promote Health, https://www.thecommunityguide.org

US Preventive Services Task Force, https://www.uspreventiveservicestaskforce.org/uspstf/

Youth Risk Behavior Surveillance System, http://www.cdc.gov/HealthyYouth/yrbs/index.htm

Risk Estimators

- **Atherosclerotic cardiovascular disease (ASCVD) Risk Estimator:** ASCVD Risk Estimator (acc.org)
  For estimation of 10-year ASCVD risk for primary prevention patients (those without ASCVD) only. Estimator includes the following variables: sex, age, race, TC, HDL-C, SBP, diabetes, smoking status, and treatment for hypertension
- **ASCVD Risk Estimator Plus:** ASCVD Risk Estimator + (acc.org)
  For estimation of 10-year ASCVD risk for primary prevention patients (those without ASCVD) only. In addition to the variables included in the ASCVD risk estimator, it additionally includes: LDL-C, DBP, statin use, and aspirin therapy

Contributors

Claudia Aguado Loi, PhD, MPH
Department of Health Sciences and Human Performance
The University of Tampa
Tampa, FL
Chapter 4: Community-Based Interventions

Barbara E. Ainsworth, PhD, MPH
College of Health Solutions
Arizona State University
Phoenix, AZ
Chapter 9: Physical Activity

Siddique Akram, MD
Department of Medicine
Larner College of Medicine
University of Vermont
Burlington, VT
Chapter 22: Chronic Liver Disease

Madison N. Alvarez, BS
Tobacco Prevention and Control Program
Wisconsin Department of Health Services
Madison, WI
Chapter 7: Tobacco Use

Henry A. Anderson, MD
Nelson Institute of Environmental Studies
School of Medicine and Public Health
University of Wisconsin-Madison
Madison, WI
Chapter 18: Chronic Respiratory Diseases

Jon Arnason, MD
Department of Medicine
School of Medicine and Public Health
University of Wisconsin-Madison
Madison, WI
Chapter 21: Arthritis and Other Musculoskeletal Diseases

Brad C. Astor, PhD, MPH
Departments of Medicine and Population Health Sciences
School of Medicine and Public Health
University of Wisconsin-Madison
Madison, WI
Chapter 23: Chronic Kidney Disease

Karina A. Atwell, MD, MPH
Department of Family Medicine and Community Health
School of Medicine and Public Health
University of Wisconsin-Madison
Madison, WI
Chapter 5: The Role of Health Care Systems in Chronic Disease Prevention and Control

John Auerbach, MBA
ICF International Inc.
Reston, VA
Foreword

Christie M. Bartels, MD, MS
Department of Medicine
School of Medicine and Public Health
University of Wisconsin-Madison
Madison, WI
Chapter 21: Arthritis and Other Musculoskeletal Diseases

Leonelo E. Bautista, MD, DrPH, MPH
Department of Population Health Sciences
School of Medicine and Public Health
University of Wisconsin-Madison
Madison, WI
Chapter 13: Hypertension

Peter A. Briss, MD, MPH
National Center for Chronic Disease Prevention and Health Promotion
Office of Medicine and Science
Centers for Disease Control and Prevention
Atlanta, GA
Chapter 1: Current Issues and Challenges in Chronic Disease Prevention and Control

Randall Brown, MD, PhD
Department of Family Medicine and Community Health
School of Medicine and Public Health
University of Wisconsin-Madison
Madison, WI
Chapter 10: Alcohol Use

Alyssa Bruehlman, MD
Department of Family Medicine and Community Health
School of Medicine and Public Health
University of Wisconsin-Madison
Madison, WI
Chapter 10: Alcohol Use

Juliana F. W. Cohen, ScD, ScM
Department of Nutrition and Public Health
Merrimack College
Andover, MA
Chapter 8: Diet and Nutrition

Ann Chodara, MD
Department Medicine
School of Medicine and Public Health
University of Wisconsin-Madison
Madison, WI
Chapter 21: Arthritis and Other Musculoskeletal Diseases

Donita R. Croft, MD, MS
Department of Medicine
School of Medicine and Public Health
University of Wisconsin-Madison
Madison, WI
Chapter 18: Chronic Respiratory Diseases

Emily C. Davis, BS
Vanderbilt Institute for Global Health
Vanderbilt University Medical Center
Nashville, TN
Chapter 20: Neurological Disorders

Bri Deyo, MPH
Department of Family Medicine and Community Health
School of Medicine and Public Health
University of Wisconsin-Madison
Madison, WI
Chapter 10: Alcohol Use

Melissa Doud, BBM
Tobacco Prevention and Control Program
Division of Public Health
Wisconsin Department of Health Services
Madison, WI
Chapter 7: Tobacco Use

Sara Doyle, MD, MPH
Department of Population Health Sciences
School of Medicine and Public Health
University of Wisconsin-Madison
Madison, WI
Chapter 20: Neurological Disorders

Russell Dunkel, DDS
Marquette University School of Dentistry
Wisconsin Department of Health Services
Madison, WI
Chapter 24: Chronic Oral Diseases

Mara Meyer Epstein, ScD, ScM
Department of Medicine
University of Massachusetts Chan Medical School
Worcester, MA
Chapter 17: Cancer

Michael Fang, PhD, MHS
Department of Epidemiology
Johns Hopkins Bloomberg School of Public Health
Baltimore, MD
Chapter 12: Diabetes

Deborah A. Galuska, PhD, MPH
Division of Nutrition, Physical Activity, and Obesity
National Center for Chronic Disease Prevention and Health Promotion
Centers for Disease Control and Prevention
Atlanta, GA
Chapter 11: Obesity

Shivani Garg, MD, MS
Department of Medicine
School of Medicine and Public Health
University of Wisconsin-Madison
Madison, WI
Chapter 21: Arthritis and Other Musculoskeletal Diseases

Yara Gholmie, PhD, RD
Department of Nutrition
Simmons University
Boston, MA
Chapter 8: Diet and Nutrition

Ingrid Glurich, PhD
Marshfield Clinic Research Institute,
Marshfield, WI
Chapter 24: Chronic Oral Diseases

Karen A. Hacker, MD, MPH
National Center for Chronic Disease Prevention and Health Promotion
Centers for Disease Control and Prevention
Atlanta, GA
Chapter 1: Current Issues and Challenges in Chronic Disease Prevention and Control

Erika W. Hagen, PhD
Department of Population Health Sciences
School of Medicine and Public Health
University of Wisconsin-Madison
Madison, WI
Chapter 15: Sleep Behaviors and Disorders

Lauren Hale, PhD
Department of Family, Population and Preventive Medicine
Renaissance School of Medicine
Stony Brook University
Stony Brook, NY
Chapter 15: Sleep Behaviors and Disorders

Jerry Halverson, MD
Rogers Behavioral Health
Madison, WI
Chapter 19: Mental Disorders

Karen Hansen, MD, MS
Department of Medicine
School of Medicine and Public Health
University of Wisconsin-Madison
Madison, WI
Chapter 21: Arthritis and Other Musculoskeletal Diseases

Julie Hildebrand, MD
Department of Rheumatology
William S. Middleton Memorial Veterans Hospital
Madison, WI
Chapter 21: Arthritis and Other Musculoskeletal Diseases

Carlyn M. Hood-Ronick, MPA, MPH
Project Access NOW
Portland, OR
Chapter 6: The Social Determinants of Chronic Disease

Vicki Huntington, BA
Tobacco Prevention and Control Program
Division of Public Health
Wisconsin Department of Health Services
Madison, WI
Chapter 7: Tobacco Use

Adrienne L. Johnson, PhD
Center for Tobacco Research and Intervention
School of Medicine and Public Health
University of Wisconsin-Madison
Madison, WI
Chapter 7: Tobacco Use

Corinne Joshu, PhD, MPH, MA
Department of Epidemiology
Johns Hopkins School of Public Health
Baltimore, MD
Chapter 17: Cancer

Paula M. Lantz, PhD, MS
Gerald R. Ford School of Public Policy and School of Public Health
University of Michigan
Ann Arbor, MI
Chapter 6: The Social Determinants of Chronic Disease

Tiffany Lin, MD
Department of Medicine
School of Medicine and Public Health
University of Wisconsin-Madison
Madison, WI
Chapter 21: Arthritis and Other Musculoskeletal Diseases

Longjian Liu, MD, PhD, MSc
Department of Epidemiology and Biostatistics
Dornsife School of Public Health
Drexel University
Philadelphia, PA
Chapter 16: Cardiovascular Disease

Fleetwood Loustalot, PhD, FNP
Division for Heart Disease and Stroke Prevention
National Center for Chronic Disease Prevention and Health Promotion
Centers for Disease Control and Prevention
Atlanta, GA
Chapter 14: Dyslipidemia

Carolina A. Macera, PhD
Graduate School of Public Health
San Diego State University
San Diego, CA
Chapter 9: Physical Activity

Ron Manderscheid, PhD
National Association of County Behavioral Health and Developmental Disability Directors
Johns Hopkins Bloomberg School of Public Health
Baltimore, MD
Chapter 19: Mental Disorders

Mary P. Martinasek, PhD, MPH
Department of Health Sciences and Human Performance
The University of Tampa
Tampa, FL
Chapter 4: Community-Based Interventions

Alyssa B. Mayer, PhD, MPH
Department of Public Health and Human Service
University of South Carolina Beaufort
Beaufort, SC
Chapter 4: Community-Based Interventions

Rozalina G. McCoy, MD, MS
Department of Medicine
University of Maryland School of Medicine
Baltimore, MD
Chapter 12: Diabetes

Justin T. McDaniel, PhD, MBA
Public Health Program
School of Human Sciences
Southern Illinois University Carbondale
Carbondale, IL
Chapter 4: Community-Based Interventions

Robert J. McDermott, PhD, MS
Department of Population Health Sciences
University of Wisconsin School of Medicine and Public Health,
Madison, WI
Chapter 4: Community-Based Interventions

Jordan Mills, DO, PhD
Southern California Permanente Medical Group
Fontana, CA
Chapter 10: Alcohol Use

Julianne Nelson, PhD, MPH
Department of Epidemiology and Biostatistics
Dornsife School of Public Health
Drexel University
Philadelphia, PA
Chapter 16: Cardiovascular Disease

Craig J. Newschaffer, PhD
College of Health and Human Development
Pennsylvania State University
State College, PA
Chapter 16: Cardiovascular Disease

Margaret B. Nolan, MD, MS
Center for Tobacco Research and Intervention
School of Medicine and Public Health
University of Wisconsin-Madison
Madison, WI
Preface
Chapter 7: Tobacco Use

Greg Nycz, BS
Family Health Center of Marshfield
Marshfield, WI
Chapter 24: Chronic Oral Diseases

Patrick J. O'Connor, MD, MA, MPH
HealthPartners Institute
Minneapolis, MN
Chapter 12: Diabetes

Deborah Olarte, PhD, RD
Center for Health Inclusion, Research and Practice
Merrimack College
North Andover, MA
Chapter 8: Diet and Nutrition

Mahmooda K. Pasha, PhD, MPH
WHO Collaborating Centre on Social Marketing and Social Change
University of South Florida College of Public Health
Tampa, FL
Chapter 4: Community-Based Interventions

Kathryn L. Penney, ScD
Channing Division of Network Medicine
Brigham and Women's Hospital
Harvard Medical School
Boston, MA
Chapter 17: Cancer

Paul E. Peppard, PhD
Department of Population Health Sciences
School of Medicine and Public Health
University of Wisconsin-Madison
Madison, WI
Chapter 15: Sleep Behaviors and Disorders

Parvathy Pillai, MD, MPH
Department of Population Health Sciences
School of Medicine and Public Health,
University of Wisconsin-Madison
Madison, WI
Chapter 6: The Social Determinants of Chronic Disease

Patrick L. Remington, MD, MPH
Department of Population Health Sciences
School of Medicine and Public Health
University of Wisconsin-Madison
Madison, WI
Preface
Chapter 2: Epidemiologic Methods for Chronic Disease Prevention and Control
Chapter 3: Chronic Disease Surveillance

Oscar L Rueda, MD, PhD
Department of Basic Sciences
School of Medicine
Universidad Industrial de Santander
Bucaramanga, Colombia
Chapter 13: Hypertension

Megan Ryan, DDS
Family Health Center of Marshfield
Marshfield, WI
Chapter 24: Chronic Oral Diseases

Adnan Said, MD, MS
Department of Medicine
School of Medicine and Public Health
University of Wisconsin-Madison
Madison, WI
Chapter 22: Chronic Liver Disease

Ahlia Sekkarie, PhD, MPH
Division for Heart Disease and Stroke Prevention
National Center for Chronic Disease Prevention and Health Promotion
Centers for Disease Control and Prevention
Atlanta, GA
Chapter 14: Dyslipidemia

Elizabeth Selvin, PhD, MPH
Department of Epidemiology
Johns Hopkins Bloomberg School of Public Health
Baltimore, MD
Chapter 12: Diabetes

Neel Shimpi, PhD, MM, BDS
Center for Clinical Epidemiology and Population Health
Marshfield Clinic Research Institute
Marshfield, WI
Chapter 24: Chronic Oral Diseases

Tripti Singh, MD
Department of Medicine
School of Medicine and Public Health
University of Wisconsin-Madison
Madison, WI
Chapter 23: Chronic Kidney Disease

Maureen A. Smith, MD, PhD, MPH
Departments of Population Health Sciences and Family Medicine and Community Health
School of Medicine and Public Health
University of Wisconsin-Madison
Madison, WI
Chapter 5: The Role of Health Care Systems in Chronic Disease Prevention and Control

Tena Springer, MA
Dental Division
Family Health Center of Marshfield
Marshfield, WI
Chapter 24: Chronic Oral Diseases

Elizabeth Stein, MD, MS
Occupational Medicine Physician
Ithaca, NY
Chapter 19: Mental Disorders

Ellen W. Stowe, PhD, MPH
Division of Nutrition, Physical Activity, and Obesity
National Center for Chronic Disease Prevention and Health Promotion
Centers for Disease Control and Prevention
Atlanta, GA
Chapter 11: Obesity

Lena C. Swander, MPH
Division of Public Health
Wisconsin Department of Health Services
Madison, WI
Chapter 3: Chronic Disease Surveillance

Angela M. Thompson-Paul, PhD, MSPH
Division of Heart Disease and Stroke Prevention
National Center for Chronic Disease Prevention and Health Promotion
Centers for Disease Control and Prevention
Atlanta, GA
Chapter 14: Dyslipidemia

Edwin Trevathan, MD, MPH
Vanderbilt Institute for Global Health
Departments of Pediatrics and Neurology
Vanderbilt University Medical Center
Nashville, TN
Chapter 20: Neurological Disorders

Shelby L. Vadjunec, MPH
Division of Public Health
Wisconsin Department of Health Services
Madison, WI
Chapter 3: Chronic Disease Surveillance

Monica Valdes-Lupi, JD, MPH
Kresge Foundation
Troy, MI
Foreword

Sandra D. Vamos, EdD
School of Interdisciplinary Health Programs
Western Michigan University
Kalamazoo, MI
Chapter 4: Community-Based Interventions

Mark V. Wegner, MD, MPH
Division of Public Health
Wisconsin Department of Health Services
Madison, WI
Preface
Chapter 3: Chronic Disease Surveillance

Lin Zhao, MD, MPH
Department of Population Health Sciences
School of Medicine and Public Health
University of Wisconsin-Madison
Madison, WI
Chapter 2: Epidemiologic Methods for Chronic Disease Prevention and Control

Index

Italicized page references indicate Figures or Tables.

A

D

E

F

G

J

K

N

O

P

Q

R

T

Y

Z